Functional Foods and Nutrition

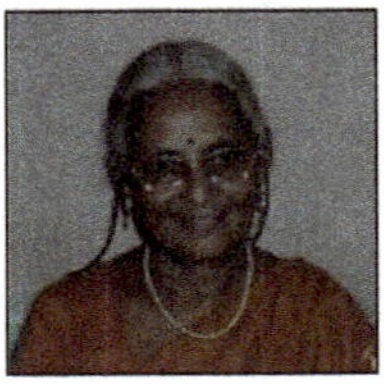

Dr. G. Subbulakshmi is an eminent nutritionist with over 45 years of teaching, research and administrative experience. She has a Ph.D in Food Science and Nutrition and has also worked as a post doctoral fellow in CFTRI, Mysore in early 1970s. She has worked as the First Principal of the S.M. Patel College of Home Science in Vallabh Vidyanagar, Gujarat and Indramani Mandelia College of Home Science in Pilani, Rajasthan. She has been instrumental in introducing internship for the students in Home Science Colleges and Sports Nutrition and Food Science and Technology in the Nutrition curriculum.

She has published several research papers and her book on Food Processing and Preservation has been widely used in the colleges. She has guided more than 25 PhD students in Food Science and Nurition apart from more than 60 M.Sc. students in their Dissertations. She has published more than 70 Research Papers in National and International Journals of repute. Dr. Subbulakshmi has worked towards the improvement of community Health and Nutrition. Having worked on research projects funded by National and International Agencies, she has prepared a number of booklets and pamphlets on nutrition related topics for educating the common man.

She has received Fulbright award for studying the college administration in USA, PL480 Research Scholarship for doing PhD, UGC's National Research Associateship award as well as Hari Om Ashram Prizes for 3 different best Research papers in Nutrition. The various awards received by Dr. Subbulakshmi speak of her abilities. She has been awarded M.L. Khurana Memorial Award – 2002; T.K. Basu Award for excellent contributions to Nutritional Sciences from International College of Nutrition USA; Life Time Achievement Award from Alumni Association of the M.S. University of Baroda; Life Time Achievement Award from Nutrition Society of India, Mumbai Chapter.

She is an active life member of many Professional Organizations like Nutrition Society of India, Association of Food Scientists and Technologists of India, Indian Dietetic Association, Home Science Association of India, Association for Women Scientists, Indian Association for Preschool Education and many others.

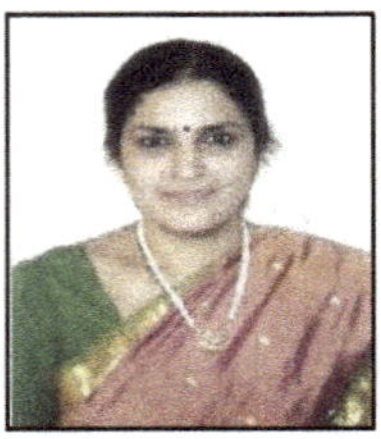

Dr. Mandalika Subhadra is an expert in Food Science and Nutrition. She is a post graduate of Sri Satya Sai Institute of Higher Learning, Anantapur,(A.P., India) and awarded gold medal for securing first rank. She has received her PhD in Food Science and Nutrition from SNDT Women's University, Mumbai, India. She has contributed her valuable expertise to various institutions during her 20 years of service as an academician and researcher. Her contribution was appreciated with a best teacher award by the Rajamahendri Degree College for Women, Andhra Pradesh. She is also a recognised PhD guide of the University of Mumbai and selected as PhD referee by various other reputed Universities. She has been actively involved in teaching and research guidance at under graduate and post-graduate levels. She has guided around 25 post-graduate students and 6 PhD scholars on research topics from various branches of nutrition including Clinical Nutrition, Community Nutrition, Nutritional Food Product Development, Food Science and Technology, Biochemistry, Micronutrients, Antioxidants, Sports and exercise Nutrition. She has got several research publications to her credit in various peer reviewed journals and has been a co-editor of a book on Methodologies of Nutritional Assessment. She has shared her research achievements in various national and international conferences. Her deep interest in research is evident through a Patency (No. 225689) she has Obtained on 'Antiestrogenic activity of phytosterols from fenugreekseeds'. She has coordinated major and minor research projects sponsored by DAE/BRNS, UGC, University of Mumbai, and reputed food industries.

Dr.Subhadra has been invited as a resource person at various seminars and conferences. She was honoured with an Ambassadorial Scholarship of Good Will by the Rotary International to take up an academic assignment at the University of Mauritius for 3 and half months in Mauritius which was highly appreciated. Besides being an academician, she is also actively involved in community outreach programmes. Currently she is working as a faculty of Home Science in the specialisation of Foods, Nutrition and Dietetics of College of Home Science, Nirmala Niketan, Mumbai.

Functional Foods and Nutrition

— *Authors* —

G. Subbulakshmi

Nutrition Consultant,
Former Director,
Department of PGSR in Home Science,
SNDT Women's University, Mumbai

and

M. Subhadra

Associate Professor,
Department of Food, Nutrition and Dietetics,
College of Home Science, Nirmala Niketan, Mumbai

2014

Daya Publishing House®

A Division of

Astral International Pvt. Ltd.

New Delhi – 110 002

ISBN 9789351301974

Published by : **Daya Publishing House®**
A Division of
Astral International Pvt. Ltd.
– ISO 9001:2008 Certified Company –
4760-61/23, Ansari Road, Darya Ganj
New Delhi-110 002
Ph. 011-43549197, 23278134
E-mail: info@astralint.com
Website: www.astralint.com

Laser Typesetting : **Classic Computer Services**, Delhi - 110 035

Printed at : **Replika Press Pvt. Ltd.**

PRINTED IN INDIA

Acknowledgements

The exciting scientific evidence on the health benefits of foods has strengthened the deep desire in our heart to emphasize the food based approach in the prevention as well as management of various clinical conditions. We tried to the best of our efforts and abilities to compile the documented scientific information and publish this book.

We are immensely grateful to Dr. C. Gopalan, whom we perceive as 'Father of Nutrition' in India for encourageing us through his highly inspiring foreword. We sincerely thank all the authors of documented research for sharing their valuable work through print and soft media. We thank Dr. Reinagel for kindly permitting us to include some information from her research in the book. The valuable contribution of all the scientists has been duly acknowledged both in the text as well as in the references given towards the end of each chapter. The copyright of the sources of information remains with the original authors. However, if reference to any author/s is missing in the book, it is purely unintentional and inadvertent and deeply regretted. We also whole heartedly thank the web search engines for providing us access to the required information without which this venture would have been impossible.

We highly appreciate and acknowledge our beloved students and research scholars, Dr. Mrudula Naik, Dr. Jyoti Amin, Mrs. Priyadarshini Lotankar, Ms. Minelly Rodrigues and Ms. Neha Vaidya for their valuable contribution and support in various ways to this compilation. We also thank all our friends and well wishers for their constant encouragement.

Dr. G. Subbulakshmi

Dr. M. Subhadra

Foreword

It is often said that "we are what we eat". Nothing has a greater or more direct bearing on our health and well-being, longevity and livelihood, than the diets we consume.

Nutrition is therefore the corner-stone of all health sciences.

India continues to carry the burden of malnutrition, especially among women and children. Vigorous efforts are continuing, in terms of both research and dissemination of knowledge, to bring about improvements. As we explore all avenues in this endeavour, we should not ignore the treasure-house of our traditional knowledge of foods and diets, and of indigenous plants that have been proved to be rich sources of essential nutrients.

Throughout the several decades of my research career as a nutrition scientist I have always emphasized the importance of using "farm solutions" rather than "pharmacy solutions" to tackle the nation's malnutrition problems. The food-based approach is the only viable, long-term, sustainable path towards nutrition for all.

Nowadays, lifestyle diseases such as diabetes and cardiovascular diseases are adding to the health care burden of our nation. As people live longer and as lifestyles and environments change, we must bestow ever-greater attention on quality of life and avoidance of disease.

The difficult but rewarding task of compiling this book has been undertaken by two distinguished nutrition scientists. I have a long acquaintance with Dr. Subbulakshmi Gurumurthy and I am familiar with her valuable contributions to nutrition science over several decades. I am very pleased with the theme of this book for three reasons. First, it brings out the value of traditional food items and sources.

Second it places emphasis on the food-based approach to nutritional well-being. Third, it focuses on promoting health by avoiding disease.

I am sure this book will be of immense interest and value to a wide variety of health scientists, teachers and researchers, and I commend the authors for their excellent work.

Dr. C. Gopalan, ***M.D., Ph.D., D.Sc, FRS.***

President, Nutrition Foundation of India, New Delhi

Former Director General, Indian Council of Medical Research, New Delhi

Preface

The changing lifestyle has resulted in various types of diseases which were less common in earlier days. Modern medicine, despite offering a variety of effective treatment options, can have several adverse effects. The value of an "alternative" therapy is now being discovered by many scientists. The only way to meet the challenge of the changing health needs is by preventive rather than curative therapy. A natural approach to prevent a disease is always better than depending on its cure.

"Let your food be your medicine" said Hippocrates, the Father of Medicine. Diet and nutrition is supportive in drug treatment of a disorder. From a dietary perspective, the functionality of foods depends on their properties. It is only if the foods are clinically proved of their preventive or curative efficacy that the present generation would develop faith in them.

It is well established that several metabolic diseases and age-related degenerative disorders are closely associated with oxidative processes in the body. Diet plays a great role in modifying the patho-physiological processes of various metabolic disorders most of which are known to involve oxidative damage. The antioxidant benefits of certain nutrients are well known. Most of these foods have now been clinically tried out *in-vitro* and *in-vivo* and quite a few have been confirmed as effective and some of them have been even proved as equal as or better than the standard medicines in use. Current research is focussed on validating the anti-oxidant capacity of foods and spices, as well as their effects on markers of oxidation. Parallel clinical trials should also aim at establishing foods as mediators of disease prevention. Moreover, the physiologically important phytochemicals such as flavonoids, phenolic acids, etc. present in foods need special attention for their role in the prevention of diseases.

Parts of certain edible plants including seeds, leaves, barks, rhizomes, latex, floral buds and stems have all been found to possess disease preventive and curative properties. Active ingredients of these plants are used to develop several life saving drugs by the pharmaceutical industries. But there are also a few studies which have shown that whole foods are more beneficial than the isolates, as the possibility of other components acting either as a catalyst or otherwise exists. This supports the views of Father of Nutrition, (India)-Dr.C.Gopalan regarding preference for 'Farm Foods' rather than 'Pharmaceutical Foods' for health.

This book is a sincere effort of the authors to compile the documented scientific evidence for the benefits of various foods in clinical conditions such as diabetes, CVD, cancer, obesity etc. which are highly prevalent globally. In addition, foods that would address some of the major etiological factors of these degenerative diseases such as inflammation, oxidative stress, infections have also been discussed. The book also covers the foods that counteract the side effects of certain drugs used in the treatment. Thus the book strongly emphasizes the need for food based approach in the light of scientific evidence and acts as tool for supportive medical nutrition therapy.

The availability of scientific proof for the therapeutic benefits of various foods, facilitates inclusion of the same in diet planning and/or counseling. This book could serve as a ready reckoner for dietitians, nutritionists, medical practitioners, researchers, academicians, students, patients and also for those who are enthusiastic in preserving health.

Dr. G. Subbulakshmi

Dr. M. Subhadra

Contents

Chapter 1
Anti-Ageing Foods

"The longer I live the less confidence I have in drugs and the greater is my confidence in the regulation and administration of diet and regimen".

– **John Redman Coxe, 1800**

Looking younger with smooth wrinkleless skin, having more flexibility, stamina, and endurance for performing both physical and mental tasks efficiently and independently is the desire of everyone.

Maintenance of age appropriate fitness helps in postponing the physiological loss of functional capacity of the body organs to lead a high quality of life for as long as possible (Wahlqvist *et al.*, 2003). Apart from the fact that individual predisposition depends on genetic variables (Klotz, 2002), food patterns and environment too have a strong influence on the ageing process.

Physical appearance of the individual is believed to be the most important marker of ageing process. Understanding that it is far more difficult to reverse the signs of ageing than to control them, several cosmetics and beauty products are developed claiming to delay the process of ageing. Everything from papaya to strawberry is being incorporated in creams, soaps and shampoos. However, it is to be noted that the developing countries cannot afford to waste food in cosmetics with majority of population going with one meal a day. Moreover, the external application of food on the skin alone cannot become a substitute for its consumption as food when consumed nourishes the whole body including skin. In fact, healthy-ageing is considered to be a beauty all by itself.

Ageing is accompanied by a variety of physiological, psychological, economic and social changes that compromise nutritional status and/or affect nutritional requirements (Munro *et al.*, 1987). For these reasons, the diets of many older adults currently do not meet the recommended levels of several essential vitamins and minerals (USDA, 1997; Cid-Rufaza, 1999). Thus, low micronutrient status is often reported in this population (Wright *et al.*, 1998; Institute of Medicine, 1997; NHANEs, 1997). Nutritional surveys of the elderly indicate a low to moderate prevalence of frank nutrient deficiencies. However, an increased risk of malnutrition, including evidence of subclinical deficiencies would have a direct impact on physiological functions of the body (Saltzman and Russell, 1998; Blumberg, 1997; Rosenberg, 1995; Munro *et al.*, 1987).

Inflammation and Oxidative Stress in Ageing

There is growing scientific agreement that anti-oxidants, particularly the polyphenolic forms, may help lower the incidence of disease, such as certain cancers, cardiovascular and neurodegenerative diseases, DNA damage, or even have anti-ageing characteristics (Obrenovich *et al.*, 2011). The lower rate of mitochondrial oxygen radical generation of long-lived animals in relation to that of short-lived ones can be a primary cause of their slow ageing rate. This is secondarily complemented in long-lived animals with low rates of lipid peroxidation due to their low degrees of fatty acid unsaturation. According to Barja (2002 a; b) these two traits suggest that the rate of generation of endogenous oxidative damage determines, at least in part, the rate of ageing in animals. These results suggest that similar mechanisms have been used to extend longevity through decreases in oxidative stress in caloric restriction and during the evolution of species with different longevities.

Chronic low-grade inflammation is a major risk factor for ageing and age-related diseases, such as Alzheimer's disease and type II diabetes. The prevention of inflammageing seems to be one of the most effective approaches to increase longevity. Ma *et al.* (1992) explained that lifespan can be extended by the inhibition of chronic low-grade inflammation via the control of intestinal microbiota for the following reasons: intestinal microbiota undergoes alterations by ageing (Biagi *et al.*, 2010; Claesson *et al.*, 2011); intestinal microbiota stimulates host mucosal and systemic immunity (Macpherson and Harris, 2004); and ageing-associated deterioration in intestinal barrier functions may permit increased systemic absorption of intestinal luminal antigens. In order to have healthy, productive and graceful maturing, it is necessary to maintain a dynamic balance between pro-inflammatory and anti-inflammatory loads (Lien *et al.*, 2010).

Traditional dietary patterns that focus on plant-based, unprocessed, seasonal and organic foods have been shown to prevent disease, delay ageing and promote optimal health.

Traditional Anti-ageing Food Practices (Global Scenario)

In some of the countries people have better longevity with low incidence of degenerative health problems such as Diabetes, CVD and Cancer. The Kuna people of the San Blas islands, off the coast of Panama, have a rate of heart disease that is nine times less than that of mainland Panamanians and is thought to be due to the cocoa drink, which is unusually rich in flavanols that help preserve the healthy function of blood vessels.

The Japanese diet includes foods with very low cholesterol content and abounds in fishes rich in polyunsaturated fats (in particular, eicosopentanoic acid), and the seaweeds Kombu (from warm waters) and Nori (from cold waters) in addition to rice, miso (paste from fermented soybeans used as seasoning in soups), tofu, mushroom and specially cultivated seaweeds. Among the Japanese, Okinawan people live about 7 years longer than Americans and have 80 per cent fewer cases of cancer and heart attacks. Extremely low death-rates in Okinawa could be due to the specific features of the Okinawan diet. In Okinawa, the consumption of sugar and salt constitutes only 25 per cent and 20 per cent (respectively) of the average amount consumed in Japan, the vegetable consumption is 3 times more, and fish is twice that of other Japanese while the energy consumption is 20 per cent lower. They also believe in eating from small plates and stop eating when they are about 80 per cent full. In Okinawa, it is believed that the diet of soya, sweet potato, green leafy vegetables and turmeric tea are some of the contributors of natives' longevity beyond 90's.

Even though Japan continues to have the highest life expectancy in the world, it is expected to be overtaken by other high longevity countries, like Sweden (which has high male and female life expectancy), Italy and Australia (with high male life expectancy). The lowered life expectancy of Japanese is believed to be due to the high amount of tobacco usage and dietary changes that have elevated the body mass index. Recently, young Japanese, particularly young men in Okinawa, have shown a tendency to avoid the traditional dishes of stewed meat and champuru (Miyagi *et al.*, 2003).

Studies among the elderly in Greece, Denmark, Australia, Spain and China have shown that the overall Mediterranean dietary pattern is more important for longevity than single nutrients thus proving that a Mediterranean diet is associated with longer survival. The Mediterranean diet consists of Olive oil, large quantities of vegetables and legumes in the form of salads and of cooked foods along with wheat, grapes and their derived products. Antioxidants represent a common element in these foods which provides a plausible explanation for the apparent health benefits (Trichopoulou and Vasilopoulou, 2000). Total lipid consumption of mediterraneans may be high, around 40 per cent of total energy intake as in Greece, or moderate, around 30 per cent of total energy intake as in Italy. But the ratio of monounsaturated to saturated dietary lipids is much higher than that in other places of the world, including northern Europe and North America (Trichopoulou, 2001) thus making a positive contribution to their health status.

Besides reducing the cardiovascular events, the risk of mortality due to myocardial infarction, and peripheral arterial disease, etc., there is some evidence that Mediterranean diet is also beneficial in relation to bone metabolism, rheumatoid arthritis, neurodegenerative age-related diseases (cognitive deficit, Alzheimer's disease, Parkinson's disease) (Pérez-López *et al.*, 2009).

A Healthy Traditional Dutch diet appears more beneficial for longevity and feasible for health promotion in older Dutch women than a Mediterranean diet. This diet is comparable with other reported healthy or prudent diets which are protective against morbidity or mortality (Waijers *et al.*, 2006).

In Korean diet, some traditional soybean-fermented foods such as Doenjang, Chunggukjang, kimchi and seaweeds were found to contain considerable amounts of vitamin B_{12} (Kwak *et al.*, 2010 a, b) contributing significantly to good vitamin B_{12} status in very old elderly Koreans.

Several dietary practices were examined for their influence on ageing process such as modification in the total energy consumption, fat and protein content in the diet. Caloric restriction by 20-30 per cent was first shown to extend life in rats nearly 80 years ago. As early as 1979 Young has reported on the basis of his review on the subject that feeding ad-libitum throughout life does not promote maximal survival and food restriction increases mean life span. Composition of energy restricted diet for its benefits on longevity was further explored. Although energy restriction provides significant influence on longevity, very high fat diets do not give the same protection as high carbohydrate diets do (Kubo *et al.*, 1987). Caloric restriction has many positive effects on health and longevity. But quality of life on a restricted diet as well as the ability to maintain that diet long term is a great concern (Roth and Polotsky, 2012). The possible importance of total energy, carbohydrate, and protein intake as well as the influence of mode of feeding need to be considered.

Recent data indicate that the decrease in mitochondrial ROS generation is due to protein restriction rather than calorie restriction, and more specifically to dietary methionine restriction. Greater longevity would be partly achieved not only by a low rate of endogenous oxidative degeneration, but also by a macromolecular composition highly resistant to oxidative modification, as is the case for lipids and proteins (López-Torres and Barja, 2008; Pamplona and Barja, 2007).

In recent years there is growing interest in the role of specific nutrients, whole foods, and also phytochemicals in the process of ageing.

Anti-ageing Nutrients

"Nutrition plays an important role in limiting the ageing process and helping to protect against damage from UV rays, the number one cause of lines and wrinkles"

– Adam Friedman, M.D.,
Director of Dermatologic Research at
Albert Einstein College of Medicine in New York City

Energy

Limiting food intake for longevity has been investigated in species from yeast to humans. In yeast and lower animals, caloric restriction has repeatedly been demonstrated to lengthen the life span. Studies of caloric restriction in non-human primates and in humans are ongoing and initial results suggest prolongation of life as well as prevention of age-related diseases (Roth and Polotsky, 2012).

It was first noted during the 1930s that dietary restriction significantly extended the lifespan of rodents (McKay *et al.*, 1935) which was also confirmed later by Ozdemir (2009); Oo *et al.* (2010) and Kailasam *et al.* (2011). The physiological explanation for the same involved significant increase in mRNA expression level of catalase, manganese superoxide dismutase (MnSOD) and copper zinc superoxide dismutase (CuZnSOD) which are likely to reflect the ability of mitochondria to eliminate ROS and delay the ageing process, on energy restriction (Yang *et al.*, 2013).

Carbohydrate

Calorie-restricted starch-fed rats had poorer early life survival, and no significant increase in mean lifespan compared to ad libitum corn starch-fed animals (726 vs 720 days). Mean life span of calorie-restricted sucrose-fed rats was significantly greater than that of all other groups (890 ±18 days) supporting the hypothesis that the dietary source of carbohydrate, *i.e.*, sucrose vs corn starch, can significantly affect lifespan independently of caloric intake (Murtagh-Mark *et al.*, 1995).

Omega 3 Fatty Acids

Many scientific studies have focused on the role of diet in protecting the brain cells from oxidative stress. Cytokines and prostaglandins may act as extracellular signals in generating additional reactive oxygen species that are associated with decrements in neuronal function or glial neuronal interactions (Rosenman *et al.*, 1995; Schipper, 1996; Steffen *et al.*, 1996; Stella *et al.*, 1997; Woodroofe, 1995) and ultimately the deficits in behavior that have been observed in ageing.

Memory loss is a prominent health concern, second only to heart disease for older individuals. Docosa-hexaenoic acid (DHA), the predominant Δ-3 fatty acid in brain and heart, plays an important role in neural and cardiac function. Reduction in plasma DHA is associated with cognitive decline in healthy elderly and Alzheimer's patients. Higher DHA intake and plasma levels are inversely correlated with increased relative risk of Alzheimer's disease (AD) and fatal coronary heart disease. Clinical studies with combined supplementation of DHA and EPA have shown some positive effects in mild cognitive impairment but not in AD, suggesting that early intervention may be a key factor to providing effective therapies. Yurko-Mauro (2010) provided data that reveal a potentially beneficial role for DHA in preventing or ameliorating cognitive decline and cardiovascular disease in the aged.

The age-related reduction of hepatic desaturase activities (which participates in the synthesis of long chains, together with elongases) can impair turnover of cerebral membrane lipids. In many structures, especially in the frontal cortex, a reduction of cervonic and arachidonic acids (synthesized from EFA) is observed during ageing, predominantly associated with a reduction of phosphatidyl-ethanolamines (mainly in the form of plasmalogens). Peroxisomal oxidation of polyunsaturated fatty acids decreases in the brain during ageing, resulting in decreased turnover of membrane fatty acids, which are also less effectively protected against peroxidation by free radicals (Bourre, 2004). These findings indicate the need for supplementation of PUFA along with antioxidants.

According to Willis *et al.* (2009 a) inclusion of PUFAs in the animal diet has been found to improve cholinergic transmission in the brain, possibly leading to improvements in cognitive functioning. The n-6/n-3 polyunsaturated fatty acid ratio was positively related to the global cognitive functions (Mini-Mental State Examination) score in the institutionalized elderly (González *et al.*, 2010). Thus, age-related cognitive and behavioral decline can be ameliorated with polyphenol or PUFA-rich plant foods supplementation (Willis *et al.*, 2009 b).

Protein and Amino Acids

Moreover, energy restricted diets if deficient in protein might induce body muscle loss. Hence, high proportion of protein in the energy restricted diets may be beneficial for stimulating protein synthesis in the muscles of ageing individuals (Paddon-Jones and Rasmussen, 2009).

Methionine

It is known that decrease in food ingestion lowers mitochondrial ROS generation and oxidative stress in young immature rats probably due to the decreased methionine ingestion. Sanchez-Roman *et al.* (2012) reported that the aged rats maintain the capacity to lower mitochondrial ROS generation and oxidative stress in response to a short-term methionine restriction. Whole-food vegan diets with moderate bean and soy intake, along with ample amounts of fruit and wine or beer, can be nutritious while being quite low in methionine (assuming concurrent B_{12} supplementation).

Low-fat vegan diets, coupled with exercise training, can be expected to promote longevity by decreasing systemic levels of insulin and free IGF-I; the latter effect would be amplified by methionine restriction - though it is not clear whether IGF-I down-regulation is the sole basis for the impact of low-methionine diets on longevity in rodents (McCarty, 2003; McCarty *et al.*, 2009).

Creatine

Creatine supplementation in elderly populations is of interest because of its potential in increasing energy production, fat-free mass, and muscle mass (Tarnopolsky, 2000). Combining the effects of creatine with protein supplementation, there would be an increase in the ability of the elderly to perform everyday tasks such as rising from a seated position and walking. However, Rawson *et al.* (2002) found that the older individuals respond differently from young individuals to creatine supplementation. Short durations of creatine supplementation for five days in ageing population had no effect on isometric strength (Rawson and Clarkson, 2000; Jakobi *et al.*, 2001) and on pedaling performance in cycling-trained elderly subjects. But creatine supplementation for the same duration was reported to increase anaerobic power and work capacity of sedentary elderly subjects (Wiroth *et al.*, 2001). Creatine supplementation for 7 days was found to be effective in increasing several indices of muscle performance, including functional tests without adverse side effects in older men (Gotshalk *et al.*, 2002) and women (Gotshalk *et al.*, 2008).

On the other hand, creatine and protein supplementation resulted in small increase in muscle strength only after 12 weeks (Chrusch *et al.*, 2001) and moderate increase after 14 weeks (Brose *et al.*, 2003). Low-dose creatine supplementation combined with protein supplementation and resistance training for 10 weeks increased lean tissue mass but not leg press strength (Candow *et al.*, 2008) than creatine alone or placebo. Therefore, Gotshalk *et al.* (2002) suggested that creatine supplementation may be a useful therapeutic strategy for older adults to attenuate loss in muscle strength and performance of functional living tasks. Dalbo *et al.* (2009) recommended that physicians should strongly consider advising older adults to supplement with creatine and to begin a resistance training regime in an effort to enhance skeletal muscle strength and hypertrophy, resulting in enhanced quality of life. But later Candow and Chilibeck (2010) reported that creatine supplementation, with and without resistance training, has the potential to influence bone biology.

More recently, Klopstock *et al.* (2011) reported that the median healthy life span of creatine-fed mice was 9 per cent higher than their control littermates and they performed significantly better in neuro-behavioral tests. In brains of creatine-treated mice, there was a trend toward a reduction of reactive oxygen species and significantly lower accumulation of the "ageing pigment" lipofuscin. Expression profiling showed an up-regulation of genes implicated in neuronal growth, neuro-protection, and learning. Thus they showed that creatine improves health and longevity in mice. Creatine supplementation has also been shown to increase brain creatine and phosphor-creatine along with improvement in sleep problems in ageing. Hence, Rawson and Venezia (2011) recommended creatine supplementation for older adults as it is inexpensive and safe and has both peripheral and central effects.

Micronutrients and Ageing

McKay *et al.* (2000) reported on the basis of their observations that supplementation with a multivitamin formulated at about 100 per cent Daily Value can decrease the prevalence of suboptimal vitamin status in older adults and improve their micronutrient status to levels associated with reduced risk for several chronic diseases.

A multi-nutrient supplement is also effective in improving inflammatory status in both men and women. However, improvement was observed to be gender specific *i.e.* markers of pain, joint pain, strength, and power in men only whereas both anxiety and balance (a risk factor for hip fracture) in women. Thus, a multi-nutrient supplement may help middle-aged individuals to prolong physical function and maintain a healthy, active lifestyle (Dunn-Lewis *et al.*, 2011).

Carotenoids

Low dietary intake of beta-carotene has been associated with poor grip, hip, and knee strength in older women and impaired lower extremity performance in older community-dwelling adults in Italy (Cesari *et al.*, 2004; Semba *et al.*, 2003). Associations between total plasma carotenoids and mortality risk remained statistically significant after taking into account: (1) plasma selenium level, which previously was found associated with mortality in this population and (2) level of thiobarbituric acid-reactive substances. By showing, prospectively, in a general healthy elderly population, that total plasma carotenoid levels were independently associated with mortality risk in men, Akbaraly *et al.* (2008; 2009) suggested that total plasma carotenoid levels could be a health indicator in elderly populations and has an independent relationship with onset of dysglycemia. According to Lauretani *et al.* (2008) low plasma carotenoids are an independent risk factor for mortality among older adults living in the community. Low plasma carotenoid levels are also associated with depressive symptoms and indicate the development of new depressive symptoms in older persons (Milaneschi *et al.*, 2012).

Semba *et al.* (2006a) observed that women in the lowest quartile of serum carotenoids had a higher risk of becoming frail (Hazard Ratio = 1.54) and the authors reported later (Semba *et al.*, 2007b) that the low serum carotenoids as indicated by low intake of fruits and vegetables were independent predictors of the progression towards severe walking disability among older women living in the community. Alipanah *et al.* (2009) indicated that higher total serum carotenoid concentrations may be protective against a decline in walking speed in older women.

Vitamin E

Considering the biological function of vitamin E as an important preventive factor, for lipid peroxidation, and on the basis of existing parallelisms between some characteristics of ageing and different symptoms of tocopherol deficiency, a possible influence of this vitamin on the ageing process was postulated. Vitamin E has been shown to enhance T cell-mediated functions in aged animals and humans. Vitamin E supplementation in animal and human subjects resulted in increased lymphocyte proliferation, IL-2 production, and decreased production of the immuno-suppressive factor PGE_2 (Meydani *et al.*, 1986; 1990). Furthermore, vitamin E supplementation was shown to reduce the risk of acquiring upper respiratory infection in the elderly (Meydani *et al.*, 2004) and influenza infection in old mice (Han *et al.*, 2000). Vitamin E exerts its effect on immune function in part by reducing macrophage PGE_2 production (Meydani *et al.*, 1986). However, recent studies indicated a direct effect of vitamin E on T cells independent of its effect on macrophages (Beharka *et al.*, 1997; Adolfsson *et al.*, 2001). This immuno-enhancing effect of vitamin E on T cells was shown to be mediated through increasing the ability of T cells from ageing mice to progress through cell division cycles and to produce IL-2 (Adolfsson *et al.*, 2001).

Han *et al.* (2006) reported that ageing has significant effects on the expression of genes associated with signal transduction, transcriptional regulation, and apoptosis pathways in T cells, and vitamin E has a significant impact on the expression of genes associated with cell cycle and T_h1/T_h2 balance in old T cells.

Vitamin D

An association between low concentrations of vitamin D and inflammation, impairments in cognitive functions such as memory and orientation, executive function as well as dementia and Alzheimer's disease is reported (Llewellyn *et al.*, 2009 and 2011; Oudshorn *et al.*, 2008; Annweiler *et al.*, 2009, 2010 and 2012). Evidence also shows that vitamin D supplementation improves age-related cognitive decline. The neuroprotective effects of vitamin D involves the modulation of inflammatory state resulting in decreased formation of amyloid beta (Aβ) oligomers, a pathological consequence of chronic inflammation (Briones and Darwish, 2012). Moore *et al.* (2005)

provided evidence to suggest that vitamin D_3 acts as an anti-inflammatory agent and reverses the age-related increase in microglial activation and the accompanying increase in IL-1beta (interleukin-1beta) concentration. In addition, Phillips *et al.* (2006) recommended that rheumatoid arthritis patients with documented osteoporosis or those at high risk for the development of this potentially devastating complication should receive calcium and vitamin D supplementation as well as an anti-resorptive agent. Briones and Darwish (2012) concluded from their study that vitamin D supplementation modulated age-related increase in pro-inflammatory state and amyloid burden. It is possible that these effects of vitamin D decreased the memory impairment seen in the aged rats making it a useful therapeutic option to alleviate the effects of ageing on cognitive function.

Vitamin C

If acute administration of ascorbic acid can improve/restore brachial artery flow-mediated dilatation in sedentary older adults, it is possible that longer-term ascorbic acid supplementation could be used therapeutically to sustain the improvement and this effect has been reported in patients with coronary artery disease and congestive heart failure (Hornig *et al.*, 1998; Gokce *et al.*, 1999). Eskurza *et al.* (2004) provided the first evidence for an important role of oxidative stress in both the impairment in peripheral conduit artery flow-mediated dilatation with sedentary human ageing and the preservation of flow-mediated dilatation with physically active ageing. Thus, the benefit of ascorbic acid supplementation has been reinforced.

In recent years, because of the presence of high concentrations of ascorbate in the human lens, considerable interest has been focused on the potential role of ascorbate as a mediator of post-synthetic modifications of crystallins in the ageing lens. It was found that many phenomena observed in ageing and cataractous lenses could be duplicated by the reaction of lens crystallins with ascorbate (Cheng *et al.*, 2002; Atalay *et al.*, 1998). Fan and Monnier (2008) have shown that pharmacologically blocking protein ascorbylation with absorbable guanidino compounds is feasible and may represent a new strategy for the delay of age-related nuclear sclerosis of the lens.

Folic Acid and Vitamin B_{12}

The diagnosis of a vitamin B_{12} deficiency, which is more prevalent in the elderly than younger individuals may be masked by intake of Folic acid (not food folate) beyond Tolerable Upper Limit. When folic acid supplements are recommended, a multi-vitamin that includes vitamin B_{12} should also be advised. The safe and effective increase in folate intake in the elderly should be promoted through naturally occurring folate-rich food sources such as orange, dark green leafy vegetables, asparagus, strawberries and legumes that are also associated with risk reduction of chronic disease.

The evidence suggests that, at the folate fortification level of 140 mcg/100 g of cereal-grain product mandated by the Food and Drug Administration, the benefits through projected decreases in homocysteine level and heart disease risk, greatly outweigh the expected risks (Tucker *et al.*, 1996). But there was no beneficial effect of 750 mcg of folic acid per day on measures of cognition or mood in older healthy women. In patients with mild to moderate cognitive decline and different forms of dementia there was no benefit from folic acid on measures of cognition or mood. Folic acid plus vitamin B_{12} was effective in reducing the serum homocysteine concentrations. (Malouf *et al.*, 2003).

Minerals and Ageing

Selenium

In older adults, low serum selenium concentrations have been associated with poor muscle strength (Beck *et al.*, 2007; Lauretani *et al.*, 2007), increased mortality (Ray *et al.*, 2006), as well as anemia (Semba *et al.*, 2006b; 2007a). These findings suggest that selenium could potentially play a role in ageing-related outcomes, including walking speed. Ray *et al.* (2006) found women living in the community who have higher serum selenium and carotenoids are at a lower risk of death.

Red cell distribution width (RDW), a measure of heterogeneity in the size of circulating erythrocytes, is associated with some chronic diseases and predicts mortality. Oxidative damage and inflammation have been theorized to affect RDW. Serum selenium is an independent predictor of RDW and may potentially mediate effects on RDW through IL-6 (Semba *et al.*, 2010).

Lower serum selenium levels are associated with greater risk of depression (Benton and Cook, 1991; Hawkes and Hornbostel, 1996; Finley and Penland, 1998; Gosney *et al.*, 2008). Research has shown that the brain has a unique feature in selenium metabolism by storing selenium so that glutathione peroxidase activity in the brain does not decrease as fast as in the liver after a low selenium diet (Buckman *et al.*, 1993; Behne and Kyriakopoulos, 2001). Based on this observation, it has been hypothesized that long-term exposure to low selenium may impact brain function such as mood or cognitive function (Gao *et al.*, 2007). As expected, higher selenium levels were associated with lower scores in Geriatric Depression Scale adjusting for demographic and medical conditions ($p = 0.0321$). However, the association between selenium and depressive symptoms was no longer significant when Cognitive Function score was adjusted in the model ($p = 0.2143$) (Gao *et al.*, 2012).

Zinc

Ageing is an inevitable biological process with gradual and spontaneous biochemical and physiological changes and increased susceptibility to diseases.

The nutritional factor, zinc, may remodel these changes with subsequent healthy ageing, because zinc improves the inflammatory/immune response as shown by *in vitro* and *in vivo* studies. Both zinc deficiency and the ageing process are characterized by impaired immune responses and systemic low grade chronic inflammation. It has been hypothesized that age-related zinc deficiency may be an important factor contributing to immune dysfunction and chronic inflammation during the ageing process (Wong and Ho, 2012). Zinc supplementation in old C-carriers restores natural killer cell cytotoxicity and zinc status (Mocchegiani *et al.*, 2010). Physiological zinc supply (12 mg Zn^{++}/day) for 1 month in elderly and in old infected patients (remission phase) restores NK cells activity comparable with values observed in healthy centenarians (Mocchegiani *et al.*, 2003).

In fact, old people aged 60-65 years or older have zinc intakes below 50 per cent of the recommended daily allowance on a given day. Old subjects with specific IL-6 polymorphism (GG allele carriers; named C-) are more suitable for zinc supplementation than the entire old population, in whom correct dietary habits with foods containing zinc (Mediterranean diet) may be sufficient in restoring zinc deficiency and impaired immune response (Mocchegiani *et al.*, 2012).

Wong *et al.* (2013) observed that age-related epigenetic dysregulation in zinc transporter expression may influence cellular zinc levels and contribute to increased susceptibility to inflammation with age. Zinc supplementation may remodel the immune alterations in elderly leading to healthy ageing.

Anti-ageing Phytonutrients

Recent studies suggest that consumption of diets rich in antioxidants and anti-inflammatory components found in fruits, nuts, vegetables, and spices may lower age-related cognitive declines and the risk of developing neurodegenerative disease (Joseph *et al.*, 2009 a). Several phytonutrients are proved to contribute to healthy ageing. Some of these are discussed below.

Astaxanthin

Astaxanthin, a xanthophyll carotenoid, has a unique cell membrane actions and diverse clinical benefits with excellent safety and tolerability. In double-blind, randomized controlled trials, astaxanthin lowered oxidative stress in overweight and obese subjects, and in smokers. The improvement in self-reported scores of pain and satisfaction for the astaxanthin group was significantly better than that for the placebo group suggesting a possible anti-inflammatory effect in rheumatoid arthritis subjects (Nir *et al.*, 2002). Ten healthy men aged 50-69, who had been complaining of forgetfulness, received astaxanthin (12 mg/day) for 12 weeks showed improvement on measures of reaction time, attention, and working memory (Satoh *et al.*, 2009). Supplementation with astaxanthin significantly improved pupillary constriction, and more than 60 per cent of the subjects indicated an improvement in the categories of difficulty to see near objects, eye strain, blurred vision, and shoulder and low-back stiffness (Kajita *et al.*, 2009). Astaxanthin's clinical success extends beyond protection against oxidative stress and inflammation, to demonstrable promise for slowing age-related functional decline (Fassett and Coombes, 2009; Kidd, 2011).

Resveratrol

Resveratrol, a stilbene type compound identified in red wine, ground nuts and fruit juices, have been found to exhibit various pharmacological activities such as anti-oxidative, anti-cancerous, anti-inflammatory and anti-ageing effects (Kim *et al.*, 2011). Interesting insights into the effect of this dietary polyphenolic compound on the lifespan of yeast and flies, implicated the potential of resveratrol as an anti-ageing phytonutrient in treating age-related human diseases. The phenolic compound possesses a low bioavailability and rapid clearance from the plasma. The positive effects of resveratrol on inflammatory response regulation may comprise relevant clinical implications (de la Lastra and Villegas, 2005).

Resveratrol (RSV) has several positive effects on metabolic functions and longevity. Joseph *et al.* (2008) reported that RSV (Pterostilbene) to be effective in reversing cognitive behavioral deficits, as well as dopamine release, and the pterostilbene levels in the hippocampus correlated with working memory.

Pifferi *et al.* (2012) found from their study on gray mouse lemur that RSV may be a potent regulator of sleep-wake rhythms and could be of major interest in the study of sleep perturbations associated with ageing and neuropathology. Resveratrol in red wine may activate genes that slow cellular ageing as proved in animal trials.

Anti-ageing Foods

According to Gladyshev (2008) the food particles first react with hydrochloric acid and enzymes in the stomach to break-down into smaller particles and then each migrate to different parts of the human molecular structure based on their relative thermodynamic stability and their relative chemical affinities for different intra-molecular attachment sites within the human body. Hence, by way of correlating these theories and subsequent data to longevity statistics the author wishes to assign gerontological values to food-stuffs based on enthalpy or heats (Gibbs function) of supramolecular interaction measurements.

Soya (*Glycine max*)

Dietary supplement with fermented soy skim milk can attenuate ageing-induced bone loss in BALB/c mice and possibly lower the risk of osteopenia or osteoporosis in ageing. The beneficial effect may be due to isoflavones as well as higher amounts of polysaccharide and peptide in freeze-dried powder of soy skim milk fermented by *Lactobacillus paracasei* subsp. paracasei NTU 101F milk (Chiang *et al.*, 2012). Dietary consumption of isoflavones in rats controlled body weight. Blake *et al.* (2011) demonstrated that isoflavonoid molecules modulate the brain's influence on behavior.

Sesame Seeds (*Sesamum indicum*)

The anti-ageing effect of sesame was elucidated to be due to the strong vitamin E activity resulting from a novel synergistic effect of sesame lignans with tocopherols. The specific inhibitory action of sesame lignans on Delta5 desaturase in polyunsaturated fatty acid synthesis was reported in studies on the microbial production of polyunsaturated fatty acids (Namiki, 2007). Activities of sesame seed lignans include inter alias modulation of fatty acid metabolism, inhibition of cholesterol absorption and biosynthesis, anti-oxidant and vitamin E-sparing effects, hypotensive effects, improvement of liver functions in connection with alcohol metabolism, and anti-ageing effects (Kamal-Eldin *et al.*, 2011).

Walnut (*Juglans regia*)

Aged rats show decrements in performance on motor and cognitive tasks that require the use of spatial learning and memory. Two per cent walnut diet improved performance on rod walking, while the 6 per cent walnut diet improved performance on the medium plank walk. Both the walnut diets improved working memory in the Morris water maze. Thus, Willis *et al.* (2009b) showed that moderate dietary walnut supplementation can improve cognitive and motor performance in aged rats. *Joseph et al.* (2009b) showed that walnut supplementation in the old rats had similar effects on cognitive function as those seen with berry fruit. *J. regia* had good anti-glycation ability, with a minimum inhibitory concentration (MIC50) of 23 microg/mL and inhibited the Maillard reaction and prevented oxidation *in vitro*. Hence, the extracts of these plants could have therapeutic uses in curbing chronic diabetic complications and slowing down ageing (Ahmad *et al.*, 2012).

Olive Oil

Four decades ago, researchers from the Seven Countries Study concluded that the mono-unsaturated fats in olive oil were largely responsible for the low rates of heart disease and cancer on the Greek island of Crete. Now it is known that olive oil also contains polyphenols, powerful anti-oxidants that may help prevent age-related diseases. Several lines of evidence point to olive oil and the olive oil-centered Mediterranean diet as conducive to longevity (Trichopoulou and Dilis, 2007). Loued *et al.* (2013) observed consumption of extra-virgin olive oil to increase the anti-inflammatory effect of high density lipoprotein and to reduce the age-related decrease in anti-atherogenic activity. Although olive oil phenols cannot reverse the detrimental effects of a prolonged intake of high amounts of fat, improving the quality of olive oil in terms of anti-oxidant content can be beneficial (Jacomelli *et al.*, 2010).

Ageing can be viewed as a quasi-programmed phenomenon driven by the over-activation of the nutrient-sensing mammalian target of rapamycin (mTOR) gerogene. mTOR-driven ageing can be triggered or accelerated by a decline or loss of responsiveness to activation of the energy-sensing protein 5' adenosine monophosphate-activated protein kinase (AMPK), a critical gerosuppressor of mTOR. Extra virgin olive oil secoiridoids constitute a new family of plant-produced gerosuppressant agents similar to resveratrol that molecularly "repair" the aimless (and harmful) AMPK/mTOR-driven quasi-program that leads to ageing and ageing-related diseases, including cancer (Menendez *et al.*, 2013).

An interesting finding by Pitozzi *et al.* (2010) was a reduced step-through latency in the light-dark box test, found in the older animals upon treatment with the oil rich in anti-oxidant phenols, possibly indicating an anxiety-lowering effect. This effect was associated with decreased glutathione reductase activity and expression in the brain, a phenomenon previously associated with decreased anxiety in rodents. Later, in 2012, Pitozzi *et al.*, reported that the treatment with olive oil phenols improved contextual memory in the step-down test to levels similar to young animals and prevented the age-related impairment in motor coordination in the rotarod test. This motor effect was correlated with reduced lipid peroxidation in the cerebellum ($p<0.05$), whereas the memory effect did not correlate with oxidation or inflammation parameters. Thus, natural polyphenols contained in extra-virgin olive oil can improve some age-related dysfunctions by differentially affecting different brain areas. Such a modulation can be obtained with an olive oil possessing sufficiently high content of polyphenols as seen in Mediterranean area.

Fish

Seafood is the only class of food that provides major fractions of DHA, vitamins B_{12} and D, iodine and selenium. Fish consumption was found to result in significantly less cognitive decline compared to the non-consumers with a linear trend between the intake of EPA+DHA and cognitive decline. An average difference of approximately 380 mg/d in EPA+DHA intake was associated with a 1.1-point difference in cognitive decline (van Gelder *et al.*, 2007). Low seafood intake due to socio-economic positions or life styles, would benefit greatly from an increased intake of omega-3 polyunsaturated fatty acid (Bourre and Paquotte, 2008) as a supplement.

Fruits and Vegetables

> *"An apple a day prevents Parkinson's disease."*
>
> *(Kukull, 2012)*

The associations between the dietary patterns and overall mortality were evaluated by Cox models adjusted for potential confounders. The 'Olive Oil and Salad' pattern, characterized by a high consumption of olive oil, raw vegetables, soups and poultry, emerged as being inversely associated with overall mortality in both crude and adjusted models (Masala *et al.*, 2007). Oxidative stress contributes to age-related cognitive decline. In some instances, consumption of fruits and vegetables rich in anti-oxidants can provide superior protection than supplementation with purified anti-oxidants. Fruit or vegetable extracts high in anti-oxidants (*e.g.* blueberry or spinach extracts) might decrease the enhanced vulnerability to oxidative stress that occurs in ageing. Apart from improvements in motor and cognitive behavior, anti-inflammatory activities might be involved in the beneficial effects of these extracts; the most important of these might be their ability to increase cellular signaling and neuronal communication (Joseph *et al.*, 2005). Gao *et al.* (2012) after adjusting for multiple confounders reported that men in the highest quintile of total intake of flavonoids had a 40 per cent lower risk of Parkinson's disease than those in the lowest quintile.

Increasing dietary intake of fruits and vegetables can retard and even reverse age-related declines in brain function and in cognitive and motor performance in rats (Galli *et al.*, 2002). A prospective study conducted in USA revealed that women with high green leafy vegetable intake experienced slower decline than women consuming the least amount (Kang *et al.*, 2005). All berries such as blackberries, blueberries, blackcurrants and black grapes contain phytochemicals - flavonoids, powerful anti-oxidants which help to protect the body against damage caused by free radicals and ageing. Intake of energy-adjusted folate, lycopene, vitamin C and E explained 28 per cent of the protective effect of fruits, berries and vegetables against all-cause mortality, and intake of vitamin C, folate and vitamin E explained 36 per cent of the protective effect against adjusted CVD mortality (Rissanen *et al.*, 2003).

Amla (*Phyllanthus emblica/Emblica officinalis/Phyllanthus niruri*)

Amla significantly reduced thiobarbituric acid-reactive substance levels of serum, renal homogenate, and mitochondria in aged rats, suggesting that amla would ameliorate oxidative stress resulting due to the process of ageing. Yokozawa *et al.* (2007a) observed that amla may prevent age-related hyper-lipidemia through attenuating oxidative stress in the ageing process. Again, Yokozawa *et al.* (2007b) found amla extract to reduce the elevated levels of serum creatinine and urea nitrogen in the aged rats. Amla extract has no pro-oxidation activity induced by iron and/or copper because of its iron and copper chelating ability. According to Chaudhuri (2002) amla helps protect the skin from the damageing effects of free radicals, non-radicals and transition metal-induced oxidative stress. It is thus suitable for use in anti-ageing, sunscreen and general purpose skin care products.

Berries

Berries are rich sources of a wide variety of anti-oxidant phenolics and the phytochemicals including flavonoids, stilbenes, tannins, and phenolic acids, which are powerful anti-oxidants and help to protect the body against damage caused by free radicals and ageing. The isolation and characterization of compounds that may delay the onset of ageing is receiving intense research attention. Some berry phenolics are being associated with this functional performance (Paredes-Lópeze *et al.*, 2010). Higher intake of flavonoids, particularly from berries, appears to reduce rates of cognitive decline in older adults. Additionally, greater intakes of anthocyanidins and total flavonoids were associated with slower rates of cognitive decline (p-trends = 0.015 and 0.053, respectively, for the global score) (Devore *et al.*, 2012).

According to Andres-Lacueva *et al.* (2005) polyphenolic compounds are able to cross the blood brain barrier and localize in various brain regions important for learning and memory. A relationship between Morris water maze performance in blue berry supplemented rats and the total number of anthocyanin compounds found in the cortex suggest that these compounds may deliver their anti-oxidant and signaling modifying capabilities centrally. According to Joseph *et al.* (2007) and Lau *et al.* (2007) polyphenols found in blue berries may exert their beneficial effects by altering stress signaling and neuronal communication.

A considerable degree of age-related object memory decline can be prevented and reversed by brief maintenance on blueberry diets (Malin *et al.*, 2011; Lau *et al.*, 2005; Joseph *et al.*, 1999). So far, strawberry (Shukitt-Hale *et al.*, 2006b), concord grape juice (Shukitt-Hale *et al.*, 2006a), black berry (Shukitt-Hale *et al.*, 2009a), or walnut supplementations (Willis *et al.*, 2009b) have been shown to be effective in reversing motor behavioral deficits. Additionally, it also appears that blue berry (BB) supplementation may inactivate stress signals and increase protective signals, because aged male rats fed a BB-supplemented diet had reduced age-induced increases in NFκB expression in the frontal cortex, hippocampus, and the striatum compared with those of aged un-supplemented controls (Goyarzu *et al.*, 2004).

Blueberry supplementation may protect against neuro-degeneration and cognitive impairment mediated by excite-toxicity and oxidative stresses (Duffy *et al.*, 2008). *B*lueberry polyphenols were able to augment the increased IGF-1 expression and attenuate learning impairments following neuro-toxic insult and exert anti-inflammatory actions, perhaps via alteration of gene expression (Shukitt-Hale *et al.*, 2008a).

Shukitt-Hale *et al.* (2008b) opined that the beneficial effects of blue berries must be through their ability to lower oxidative stress and inflammation, calcium buffering ability, neuro-protective stress shock proteins and plasticity. Besides, the beneficial effects of the berry fruit may involve 4 factors: (1) increase in the activation of protein pathways involved in cognitive function, (2) free radical scavenging, (3) activation of protective signals, and (4) inhibition of stress signals. Straw berries and blue berries and most recently, black berries (Shukitt-Hale *et al.*, 2009a) also enhanced cognitive and motor behavior in aged rats on long term supplementation. Joseph *et al.* (2009) reported similar findings when they supplemented the berries for long term (from 6 to 15 m of age; F344 rats) (BB or strawberry extract at 2 per cent of the diet). They retarded age-related decrements in cognitive or neuronal function. The supplemented diets prevented the onset of age-related deficits in several indices (*e.g.* Morris water maze performance) (Joseph *et al.*, 1998).

Transplantation of central nervous tissue has been proposed as a therapeutic intervention for age-related neuro-degenerative diseases and stroke. However, survival of embryonic neuronal cells is hampered by detrimental factors in the aged host brain such as circulating inflammatory cytokines and oxidative stress. Previously Willis *et al.* (2005) reported that supplementation with 2 per cent Blueberry in the diet increases graft growth and neuronal survival in intraocular hippocampal grafts to aged hosts. Recently, Willis *et al.* (2010) demonstrated direct effects of Blueberry upon microglial activation both during isolated conditions and in the aged host brain and suggest that this nutraceutical can attenuate age-induced inflammation. Blue berry treatment increased survival during acute heat stress, but was not protective against acute oxidative stress. The blue berry extract consists of three major fractions that all contain anti-oxidant activity. However, only one fraction, enriched in proanthocyanidin compounds, increased C. elegans lifespan and thermotolerance (Wilson *et al.*, 2006).

Wolf Berries (*Lycium barbarum*)

Lycium barbarum polysaccharides (LBP), extracts from the wolfberries, a Chinese anti-ageing medicine have been established for their antioxidant potency (Li *et al.*,, 2007). LBP showed neuro-protective function in the retina when given prophylactically. LBP treatment for 1 week effectively protected the retina from neuronal death, apoptosis, glial cell activation, aquaporin water channel up-regulation, disruption of blood-retinal barrier and oxidative stress (Li *et al.*, 2011) thus LBP may have a neuro-protective role to play in ocular diseases for which retinal ischemia/reperfusion is a feature. A new arabinogalactan-protein (LBP-III) isolated from LBP attenuated A beta peptide-activated caspase-3-like activity. LBP-III markedly reduced the phosphorylation of PKR triggered by A beta peptide. Since the phosphorylation state of PKR increased with age, reduction of its phosphorylation triggered by A beta peptide may implicate that LBP-III from *Lycium barbarum* is a potential neuro-protective agent in AD opening a window for the development of a neuro-protective agent for anti-ageing from Chinese medicine (Yu *et al.*, 2005; 2007). Chang and So (2008) have accumulated scientific evidence for its anti-ageing effects of Wolf Berries that should be utilized in modern preventive medicine.

Concord Grape Juice

Rats that drank the 10 per cent grape juice from age 19 to 21 months had improvements in oxotremorine enhancement of K^+-evoked release of dopamine from striatal slices and in cognitive performance on the Morris water maze, and the 50 per cent grape juice produced improvements in motor function (Shukitt-Hale *et al.*, 2006a). Interestingly, a preliminary investigation conducted by Krikorian *et al.* (2008) on the cognitive benefits of grape juice in aged humans has shown that older adults with memory declines, but not dementia, had significant improvements in several measures of cognitive function when supplemented with Concord grape juice for 12 wk as compared to the placebo. Collaborative findings indicate that blue berry or Concord grape juice supplementation in humans with mild cognitive impairment increased verbal memory performance, thus translating the animal findings to humans. Concord grapes thus may increase "health span" and enhance cognitive and motor function in ageing (Joseph *et al.*, 2009 b).

Apple (*Malus domestica/Malus communis/Malus pumila*)

Tchantchou *et al.* (2005) demonstrated that consumption of anti-oxidant-rich foods such as apples prevent the decline in cognitive performance that accompanies normal ageing. Plant-derived polyphenols, which are found in commonly consumed food plants such as tea, cocoa, blueberry and grape, have been proposed to have many health benefits, including slowing ageing. *In vivo* studies have demonstrated the lifespan-extending ability of polyphenol-containing plants (tea, blue berry, cocoa, apple, and pomegranate). These and multiple other plant polyphenols have been shown to have beneficial effects on ageing-associated changes across a variety of organisms from worm and fly through rodent and human (Uysal *et al.*, 2013). Phloridzin, an apple polyphenol notably increased the activity of superoxide dismutase (SOD) and SIRT1 suggesting that SOD and SIR2 have important roles in phloridzin-regulated lifespan extension of yeast, and potentially anti-ageing effects for mammalian cells via SIRT1 (Xiang *et al.*, 2011).

Plums (*Prunus salicina/Prunus domestica*)

Rats from 19 to 21 mo of age fed plum juice had improved working memory in the Morris water maze, whereas rats fed dried plum powder were not different from the control group, possibly due to the smaller quantity of phenolics consumed in the powder group compared with the juice group (Shukitt-Hale *et al.*, 2009b).

Ash Gourd (*Benincasa hispida*)

Ash gourd, belonging to the family Cucurbitaceae, is employed as a main ingredient in kusmanda lehyam, which is used in numerous nervous disorders in the Ayurvedic system of medicine (Aslokar *et al.*, 1992). The major constituents of this fruit are triterpenoids, flavanoids, glycosides, saccharides, carotenes, vitamins, β sitosterin and uronic acid (Kirtikar and Basu, 1918; Nadkarni, 1976; Anil Kumar and Ramu, 2002). The *in vitro* evaluation of a topical cream containing the extract of ash gourd showed skin renewal activity and thus the *Benincasa* fruit extract may prove as an anti-ageing preparation that can be used for retarding the symptoms of ageing (Sabale *et al.*, 2011).

Mandal *et al.* (2009; 2010) reported that *B. hispida* T. has anti-hypochlorhydric activity that prevents the experimental hypochlorhydria and age-induced hypochlorhydria in rat. Pre-administration followed by co-administration of aqueous extract of *B. hispida* (ABH) resulted in significant correction of ranitidine-induced hypochlorhydria in rat. This aqueous extract-treated group showed significantly ($P<0.05$) increased levels of vitamin C, pepsin, and chloride concentration in gastric juice as well as the antioxidant status in respect to other extract-treated groups. Thus Mandal *et al.* (2012) concluded that aqueous extract of ash gourd has a very effective anti-hypochlorhydric and anti-oxidative property.

Spices

The beneficial role of spices (turmeric, curry leaves, ginger, nutmeg etc) which are used generously in Indian cuisine may partly explain the reason for the low incidence of Alzheimer's disease in India (Balenahalli *et al.*, 2010).

Turmeric (*Curcuma longa*)

Turmeric for example, has been prescribed in the literature of Ayurveda ("science of long life") for a wide variety of ailments including obesity, dating from about 3000 BC. In addition to the polyphenols found in walnuts and berry fruits, curcuminoids found in the curry spice turmeric may have similar effects. The biophenolic curcumin, a food preservative, inhibitor of lipid peroxidation with potent anti-inflammatory and anti-cancer activities has a long history of use in Asian traditional medicines (Aggarwal *et al.*, 2007). Curcumin induces cellular stress responses in normal human skin fibroblasts through phosphatidylinositol 3-kinase/AKT pathway and redox signaling, supporting the view that curcumin-induced hormetic stimulation of cellular antioxidant defenses can be a useful approach toward anti-ageing intervention (Lima *et al.*, 2011).

Curcumin from turmeric reduces the elevated oxidative and lipid-mediated stress associated with inflammation, obesity, and atherosclerosis. Zingg *et al.* (2013) are of the opinion that at the cellular level, curcumin may induce a mild oxidative and lipid-metabolic stress leading to an adaptive cellular stress response by hormetic stimulation of cellular antioxidant defense systems and lipid metabolic enzymes. The resulting lower oxidative and lipid-mediated stress may not only explain the beneficial effects of curcumin on inflammation, cardiovascular, and neurodegenerative disease, but may also contribute to the increase in maximum life-span observed in animal models.

Cinnamon (*Cinnamomum zeylanicum*)

Cinnamomum cassia bark (Chinese pharmaceutical name: *Cinnamomi Cortex*, CIN) significantly extended life span in *C. elegans*. CIN in both SQDB and HLXL formula extended life span via modulation of multiple longevity assurance genes, including genes involved in insulin signaling and stress response pathways (Yu *et al.*, 2010). Cinnamon extract facilitates collagen biosynthesis. Cinnamaldehyde significantly increased the phosphorylation levels of the IGF-I receptor and its downstream signaling molecules such as insulin receptor substrate-1 and Erk1/2 in an IGF-I-independent manner. These results suggested that cinnamon extract is useful in anti-ageing treatment of skin (Takasao *et al.*, 2012). Peng *et al.* (2010) observed that cinnamon bark proanthocyanidins exerted protective effects on glucose consumption impaired by methylglyoxal in 3T3-L1 fat cells.

Curry Leaves (*Murraya koenigii*)

Dementia is a syndrome of gradual onset and continuous decline of higher cognitive functioning. It is a common disorder in older persons and has become more prevalent today. Significant improvement in memory scores of young and aged mice fed curry leaves (20 and 30 mg/kg, p.o.) was demonstrated by Mani *et al.* (2012). The alkaloidal extract of curry leaves improved the level of protective antioxidants such as glutathione peroxidase, reduced glutathione, glutathione reductase, superoxide dismutase and catalase in brain homogenate at higher doses (20 and 40mg/kg, p.o.). Moreover, a dose dependent decline was noted in lipid peroxidation and the nitric oxide assay at all doses (10, 20 and 40mg/kg, p.o.). Interestingly, significant progress was noted with the supplementation of curry leaves by an improvement of the acetylcholine levels and a reduction in the acetylcholinesterase activity in aged mouse brain. In addition, a significant elevation of serum albumin, alkaline phosphatase, alanine transaminase, aspartate transaminase and total protein as well as a decline in creatinine, total cholesterol, urea nitrogen and glucose levels with curry leaves also ameliorated the hepatic and renal functions in normal ageing process. Thus Mani *et al.* (2012; 2013) showed the possible utility of *Murraya koenigii* leaves in neuro-protection against neurodegenerative disorders such as Alzheimer's disease.

Green Tea

Epigallocatechin gallate (EGCG) is a main active ingredient of green tea. The significant longevity-extending effects of EGCG on *Caenorhabditis elegans* demonstrated by some studies could be attributed to its *in vitro* and *in vivo* free radical-scavenging effects and its up-regulating effects on stress-resistance-related proteins, including (1) superoxide dismutase-3 (SOD-3), (2) heat shock protein-16.2 (HSP-16.2) and (3) HSP-16:GFP expression (Zhang *et al.*, 2009; Abbas and Wink, 2009). The survival-enhancing effects of EGCG on *C. elegans* under stress are very important for anti-ageing research. Unno *et al.* (2007) found that daily consumption of green tea catechin (GT-catechin) prevented memory regression and DNA oxidative damage in the mice. GT-catechin did not prolong the lifetime of senescence-accelerated mice, but it did delay brain senescence. These findings suggested that continued intake of GT-catechin might promote healthy ageing of the brain in older persons. Unno *et al.* (2008) found that even when ingestion started at the adult age, GT-catechin is helpful in suppressing brain dysfunction with ageing.

The decline in the activity of glutathione peroxidase (GPx), an essential enzyme for reduction of hydrogen and lipid peroxides was prevented in aged mice that had consumed GT-catechin. The increased level of carbonyl proteins, a marker of oxidative damage in proteins, was also significantly reduced in aged mice that had consumed GT-catechin (Kishido *et al.*, 2007).

Other Anti-ageing Agents

Rice [*Oryza sativa* L. (Gramineae)] bran is a rich source of phytochemicals. Its oil also contains several bioactive components that exhibit anti-oxidative properties such as ferulic acid (F), γ-oryzanol (O), and phytic acid (P) which can be a new source of cosmetic raw materials. The formulations containing niosomes entrapped with the rice bran bioactive compounds gave superior clinical anti-ageing activity which can be applied as a novel skin product (Manosroi *et al.*, 2012).

Probiotics

In the 1970s, Soviet Georgia was reported to have more centenarians per capita than any other country claiming that the secret of their long lives was yogurt, a food ubiquitous in their diets. Matsumoto *et al.* (2011) demonstrated increased longevity in mice following probiotic (yogurt) treatment, possibly due to the suppression of chronic low-grade inflammation in the colon induced by higher intestinal luminal polyamine levels (Matsumoto and Kurihara, 2011) and decreased levels of acute inflammation markers in hospitalized elderly patients (Matsumoto *et al.*, 2001). While the age-defying powers of yogurt never have been proved directly, yogurt being rich in calcium and good bacteria, helps stave off osteoporosis and maintain gut health, and also diminish the incidence of age-related intestinal illness.

Conclusions

From the foregoing it is clear that restriction of dietary energy, consumption of foods rich in certain nutrients, polyphenols and anti-oxidants could delay the process of ageing and/or support healthy ageing by increasing the protective signaling against oxidative and inflammatory stressors, and preventing the age related degenerative diseases. Moreover, the beneficial role of foods in cognitive failure and problems associated with cognitive performance in the aged were also addressed by several scientists. More studies on the role of probiotics in healthy ageing is recommended.

References

Abbas S, Wink M (2009). Epigallocatechin gallate from green tea (*Camellia sinensis*) increases lifespan and stress resistance in *Caenorhabditis elegans*. Planta. Med. 75 (3): 216 - 21.

Adolfsson, O., B. T. Huber, S. N. Meydani (2001). Vitamin E-enhanced IL-2 production in old mice: naive but not memory T cells show increased cell division cycling and IL-2-producing capacity. J. Immunol. 167: 3809 - 17.

Aggarwal BB, Sundaram C, Malani N, Ichikawa H (2007). Curcumin: the Indian solid gold. Adv. Exp. Med. Biol. 595: 1 - 75.

Ahmad H, Khan I, Wahid A (2012). Antiglycation and anti-oxidation properties of *Juglans regia* and *Calendula officinalis*: possible role in reducing diabetic complications and slowing down ageing. J. Tradit. Chin. Med. 32 (3): 411 - 14.

Akbaraly TN, Favier A, Berr C (2009). Total plasma carotenoids and mortality in the elderly: results of the Epidemiology of Vascular Ageing (EVA) study. Br. J. Nutr. 101 (1): 86 - 92.

Akbaraly TN, Fontbonne A, Favier A, Berr C (2008). Plasma carotenoids and onset of dysglycemia in an elderly population: results of the Epidemiology of Vascular Ageing Study. Diabetes Care. 31 (7): 1355 - 59.

Alipanah N, Varadhan R, Sun K, Ferrucci L, Fried LP, Semba RD (2009). Low serum carotenoids are associated with a decline in walking speed in older women. J. Nutr. Health. Ageing. 13 (3): 170 - 75.

Andres-Lacueva C, Shukitt-Hale B, Galli RL, Jauregui O, Lamuela-Raventos RM, Joseph JA (2005). Anthocyanins in aged blueberry-fed rats are found centrally and may enhance memory. Nutr. Neurosci. 8 (2): 111 - 20.

Anil Kumar D, Ramu P (2002). Effect of methanolic extract of *Benin-casa hispida* against histamine and acetylcholine induced bron-chospasm in guniea pigs. Indian J. Pharmacol. 34: 365 - 66.

Annweiler C, Allali G, Allain P, Bridenbaugh S, Schott AM, Kressig RW, Beauchet O (2009). Vitamin D and cognitive performance in adults: a systematic review. Eur. J. Neurol. 6: 1083 - 89.

Annweiler C, Fantino B, Schott AM, Krolak-Salmon P, Allali G, Beauchet O (2012). Vitamin D insufficiency and mild cognitive impairment: cross-sectional association. Eur. J. Neurol. 19: 1023 - 29.

Annweiler C, Schott AM, Rolland Y, Blain H, Herrmann FR, Beauchet O (2010). Dietary intake of vitamin D and cognition in older women: a large population-based study. Neurology. 75: 1810 - 16.

Aslokar LV, Kakkar KK, Chakre OJ (1992). Glossary, Indian medicinal plants with active principles. Part I. 1st ed. CSIR. New Delhi. p. 119.

Atalay A, Ogus A, Bateman O, Slingsby C (1998). Vitamin C induced oxidation of eye lens gamma crystallins. Biochimie. 80: 283 - 88.

Balenahalli NR, Sathyanarayana Rao TS, Annamalai P, Kumar S, Jagannatha Rao KS (2010). Neuronutrition and Alzheimer's disease. J. Alzheimers Dis. 19: 1123 - 39.

Barja G (2002 a). Rate of generation of oxidative stress-related damage and animal longevity. Free Radic. Biol. Med. 33 (9): 1167 - 72.

Barja G (2002 b). Endogenous oxidative stress: relationship to ageing, longevity and caloric restriction. Ageing Res. Rev. (3): 397 - 411.

Beharka, A. A., D. Wu, S. N. Han, S. N. Meydani (1997). Macrophage prostaglandin production contributes to the age-associated decrease in T cell function which is reversed by the dietary antioxidant vitamin E. Mech. Ageing Dev. 93: 59 - 77.

Beck J, Ferrucci L, Sun K, Walston J, Fried LP, Varadhan R, Guralnik JM, Semba RD (2007). Low serum selenium concentrations are associated with poor grip strength among older women living in the community. Biofactors. 29: 37 - 44.

Behne D, Kyriakopoulos A (2001). Mammalian selenium-containing proteins. Annu. Rev. Nutr. 21: 453 - 53.

Benton D, Cook R(1991). The impact of selenium supplementation on mood. Biol. Psychiatry. 29 (11): 1092 - 98.

Biagi E, Nylund L, Candela M, Ostan R, Bucci L, *et al.* (2010). Through ageing, and beyond: gut microbiota and inflammatory status in seniors and centenarians. PLoS One. 5: e10667.

Blake C, Fabick KM, Setchell KD, Lund TD, Lephart ED (2011). Neuro-modulation by soy diets or equol: anti-depressive and anti-obesity-like influences, age- and hormone-dependent effects. BMC. Neurosci. 12 : 28.

Blumberg J (1997). Nutritional needs of seniors. J. Am. Coll. Nutr 16: 517 - 23.

Bourre JM (2004). Roles of unsaturated fatty acids (especially omega-3 fatty acids) in the brain at various ages and during ageing. J. Nutr. Health. Ageing. 8 (3): 163 - 74.

Bourre JM, Paquotte P (2008). Seafood (wild and farmed) for the elderly: contribution to the dietary intakes of iodine, selenium, DHA and vitamins B_{12} and D. J. Nutr. Health. Ageing. 12 (3): 186 - 92.

Briones TL, Darwish H (2012). Vitamin D mitigates age-related cognitive decline through the modulation of pro-inflammatory state and decrease in amyloid burden. J. Neuroinflammation. 9: 244.

Brose A, Parise G, Tarnopolsky MA (2003). Creatine supplementation enhances isometric strength and body composition improvements following strength exercise training in older adults. *The Journal of Gerontology: Series A.* 58 (1): 11 - 19.

Buckman TD, Sutphin MS, Eckhert CD (1993). A comparison of the effects of dietary selenium on selenoprotein expression in rat brain and liver. Biochim. Biophys. Acta. 1163 (2): 176 - 84.

Candow DG, Chilibeck PD (2010). Potential of creatine supplementation for improving ageing bone health. J. Nutr. Health. Ageing. 14 (2): 149 - 53.

Candow DG, Little JP, Chilibeck PD, *et al.* (2008). Low-dose creatine combined with protein during resistance training in older men. *Medicine and Science in Sports and Exercise.* 40 (9): 1645 - 52.

Cesari M, Pahor M, Bartali B, Cherubini A, Penninx BW, Williams GR, Atkinson H, Martin A, Guralnik JM, Ferrucci L (2004). Antioxidants and physical performance in elderly persons: the Invecchiare in Chianti (InCHIANTI) study. Am. J. Clin. Nutr. 79: 289 - 94.

Chang RC, So KF (2008). Use of anti-ageing herbal medicine, *Lycium barbarum*, against ageing-associated diseases. What do we know so far? Cell. Mol. Neurobiol. 28 (5): 643 - 52.

Chaudhuri RK (2002). Emblica cascading antioxidant: a novel natural skin care ingredient. Skin Pharmacol. Appl. Skin Physiol. 15 (5): 374 - 80.

Cheng R, Lin B, Ortwerth BJ (2002). Rate of formation of AGEs during ascorbate glycation and during ageing in human lens tissue. Biochim. Biophys. Acta. 1587: 65 - 74.

Chiang SS, Liao JW, Pan TM (2012). Effect of bioactive compounds in lactobacilli-fermented soy skim milk on femoral bone microstructure of ageing mice. J. Sci. Food Agric. 92 (2): 328 – 35.

Chrusch MJ, Chilibeck PD, Chad KE, Davison KS, Burke DG (2001). Creatine supplementation combined with resistance training in older men. *Medicine and Science in Sports and Exercise.* 33 (12): 2111 - 17.

Cid-Rufaza J, Caulfield L, Barron Y, West S (1999). Nutrient intakes and adequacy among an older population on the eastern shore of Maryland: The Salisbury Eye Evaluation. J. Am. Diet. Assoc. 99: 564 - 71.

Claesson MJ, Cusack S, O'Sullivan O, Greene-Diniz R, de Weerd H, *et al.* (2011). Composition, variability, and temporal stability of the intestinal microbiota of the elderly. Proc. Natl. Acad. Sci. U S A. 108 (Suppl 1): 4586 - 91.

de la Lastra CA, Villegas I (2005). Resveratrol as an anti-inflammatory and anti-ageing agent: mechanisms and clinical implications. Mol. Nutr. Food Res. 49 (5): 405 - 30.

Devore EE, Kang JH, Breteler MM, Grodstein F (2012). Dietary intakes of berries and flavonoids in relation to cognitive decline. Ann. Neurol. 72 (1): 135 - 43.

Dalbo VJ, Roberts MD, Lockwood CM, Tucker PS, Kreider RB, Kerksick CM (2009). The effects of age on skeletal muscle and the phosphocreatine energy system: can creatine supplementation help older adults. Dyn. Med. 8: 6.

Duffy KB, Spangler EL, Devan BD, Guo Z, Bowker JL, Janas AM, Hagepanos A, Minor RK, DeCabo R, Mouton PR, Shukitt-Hale B, Joseph JA, Ingram DK. (2008) A blueberry-enriched diet provides cellular protection against oxidative stress and reduces a kainate-induced learning impairment in rats. Neurobiol Ageing. 29 (11): 1680 - 89.

Dunn-Lewis C, Kraemer WJ, Kupchak BR, Kelly NA, Creighton BA, Luk HY, Ballard KD, Comstock BA, Szivak TK, Hooper DR, Denegar CR, Volek JS (2011). A multi-nutrient supplement reduced markers of inflammation and improved physical performance in active individuals of middle to older age: a randomized, double-blind, placebo-controlled study. Nutr. J. 10: 90.

Eskurza I, Monahan KD, Robinson Ja, Seals DR (2004). Effect of acute and chronic ascorbic acid on flow-mediated dilatation with sedentary and physically active human ageing. J. Physiol. 556 (Pt 1): 315 – 24.

Fan X, Monnier VM (2008). Nucleophilic compounds decrease advanced glycation end products (AGEs) from ascorbic acid in the hSVCT2 transgenic mouse model of lenticular ageing. Invest. Ophthalmol. Vis. Sci. 49 (11): 4945 - 52.

Fassett RG, Coombes JS (2009). Astaxanthin, oxidative stress, inflammation and cardiovascular disease. Future Cardiol. 5 (4): 333 - 42.

Finley JW, Penland JG (1998). Adequacy or deprivation of dietary selenium in healthy men clinical and psychological findings. J Trace Elem Exp Med. 11: 1 – 27.

Galli RL, Shukitt-Hale B, Youdim KA, Joseph JA (2002). Fruit polyphenolics and brain ageing: nutritional interventions targeting age-related neuronal and behavioral deficits. Ann. N.Y. Acad. Sci. 959: 128 - 32.

Gao S, Jin Y, Hall KS, Liang C, Unverzagt FW, Ji R *et al.* (2007). Selenium level and cognitive function in rural elderly Chinese. Am. J. Epidemiol. 165 (8): 955 - 65.

Gao S, Jin Y, Unverzagt FW, Liang C, Hall KS, Cao J, Ma F, Murrell JR, Cheng Y, Li P, Bian J, Hendrie HC (2012). Selenium level and depressive symptoms in a rural elderly Chinese cohort. BMC Psychiatry. 2012; 12: 72.

Gao X, Cassidy A, Schwarzschild MA, Rimm EB, Ascherio A (2012). Habitual intake of dietary flavonoids and risk of Parkinson disease. Neurology. 78 (15): 1138 – 45.

Gladyshev GP (2008). [Effect of foodstuff on healthy longevity]. Adv Gerontol. 21 (1): 34 - 36. [Article in Russian].

Gokce N, Keaney JF, Jr, Frei B, Holbrook M, Olesiak M, Zachariah BJ, Leeuwenburgh C, Heinecke JW, Vita JA (1999). Long-term ascorbic acid administration reverses endothelial vasomotor dysfunction in patients with coronary artery disease. Circulation. 99: 3234 - 40.

González S, Huerta JM, Fernández S, Patterson AM, Lasheras C (2010). The relationship between dietary lipids and cognitive performance in an elderly population. Int. J, Food Sci, Nutr. 61 (2): 217 – 25.

Gosney MA, Hammond MF, Shenkin A, Allsup S (2008). Effect of micronutrient supplementation on mood in nursing home residents. Gerontology. 54 (5): 292 - 99.

Gotshalk LA, Kraemer WJ, Mendonca MAG, *et al.* (2008). Creatine supplementation improves muscular performance in older women. *European Journal of Applied Physiology.* 102 (2): 223 - 31.

Gotshalk LA, Volek JS, Staron RS, Denegar CR, Hagerman FC, Kraemer WJ (2002). Creatine supplementation improves muscular performance in older men. Med. Sci. Sports Exerc. 34 (3): 537 - 43.

Goyarzu P, Malin DH, Lau FC, Taglialatela G, Moon WD, Jennings R, Moy E, Moy D, Lippold S et al. (2004). Blueberry supplemented diet: effects on object recognition memory and nuclear factor-kappa B levels in aged rats. Nutr. Neurosci. 7: 75 - 83.

Han SN, Adolfsson O, Lee CK, Prolla TA, Ordovas J, Meydani SN (2006). Age and vitamin E-induced changes in gene expression profiles of T cells. J. Immunol. 177 (9): 6052 - 61.

Han SN, Wu D,. Ha WK, Beharka A, Smith DE,. Bender BS, Meydani SN (2000). Vitamin E supplementation increases T helper 1 cytokine production of old mice infected with influenza virus. Immunology. 100: 487 - 93.

Hawkes WC, Hornbostel L (1996). Effects of dietary selenium on mood in healthy men living in a metabolic research unit. Biol Psychiatry. 39 (2): 121 - 28.

Hornig B, Arakawa N, Kohler C, Drexler H (1998). Vitamin C improves endothelial function of conduit arteries in patients with chronic heart failure. Circulation. 97: 363 - 68.

Institute of Medicine (1997). Dietary Reference Intakes: Calcium, Phosphorus, Magnesium, Vitamin D, and Fluoride. Washington, DC: National Academy Press.

Jacomelli M, Pitozzi V, Zaid M, Larrosa M, Tonini G, Martini A, Urbani S, Taticchi A, Servili M, Dolara P, Giovannelli L (2010). Dietary extra-virgin olive oil rich in phenolic antioxidants and the ageing process: long-term effects in the rat. J. Nutr. Biochem. 21 (4): 290 - 96.

Jakobi JM, Rice CL, Curtin SV, Marsh GD (2001). Neuromuscular properties and fatigue in older men following acute creatine supplementation. *European Journal of Applied Physiology*. 84 (4): 321 - 28.

Joseph J, Cole G, Head E, Ingram D (2009a). Nutrition, brain ageing, and neurodegeneration. J. Neurosci. 29 (41): 12795 - 801.

Joseph JA, Fisher DR, Cheng V, Rimando AM, Shukitt-Hale B (2008). Cellular and behavioral effects of stilbene resveratrol analogues: implications for reducing the deleterious effects of ageing. J. Agric. Food Chem. 56 (22): 10544 - 51.

Joseph JA, Shukitt-Hale B, Casadesus G (2005). Reversing the deleterious effects of ageing on neuronal communication and behavior: beneficial properties of fruit polyphenolic compounds. Am. J. Clin. Nutr. 81 (1 Suppl): 313S - 316S.

Joseph JA, Shukitt-Hale B, Denisova NA, Prior RL, Cao G, Martin A, Taglialatela G, Bickford PC (1998). Long-term dietary strawberry, spinach, or vitamin E supplementation retards the onset of age-related neuronal signal-transduction and cognitive behavioral deficits. J. Neurosci. 18: 8047 - 55.

Joseph JA, Shukitt-Hale B, Lau FC (2007). Fruit polyphenols and their effects on neuronal signaling and behavior in senescence. Ann. N. Y. Acad. Sci. 1100: 470 - 85.

Joseph JA, Shukitt-Hale B, Willis LM (2009b). Grape Juice, Berries, and Walnuts Affect Brain Ageing and Behavior. Journal of Nutrition. 139 (9): 1813S - 17S.

Joseph JA, Shukitt-Hale B, Denisova NA, Bielinski D, Martin A, McEwen JJ, Bickford PC (1999). Reversals of age-related declines in neuronal signal transduction, cognitive, and motor behavioral deficits with blueberry, spinach, or strawberry dietary supplementation. J. Neurosci. 19: 8114 - 21.

Kailasam M, Kaneko G, Oo AKS, Ozaki Y, Thirunavukkarasu AR, *et al*. (2011). Effects of calorie restriction on the expression of manganese superoxide dismutase and catalase under oxidative stress conditions in the rotifer *Brachionus plicatilis*. Fisheries Science. 77: 403 - 409.

Kajita M, Tsukahara H, Kato M (2009). The effects of a dietary supplement containing astaxanthin on the accommodation function of the eye in middle-aged and older people. Med. Consult. New Remedies. 46: 89 - 93.

Kamal-Eldin A, Moazzami A, Washi S (2011). Sesame seed lignans: potent physiological modulators and possible ingredients in functional foods and nutraceuticals. Recent Pat. Food Nutr. Agric. 3 (1): 17 - 29.

Kang JH, Ascherio A, Grodstein F (2005). Fruit and vegetable consumption and cognitive decline in ageing women. Ann. Neurol. 57 (5): 713 - 20.

Kidd P (2011). Astaxanthin, cell membrane nutrient with diverse clinical benefits and anti-ageing potential. Altern. Med. Rev. 16 (4): 355 - 64.

Kim MH, Yoo DS, Lee SY, Byeon SE, Lee YG, Min T, Rho HS, Rhee MH, Lee J, Cho JY (2011). The TRIF/TBK1/IRF-3 activation pathway is the primary inhibitory target of resveratrol, contributing to its broad-spectrum anti-inflammatory effects. Pharmazie. 66(4): 293 - 300.

Kirtikar KR, Basu BD (1918). Indian medicinal plants. 2nd ed. Vol. 2. Allahabad: Lalit Mohan Basu; p. 883.

Kishido T, Unno K, Yoshida H, Choba D, Fukutomi R, Asahina S, Iguchi K, Oku N, Hoshino M (2007). Decline in glutathione peroxidase activity is a reason for brain senescence: consumption of green tea catechin prevents the decline in its activity and protein oxidative damage in ageing mouse brain. Biogerontology. 8 (4): 423 - 30.

Klopstock T, Elstner M, Bender A (2011). Creatine in mouse models of neurodegeneration and ageing. Amino Acids. 40 (5): 1297 - 303.

Klotz T (2002). [Fitness in the elderly]. Urologe A. 41 (4): 315 - 17. [Article in German].

Krikorian R, Nash TA, Shidler MD, Shukitt-Hale B, Joseph JA (2008). Concord grape juice supplementation improves memory function in older adults. American Ageing Association Annual Meeting; June 1, 2008. Boulder (CO): American Ageing Association.

Kubo C, Johnson BC, Gajjar A, Good RA (1987). Crucial dietary factors in maximizing life span and longevity in autoimmune-prone mice. J Nutr. 117 (6): 1129 - 35.

Kukull WA (2012). An apple a day to prevent Parkinson disease: reduction of risk by flavonoids. Neurology. 78 (15): 1112 - 13.

Kwak CS, Lee MS, Lee HJ, Whang JY, Park SC (2010 a). Dietary source of vitamin B(12) intake and vitamin B(12) status in female elderly Koreans aged 85 and older living in rural area. Nutr. Res. Pract. 4 (3): 229 - 34.

Kwak CS, Lee MS, Se In Oh, and Sang Chul Park (2010 b). Discovery of Novel Sources of Vitamin B_{12} in Traditional Korean Foods from Nutritional Surveys of Centenarians. Curr. Gerontol. Geriatr. Res. 2010: 374897.

Lau FC, Shukitt-Hale B, Joseph JA (2005). The beneficial effects of fruit polyphenols on brain ageing. Neurobiol. Ageing. 26 (Suppl 1): 128 - 32.

Lau FC, Shukitt-Hale B, Joseph JA (2007). Nutritional intervention in brain ageing: reducing the effects of inflammation and oxidative stress. Subcell. Biochem. 42: 299 - 318.

Lauretani F, Semba RD, Bandinelli S, Ray AL, Guralnik JM, Ferrucci L (2007). Association of low plasma selenium concentrations with poor muscle strength in older community-dwelling adults: the InCHIANTI study. Am. J. Clin. Nutr. 86: 347 - 52

Lauretani F, Semba RD, Dayhoff-Brannigan M, Corsi AM, Di Iorio A, Buiatti E, Bandinelli S, Guralnik JM, Ferrucci L (2008). Low total plasma carotenoids are independent predictors of mortality among older persons: the InCHIANTI study. Eur. J. Nutr. 47 (6): 335 - 40.

Li SY, Yang D, Yeung CM, Yu WY, Chang RC, So KF, Wong D, Lo AC (2011). Lycium barbarum polysaccharides reduce neuronal damage, blood-retinal barrier disruption and oxidative stress in retinal ischemia/reperfusion injury. PLoS One. 6: e16380.

Li XM, Ma YL, Liu XJ (2007). Effect of the *Lycium barbarum* polysaccharides on age-related oxidative stress in aged mice. J. Ethnopharmacol. 111: 504 - 511.

Lien EJ, Lien LL, Wang J (2010). Longevity depends on a balance between pro-inflammatory and anti-inflammatory factors: use of TCMS and natural products. Curr. Drug Discov. Technol. 7 (1): 13 - 21.

Lima CF, Pereira-Wilson C, Rattan SI (2011). Curcumin induces heme oxygenase-1 in normal human skin fibroblasts through redox signaling: relevance for anti-ageing intervention. Mol. Nutr. Food Res. 55 (3): 430 - 42.

Llewellyn DJ, Lang IA, Langa M, Melzer D (2011). Vitamin D and cognitive impairment in the elderly U.S. population. J. Gerontol. A Biol. Sci. Med. Sci. 66: 59 - 65.

Llewellyn DJ, Langa KM, Lang IA (2009). Serum 25-hydroxyvitamin D concentration and mild cognitive impairment. J. Geriatr. Psychiatry Neurol. 22: 188 - 95.

López-Torres M, Barja G (2008). [Calorie restriction, oxidative stress and longevity]. Rev. Esp. Geriatr. Gerontol. 43 (4): 252 - 60. [Article in Spanish].

Loued S, Berrougui H, Componova P, Ikhlef S, Helal O, Khalil A (2013). Extra-virgin olive oil consumption reduces the age-related decrease in HDL and paraoxonase 1 anti-inflammatory activities. Br. J. Nutr. 19: 1 - 13.

Ma TY, Hollander D, Dadufalza V, Krugliak P (1992). Effect of ageing and caloric restriction on intestinal permeability. Exp. Gerontol. 27: 321 - 33.

Macpherson AJ, Harris NL (2004). Interactions between commensal intestinal bacteria and the immune system. Nat. Rev. Immunol. 4: 478 - 85.

Malin DH, Lee DR, Goyarzu P, Chang YH, Ennis LJ, Beckett E, Shukitt-Hale B, Joseph JA. (2011) Short-term blueberry-enriched diet prevents and reverses object recognition memory loss in ageing rats. Nutrition. 27 (3): 338 - 42.

Malouf M, Grimley EJ, Areosa SA (2003). Folic acid with or without vitamin B_{12} for cognition and dementia. Cochrane Database Syst. Rev. 4: CD004514.

Mani V, Ramasamy K, Ahmad A, Parle M, Shah SA, Majeed AB (2012). Protective effects of total alkaloidal extract from *Murraya koenigii* leaves on experimentally induced dementia. Food Chem. Toxicol. 50 (3-4): 1036 - 44.

Mani V, Ramasamy K, Ahmad A, Wahab SN, Jaafar SM, Kek TL, Salleh MZ, Majeed AB (2013). Effects of the total alkaloidal extract of *Murraya koenigii* leaf on oxidative stress and cholinergic transmission in aged mice. Phytother. Res. 27 (1): 46 - 53.

Mandal U, De D, Nandi DK, Biswas A, Ghosh D (2009). Anti-hypochlorhydric and anti-lipidperoxidative activity of composite extract of whole plant of *Fumaria vaillatii* and ripe fruit of *Benincasa hispida* on aged male albino rat. Pharmacologyonline. 1: 573 - 77.

Mandal U, Nandi D, Chatterjee K, Biswas A, Ghosh D (2010). Remedial effect of aqueous extract of whole plant of *Fumaria vaillantii* Loisel and ripe fruit of *Benincasa hispida* Thunb in ranitidine induced-hypochlorhydric male rat. Int. J. Appl. Res. Nat. Prod. 3: 37 - 47.

Mandal U, De D, Ali KM, Biswas A, Ghosh D (2012). Effect of different solvent extracts of *Benincasa hispida* T. on experimental hypochlorhydria in rat. J. Adv. Pharm. Technol. Res. 3 (1): 41 - 46.

Manosroi A, Chutoprapat R, Abe M, Manosroi W, Manosroi J (2012). Anti-ageing efficacy of topical formulations containing niosomes entrapped with rice bran bioactive compounds. Pharm. Biol. 50 (2): 208 - 24.

Masala G, Ceroti M, Pala V, Krogh V, Vineis P, Sacerdote C, Saieva C, Salvini S, Sieri S, Berrino F, Panico S, Mattiello A, Tumino R, Giurdanella MC, Bamia C, Trichopoulou A, Riboli E, Palli D (2007). A dietary pattern rich in olive oil and raw vegetables is associated with lower mortality in Italian elderly subjects. Br. J. Nutr. 98 (2): 406 - 15.

Matsumoto M, Kurihara S (2011). Probiotics-induced increase of large intestinal luminal polyamine concentration may promote longevity. Med. Hypotheses. 77 (4): 469 - 72.

Matsumoto M, Kurihara S, Kibe R, Ashida H, Benno Y (2011). Longevity in mice is promoted by probiotic-induced suppression of colonic senescence dependent on upregulation of gut bacterial polyamine production. PLoS One. 6 (8): e23652.

Matsumoto M, Ohishi H, Benno Y (2001). Impact of LKM512 yogurt on improvement of intestinal environment of the elderly. FEMS Immunol. Med. Microbiol. 31: 181 - 186.

McCay, C., Crowell, M., Maynard, L., 1935. The effect of retarded growth upon the length of life and upon ultimate size. J. Nutr. 10, 63–79.

McKay DL, Perrone G, Rasmussen H, Dallal G, Hartman W, Cao G, Prior RL, Roubenoff R, Blumberg JB (2000). The effects of a multivitamin/mineral supplement on micronutrient status, antioxidant capacity and cytokine production in healthy older adults consuming a fortified diet. J. Am. Coll. Nutr. 19 (5) 613 - 21.

McCarty MF (2003). A low-fat, whole-food vegan diet, as well as other strategies that down-regulate IGF-I activity, may slow the human ageing process. Med. Hypotheses. 60 (6): 784 - 92.

McCarty MF, Barroso-Aranda J, Contreras F (2009). The low-methionine content of vegan diets may make methionine restriction feasible as a life extension strategy. Med. Hypotheses. 72 (2): 125 - 28.

Menendez JA, Joven J, Aragonès G, Barrajón-Catalán E, Beltrán-Debón R, Borrás-Linares I, Camps J, Corominas-Faja B, Cufí S, Fernández-Arroyo S, Garcia-Heredia A, Hernández-Aguilera A, Herranz-López M, Jiménez-Sánchez C, López-Bonet E, Lozano-Sánchez J, Luciano-Mateo F, Martin-Castillo B, Martin-Paredero V, Pérez-Sánchez A, Oliveras-Ferraros C, Riera-Borrull M, Rodríguez-Gallego E, Quirantes-Piné R, Rull A, Tomás-Menor L, Vazquez-Martin A, Alonso-Villaverde C, Micol V, Segura-Carretero A (2013). Xenohormetic and anti-ageing activity of secoiridoid polyphenols present in extra virgin olive oil: a new family of gero-suppressant agents. Cell. Cycle. 12 (4): 555 - 78.

Meydani, S. N., M. Meydani, C. P. Verdon, A. A. Shapiro, J. B. Blumberg, K. C. Hayes. 1986. Vitamin E supplementation suppresses prostaglandine E_2 synthesis and enhances the immune response of aged mice. Mech. Ageing Dev. 34: 191-201.

Meydani, S. N., M. P. Barklund, S. Liu, M. Meydani, R. A. Miller, J. G. Cannon, F. D. Morrow, R. Rocklin, J. B. Blumberg. 1990. Vitamin E supplementation enhances cell-mediated immunity in healthy elderly subjects. Am. J. Clin. Nutr. 52:557-563.

Meydani, S. N., L. S. Leka, B. C. Fine, G. E. Dallal, G. T. Keusch, M. F. Singh, D. H. Hamer. 2004. Vitamin E and respiratory tract infections in elderly nursing home residents: a randomized controlled trial. J. Am. Med. Assoc. 292: 828-836.

Milaneschi Y, Bandinelli S, Penninx BW, Corsi AM, Lauretani F, Vazzana R, Semba RD, Guralnik JM, Ferrucci L (2012). The relationship between plasma carotenoids and depressive symptoms in older persons. World J. Biol. Psychiatry. 13 (8): 588 - 98.

Miyagi S, Iwama N, Kawabata T, Hasegawa K (2003). Longevity and diet in Okinawa, Japan: the past, present and future. Asia Pac. J. Public Health. 15 Suppl: S3-9.

Mocchegiani E, Malavolta M, Costarelli L, Giacconi R, Cipriano C, Piacenza F, Tesei S, Basso A, Pierpaoli S, Lattanzio F (2010). Zinc, etallothioneins and immuno-senescence. Proc. Nutr. Soc. 69 (3): 290 - 99.

Mocchegiani E, Muzzioli M, Giacconi R, Cipriano C, Gasparini N, Franceschi C, Gaetti R, Cavalieri E, Suzuki H (2003). Metallothioneins/PARP-1/IL-6 interplay on natural killer cell activity in elderly: parallelism with nonagenarians and old infected humans. Effect of zinc supply. Mech. Ageing Dev. 124 (4): 459 - 68.

Mocchegiani E, Romeo J, Malavolta M, Costarelli L, Giacconi R, Diaz LE, Marcos A (2012). Zinc: dietary intake and impact of supplementation on immune function in elderly. Age (Dordr). 2012 Jan 6. [Epub ahead of print].

Moore ME, Piazza A, McCartney Y, Lynch MA (2005). Evidence that vitamin D_3 reverses age-related inflammatory changes in the rat hippocampus. Biochem. Soc. Trans. 33 (Pt 4): 573 - 77.

Munro H, Suter P, Russell R (1987). Nutritional requirements of the elderly. Ann. Rev. Nutr. 7: 23 - 49.

Murtagh-Mark CM, Reiser KM, Harris R Jr, McDonald RB (1995). Source of dietary carbohydrate affects life span of Fischer 344 rats independent of caloric restriction. J Gerontol A Biol. Sci.Med. Sci. 50 (3): B148 - 54.

Nadkarni AK (1976). The Indian Materia Medica. Popular Prakashan Pvt. Ltd. Mumbai, India. pp. 185 - 86.

Namiki M (2007). Nutraceutical functions of sesame: a review. Crit. Rev. Food Sci. Nutr. 47 (7): 651 - 73.

NHANES (National Health and Nutrition Examination Survey III) 1988 - 94. CD Rom Series 11, No. 1, 1A, 1997.

Nir Y, Spiller G, Multz C (2002). Effect of an astaxanthin containing product on rheumatoid arthritis. J. Am. Coll. Nutr. 21: 490.

Obrenovich ME, Li Y, Parvathaneni K, Yendluri BB, Palacios HH, Leszek J, Aliev G (2011). Antioxidants in health, disease and ageing. CNS Neurol Disord Drug Targets. 10 (2): 192 - 207.

Oo AKS, Kaneko G, Hirayama M, Kinoshita S, Watabe S (2010). Identification of genes differentially expressed by calorie restriction in the rotifer (*Brachionus plicatilis).* Journal of Comparative Physiology. B: Biochemical, Systemic, and Environmental Physiology. 180: 105 - 116.

Oudshorn C, Mattace-Raso FUS, Van der Velde N, Colin EM, Van der Cammen TJM (2008). Higher serum vitamin D3 levels are associated with better cognitive test performance in patients with Alzheimer's disease. Dement. Geriatr. Cogn. Disord. 25: 539 - 43.

Ozdemir N (2009). The Effect of Caloric Restriction on the Life Span and Reproduction of Fresh Water Rotifer (*Brachionus calyciflorus*). Journal of Animal and Veterinary Advances. 8: 669 - 673.

Paddon-Jones D, Rasmussen BB (2009). Dietary protein recommendations and the prevention of sarcopenia.*Current Opinion in Clinical Nutrition and Metabolic Care.* 12 (1): 86 - 90.

Pamplona R, Barja G (2007). Highly resistant macromolecular components and low rate of generation of endogenous damage: two key traits of longevity. Ageing Res. Rev. 6 (3): 189 - 210.

Peng X, Ma J, Chao J, Sun Z, Chang RC, Tse I, Li ET, Chen F, Wang M (2010). Beneficial effects of cinnamon proanthocyanidins on the formation of specific advanced glycation endproducts and methylglyoxal-induced impairment on glucose consumption. J. Agric. Food Chem. 58 (11): 6692 - 96.

Pérez-López FR, Chedraui P, Haya J, Cuadros JL (2009). Effects of the Mediterranean diet on longevity and age-related morbid conditions. Maturitas. 64 (2): 67-79.

Paredes-López O, Cervantes-Ceja ML, Vigna-Pérez M, Hernández-Pérez T (2010). Berries: improving human health and healthy ageing, and promoting quality life–a review. Plant. Foods Hum. Nutr. 65 (3): 299 - 308.

Phillips K, Aliprantis A, Coblyn J (2006). Strategies for the prevention and treatment of osteoporosis in patients with rheumatoid arthritis. Drugs Ageing. 23 (10): 773 - 79.

Pifferi F, Rahman A, Languille S, Auffret A, Babiloni C, Blin O, Lamberty Y, Richardson JC, Aujard F (2012). Effects of dietary resveratrol on the sleep-wake cycle in the non-human primate gray mouse lemur (*Microcebus murinus*). Chronobiol. Int. 29 (3): 261 - 70.

Pitozzi V, Jacomelli M, Catelan D, Servili M, Taticchi A, Biggeri A, Dolara P, Giovannelli L (2012). Long-term dietary extra-virgin olive oil rich in polyphenols reverses age-related dysfunctions in motor coordination and contextual memory in mice: role of oxidative stress. Rejuvenation Res. 15 (6): 601 - 612.

Pitozzi V, Jacomelli M, Zaid M, Luceri C, Bigagli E, Lodovici M, Ghelardini C, Vivoli E, Norcini M, Gianfriddo M, Esposto S, Servili M, Morozzi G, Baldi E, Bucherelli C, Dolara P, Giovannelli L (2010). Effects of dietary extra-virgin olive oil on behaviour and brain biochemical parameters in ageing rats. Br. J. Nutr. 103 (11): 1674 - 83.

Rawson ES, Clarkson PM (2000). Acute creatine supplementation in older men. *International Journal of Sports Medicine*. 21 (1): 71 - 75.

Rawson ES, Clarkson PM, Price TB, Miles MP (2002). Differential response of muscle phosphocreatine to creatine supplementation in young and old subjects. *Acta. Physiologica. Scandinavica*. 174 (1): 57 – 65.

Rawson ES, Venezia AC (2011). Use of creatine in the elderly and evidence for effects on cognitive function in young and old. Amino Acids. 40 (5): 1349 - 62.

Ray AL, Semba RD, Walston J, Ferrucci L, Cappola AR, Ricks MC, Xue QL, Fried LP (2006). Low serum selenium and total carotenoids are independent predictors of mortality among older women living in the community: the Women's Health and Ageing Studies. J. Nutr. 136: 172 - 76.

Rissanen TH, Voutilainen S, Virtanen JK, Venho B, Vanharanta M, Mursu J, Salonen JT (2003). Low intake of fruits, berries and vegetables is associated with excess mortality in men: the Kuopio Ischaemic Heart Disease Risk Factor (KIHD) Study. J. Nutr. 133 (1): 199 - 204.

Rosenberg I (1995). Nutritional Assessment of Elderly Populations, Bristol-Myers Squibb/Mead Johnson Nutrition Symposia. vol 13. Raven Press. New York.

Rosenman SJ, Shrikant P, Dubb L, Benveniste E, Ransohoff R (1995). Cytokine-induced expression of vascular cell adhesion molecule-1 (VCAM-1) by astrocytes and astrocytoma cell lines. J. Immunol. 154: 1888 - 99.

Roth LW, Polotsky AJ (2012). Can we live longer by eating less? A review of caloric restriction and longevity. Maturitas. 71 (4): 315 - 19.

Sabale V, Kunjwani H, Sabale P (2011). Formulation and *in vitro* evaluation of the topical antiageing preparation of the fruit of *Benincasa hispida*. J. Ayurveda. Integr. Med. 2 (3): 124 - 48.

Saltzman J, Russell R (1998). The ageing gut: nutritional issues. Gastroenterology Clinics of North America 27: 309 - 324.

Sanchez-Roman I, Gómez A, Pérez I, Sanchez C, Suarez H, Naudí A, Jové M, Lopez-Torres M, Pamplona R, Barja G (2012). Effects of ageing and methionine restriction applied at old age on ROS generation and oxidative damage in rat liver mitochondria. Biogerontology. 2012 May 13. [Epub ahead of print].

Satoh A, Tsuji S, Okada Y *et al.* (2009). Preliminary clinical evaluation of toxicity and efficacy of a new astaxanthin-rich *Haematococcus pluvialis* extract. J. Clin. Biochem. Nutr. 44: 280 - 84.

Schipper HM (1996). Astrocytes, brain ageing, and neurodegeneration. Neurobiol Ageing. 17: 467–80.

Semba RD, Bartali B, Zhou J, Blaum C, Ko CW, Fried LP (2006a). Low serum micronutrient concentrations predict frailty among older women living in the community. J. Gerontol. A Biol. Sci. Med. Sci. 61 (6): 594 - 99.

Semba RD, Blaum C, Guralnik JM, Totin D, Ricks MO, Fried LP (2003). Low carotenoid and vitamin E status are associated with indicators of sarcopenia among older women living in the community. Ageing Clin. Exp. Res. 15: 482 - 87.

Semba RD, Ferrucci L, Cappola AR, Ricks MO, Ray AL, Xue QL, Guralnik JM, Fried LP (2006b). Low serum selenium is associated with anemia among older women living in the community: the Women's Health and Ageing Studies I and II. Biol. Trace Elem. Res. 112 (2): 97 - 107.

Semba RD, Patel, KV, Ferrucci L, Sun K, Roy CN, Guralnik JM, Fried LP (2010). Serum antioxidants and inflammation predict red cell distribution width in older women: the Women's Health and Ageing Study I. Clin. Nutr.9 (5): 600 - 604.

Semba RD, Ricks MO, Ferrucci L, Xue QL, Guralnik JM, Fried LP (2007a). Low serum selenium is associated with anemia among older adults in the United States. Eur J Clin Nutr. 2007 Sep 5; [Epub ahead of print].

Semba RD, Varadhan R, Bartali B, Ferrucci L, Ricks MO, Blaum C, Fried LP (2007b). Low serum carotenoids and development of severe walking disability among older women living in the community: the women's health and ageing study I. Age Ageing. 36 (1): 62 - 67.

Shukitt-Hale B, Carey A, Simon L, Mark DA, Joseph JA (2006 a). The effects of Concord grape juice on cognitive and motor deficits in ageing. Nutrition. 22: 295 - 302.

Shukitt-Hale B, Cheng V, Bielinski D, Carey AN, Lau FC, Seeram NP, Heber D, Joseph JA (2006 b). Differential brain regional specificity to blueberry and strawberry polyphenols in improved motor and cognitive function in aged rats. Soc. Neurosci. Abstr. 32: 81 - 15.

Shukitt-Hale B, Cheng V, Joseph JA (2009a). Effects of blackberries on motor and cognitive function in aged rats. Nutritional Neuroscience. 12: 135 - 40.

Shukitt-Hale B, Kalt W, Carey AN, Vinqvist-Tymchuk M, McDonald J, Joseph JA (2009b). Plum juice, but not dried plum powder, is effective in mitigating cognitive deficits in aged rats. Nutrition. 25 (5): 567 - 73.

Shukitt-Hale B, Lau FC, Carey AC, Galli RL, Spangler EL, Ingram DK, Joseph JA (2008a). Blueberry polyphenols prevent kainic acid-induced decrements in cognition and alter inflammatory gene expression in rat hippocampus. Nutr. Neurosci. 11: 172 - 82.

Shukitt-Hale B, Lau FC, Joseph JA (2008b). Berry fruit supplementation and the ageing brain. J Agric Food Chem. 56 (3): 636 - 41.

Steffen BJ, Breier G, Butcher E, Schulz M, Engelhardt B (1996). ICAM-1, VCAM-1, and MAdCAM-1 are expressed on choroid plexus epithelium but not endothelium and mediate binding of lymphocytes *in vitro*. Am. J. Pathol. 148: 1819 - 38.

Stella N, Estelles A, Siciliano J, Tence M, Desagher S, Piomelli D, Glowinski J, Premont J (1997). Interleukin-1 enhances the ATP-evoked release of arachidonic acid from mouse astrocytes. J. Neurosci. 17: 2939 - 46.

Takasao N, Tsuji-Naito K, Ishikura S, Tamura A, Akagawa M (2012). Cinnamon extract promotes type I collagen biosynthesis via activation of IGF-I signaling in human dermal fibroblasts. J. Agric. Food Chem. 60 (5): 1193 - 200.

Tarnopolsky MA (2000). Potential benefits of creatine monohydrate supplementation in the elderly. *Current Opinion in Clinical Nutrition and Metabolic Care.* 3 (6): 497 - 502.

Tchantchou F, Chan A, Kifle L, Ortiz D, Shea TB (2005). Apple juice concentrate prevents oxidative damage and impaired maze performance in aged mice. J. Alzheimers Dis. 8 (3) 283 - 87.

Trichopoulou A (2001). Mediterranean diet: the past and the present. Nutr. Metab. Cardiovasc. Dis. 11 (4 Suppl): 1 - 4.

Trichopoulou A, Dilis V (2007). Olive oil and longevity. Mol. Nutr. Food Res. 51 (10): 1275 - 78.

Trichopoulou A, Vasilopoulou E (2000). Mediterranean diet and longevity. Br. J. Nutr. 84 Suppl 2: S205 - 209.

Tucker KL, Mahnken B, Wilson PW, Jacques P, Selhub J (1996). Folic acid fortification of the food supply. Potential benefits and risks for the elderly population. JAMA. 276 (23): 1879 - 85.

Unno K, Ishikawa Y, Takabayashi F, Sasaki T, Takamori N, Iguchi K, Hoshino M (2008). Daily ingestion of green tea catechins from adulthood suppressed brain dysfunction in aged mice. Biofactors. 34 (4): 263 - 71.

Unno K, Takabayashi F, Yoshida H, Choba D, Fukutomi R, Kikunaga N, Kishido T, Oku N, Hoshino M (2007). Daily consumption of green tea catechin delays memory regression in aged mice. Biogerontology. 8 (2): 89 - 95.

USDA (1997). Agricultural Research Service: Data tables: Results from USDA's 1994 - 96 Continuing Survey of Food Intakes by Individuals and 1994 - 96 Diet and Health Knowledge Survey, ARS Food Surveys Research Group.

Uysal U, Seremet S, Lamping JW, Adams JM, Liu DY, Swerdlow RH, Aires DJ (2013). Consumption of polyphenol plants may slow ageing and associated diseases. Curr. Pharm. Des. 2013 Feb 19. [Epub ahead of print].

van Gelder BM, Tijhuis M, Kalmijn S, Kromhout D (2007). Fish consumption, n-3 fatty acids, and subsequent 5-y cognitive decline in elderly men: the Zutphen Elderly Study. Am. J. Clin. Nutr. 85 (4): 1142 - 47.

Waijers PM, Ocké MC, van Rossum CT, Peeters PH, Bamia C, Chloptsios Y, van der Schouw YT, Slimani N, Bueno-de-Mesquita HB. (2006). Dietary patterns and survival in older Dutch women. Am. J. Clin. Nutr. 83 (5): 1170 - 76.

Wahlqvist ML, Darmadi-Blackberry I, Savige GS, Kouris-Blazos A, Trichopoulos D (2003). Age-fitness. How achievable with food? Forum Nutr. 56: 258 - 61.

Willis L, Bickford P, Zaman V, Moore A, Granholm AC (2005). Blueberry extract enhances survival of intraocular hippocampal transplants. Cell Transplant. 14 (4): 213 - 23.

Willis LM, Freeman L, Bickford PC, Quintero EM, Umphlet CD, Moore AB, Goetzl L, Granholm AC (2010). Blueberry supplementation attenuates microglial activation in hippocampal intraocular grafts to aged hosts. Glia. 58 (6): 679 - 90.

Willis LM, Shukitt-Hale B, Cheng V, Joseph JA (2009 b). Dose-dependent effects of walnuts on motor and cognitive function in aged rats. Br. J. Nutr. 101 (8): 1140 - 44.

Willis LM, Shukitt-Hale B, Joseph JA (2009a). Dietary polyunsaturated fatty acids improve cholinergic transmission in the aged brain. Genes Nutr. 4 (4): 309 - 14.

Wilson MA, Shukitt-Hale B, Kalt W, Ingram DK, Joseph JA, Wolkow CA (2006). Blueberry polyphenols increase lifespan and thermotolerance in *Caenorhabditis elegans*. Ageing Cell. 5 (1): 59 - 68.

Wiroth JB, Bermon S, Andreï S, Dalloz E, Hébuterne X, Dolisi C (2001). Effects of oral creatine supplementation on maximal pedalling performance in older adults. *European Journal of Applied Physiology*. 84 (6): 533 - 39.

Wong CP, Ho E (2012). Zinc and its role in age-related inflammation and immune dysfunction. Mol. Nutr. Food Res. 56 (1): 77 - 87.

Wong CP, Magnusson KR, Ho E (2013). Increased inflammatory response in aged mice is associated with age-related zinc deficiency and zinc transporter dysregulation. J. Nutr. Biochem. 24 (1): 353 - 59.

Woodroofe MN (1995). Cytokine production in the central nervous system. Neurology. 45 (Suppl 6): S6 - 10.

Wright J, Bialostosky K, Gunter E, Carroll M, Najjar M, Bowman B, Johnson C (1998). Blood Folate and vitamin B12: United States, 1988 - 94. Vital Health Stat 11: 1 - 78,

Yang J, Dong S, Jiang Q, Kuang T, Huang W, Yang J (2013). Changes in Expression of Manganese Superoxide Dismutase, Copper andZinc Superoxide Dismutase and Catalase in *Brachionus calyciflorus* during the Ageing Process. PLoS One. 8 (2): e57186.

Yokozawa T, Kim HY, Kim HJ, Okubo T, Chu DC, Juneja LR (2007a). Amla (*Emblica officinalis* Gaertn.) prevents dyslipidaemia and oxidative stress in the ageing process. Br. J. Nutr. 97 (6): 1187 - 95.

Yokozawa T, Kim HY, Kim HJ, Tanaka T, Sugino H, Okubo T, Chu DC, Juneja LR. *et al*. (2007b). Amla (*Emblica officinalis* Gaertn.) attenuates age-related renal dysfunction by oxidative stress. J. Agric. Food Chem. 55 (19): 7744 - 52.

Young VR (1979). Diet as a modulator of ageing and longevity. Fed. Proc. 38 (6): 1994 - 2000.

Yu MS, Leung SK, Lai SW, Che CM, Zee SY, So KF, Yuen WH, Chang RC (2005). Neuro-protective effects of anti-ageing oriental medicine *Lycium barbarum* against beta-amyloid peptide neurotoxicity. Exp. Gerontol. 40: 716 - 27.

Yu MS, Lai CS, Ho YS, Zee SY, So KF, Yuen WH, Chang RC (2007). Characterization of the effects of anti-ageing medicine *Fructus lycii* on beta-amyloid peptide neurotoxicity. Int. J. Mol.Med. 20: 261 - 68.

Yu Young-Beob, Dosanjh L, Lao L, Tan M, Shim BS, and Luo Y (2010). *Cinnamomum cassia* Bark in Two Herbal Formulas Increases Life Span in *Caenorhabditis elegans* via Insulin Signaling and Stress Response Pathways. PLoS One. 5 (2): e9339.

Yurko-Mauro K (2010). Cognitive and cardiovascular benefits of docosahexaenoic acid in ageing and cognitive decline. Curr. Alzheimer. Res. 7 (3): 190 - 96.

Zhang L, Jie G, Zhang J, Zhao B (2009). Significant longevity-extending effects of EGCG on Caenorhabditis elegans under stress. Free Radic. Biol. Med. 46 (3): 414 - 21.

Zingg JM, Hasan ST, Meydani M (2013). Molecular mechanisms of hypo-lipidemic effects of curcumin. Biofactors. 39 (1): 101 - 121.

Xiang L, Sun K, Lu J, Weng Y, Taoka A, Sakagami Y, Qi J (2011). Anti-ageing effects of phloridzin, an apple polyphenol, on yeast via the SOD and Sir2 genes. Biosci. Biotechnol. Biochem. 75 (5): 854 - 58.

Chapter 2

Anti-Allergic Foods

The term "food hypersensitivity" is referred to any pathological manifestation due to consumption of a specific food. As per the molecular mechanism of action it is termed as "food intolerance" or "food allergy". Food allergy is a common widespread problem globally and is on the rise in recent years. It is also termed type I hypersensitivity, and is defined as " a disease following a response by the immune system to an otherwise innocuous antigen" or "an allergic reaction provoked by re exposure to a specific type of antigen referred to as an allergen" which involves IgE antibody (en.wikipedia.org/wiki).

Allergen could be a substance of any chemical nature in the environment, capable of inducing allergy or specific hypersensitivity. The route of entry of an allergen can be through inhalation, food, touch or injection. Hypersensitivity occurs upon re exposure to an allergen. Allergy may be immediate or delayed, local or systemic and include anaphylaxis and contact dermatitis.

Though the exact prevalence of food allergy in the general population is unknown, its incidence is reported to be 20 per cent in general population and 12 per cent among children (Castellazzi *et al.,* 2013). The increasing occurrence of food allergies and eczema are now adding to the already existing substantial burden of asthma and respiratory allergic diseases (Prescott and Nowak-Wêgrzyn, 2011). Since, the consequences of food allergy could be dangerous and sometimes life threatening, it has become a growing food safety concern.

Several treatment strategies have been developed depending on the nature of allergens and the kind of the immunological mechanisms involved (Burks *et al.,* 2001; Pons *et al.,* 2005). Ribeiro *et al.* (2013) from a descriptive, cross-sectional self-administered questionnaire concerning the current recommendations of pediatricians, pediatric gastroenterologists, allergists and nutritionists revealed that there are gaps in the knowledge of professionals about the primary prevention of food allergy. The professionals recommended modifying the age of introduction of complementary feeding to prevent the development of food allergy.

Based on extensive characterization of food allergens and a better understanding of the immunological mechanisms underlying allergic disease, promising therapeutic modalities for the treatment and eventual prevention of food allergy are being developed. Currently, strict avoidance of the allergenic food and ready access to self-injectable epinephrine is the 'standard of care' for food allergy.

Novel immunotherapeutic strategies include peptide immunotherapy, traditional Chinese medicine, mutated or homologous protein immunotherapy, DNA immunization and immunization with immuno-stimulatory sequences, of which all strive to elicit a decreased T helper cell type 2-like response or tolerance by the immune system in response to a specific food allergen. Other approaches such as the anti-IgE therapy or the Fcgamma-Fcepsilon fusion protein aim at preventing the release of mediators by mast cells. The combination of these different approaches would probably offer the best treatment for food-allergy in future (Wild and Leherer, 2001; Pons and Burks, 2005; Burks *et al.*, 2001; 2008).

Quite a few food immuno-therapies are being developed that involve oral, sublingual, epicutaneous, or subcutaneous administration of small amounts of native or modified allergens to induce immune tolerance followed by a maintenance phase with regular intake of a maximum tolerated amount of food. Oral immuno-therapy seems to be a promising approach for food allergic patients based on results from small uncontrolled and controlled studies. For example, diet containing heated milk and egg may represent an alternative approach to oral immuno-modulation for cow's milk and egg allergic subjects (Martinolli *et al.*, 2013).

There is increasing evidence that the unbalanced composition of the human microbiome on human skin and mucosal surfaces may be a key player in the development of inflammatory diseases like allergy and asthma. However, this concept has not yet been verified in the recent past. There are few studies using bacterial lysates to cure food allergy, for example, *Escherichia coli* plus *Enterococcus faecalis* in an inactive form through a preparation-ProSymbioflor, and heat-killed *Bifidobacterium breve* and *Streptococcus thermophilus*. However, prevalence of food allergy could not be reduced by such interventions (Lau, 2013).

Foods that can prevent the development of wheezing through their antioxidant effects contain vitamin C and selenium; blood levels of these elements correlate negatively with the risk of wheezing. Intake of vitamin E during pregnancy also appears to be correlated with a reduced risk of wheezing in the offspring. Similarly, low intake of zinc and carotenoids by pregnant women is associated with an increased risk of wheezing and asthma in childhood. Fiber also has anti-inflammatory properties and protective effects against allergic diseases such as atopic dermatitis and asthma (Peroni *et al.*, 2012).

Several attempts are made towards decreasing or alleviating the allergeniciy of certain foods as discussed below.

Cow's Milk Allergy

The first adverse reactions to cow's milk were already described 2000 years ago. However, the analysis of cow's milk allergens started only 50 years ago (Hochwallner *et al.*, 2013). Administration of probiotics in addition to elimination diet and base treatment to infants improved gastrointestinal manifestations of cow's milk allergy (Ivakhnenko and Nyankovskyy, 2013).

Exclusive breastfeeding may help to prevent allergic disease among infants by decreasing exposure to exogenous antigens, protecting against infections, promoting gastrointestinal mucosal maturation and the development of gut microbiota, and conferring immuno-modulatory and anti-inflammatory benefits (Szajewska, 2012). Promotion of breastfeeding, the use of hydrolysed formula for lactose intolerant infants in the first 6 months of life and introduction of solid foods between 4 and 6 months are recommended.

Egg White Allergy

Egg allergy has been shown to be the most common food allergy in children with atopic dermatitis (Sampson and McCaskill, 1985; Niggemann *et al.*, 1999). Hen eggs are one of the most frequent causes for adverse reactions (Bock and Atkins, 1990; Boyano-Martínez *et al.*, 2002) affecting approximately 1.6 per cent of children (Sicherer and Sampson, 2006; Eggesbø *et al.*, 2001).

Heated foods often present low allergenicity, and have recently been used in specific oral immunotherapy for food allergies. Since, the intact proteins in raw egg are responsible for their allergenicity (Escudero *et al.*, 2013), denaturation of the same could be a preventive strategy. The effectiveness of heat treatment at various levels and duration on the allegenicity of egg white has been tested by several scientists. The ovalbumin (OVA, a major allergen) in egg white heated at 100°C for 5 min lost allergenicity, but demonstrated higher digestive stability and slower absorption in intestine, without causing inflammation while untreated egg white presented intestinal inflammation (Watanabe *et al.*, 2013). The loss of potential allergenicity of OVA was at the expense of increased IgG reactivity. Glycation of OVA on heating also significantly reduced its potential allergenicity (Ma *et al.*, 2013).

Whereas baking or boiling of egg white for 30 minutes rather than 10 minutes resulted in a significant reduction in allergenicity as evident from the decreased intensity of the protein band at 45 kD (corresponding to ovalbumin). Thus the duration rather than the temperature in heat treatment was shown to influence the composition and reduce allergenicity of egg white proteins (Shin *et al.*, 2013).

Many children with IgE-mediated allergy to egg can tolerate egg in baked foods. Out of 236 egg-allergic children who had been strictly avoiding egg in their diet and put on open food challenge to baked egg, 64 per cent passed and successfully incorporated baked egg into their diet. Only 36 per cent reacted to this challenge. However, Turner *et al.* (2013) therefore recommended that open food challenge to baked egg should take place under medical supervision.

On the other hand observational studies suggest that early regular ingestion of allergenic foods might reduce the risk of food allergy. Palmer *et al.* (2013) confirmed that induction of immune tolerance pathways and reduction in egg allergy incidence can be achieved by early regular oral egg exposure in infants with eczema but cautioned that these high-risk infants when first exposed to egg may have sensitization already by 4 months of age.

Peanut Allergy

Among food allergies, peanut allergy is frequently associated with severe anaphylactic reactions. The only preventive measure for peanut allergy is strict avoidance of the incriminating food (Burks *et al.*, 2004). The use of the anti-IgE therapy in conjunction with other immunotherapy has been recommended by Pons *et al.* (2005). Recently, it was reported that Transforming growth factor beta (TGF-β) induced in the gut by VSL#3 (A probiotic medical food) supplementation, is capable of reducing the Th2 inflammation associated with food anaphylaxis in a mouse model of peanut sensitization. TGF-β acts through the induction/maintenance of regulatory T cells expressing FOXP3 and/or latency-associated peptide (Barletta *et al.*, 2013).

Despite that during childhood natural tolerance development is frequent, some children with cow's milk or hen's egg allergy and the majority of children with peanut allergy remain allergic until adulthood, limiting not only the diet of patients but also their quality of life (Martinolli *et al.*, 2013).

Certain foods, food hydrolysates, phytochemicals and probiotic organisms have been identified with anti allergic properties, emphasizing the food based approach as a remedial measure to food allergies.

Foods

Vegetable and Fruit Concentrate

Current therapies such as inhaled steroids, long-acting beta-agonist bronchodilators, antihistamines and immuno-modulators may control the symptoms of allergic asthma but fail to modify the underlying disease. Excessive use of steroids and other immuno-suppresents alter the patient's quality of life, produce undesirable toxicities, and increase the risk of other pathologies such as diabetes. Hence novel therapeutic options to manage asthma are desirable (Ramana *et al.*, 2011). A combination of fruit plus vegetable concentrate, fish oil and probiotics (FVFP supplement) was found to be effective in controlling improved pulmonary function in asthmatic children in a 16-week school-based double-blind placebo-controlled randomised trial (Lee *et al.*, 2013).

A reduction in the levels of IgE, histamine, and interleukin (IL)-1β in serum by bamboo salt (BS -a specially processed salt prepared from sun-dried salt (SDS) and bamboo in Korea) was reported by Kim *et al.* (2012). The number of eosinophils and infiltration of mast cells also decreased on BS treatment in ovalbumin sensitised mice. The other benefits of BS treatment included inhibition of caspase-1 activity, production of IL-1β and thymic stromal lymphopoietin in the nasal mucosa tissue. Thus the authors confirmed the *in vitro* anti-allergic and anti-inflammatory effects of BS in allergic rhinitis mice models.

Though numerous synthetic aldose reductase inhibitors have been tested, these have not been very successful clinically. In the course of identifying and testing new and effective ARIs, Reddy *et al.* (2011) have evaluated a number of traditional and common dietary sources and found that some spice principles and fruits & vegetables have the potential to inhibit aldose reductase (ALR2) under *in vitro* conditions and in animal models. Flavonoids are abundantly found in fruits, vegetables, herbs and spices, and some flavonoids have been shown to inhibit ALR2 (Kawanishi *et al.*, 2003; Zenon *et al.*, 1990; Fernández *et al.*, 2005; Matsuda *et al.*, 2005; Varma *et al.*, 1975). Rutin is one of the commonly found dietary flavonols. Varma *et al.* (1975) demonstrated that rutin may have ARI activity. Prominent inhibitory property was found in spinach, cumin, fennel, lemon, basil and black pepper with an approximate IC50 of 0.2 mg/mL with an excellent selectivity towards aldose reductase. As against this, 10 to 20 times higher concentrations were required for 50 per cent inhibition of aldehyde reductase (Saraswat *et al.*, 2008).

Fenugreek

Fenugreek extract was found to reduce ear thickness as well as the infiltration of eosinophils and mast cells. In homogenized ear, the production of IL-4, IL-5, IL-13, and IL-1β was suppressed. Their differentiation into Th2 cells was also prevented in the splenocytes of OVA-induced allergic mice. This confirms the traditional practice of fenugreek being useful in treating allergic inflammatory diseases (Bae *et al.*, 2012).

Date Palm (*Phoenix dactylifera* L.)

Oral administration of a hot water extract of matured fruit of the date palm resulted in significantly lower sneezing and nose rubbing events in mice than in controls. Karasawa and Otani (2012) proposed that some polyphenols in the date may reduce mite-induced allergic symptoms in mice *via* a decrease in the number of IgE-producing plasma cells and high-affinity IgE receptor-expressing mast cells.

Turmeric (*Curcuma longa*)

Turmeric is known for its multiple health benefits and has been used in treating several diseases including respiratory disorders. The active component of turmeric is curcumin, a polyphenolic phytochemical, with anti-inflammatory, anti-amyloid, antiseptic, anti-tumor, and anti-oxidative properties.

In the last two decades curcumin has been shown to be a potent immunomodulatory agent that can modulate the activation of T cells, B cells, macrophages, neutrophils, natural killer cells, and dendritic cells. Curcumin can also down-regulate the expression of various pro-inflammatory cytokines including TNF, IL-1, IL-2, IL-6, IL-8, IL-12, and chemokines, most likely through inactivation of the transcription factor NF-kappaB. The inhibitory effect of curcumin on histamine release from mast cells is responsible for its anti-allergic properties (Jagetia and Aggarwal, 2007). Intragastric treatment of latex-sensitized mice with curcumin demonstrated a diminished Th2 response with a concurrent reduction in lung inflammation. Eosinophilia was markedly reduced along with a reduction in the co-stimulatory molecule expression (CD80, CD86, and OX40L) on antigen-presenting cells, and expression of MMP-9, OAT, and TSLP genes (Kurup *et al.*, 2007; Kurup and Barrios, 2008).

Oh *et al.* (2011) also observed that treatment with curcumin significantly attenuated airway hyper responsiveness (AHR) and reduced the numbers of total leukocytes and eosinophils in broncho-alveolar lavage (BAL) fluid. Infiltration of inflammatory cells and mucus occlusions in lung tissue were also significantly ameliorated, along with a decreased level of IgE in BAL fluid. Curcumin attenuates the development of allergic airway inflammation and development of asthma possibly through inhibition of NF-κB activation in the asthmatic lung tissue.

Mango-ginger (*Curcuma amada* Roxb.)

Anti-inflammatory activity, platelet aggregation inhibitory activity, cytotoxicity and anti-allergic activity are some of the biological activities of mango ginger. The major chemical components that might be responsible to these benefits include phytochemicals such as phenolic acids, volatile oils, curcuminoids and terpenoids like difurocumenonol, amadannulen and amadaldehyde (Policegoudra *et al.*, 2011).

Mangosteen *(Garcinia mangostana)*

Alpha- and γ-mangostin, which are the major xanthones purified from a mangosteen exhibit a wide range of anticancer, antioxidant, and anti-inflammatory activities. In addition, administration of α- and γ-mangostins significantly reduced the major patho-physiological features of allergic asthma, including inflammatory cell recruitment into the airway, AHR and increased levels of Th2 cytokines suggesting the therapeutic potential of α- and γ-mangostin in the treatment of allergic asthma (Jang *et al.*, 2012).

Picholine Olive Oil

Picholine olive oil from Montpellier in Southern France showed an inhibitory effect on the chemical mediator release and decreased expressions of genes related to type I allergy in RBL-2H3 cells as Picholine olive oil has high content of flavonoids, especially apigenin (Isoda *et al.*, 2012).

Bilberry (*Vaccinium myrtillus* L.)

Bilberry is one of the best sources of anthocyanins and provides 15 anthocyanin analogues, each composed of one of five anthocyanidins and one of three glucosides. (Ichiyanagi *et al.*, 2004). In addition, it was recently shown that oral administration of cyanidin-3-o-β-D-glucoside, an anthocyanin found in black rice, as well as its metabolite cyanidin, promotes anti-scratching behavior in pruritogen-induced acute pruritus in mice (Han *et al.*, 2009). Treatment with Bilberon-25 significantly attenuated the TNCB-induced increase in scratching behaviour, but dexamethasone did not. In contrast, ear swelling was ameliorated by dexamethasone treatment, and significantly decreased by Bilberon-25. Hence, Yamaura *et al.* (2011) reported that anthocyanins from bilberry might be beneficial for the treatment of chronic allergic contact dermatitis. It has been reported that anthocyanins are particularly sensitive to thermal treatment and are easily hydrolyzed to anthocyanidins when exposed to high temperatures. So, Yamaura *et al.* (2012) on further experimentation concluded that the anthocyanin-rich but not anthocyanidin-rich bilberry extract may be a useful dietary supplement for skin diseases involving pruritic symptoms, such as chronic allergic contact dermatitis, atopic dermatitis, and rhinitis.

Vitamin D

Vitamin D deficiency has been reported to be a risk factor for allergic asthma in children (Litonjua, 2012). Vitamin D supplementation was found to ameliorate clinical signs of mild, moderate and severe atopic dermatitis according to SCORAD (Scoring Atopic Dermatitis) and TIS value index (Three Item Severity score) and it is also said to be a safe and well-tolerated form of therapy (Samochocki *et al.*, 2013; Amestejani *et al.*, 2012). Similarly, Hart (2013) and Agrawal *et al.* (2013) found vitamin D supplementation to reduce airway hypersensitivity and allergic airway inflammation in animals. In children cow's milk allergy, adequate intake of vitamin D showed a positive correlation with serum concentration of 25-hydroxy vitamin D (Rowicka *et al.*, 2012). Hartmann *et al.* (2012) provided evidence that systemic Vitamin D Receptor (VDR) agonist treatment may improve allergen-triggered eczema *in vivo.*

Food Hydrolysates: Whey/Casein Hydrolysate

The whey hydrolysate as well as casein hydrolysate was found to be equally effective in food allergies. The symptom-based score (a tool useful to evaluate the efficacy of dietary treatment in infants with cow's milk protein allergy) developed by Vandenplas *et al.* (2013) showed statistically significant reductions in both groups. The total and specific IgE and skin prick test results were similar. Further, the whey hydrolysate standard formula sequence led to better growth at the age of 1 year than the other three feeding regimens tested.

A follow up study of infants upto 5 years of age showed a significant lowering in the cumulative incidence of atopic disease in the breast-fed as well as the whey hydrolysate group of children; but soy formula was not effective. Similarly, in the 18-60 month period, prevalence of eczema and severity were less in the whey hydrolysate group compared with the other groups. Exclusive breast-feeding or feeding with a partial whey hydrolysate formula is associated with lower incidence of atopic disease and food allergy. This is a cost-effective approach to the prevention of allergic disease in children (Chandra, 1997).

Phytochemicals

Currently, there is a renewed interest in the use of phytochemicals in inflammation and allergic diseases. Fisetin (3,7,3',4'-tetrahydroxyflavone), a naturally occurring bioactive flavonol, has been shown to inhibit NF-κB activity (Goh *et al.*, 2012). Phenolic acids and polyphenols, such as flavonoids, are the best studied natural substances known to possess an anti-inflammatory and anti-allergic (Manach *et al.*, 2004; Williams and Grayer, 2004; Chirumbolo, 2010; 2013; Visioli *et al.*, 2011; Calderon-Montano *et al.*, 2011; Russo *et al.*, 2012; Magrone and Jirillo, 2012; Singh *et al.*, 2011) as well as immune-modulating potential (Hollman and Katan, 1999; Middleton *et al.*, 2000). Though several phytochemicals have been investigated for their anti-allergic activity, the mechanism of action could not be elucidated so far which has limited their therapeutic application (Bellik *et al.*, 2012).

Probiotics

In patients suffering from multiple food allergies, induction of oral tolerance by specific probiotics continues to attract research interest (Nermes *et al.*, 2013).

Due to their immuno-modulatory properties, several probiotic organisms have been found to be effective and safe in controlling the food allergies. The benefits of probiotics in various types of food allergies and the mode of action are discussed below.

Probiotics are nonpathogenic microorganisms which, when ingested, exert a positive influence on the health or physiology of the host. Their mechanism of action and effects are now studied using the same pharmacological approach as for drugs. Randomized double-blind studies have provided evidence of probiotic effectiveness for the treatment and prevention of acute diarrhea and antibiotic-induced diarrhea, as well as for the prevention of cow milk–induced food allergy in infants and young children (Goldin and Gorbach, 2008).

Gut microbiota composition can be used to discriminate between allergic and healthy children, and the distinction may precede clinical manifestations of disease. Breast milk provides the first inoculum of bacteria, which influences the risk of becoming allergic later in life. Bifidobacterium species are major determinants of disease risk. Specific probiotics may modulate early microbial colonization, which represents the first intervention target in allergic disease, together with their ability to reverse the increased intestinal permeability, characteristic of children with atopic eczema and food allergy. A balanced gut microbiota is crucial for the development of healthy immuno-regulation and gut barrier function to allow brisk immune responses to pathogens and systemic hypo-responsiveness to harmless antigens such as food (Nermes *et al.*, 2013).

The clinical situations studied include prevention or treatment of lactose intolerance and allergy (especially atopic eczema), apart from other antibiotic-associated disorders (Marteau, 2002). The potential application of probiotics on many other effects is under investigation. However, according to Singh *et al.* (2013) many of these clinical studies require validation before applying these results to clinical realm. Analyzing the results from meta-analyses and systematic reviews that combine results of studies from different types of probiotics to examine the effects in any disease state, Minocha (2009) said that specific strains are effective only in specific disease states.

A large number of people, as they age, experience a decline in the level of lactase (β-galactosidase) in the intestinal brush border mucosa. This decline causes lactose to be incompletely absorbed, resulting in flatus, bloating, abdominal cramps, and moderate-to-severe diarrhoea *i.e. Lactose mal-absorption* (Goldin and Gorbach, 2008). Several studies have demonstrated that, during the fermentative process in the production of yogurt, lactase is produced, which can exert its influence in the intestinal tract (deVrese *et al.*, 2001; Kolars *et al.*, 1984). The organisms commonly used for the production of yogurt are *Lactobacillus bulgaricus* and *Streptococcus salivarius* subsp. *Thermophilus*. Kim and Gilliland (1983) found that feeding yogurt to lactose-intolerant individuals caused a significant reduction in the level of breath hydrogen compared with that in subjects who were fed milk, thus proving its benefit.

Supplementation with the probiotic *Lactobacillus reuteri* reduced the incidence of IgE-associated allergic disease in infancy, but did not lead to a lower prevalence of respiratory allergic disease in school age (Abrahamsson *et al.*, 2013).

Studies have reported a significant reduction in asthma and eczema from supplementation with a mixture of galacto- and fructo-oligosaccharide (GOS/FOS 9:1 ratio) (8 g/L) to infants at high risk of allergy; and in eczema from supplementation with GOS/FOS (9:1) (6.8 g/L) and acidic oligosacccharide (1.2 g/L) in infants not selected for allergy risk. But Osborn and Sinn (2013) after reviewing the available work on high risk infants concluded that further research is needed before routine use of prebiotics (oligosaccharide) can be recommended for prevention of allergy in formula fed infants. There is some evidence that a prebiotic supplement added to infant feeds may prevent eczema. It is unclear whether the use of prebiotic should be restricted to infants at high risk of allergy or may have an effect in low risk populations; or whether it may have an effect on other allergic diseases including asthma.

Though probiotic bacteria continue to represent the most promising intervention for primary prevention of allergic disease, Ismail *et al.* (2013) expressed the need for well-designed definitive intervention studies as a research priority.

Conclusions

Several strategies such as maintenance of hygienic conditions, avoidance of microbial exposure and consumption of probiotic supplements have been suggested to control food allergy. Nutrients such as polyunsaturated fatty acids, anti-oxidants, folate and vitamin D are also being investigated (Prescott and Nowak-Wêgrzyn, 2011).

However, the current evidence-based guidelines for allergy prevention still remain limited and there is a need for identification of suitable markers, risk factors and preventive mechanisms. Desirable therapeutic strategies for the treatment and prevention of the food allergies must be safe, relatively inexpensive, and easily administered.

References

Abrahamsson TR, Jakobsson T, Björkstén B, Oldaeus G, Jenmalm MC (2013). No effect of probiotics on respiratory allergies: a seven-year follow-up of a randomized controlled trial in infancy. Pediatr. Allergy. Immunol. 24 (6): 556 - 61.

Agrawal T, Gupta GK, Agrawal DK (2013). Vitamin D supplementation reduces airway hyperresponsiveness and allergic airway inflammation in a murine model. Clin. Exp. Allergy. 43 (6): 672 - 83.

Amestejani M, Salehi BS, Vasigh M, Sobhkhiz A, Karami M, Alinia H, Kamrava SK, Shamspour N, Ghalehbaghi B, Behzadi AH (2012). Vitamin D supplementation in the treatment of atopic dermatitis: a clinical trial study. J. Drugs. Dermatol. 11 (3): 327 - 30.

Bae MJ, Shin HS, Choi DW, Shon DH (2012). Anti-allergic effect of *Trigonella foenum-graecum* L. extracts on allergic skin inflammation induced by trimellitic anhydride in BALB/c mice. J. Ethnopharmacol. 144 (3): 514 - 22.

Barletta B, Rossi G, Schiavi E, Butteroni C, Corinti S, Boirivant M, Di Felice G (2013). Probiotic VSL#3-induced TGF-β ameliorates food allergy inflammation in a mouse model of peanut sensitization through the induction of regulatory T cells in the gut mucosa. Mol. Nutr. Food Res. 2013 Aug 14. doi: 10.1002/mnfr.201300028. [Epub ahead of print].

Bellik Y, Boukraâ L, Alzahrani HA, Bakhotmah BA, Abdellah F, Hammoudi SM, Iguer-Ouada M (2012). Molecular mechanism underlying anti-inflammatory and anti-allergic activities of phytochemicals: an update. Molecules. 18 (1): 322 - 53.

Bock SA, Atkins FM (1990). Patterns of food hyper-sensitivity during sixteen years of double-blind, placebo-controlled food challenges. J. Pediatr. 117: 561 - 567.

Boyano-Martínez T, García-Ara C, Díaz-Pena JM, Martín-Esteban M (2002). Prediction of tolerance on the basis of quantification of egg white-specific IgE antibodies in children with egg allergy. J. Allergy. Clin. Immunol. 110: 304 - 309.

Burks W, Bannon G, Lehrer SB (2001). Classic specific immunotherapy and new perspectives in specific immunotherapy for food allergy. Allergy. 56 Suppl. 67: 121 - 24.

Burks W, Kulis M, Pons L (2008). Food allergies and hypersensitivity: a review of pharmacotherapy and therapeutic strategies. Expert Opin Pharmacother. 9 (7): 1145 - 52.

Burks W, Lehrer SB, Bannon GA (2004). New approaches for treatment of peanut allergy: chances for a cure. Clin. Rev. Allergy. Immunol. 27 (3): 191 - 96.

Calderon-Montano JM, Burgos-Moron E, Perez-Guerrero C, Lopez-Lazaro M (2011). A review on the dietary flavonoid kaempferol. Mini Rev. Med. Chem. 11: 298 - 344

Castellazzi AM, Valsecchi C, Caimmi S, Licari A, Marseglia A, Leoni MC, Caimmi D, Miraglia del Giudice M, Leonardi S, La Rosa M, Marseglia GL (2013). Probiotics and food allergy. Ital. J. Pediatr. 39: 47.

Chandra RK (1997). Five-year follow-up of high-risk infants with family history of allergy who were exclusively breast-fed or fed partial whey hydrolysate, soy, and conventional cow's milk formulas. J Pediatr Gastroenterol Nutr. 24 (4): 380 - 88.

Chirumbolo S (2010). The role of quercetin, flavonols and flavones in modulating inflammatory cell function. Inflamm. Allergy. Drug. Targets. 9: 263 - 85.

Chirumbolo S (2013). Dietary assumption of plant polyphenols and prevention of allergy. Curr. Pharm. Des. 2013 May 16. [Epub ahead of print].

deVrese M, Stegelmann A, Richter B, Fenseau S, Love C, Schrezenneir J (2001). Probiotics compensation for lactose insufficiency. Am. J. Clin. Nutr. 73: 421 - 29.

Eggesbø M, Botten G, Halvorsen R, Magnus P (2001). The prevalence of allergy to egg: a population-based study in young children. Allergy. 56: 403 - 411.

Escudero C, Sánchez-García S, Rodríguez del Río P, Pastor-Vargas C, García-Fernández C, Pérez-Rangel I, Ramírez-Jiménez A, Ibánez (2013). MDDehydrated egg white: an allergen source for improving efficacy and safety in the diagnosis and treatment for egg allergy. Pediatr. Allergy. Immunol. 24 (3): 263 - 69.

Fernández M, Caballero J, Helguera, AM, Castro EA, González MP (2005). Quantitative structure–activity relationship to predict differential inhibition of aldose reductase by flavonoid compounds. Bioorg. Med. Chem. 13: 3269 - 77.

Goh FY, Upton N, Guan S, Cheng C, Shanmugam MK, Sethi G, Leung BP, Wong WS (2012). Fisetin, a bioactive flavonol, attenuates allergic airway inflammation through negative regulation of NF-κB. Eur. J. Pharmacol. 679 (1-3): 109 - 116.

Goldin BR, Gorbach SL (2008). Clinical indications for probiotics: an overview. Clin. Infect. Dis. 46 Suppl. 2: S96 - 100.

Han SJ, Ryu SN, Trinh HT, Joh EH, Jang SY, Han MJ, Kim DH (2009). Metabolism of cyanidin-3-O-beta-D-glucoside isolated from black colored rice and its anti-scratching behavioral effect in mice. J. Food. Sci. 74 (8): H253 - 58.

Hart PH (2013). Benefits of vitamin D for allergic airways. Clin. Exp. Allergy. 43 (6): 580 - 82.

Hartmann B, Riedel R, Jörss K, Loddenkemper C, Steinmeyer A, Zügel U, Babina M, Radbruch A, Worm M (2012). Vitamin D receptor activation improves allergen-triggered eczema in mice. J. Invest. Dermatol. 132 (2): 330 - 36.

Hochwallner H, Schulmeister U, Swoboda I, Spitzauer S, Valenta R (2013). Cow's milk allergy: From allergens to new forms of diagnosis, therapy and prevention. Methods. pii: S1046 - 2023 (13) 00303 - 304.

Hollman PC, Katan MB (1999). Health effects and bioavailability of dietary flavonols. Free Radic. Res. 31: S75 - S80.

Ichiyanagi T, Kashiwada Y, Ikeshiro Y, Hatano Y, Shida Y, Horie M, Matsugo S, Konishi T (2004). Complete assignment of bilberry (*Vaccinium myrtillus* L.) anthocyanins separated by capillary zone electrophoresis. Chem. Pharm. Bull. 52: 226 - 29.

Ismail IH, Licciardi PV, Tang ML (2013). Probiotic effects in allergic disease. J Paediatr Child Health. 2013 Apr 11. doi: 10.1111/jpc.12175. [Epub ahead of print].

Isoda H, Motojima H, Margout D, Neves M, Han J, Nakajima M, Larroque M (2012). Anti-allergic effect of Picholine olive oil-in-water emulsions through β-hexosaminidase release inhibition and characterization of their physicochemical properties. J. Agric. Food. Chem. 60 (32): 7851 - 58.

Ivakhnenko O, Nyankovskyy S (2013). [Effect of probiotics on the dynamics of gastrointestinal symptoms of food allergy to cow's milk protein in infants]. Georgian Med News. (219):46-52. [Article in Russian].

Jagetia GC, Aggarwal BB (2007). "Spicing up" of the immune system by curcumin. J. Clin. Immunol. 27 (1): 19 - 35.

Jang HY, Kwon OK, Oh SR, Lee HK, Ahn KS, Chin YW (2012). Mangosteen xanthones mitigate ovalbumin-induced airway inflammation in a mouse model of asthma. Food Chem Toxicol. 50 (11): 4042 - 50.

Karasawa K, Otani H (2012). Anti-allergic properties of a matured fruit extract of the date palm tree (*Phoenix dactylifera L.*) in mite-sensitized mice. J. Nutr. Sci. Vitaminol. (Tokyo). 58 (4): 272 - 77.

Kawanishi K, Ueda H, Moriyasu M (2003). Aldose reductase inhibitors from the nature. Curr. Med. Chem. 10: 1353 - 74.

Kim HS, Gilliland SE (1983). *Lactobacillus acidophilus* as dietary adjunct for milk to aid lactose digestion in humans. J. Dairy. Sci. 1; 66: 959 - 66.

Kim KY, Nam SY, Shin TY, Park KY, Jeong HJ, Kim HM (2012). Bamboo salt reduces allergic responses by modulating the caspase-1 activation in an OVA-induced allergic rhinitis mouse model. Food. Chem. Toxicol. 50 (10): 3480 - 88.

Kolars JC, Levitt MD, Aouj M, Savaino DA (1984). Yogurt - an anti-digesting source of lactose. N. Engl. J. Med. 310: 1 - 3.

Kurup VP, Barrios CS (2008). Immunomodulatory effects of curcumin in allergy. Mol. Nutr. Food Res. 52 (9): 1031 - 39.

Kurup VP, Barrios CS, Raju R, Johnson BD, Levy MB, Fink JN (2007). Immune response modulation by curcumin in a latex allergy model. Clin. Mol. Allergy. 5: 1.

Lau S (2013). Bacterial lysates in food allergy prevention. Curr. Opin. Allergy. Clin. Immunol. 13 (3): 293 - 95.

Lee SC, Yang YH, Chuang SY, Huang SY, Pan WH (2013). Reduced medication use and improved pulmonary function with supplements containing vegetable and fruit concentrate, fish oil and probiotics in asthmatic school children: a randomized controlled trial. Br. J. Nutr. 110 (1): 145 - 55.

Litonjua AA (2012). Vitamin D deficiency as a risk factor for childhood allergic disease and asthma. Curr. Opin. Allergy. Clin. Immunol. 12 (2): 179 - 85.

Ma XJ, Chen HB, Gao JY, Hu CQ, Li X (2013). Conformation affects the potential allergenicity of ovalbumin after heating and glycation. Food. Addit. Contam. Part A - Chem. Anal. Control. Expo. Risk. Assess. 2013. Aug 6. [Epub ahead of print].

Magrone T, Jirillo E (2012). Influence of polyphenols on allergic immune reactions: Mechanisms of action. Proc. Nutr. Soc. 71: 316 - 21.

Manach C, Scalbert A, Morand C, Remesy C, Jimenez L (2004). Polyphenols: Food sources and bioavailability. Am. J. Clin. Nutr. 79: 727 - 47.

Marteau PR (2002). Probiotics in clinical conditions. Clin. Rev. Allergy. Immunol. 22 (3): 255 - 73.

Martinolli F, Carraro S, Berardi M, Ferraro V, Baraldi E, Zanconato S (2013). Immunotherapy for food allergies in children. Curr. Pharm. Des. 2013 May 17. [Epub ahead of print].

Matsuda, H., Morikawa, T., Toguchida, I. and Yoshikawa, M (2005). Structural requirements of flavonoids and related compounds for aldose reductase inhibitory activity. Chem. Pharm. Bull. Tokyo. 50: 788 - 95.

Middleton EJ, Kandaswami C, Theoharides TC (2000). The effects of plant flavonoids on mammalian cells: Implications for inflammation, heart disease, and cancer. Pharmacol. Rev. 52: 673 - 751.

Minocha A (2009) Probiotics for preventive health. Nutr. Clin. Pract. 24 (2): 227 - 41.

Nermes M, Salminen S, Isolauri E (2013). Is There a Role for Probiotics in the Prevention or Treatment of FoodAllergy? Curr. Allergy. Asthma. Rep. 2013 Aug 10. [Epub ahead of print].

Niggemann B, Sielaff B, Beyer K, Binder C, Wahn U (1999). Outcome of double-blind, placebo-controlled food challenge tests in 107 children with atopic dermatitis. Clin. Exp. Allergy. 29: 91 - 96.

Oh SW, Cha JY, Jung JE, Chang BC, Kwon HJ, Lee BR, Kim DY (2011). Curcumin attenuates allergic airway inflammation and hyper-responsiveness in mice through NF-κB inhibition. J. Ethnopharmacol. 136 (3): 414 - 21.

Osborn DA, Sinn JK (2013). Prebiotics in infants for prevention of allergy. Cochrane. Database. Syst. Rev. 2013 Mar 28; 3: CD006474

Palmer DJ, Metcalfe J, Makrides M, Gold MS, Quinn P, West CE, Loh R, Prescott SL (2013). Early regular egg exposure in infants with eczema: A randomized controlled trial. J. Allergy. Clin. Immunol. 132 (2): 387 - 392.

Peroni DG, Bonomo B, Casarotto S, Boner AL, Piacentini GL (2012). How changes in nutrition have influenced the development of allergic diseases in childhood. Ital. J. Pediatr. 38: 22.

Policegoudra RS, Aradhya SM, Singh L (2011). Mango-ginger (*Curcuma amada* Roxb.) - a promising spice for phytochemicals and biological activities.J. Biosci. 36 (4): 739 - 48.

Pons L, Burks W (2005). Novel treatments for food allergy. Expert. Opin. Investig. Drugs. 14 (7): 829 - 34.

Pons L, Palmer K, Burks W (2005). Towards immuno-therapy for peanut allergy. Curr. Opin. Allergy. Clin. Immunol. 5 (6): 558 - 62.

Prescott S, Nowak-Wêgrzyn A (2011). Strategies to prevent or reduce allergic disease. Ann. Nutr. Metab. 59 Suppl. 1: 28 - 42.

Ramana KV, Yadav UC, Calhoun WJ, Srivastava SK (2011). Current prospective of aldose reductase inhibition in the therapy of allergic airway inflammation in asthma. Curr. Mol. Med. 11 (7): 599 - 608.

Reddy GB, Muthenna P, Akileshwari C. Saraswat M, Petrash JM (2011). Inhibition of aldose reductase and sorbitol accumulation by dietary rutin. Current Science. 101: 9 - 10.

Ribeiro CC, Leite Speridiao Pda G, de Morais MB (2013). Knowledge and practice of physicians and nutritionists regarding the prevention of food allergy. Clin. Nutr. 32 (4): 624 - 29.

Rowicka G, Strucinska M, Ambroszkiewicz J (2012). Vitamin D status in children with cow's milk allergy. Med. Wieku. Rozwoj. 16 (4): 307 - 12. [Article in Polish].

Russo M, Spagnuolo C, Tedesco I, Bilotto S, Russo GL (2012). The flavonoid quercetin in disease prevention and therapy: Facts and fancies. Biochem. Pharmacol. 83: 6 - 15.

Samochocki Z, Bogaczewicz J, Jeziorkowska R, Sysa-Jêdrzejowska A, Glinska O, Karczmarewicz E, McCauliffe DP, WoŸniacka A (2013). Vitamin D effects in atopic dermatitis. J. Am. Acad. Dermatol. 69 (2): 238 - 44.

Sampson HA, McCaskill CC (1985). Food hypersensitivity and atopic dermatitis: evaluation of 113 patients. J. Pediatr. 107: 669 - 675.

Saraswat M, Muthenna P, Suryanarayana P, Petrash JM, Reddy GB (2008). Dietary sources of aldose reductase inhibitors: prospects for alleviating diabetic complications. Asia Pac. J. Clin. Nutr. 17 (4): 558 - 65.

Shin M, Han Y, Ahn K (2013). The influence of the time and temperature of heat treatment on the allergenicity of egg white proteins. Allergy. Asthma. Immunol Res. 5 (2): 96 - 101.

Sicherer SH, Sampson HA (2006). Food allergy. J. Allergy. Clin. Immunol. 117: S470 - S475.

Singh A, Holvoet S, Mercenier A (2011). Dietary polyphenols in the prevention and treatment of allergic diseases. Clin. Exp. Allergy. 41: 1346 - 59.

Singh VP, Sharma J, Babu S, Rizwanulla, Singla A (2013). Role of probiotics in health and disease: a review. J. Pak. Med. Assoc. 63 (2): 253 - 57.

Szajewska H (2012). Early nutritional strategies for preventing allergic disease. Isr. Med. Assoc. J. 14 (1): 58 - 62.

Turner PJ, Mehr S, Joshi P, Tan J, Wong M, Kakakios A, Campbell DE (2013). Safety of food challenges to extensively heated egg in egg-allergic children: a prospective cohort study. Pediatr. Allergy. Immunol. 24 (5): 450 - 55.

Vandenplas Y, Steenhout P, Planoudis Y, Grathwohl D; Althera Study Group (2013). Treating cow's milk protein allergy: a double-blind randomized trial comparing two extensively hydrolysed formulas with probiotics. Acta Paediatr. 2013 Jul 9. doi: 10.1111/apa.12349. [Epub ahead of print].

Varma SD, Mikuni I, Kinoshita JH (1975). Flavonoids as inhibitors of lens aldose reductase. Science. 188: 1215 - 16.

Visioli F, de la Lastra CA, Andres-Lacueva C, Aviram M, Calhau C, Cassano A, D'Archivio M, Faria A, Fave G, Fogliano V, Llorach R, Vitaglione P, Zoratti M, Edeas M (2011). Polyphenols and human health: A prospectus. Crit. Rev. Food Sci. Nutr. 51: 524 - 46.

Watanabe H, Toda M, Sekido H, Wellner A, Fujii T, Henle T, Hachimura S, Nakajima-Adachi H (2013). Heat treatment of egg white controls allergic symptoms and induces oral tolerance to ovalbumin in a murine model of food allergy. Mol. Nutr. Food. Res. 2013 Aug 26. doi: 10.1002/mnfr.201300205. [Epub ahead of print].

Wild LG, Lehrer SB (2001). Immuno-therapy for food allergy. Curr. Allergy. Rep. 1 (1): 48 - 53.

Williams CA, Grayer RJ (2004). Anthocyanins and other flavonoids. Nat. Prod. Rep. 21: 539 - 73.

Yamaura K, Ishiwatari M, Yamamoto M, Shimada M, Bi Y, Ueno K (2012). Anthocyanins, but not anthocyanidins, from bilberry (*Vaccinium myrtillus* L.) alleviate pruritus via inhibition of mast cell degranulation. J. Food Sci. 77 (12): H262 - 67.

Yamaura K, Shimada M, Ueno K (2011). Anthocyanins from bilberry (*Vaccinium myrtillus* L.) alleviate pruritus in a mouse model of chronic allergic contact dermatitis. Pharmacognosy. Res. 3 (3): 173 - 77.

Zenon 3rd, GJ, Abobo CV, Carter BL, Ball DW (1990). Potential use of aldose reductase inhibitors to prevent diabetic complications. Clin. Pharm. 9: 446 - 57.

Chapter 3

Anti-Carcinogenic Foods

Cancer is a disease of regulation of tissue growth. Several types of cancers have been diagnosed affecting various organ/tissue systems of the body. These include, cancer of reproductive, gastrointestinal, renal, skeleto-muscular and respiratory systems along with endocrinal cancer and oral cancer. An estimated 12.66 million people were diagnosed with cancer across the world in 2008 (Ferlay *et al.*, 2010a). Cancer was estimated to account for 13 per cent of all deaths (due to any cause) worldwide in 2008 (Ferlay *et al.*, 2010b; WHO, 2008).

In cancer, certain cells of the body display uncontrolled growth and invasion, destroying the adjacent tissues while spreading to other body locations. Transformation of a normal cell into a cancer cell involves alteration of genes which regulate cell growth and differentiation. According to Szarc *et al.* (2010) epigenetic changes in DNA methylation patterns at CpG sites (epimutations) or corrupt chromatin states of key inflammatory genes and non-coding RNAs, has recently emerged as major governing factors in cancer, chronic inflammatory and metabolic disorders. Reciprocally, inflammation, metabolic stress and diet composition can also change activities of the epigenetic machinery and indirectly or directly change chromatin marks. It is known that lifestyle, environmental conditions and nutritional components influence gene expression.

Diet is one of the important factors in cancer etiology and prevention. Diet components may modify the risk of cancer through the influence on multiple processes, including DNA repair, cell proliferation and apoptosis. Numerous clinical, patho-physiological and epidemiological studies have underlined the detrimental as well as beneficial role of nutritional factors in complex inflammation related disorders such as allergy, asthma, obesity, type 2 diabetes, cardiovascular disease, rheumatoid arthritis, auto-immune disorders and cancer.

Recent research efforts have been greatly emphasized on the recognition of naturally occurring plant derived substances that are capable of inhibiting, retarding or reversing the development of cancer and also to avoid the problems that exist with current chemo-therapeutic regimens. Several epidemiological annotations and a number of laboratory studies have indicated cancer chemo-preventive and anti-carcinogenic potential of plant derived agents that have been traditionally used for treatment of varied human disorders in different parts of the globe.

The patterns of exposure to cancer initiators and promoters and of genetic susceptibility may determine the variations in the site-specific risks of cancer seen across populations (Potter and Steinmetz, 1996). Fruits, vegetables, spices, herbs and/or beverages are typical foods containing various phytochemicals and have been used for prevention and treatment of a variety of human ailments since time immemorial. Nowadays, a large number of individuals are motivated towards the use of phyto-chemicals in order to prevent or treat chronic diseases. Several epidemiological studies have shown that populations that consume diets rich in fruits and vegetables have an overall lower cancer incidence. Based on these encourageing observations, research efforts from across the globe have focused on identifying, characterizing, and providing scientific basis to the efficacy of various phytonutrients towards developing an effective strategy to control various human malignancies.

The unique dietary constituents like chili pepper, cloves, black pepper and black cumin have promise as chemo-preventive agents. The anti-carcinogenic benefits of selected foods have been discussed below along with the available scientific evidences.

Turmeric (*Curcuma longa*)

Turmeric has been shown to inhibit chemical carcinogenesis. Curcumin (diferuloylmethane) is an anti-oxidant extract from the spice turmeric that produces a wide range of health benefits. The activity of curcumin reported against leukemia and lymphoma, gastrointestinal cancers, genitourinary cancers, breast cancer, ovarian cancer, head and neck squamous cell carcinoma, lung cancer, melanoma, neurological cancers, and sarcoma reflects its ability to affect multiple targets (Anand *et al.*, 2008). Recently, curcumin's therapeutic potential for preventing and treating various cancers is being recognized and explored more systematically in various diseases. Due to its increased bioavailability in the gastro-intestinal tract, curcumin may be particularly suited to treat gastro-intestinal diseases.

Curcumin has been found to inhibit colon cancer cell proliferation *in vitro* mainly by accumulating cells in the G2/M phase and that this effect is independent of its ability to inhibit prostaglandin synthesis. Hanif *et al.* (1997) opined that inhibition of arachidonic acid metabolism by curcumin might be responsible for the effect. It was later confirmed by Huang *et al.* (1997) who demonstrated that curcumin is a strong inhibitor of arachidonic acid-induced edema of mouse ears *in vivo* and epidermal cyclo-oxygenase and lipoxygenase activities *in vitro*. Further, curcumin is found to suppress NF-κB activation (Singh and Aggarwal, 1995) and down-regulate the expression of NF-κB–regulated gene products involved in survival, proliferation, angiogenesis, invasion, and metastasis (Mukhoadhyay *et al.*, 2001; Kumar *et al.*, 1998; Aggarwal *et al.*, 2006) of the tumor. Nuclear transcription factor- kB (NF-kappaB) is known to regulate cell survival, proliferation, tumorigenesis, and inflammation. Plummer *et al.* (1999) showed that curcumin inhibits COX-2 expression in colon cells by inhibition of NF-κB activation via the NIK/IKK signaling complex. This phytochemical has been shown to modulate various mechanisms linked with radio-resistance, such as quenching reactive oxygen species (Das and Das, 2002), down-regulating COX-2, multi-drug resistance protein Bcl-2, and surviving expression (Aggarwal *et al.*, 2006; Limtrakul *et al.*, 2004; Tomita *et al.*, 2006), inhibiting phosphoinositide 3-kinase/AKT activation (Aoki *et al.*, 2007), suppressing growth factor signaling pathways (Sethi *et al.*, 2007), Inhibiting signal transducers and activators of transcription 3 activation (Bharti *et al.*, 2003).

Proliferation of various pancreatic cancer cell lines has been inhibited in the apoptosis induced by gemcitabine and inhibited constitutive NF-kappaB activation in the cells *in vitro*. Tumors from mice injected with pancreatic cancer cells and treated with a combination of curcumin and gemcitabine *in vivo*, showed significant reductions in volume (P = 0.008 versus control; P = 0.036 versus gemcitabine alone), Ki-67 proliferation index, NF-kappaB activation, and expression of NF-kappaB-regulated gene products compared with tumors from control mice. The combination treatment was also highly effective in suppressing angiogenesis as indicated by a decrease in CD31(+) microvessel density (Kunnumakkara *et al.*, 2007). Curcumin also potentiates the anti-tumor effects of radiation therapy in colorectal cancer by suppressing NF-kappaB and NF-kappaB-regulated gene products, leading to inhibition of proliferation and angiogenesis (Kunnumakkara *et al.*, 2008a; b)). In addition, it sensitized colorectal cancer to the anti-tumor and anti-metastatic effects of capecitabine by suppressing NF-kappaB cell signaling pathway (Kunnumakkara *et al.*, 2009).

Curcumin has also shown some promise in the prevention of oral carcinogenesis. In the 7, 12-dimethylbenz[a]anthracene (DMBA) hamster buccal pouch model of carcinogenesis, curcumin alone or when administered together with piperine significantly reduced the formation of oral carcinoma (Krishnaswamy *et al.*, 1998), probably due to its anti-lipid peroxidative and anti-oxidant potential together with its effect on modulating carcinogen detoxification.

Cancer researchers are currently focusing on agents that induce apoptosis as the next generation of cancer drugs. The most effective component available to induce apoptosis may be curcumin. Interestingly, curcumin acts like a "hypnotist" with cancer cells, tricking them into programming their own destruction. Thus, curcumin induces cancer cell apoptosis. In a wide range of cancer cells, curcumin has been shown to induce cell shrinkage, chromatin condensation, DNA fragmentation and block cellular signal transduction, all of which are characteristics of apoptosis. Curcumin inhibits tumorigenesis during both initiation and promotion (post-initiation) periods in several experimental animal models. Topical application of curcumin inhibits TPA-induced increases in the per cent of epidermal cells in synthetic (S) phase of the cell cycle (Huang *et al.*, 2007). A dose of 1.5 grams of turmeric per day for 30 days caused a significant reduction in the amount of mutagens excreted in the urine of smokers (Polasa *et al.*, 1992).

Nagabhushan and his colleagues (1987, 1988 and 1992) have shown that the curcumin in turmeric can inhibit the mutagenicity of polycyclic aromatic hydrocarbons (PAHs), inhibit radiation-induced chromosome damage, prevent the formation of harmful heterocyclic amines and nitroso compounds, which may result in the body when certain processed foods, such as processed meat products that contain nitrosamines, are eaten and irreversibly inhibit the multiplication of leukemia cells in a cell culture.

Curcumin present at micromolar concentration is able to inhibit the growth of estrogen-positive human breast MCF-7 cells induced individually or by a mixture of the pesticides endosulfane, DDT and chlordane or 17-beta estradiol. When curcumin and genistein were added together to MCF-7 cells, a synergistic effect resulting in a total inhibition of the induction of MCF-7 cells by the high estrogenic activity of endosulfane/chlordane/DDT mixtures was noted. Thus, it is evident that the combination of curcumin and genistein in the diet has the potential to reduce the proliferation of estrogen positive cells by mixtures of pesticides or 17-beta estradiol. Since it is difficult to remove pesticides completely from the environment or the diet and since both turmeric and soybeans are not toxic to humans, their inclusion in the diet in order to prevent hormone related cancers deserves consideration (Duncan *et al.*, 1999). Curcumin and catechin inhibit the invasion of B16F-10 melanoma cells in mice by inhibition of metallo-proteinases, thereby inhibiting lung metastasis (Menon *et al.*, 1999).

Curcumin significantly inhibited pulmonary and liver adenoma formation and growth in BALB/c mice. The precise mechanism by which curcumin inhibits lung and liver tumorigenesis remains to be elucidated. Thus, curcumin appears to be a promising new chemotherapeutic and preventive agent for lung and liver cancer induced by DHPN (Huang *et al.*, 2008b).

Curcumin has profound immunosuppressive effects mediated via inhibition of IL-2 synthesis; mitogen and IL-2 induced activation of human lymphocytes. This effect may be mediated via NF-kappaB inhibition (Ranjan *et al.*, 2004).

Curcumin acts upon oxidative stress in human breast epithelial cells transformed by the effect of radiation in the presence of estrogen (Calaf *et al.*, 2011). Numerous other studies have noted significant anti-prostate cancer activity by curcumin (Nakamura *et al.*, 2002, Dorai *et al.*, 2001). Curcumin is well-tolerated; the most common side effects are nausea and diarrhea. Theoretical interactions exist due to purported effects on metabolic enzymes and transport proteins, but clinical reports do not support any meaningful interactions. Nonetheless, caution, especially with chemotherapy agents, is advised. Late-phase clinical trials are still needed to confirm most beneficial effects (Asher and Spelman, 2013).

Honey

Honey was found to be a suitable alternative for wound healing, burns and various skin conditions, and to potentially have a role in cancer care. Bardy *et al.*

(2008) opine that in the cancer setting, honey may be used for radiation-induced mucositis, radiotherapy-induced skin reactions, hand and foot skin reactions in chemotherapy patients and for oral cavity and external surgical wounds. Honey applied topically to the oral mucosa of patients undergoing radiation therapy appears to provide a distinct benefit by limiting the severity of mucositis (Khanal *et al.*, 2010). Rashad *et al.* (2009) confirmed the prophylactic use of pure natural honey as effective in reducing mucositis resulting from radio-chemotherapy in patients with head and neck cancer. In the case of oral squamous cell carcinomas (OSCC) and human osteosarcoma (HOS) the treatment includes surgery and/or radiotherapy which often lead to reduced quality of life. Ghashm *et al.* (2010) proved that Tualang honey has anti-proliferative effect on OSCC and HOS cell lines by inducing early apoptosis. Tomasin and Gomes-Marcondes (2011) also confirmed that honey can modulate tumour growth by reducing cell proliferation and increasing apoptosis susceptibility.

Honey may also cause cell death in the human renal cancer cell lines (ACHN), in which apoptosis plays an important role. Most of the drugs used in the cancer treatment are apoptotic inducers, hence apoptotic nature of honey is considered vital. Samarghandian *et al.* (2011) prepared cell cultures in Dulbecco's modified Eagle's medium with 10 per cent fetal bovine serum treated with different concentrations of honey for 3 consecutive days. Cell viability was quantified by the 3-(4,5-Dimethylthiazol-2-yl)-2,5-diphenyltetrazolium bromide assay. Apoptotic cells were determined using Annexin-V-fluorescein isothiocyanate (FITC) by flow cytometry. They found a decrease in the cell viability in the malignant cells with honey in a concentration and time-dependent manner.

Ehrlich ascites carcinoma is a spontaneous murine mammary adeno-carcinoma adapted to ascites form and carried in outbred mice by serial intra-peritoneal (i/p) passages. Jagannathan's team (2010) showed that honey containing higher phenolic content significantly inhibited the growth of Ehrlich ascites carcinoma suggesting honey and eugenol (one of the phenolic constituents of honey) to be promising remedies in cancer chemo-prevention. Again, Jagannathan *et al.* (2011) demonstrated molecular mechanism of eugenol-induced apoptosis in human colon cancer cells and thus, reinforce eugenol as a potential chemo-preventive agent against colon cancer.

Jagannathan (2011) promulgates honey with common flavonoids like chrysin, genistein, biochanin, quercetin, kaempferol, and naringenin as potential components for reversing multi drug resistance (MDR). He foresees that honey, a novel chemo-sensitizer, can reduce the huge amount invested in developing new chemo-sensitizers to overcome the burden of chemoresistance. Moreover, honey is readily available, affordable and well accepted by patients. Hence, it is useful for improving the quality of life in cancer patients undergoing radiation therapy.

Shoma *et al.* (2010) demonstrated a striking regression of the mean projected coetaneous surface area of lesions among breast cancer patients undergoing radiotherapy. A shorter duration of treatment and complete recovery after 12 weeks was observed among a group of patients who were treated with honey along with standard burn treatment and pentoxifylline (PTX). Moreover, the addition of honey was associated with marked relief of pain and rescue of proper motion. Thus it is proved that combination of PTX and honey is an ideal measure for treatment of radiation-induced burn following breast conservative surgery.

One of the major stumbling blocks for cancer chemotherapy is multidrug resistance (MDR) developed by cancer cells. Since ancient times, honey has been used successfully for the treatment of a broad spectrum of infections with no risk of resistance development. MDR in nosocomial pathogens is a continually evolving and alarming problem in health care units. Majtan *et al.* (2011) proved that Honeydew honey with strong anti-bacterial activity could be used as a potential agent to eradicate multi-drug resistant clinical isolates as Slovak Honeydew honey showed exceptional anti-bacterial activity against multi-drug resistant *S. maltophilia* isolates and was more efficient than Manuka honey.

Fauzi *et al.* (2011) showed that Tualang honey (TH) has significant anti-cancer activity against human breast and cervical cancer cells as there was an increase in lactate dehydrogenase leakage from the cell membranes indicating that TH is cytotoxic to all the cancer cells with effective concentrations of 2.4 - 2.8 per cent. But when the effect of active Manuka honey was assessed on radiation-induced mucositis in 131 patients (diagnosed with head and neck cancer and undergoing radiotherapy), by Bardy *et al.* (2012) it was not found to improve mucositis. But both the honey and the syrup seemed to be associated with a reduction in bacterial infections. But, it was presumed by the authors that poor compliance after the onset of mucositis, may have affected the findings.

Honey may also cause cell death in the human renal cancer cell lines, in which apoptosis plays an important role. Most of the drugs used in the cancer treatment are apoptotic inducers, hence apoptotic nature of honey is considered vital. Samarghandian *et al.* (2011) found a decrease in the cell viability in the malignant cells with honey in a concentration and time-dependent manner.

Tomasin and Gomes-Marcondes (2011) verified the influence of *Aloe vera* and honey on tumour growth and in the apoptosis process by assessing tumour size, the cell proliferation rate (Ki67-LI) and Bax/Bcl-2 expression at 7, 14 and 20 days after Walker 256 carcinoma implant in Wistar rats. A decrease in relative weight (per cent) and Ki67-LI in tumours from the *Aloe vera* and honey group was observed as compared to those from the control group. The Bax/Bcl-2 ratio increased in tumours of the experimental group at all tested time points. These data suggest *Aloe vera* and honey can modulate tumor growth by reducing cell proliferation and increasing apoptosis susceptibility.

Garlic (*Allium sativum*)

Allium vegetables rich in flavonols and organosulfur compounds have tumor-inhibitory properties (Fenwick and Hanley, 1985; Milner, 2001a; Fukushima *et al.*, 1997; Welsh *et al.*, 1992; Ali *et al.*, 2000). Epidemiologic studies have related consumption of allium vegetables including garlic, onions, leeks, chives, scallions, and shallots to lower risks for cancers of the stomach (Dorant *et al., 1996;* Gao *et al.*, 1999; You *et al.*, 1989), gastric, colon (Fleischauer *et al., 2000;* Fleischauer and Arab, 2001) esophagus (Gao *et al.*, 1999), endometrial (Galeone *et al.*, 2009) and breast

(Challier *et al.*, 1998) (Milner, 2006; Pinto *et al.*, 2000). Large data set from southern European populations showed an inverse association between the frequency of use of allium vegetables and the risk of several common cancers (Galeone *et al.*, 2006) as well as benign prostatic hyperplasia (Galeone *et al.*, 2007). The reduced risk of prostate cancer associated with allium vegetables was independent of body size, intake of other foods, and total calorie intake and was more pronounced for men with localized than with advanced prostate cancer. Hsing *et al.*, 2002).

Several epidemiological observations and a number of laboratory studies have indicated anti-carcinogenic potential of garlic, which has been traditionally used from time immemorial for varied human ailments in different parts of the globe. Hence, in recent years, extensive research has been conducted on the anti-carcinogenic potential of allium vegetables and their constituents, *viz.*, allyl sulfides and flavonoids (particularly quercetin which is present abundantly in onion) resulting in mounting evidence that garlic extracts possess significant anti-cancer actions. Epidemiological studies have shown a dose-dependent benefit of garlic in several types of cancers. In tumor-bearing mice, significant anti-tumor effects of aged black garlic extracts (ABGE) such as growth inhibition of inoculated tumors were observed. Further investigation of serum superoxide dismutases, glutathione peroxidase, IL-2 and the increased indices of spleen and thymus indicated that the anti-cancer action of ABGE may be partly due to its anti-oxidant and immuno-modulative effects (Wang *et al.*, 2012a).

Garlic components have been found to block covalent binding of carcinogens to DNA, enhance degradation of carcinogens, have anti-oxidative and free radical scavenging properties and to regulate cell proliferation, apoptosis and immune responses. There are a number of mechanisms at work which jointly are responsible for eliciting the anti-carcinogenic effects noted in laboratory studies in a wide range of experimental systems (Das, 2002).

Sengupta *et al.* (2004) in his review article reported that organo-sulfur compounds present in allium vegetables are considered to be responsible for the beneficial effects of these herbs. Several mechanisms have been proposed to explain the cancer-preventive effects of these compounds including inhibition of mutagenesis, modulation of enzyme activities and inhibition of DNA adduct formation, free-radical scavenging, and effects on cell proliferation and tumor growth.

Miroddi *et al.* (2011) found the oil-soluble sulfur compounds to be responsible for anti-cancer effects exerted through multiple mechanisms such as: inhibition of metabolic carcinogenic activation, arrest of cell cycle, anti-oxidant and pro-apoptotic action. Kim *et al.* (2012) clearly indicated that hexane extracts of garlic cloves-induced ROS are key mediators of mitochondrial membrane potential collapse, which leads to the induction of apoptosis, followed by caspase activation. However, further research is recommended to support these findings.

Onion (*Allium cepa*)

In recent years, extensive research has focused on the anti-carcinogenic potential of onion and its organosulfur constituents (Le Bon and Siess, 2000). Phytochemical research has proved that onion is rich in flavonols and organosulfur compounds, which have exhibited tumor inhibitory properties in laboratory studies (Virtanen and Matikkala, 1976; Block, 1985; Arabbi *et al.*, 2004). In a French epidemiological study, higher onion intake was correlated with lower risk of breast cancer (Challier *et al.*, 1998). Furthermore, many experimental studies have demonstrated that organosulfur compounds and onion extracts have inhibitory effects on carcinogenesis in animals. Wang *et al.* (2012b) suggested that the apoptosis induced by ethyl acetate extract of onion (EEO) occurs via inhibition of fatty acid synthase (FAS). The authors found that EEO could suppress lipid accumulation during the differentiation of 3T3-L1 adipocytes, which was also related to its inhibition of intracellular FAS activity suggesting that onion might be useful for preventing obesity-related malignancy.

Ginger (*Zingiber officinale*)

Ginger has been shown to possess chemo-preventive and anti-carcinogenic property (Surh, 2002; Shukla and Singh, 2007) against 1,2-dimethylhydrazine-induced colon cancer by virtue of its ability to lower the activities of the microbial enzymes beta-glucuronidase and mucinase (Manju and Nalini, 2006). It is reported that [6]-, [8]-, and [10]-gingerols had little or no effect but [6]-shogaol significantly inhibited the growth of A-2780 ovarian cancer cells (Rhode *et al.*, 2007). Kim *et al.* (2008) reported that [6]-shogaol exhibited much stronger growth-inhibitory effects on A-549 human lung cancer cells, SK-OV-3 human ovarian cancer cells, SKMEL-2 human skin cancer cells, and HCT-15 human colon cancer cells than [4]-, [6]-, [8]-, and [10]-gingerols. Shogaols are metabolized extensively in mouse and human to form thiol-conjugated metabolites and glutathione might play an important role in the cancer-preventive activity of ginger (Chen *et al.*, 2013). Its metabolites are bioactive compounds, and the mercapturic acid pathway is one of the major biotransformation pathways of [6]-shogaol (Chen *et al.*, 2012).

Nausea and vomiting are among the most prevalent and disturbing side effects of chemotherapy. Addition of ginger (1.5 g/d) to standard anti-emetic therapy (granisetron plus dexamethasone) in patients with advanced breast cancer effectively reduced the prevalence of nausea 6 to 24 hours post-chemotherapy although there was no other additional advantage in reducing prevalence or severity of acute or delayed chemotherapy-induced nausea and vomiting (Panahi *et al.*, 2012). Liu *et al.* (2012) demonstrated that terpenoids from Steam Distilled Extract of Ginger mediated apoptosis by activating p53 and therefore recommended further investigations as agents for the treatment of endometrial cancer.

The results of the animal pilot study conducted by Citronberg *et al.* (2013) suggest that ginger may reduce proliferation in the normal-appearing colorectal epithelium, and increase apoptosis and differentiation relative to proliferation especially in the differentiation zone of the crypts and support a larger study to further investigate these results.

TUNEL (Terminal deoxynucleotidyl transferase dUTP nick end labeling) assay indicated that apoptosis was triggered by metabolites M2, M13 of [6]-shogaol, and its two diastereomers M13-1 and M13-2. There was no significant difference between the apoptotic effect of [6]-shogaol and the effect of M2 and M13 after 6 hour treatment.

The most active metabolite M2 had almost no toxicity to CCD-18Co and IMR-90 normal cells with IC (50)s of 99.18 and 98.30 μM, respectively (Zhu *et al.*, 2013).

Saffron (*Crocus sativus*)

One of the most promising strategies for cancer prevention today is chemo-prevention using readily available natural substances from vegetables, fruits, herbs and spices. Among the spices, saffron (*Crocus sativus*, L) a member of the large family Iridaceae, in the *in vitro* colony-forming test system, displayed a dose-dependent inhibitory effect only against human malignant cells. All isolated carotenoid ingredients of saffron demonstrated cytotoxic activity against *in vitro* tumor cells. Saffron crocin derivatives possessed a stronger inhibitory effect on tumor cell colony formation. Overall, these results suggest that saffron itself, as well as its carotenoid components, might be used as potential cancer chemo-preventive agents (Abdullaev *et al.*, 2003).

Significant reduction in papilloma formation was found with saffron application in the pre-initiation and post-initiation periods, and particularly when the agent was given both pre- and post-initiation. The inhibition appeared to be at least partly due on modulatory effects of saffron on some phase II detoxifying enzymes like glutathione-S-transferase (GST) and glutathione peroxidase (GPx), as well as catalase (CAT) and superoxide dismutase (SOD) (Das *et al.*, 2004). Das *et al.* (2010) also found saffron to inhibit DMBA-induced skin carcinoma in mice when treated early which according to them may be due at least in part, to the induction of cellular defense systems. Amin *et al.* (2011) provided evidence that saffron exerts a significant chemo-preventive effect against liver cancer through inhibition of cell proliferation and induction of apoptosis and also protects rat liver from cancer via modulating oxidative damage and suppressing inflammatory response.

Doses inducing 50 per cent cell growth inhibition (LD50) on HeLa cells were 2.3 mg/ml for an ethanolic extract of saffron dry stigmas, 3 mM for crocin, 0.8 mM for safranal and 3 mM for picrocrocin. Crocetin did not show cytotoxic effect. Cells treated with crocin exhibited wide cytoplasmic vacuole-like areas, reduced cytoplasm, cell shrinkage and pyknotic nuclei, suggesting apoptosis induction. Considering its water-solubility and high inhibitory growth effect, crocin is the more promising saffron compound to be assayed as a cancer therapeutic agent (Escribano *et al.*, 1996).

Crocin isolated from Kashmiri saffron decreased cell viability in Dalton's lymphoma cells, in a concentration and time-dependent manner. Significant increase in the lifespan of Dalton's lymphoma bearing animals was noted by 37 per cent and 44 per cent, *in vitro* and *in vivo* respectively. Animals given treatment with crocin prior to induction of cancer showed 58 per cent increase in lifespan and 95.6 per cent reduction of solid tumor on the 31st day after tumor inoculation. Crocin also showed significant impact on hematological parameters, like the hemoglobin count and numbers of lymphocytes thus proving that crocin from *Crocus sativus* has significant anti-tumor activity (Bakshi *et al.*, 2009).

Cumin Seeds (*Cuminum cyminum*)

Medicinal plants are considered as potential sources of new chemotherapeutic drugs because of their diverse phytochemicals and little or no toxic effect. Among the nine plant products tested, cumin seeds significantly decreased the incidence of both B[a]P-induced neoplasia and 3'MeDAB-induced hepatomas (Aruna and Sivaramakrishnan, 1992). They observed that cumin seed significantly decreased the incidence of both benzo [a] pyrene P-induced neoplasia and 3'-methyl-4-dimethyl-aminoazobenzene -induced hepatomas in mice and suggested that it could be attributed to its ability to modulate carcinogen metabolism and thus may prove to be valuable anti-carcinogenic agent.

Cumin seeds increased the carcinogen-detoxifying enzyme, glutathione-S-transferase activity by more than 78 per cent in the stomach, liver and oesophagus, - high enough to be considered as protective agents against carcinogenesis. Also it significantly suppressed (*in vivo*) the chromosome aberrations (CA) caused by benzo (a) pyrene in mouse bone marrow cells to be considered as protective agents against carcinogenesis (Aruna and Sivaramakrishnan, 1990). Glutathione levels were also significantly elevated in all the three tissues thus proving its anti-cancer benefit.

Colon cancer is the second most common cancer among men and women worldwide. Cumin and black pepper may protect the colon by decreasing the activity of beta-glucuronidase and mucinase. Histo-pathological studies also showed lesser infiltration into the submucosa, fewer papillae and lesser changes in the cytoplasm of the cells in the colon in cumin and black pepper treated animals (Nalini *et al.*, 1998). Nalini *et al.* (2006) confirmed that cumin suppresses colon carcinogenesis in the presence of a colon-specific carcinogen, 1,2-dimethylhydrazine (DMH) and significantly lowers the number of tumors in the colon.

According to Gagandeep *et al.* (2003) reduction in tumor burden and significant elevation of the specific activities of superoxide dismutase ($p < 0.01$) and catalase ($p < 0.05$) and other related observations strongly suggest the chemo-preventive potentials of cumin seed and its ability to modulate carcinogen metabolism.

Kalaumjî or Kaljeera (*Nigella sativum*)

Constituents of the *Nigella sativa* seed are reported to possess potent anti-oxidant effects. Treatment with anti-cancer drugs such as cyclo-phosphamide (CTX) is associated with significant toxicity due to over-production of reactive oxygen species, resulting in increased levels of oxidative stress. Alenzi *et al.* (2010) found that the administration of NSO or TQ can lower CTX-induced toxicity as shown by an up-regulation of anti-oxidant mechanisms, indicating a potential clinical application for these agents to minimize the toxic effects of treatment with anti-cancer drugs.

Salim and Fukushima (2003) demonstrated that the volatile oil of N. sativa has the ability to inhibit colon carcinogenesis of rats in the post-initiation stage, with no evident adverse side effects, and that the inhibition may be associated, in part, with suppression of cell proliferation in the colonic mucosa.

Black Pepper (*Piper nigrum*) and Hot Pepper

Black pepper (*Piper nigrum*) and hot pepper (Capsicum spp.) are widely used in traditional medicines. Hot Capsicum spp. extracts and its active principles, capsaicinoids, have been linked with anti-cancer and anti-inflammatory activities. The alkylamides and piperine from black pepper suppressed TNF-induced NF-kappa B activation. Capsaicin (trans-8-methyl-N-vanillyl-6-nonenamide) is an ingredient of chilli peppers with inhibitory effects against cancer cells of different origin. Capsaicin induces cellular apoptosis through a caspase-independent pathway in MCF-7 cells, and that reactive oxygen species and intracellular calcium ion fluctuation has a minimal role in the process. The human cancer cell proliferation inhibitory activities of piperine and alklyl amides in capsicum and black pepper were dose dependant suggesting that black pepper and its constituents like hot pepper, exhibit anti-inflammatory, anti-oxidant and anti-cancer activities (Liu *et al.*, 2010). According to Thoennissen *et al.* (2010) capsaicin is a novel modulator of the epidermal growth factor receptor (EGFR/HER-2) pathway in both ER positive and negative breast cancer cells with a potential role in the treatment and prevention of human breast cancer. The anti-inflammatory potential of capsaicin is attributed to its inhibitory effect on inducible COX-2 mRNA expression. Cytochrome P4502E1 mediates the activation of xenobiotics such as vinyl carbamate and dimethyl nitrosamine to their toxic metabolites. This metabolic activation of xenobiotics by Cytochrome P4502E1 has been shown to be inhibited by capsaicin. Capsaicin also generates reactive oxygen species in cells with resultant induction of apoptosis and cell cycle arrest, which is beneficial for cancer chemo-prevention (Oyagbemi *et al.*, 2010).

The inhibitory effects of capsaicin on cancer development in multiple organs, such as stomach, lung, and liver have been extensively documented (Surh and Lee, 1995; Bernatchez *et al.*, 1999; Kundu and Surh, 2009). These inhibitory effects of capsaicin on promoter through the inactivation of two defined eukaryotic transcription factors - Nuclear Factor-kappaB (NF-kB), and activator protein 1 (AP-1) have been reported (Surh *et al.*, 2000). Therefore, capsaicin suppresses TPA-stimulated activation of NF-kB through inhibition of IkBa degradation and blockade of the subsequent nuclear translocation of p65 in human pro-myelocytic leukemia HL-60 cells (Han *et al.*, 2002).

Majdalawieh and Carr (2010) confirmed that black pepper and cardamom exert immuno-modulatory roles and anti-tumor activities, and hence they manifest themselves as natural agents that can promote the maintenance of a healthy immune system. It is possible that black pepper and cardamom constituents can be used as potential therapeutic tools to regulate inflammatory responses and prevent/attenuate carcinogenesis.

Tea

Tea is one of the most widely consumed beverages, second only to water. Many experimental researches in laboratory animals demonstrated that tea components had an inhibitory effect on carcinogenesis at a number of organ sites. The anti-carcinogenic effects of tea have been attributed to the modulation of mitotic signal transduction by the polyphenol fraction of tea (Lin and Liang, 2000).

Tea consumption has also been shown to afford protection against chemical carcinogen-induced stomach, lung, esophagus, duodenum, pancreas, liver, breast, and colon carcinogenesis in specific bioassay models. Several epicatechin derivatives (polyphenols) present in green tea have been shown to possess anti-carcinogenic activity; the most active is (-)-epigallocatechin-3-gallate (EGCG), which is also the major constituent of Green Tea Polyphenols (GTP). Several theories have been put forward, including inhibition of UV and tumor promoter-induced ornithine decarboxylase, cyclo-oxygenase, and lipoxygenase activities, antioxidant and free radical scavenging activity; enhancement of antioxidant (glutathione peroxidase, catalase, and quinone reductase) and phase II (glutathione-S-transferase) enzyme activities; inhibition of lipid peroxidation, and anti-inflammatory activity. These properties of tea polyphenols make them effective chemo-preventive agents against the initiation, promotion, and progression stages of multistage carcinogenesis (Katiyar and Mukhtar, 1997).

A growing number of studies document EGCG-mediated induction of apoptotic pathways and inhibition of pro-survival factors when combined with chemotherapy or radiation. Ferrario *et al.* (2011) demonstrated the efficacy of EGCG in modulating photofrin (PH)-mediated photodynamic therapy responses by increasing tumor apoptosis and decreasing expression of pro-survival and angiogenic molecules within the tumor micro-environment.

Cinnamon (*Cinnamomum zeylanicum*)

Cinnamon extract inhibits vascular endothelial growth factor-induced endothelial cell proliferation, migration, and tube formation *in vitro,* sprouts formation from aortic ring *ex-vivo*, and tumor-induced blood vessel formation in mice (Lu *et al.*, 2010). *In vitro* studies also showed that components of cinnamon control angiogenesis associated with the proliferation of cancer cells (Qin *et al.*, 2010).

Wondrak *et al.* (2010) reported that cinnamon could potentially be useful in cancer prevention and/or treatment. Pharmacological experiments suggest that the cinnamon-derived dietary factor cinnamaldehyde activates the Nrf2-dependent antioxidant response in human epithelial colon cells and may therefore represent an experimental chemo-preventive dietary factor targeting colorectal carcinogenesis in humans.

Cloves (*Syzygium aromaticum*)

Banerjee and Das (2005) have shown that oral administration of aqueous infusions of clove at a dose of 100 microl/mouse/day not delayed the formation of papilloma but also reduced the incidence of papilloma as well as the cumulative number papillomas per papilloma bearing mouse. Aqueous infusion of clove effectively reduced Incidence of hyperplasia, dysplasia and carcinoma in mice. Significant reduction in the number of proliferating cells and an increased number of apoptotic cells was also noted in these benzo (a) pyrene induced lung lesions following clove treatment. Western blotting analysis revealed that clove infusion up-regulates the expression of pro-apoptotic proteins p53 and Bax, and down-regulates the expression of anti-apoptotic protein Bcl-2 in the pre-cancerous stages. Expression of caspase 3 and its activation by clove infusion were evident from a very early stage of carcinogenesis (eighth week). Clove infusion was also found to down-regulate the expression of some growth-promoting proteins, viz, COX-2, cMyc, Hras (Banerjee *et al.*, 2006).

The water, ethanol and oil extracts of cloves tested against HeLa (cervical cancer), MCF-7 (ER + ve) and MDA-MB-231 (ER - ve) (breast cancer), DU-145 (prostate cancer) and TE-13 (esophageal cancer) cell lines *in vitro*, showed different patterns of cell growth inhibition activity, with the oil extract having maximal cyto-toxic activity. Maximum cell death and apoptotic cell demise occurred in TE-13 cells within 24 hours by clove oil at 300 µl/ml with 80 per cent cell death whereas DU-145 cells showed minimal cell death. At the same time, no significant cyto-toxicity was found in human PBMC's at the same dose (Dwivedi *et al.*, 2011).

Fruits and Vegetables

Epidemiologic evidence indicates association between high fruit and vegetable intake and a reduced risk for many cancers (Vainio and Bianchini, 2003), and there are a number of biologically plausible reasons for this observation (Kirsh *et al.*, 2007). Fruit and vegetable constituents, including fiber, micronutrients (such as vitamins C and E and folate), and phytochemicals - carotenoids, phenolics, isoflavanoids, isothiocyanates, and indoles have been shown to be anti-carcinogens (Steinmetz and Potter, 1991). These substances detoxify enzymes, scavenge oxidative agents, inhibit malignant transformation, stimulate immune function, and regulate the cell cycle (Liu, 2004; Steinmetz and Potter, 1991). Cruciferous vegetables, in particular, may play a role in prostate cancer risk (Kristal and Lampe, 2002), specifically because of their high content of glucosinolate-derived compounds (Kirsh *et al.*, 2007). These compounds protect prostate cancer cells from DNA damage (Brookes *et al.*, 2001), induce apoptosis (Singh *et al.*, 2005) and inhibit prostate cancer cell proliferation (Xiao *et al.*, 2003).

The use of phytochemicals present in fruits and vegetables has gained worldwide acceptance as chemo-preventive agents against cancer cells. These non-nutrient phytochemicals either block or reverse multistage carcinogenesis. Molecular mechanisms which are involved for eliciting the effects of phytochemicals in cancerous cells are noticed in a range of experimental systems. This has opened up new avenue for researchers working in the field of chemo-prevention and merits further scrutiny to establish the role of phytochemicals in prevention of fatal human diseases like cancer (Singh *et al.*, 2012).

Onion a potent antioxidant, with flavonoids and organosulphur compounds and garlic extracts with allixin and organo-selenium compounds have been reported to possess significant anti-mutagenic activities in the bladder (Malaveille *et al.*, 1996), brain (Hu *et al.*, 1999), breast (Challier *et al.*, 1998), colon (Deschner *et al.*, 1991), lung (Khanduja *et al.*, 1999), ovary (Shen *et al.*, 1999) and stomach (Dorant *et al.*, 1996) cancers.

Pomegranate (*Punica granatum*)

Pomegranate is considered as the "nature's power fruit." In the past decade numerous studies on the antioxidant, anti-carcinogenic, and anti-inflammatory properties of pomegranate constituents have been published, focusing on treatment and prevention of cancer, cardiovascular disease, diabetes, dental conditions, erectile dysfunction, bacterial infections, antibiotic resistance, and ultraviolet radiation-induced skin damage. Other potential applications include infant brain ischemia, male infertility, Alzheimer's disease, arthritis, and obesity. The synergistic action of the pomegranate constituents appears to be superior to that of single constituents (Jurenka, 2008). All forms of pomegranate preparations were found to inhibit PC-3 cell invasion through Matrigel and also inhibited the growth of PC-3 xenograft in athymic nude mice (Lansky *et al.*, 2005).

Prostate cancer is the second leading cause of cancer-related deaths among U.S. males with a similar trend in many Western countries. Recent researches have shown that pomegranate extracts selectively inhibit the growth of breast, prostate, colon and lung cancer cells in culture. Malik and Mukhtar (2006) showed that pomegranate fruit extract through modulations in the cyclin kinase inhibitor-cyclin-dependent kinase machinery, resulted in inhibition of cell growth followed by apoptosis of highly aggressive human prostate carcinoma PC-3 cells. Components from pomegranate fruit each belonging to different representative chemical classes and showing known anti-cancer activities have been tested as potential inhibitors of *In vitro* invasion of human prostate cancer cells in an assay employing Matrigel artificial membranes (Seeram *et al.*, 2005; 2007).

In preclinical animal studies, oral consumption of pomegranate extract inhibited growth of lung, skin, colon and prostate tumors (Adhami *et al.*, 2009; Bell and Hawthorne, 2008). Sartippour *et al.* (2008) concluded from their study that an ellagitannin-rich pomegranate extract can inhibit tumor-associated angiogenesis as one of several potential mechanisms for slowing the growth of prostate cancer in chemo-preventive applications.

Colon cancer is one of the major causes of cancer-related death in the Western world. Pomegranate fruit extracts (PFEs) possess polyphenolic and other compounds with anti-proliferative, pro-apoptotic and anti-inflammatory effects in prostate, lung, and other cancers (Malik *et al.*, 2005; Hong *et al.*, 2008; Pantuck *et al.*, 2006; Khan, 2009). Further, the inhibition of motility and invasion by the fruit extracts, coincident with suppressed RhoC and RhoA protein expression, suggests a role for these defined extracts in lowering the metastatic potential of aggressive breast cancer species. Khan *et al.* (2007; 2009) found the fruit extract to be a useful chemo-preventive/chemo-therapeutic agent against human lung cancer too. Further, polyphenolic constituents in the pomegranate have been found to play an important role in the modulation of inflammatory signals in colon cancer cells also (Adams *et al.*, 2006; Kohno *et al.*, 2004).

Fermented pomegranate juice resulted in 42 per cent reduction in the number of lesions compared with control, whereas the peak separated from the fermented juice and the pomegranate seed oil each resulted in 87 per cent reduction in number of tumorigenic lesions. The results suggested enhanced potential for the purified compound as well as pomegranate seed oil both greater than pomegranate fermented juice polyphenols (Mehta and Lansky, 2004).

The inhibition and apoptosis induction were significantly higher in the combination treatments consisting of pomegranate extracts and genistein than in the single treatments with either agent although both pomegranate extract and genistein independently had significant - and time-dependent cytotoxic effects on MCF-7 cells (Jeune *et al.*, 2005).

Pomegranate seed oil has been investigated for possible skin cancer chemo-preventive efficacy in mice (Hora *et al.*, 2003; Afaq *et al.*, 2005a; 2005b; Syed *et al.*, 2006; Pacheco-Palencia *et al.*, 2008). A multicentric study was conducted by Albrecht *et al.* (2004) of the effects of pomegranate cold-pressed (Oil) or supercritical CO_2-extracted (S) seed oil, fermented juice polyphenols (W), and pericarp polyphenols (P) on human prostate cancer cell xenograft growth *in vivo*, and/or proliferation, cell cycle distribution, apoptosis, gene expression, and invasion across Matrigel, *in vitro*. Oil, W, and P each acutely inhibited *in vitro* proliferation of LNCaP, PC-3, and DU-145 human cancer cell lines showing the anti-tumor activity of pomegranate derived materials against human prostate cancer mediated by changes in both cell cycle distribution and induction of apoptosis.

Papaya (*Carica papaya* L.)

Various parts of *Carica papaya* (CP) have been traditionally used as ethnomedicine for a number of disorders, including cancer. There have been anecdotes of patients with advanced cancers achieving remission following consumption of tea extract made from CP leaves (Otsuki *et al.*, 2010). The active components of CP extract, which inhibits tumor cell growth and stimulates anti-tumor effects, is the fraction with molecular weight less than 1000.

Grape Seeds (*Vitis vinifera*)

Grape seed extract is a rich source of pro anthocyanidins. It acts against colorectal cancer and also protects the liver from oxidative damage following bile duct ligation in rats. This effect possibly involves the inhibition of neutrophil infiltration and lipid peroxidation, and thus restoration of oxidant and anti-oxidant balance in the tissue. The growth inhibitory and apoptotic effects of Grape seed extract against colorectal cancer could be mediated via an up-regulation of Cip1/p21 (Kaur *et al.*, 2006).

Pakhale *et al.* (2007) and Ramchandani *et al.* (2008) found both seedless and seeded grape seed extracts to possess anti-tumor activity in target tissues of mice as was evident from their ability to delay tumor formation along with a significant decrease in tumor multiplicity and incidence. Sharma *et al.* (2004) showed a strong possibility of synergistic efficacy of grape seed extract and doxorubicin combination for breast cancer treatment, independent of estrogen receptor status of the cancer cell. Leifert and Abeywardena (2008) observed inhibition of cholesterol uptake and pro-inflammatory 5-LOX activity to be beneficial in preventing the development of chronic degenerative diseases such as cardiovascular disease and cancer.

Singh *et al.* (2004) found that feeding grape seed extract strongly inhibited tumor growth that accounted for 59-73 per cent ($p < 0.001$) inhibition in tumor volume and 37-47 per cent ($p < 0.05$) decrease in tumor weight at the end of the experiment without affecting the body weight gain profile and diet consumption. Immunohistochemical analysis of tumors showed that grape seed extract decreases proliferation index by 51-66 per cent ($p < 0.001$) and increases apoptotic index by 3-4-fold ($p < 0.001$). CD31 staining for endothelial cells, showed decrease in intra-tumoral micro-vasculature in grape seed extract-fed group of mice. Thus, the authors suggested that grape seed possesses anticancer efficacy against hormone-refractory human PCA, which is associated with its anti-proliferative, pro-apoptotic and anti-angiogenic activities together with up-regulation of IGFBP-3. Hence it is beneficial in the treatment of chronic degenerative diseases such as cardiovascular disease and cancer.

Studies from various scientific groups conclude that both grapes and grape-based products are excellent sources of various anticancer agents and their regular consumption should thus be beneficial to the general population (Kaur *et al.*, 2009a; b). Grape waste management is one of the main problems of winery industries, but, conversely, grape waste contains a high amount of polyphenols that might protect against human diseases related to oxidative stress, such as colorectal cancer. Lazzè *et al.* (2009) by the clonogenic assay and the cell cycle distribution analysis observed that the grape extract has a significant anti proliferative effect in a tumor cell line indicating that grape extract is a promising product to be used as an anti-free radical agent and could exert a chemo-preventive action. Anter *et al.* (2011) suggested that red table grapes are potent anti-mutagens that protect DNA from oxidative damage as well as being cytotoxic toward the HL60 tumor cell line.

Interestingly, recent patents regarding grape polyphenols show a tendency to depend on a minimum use of severe extraction processes and organic solvents. (Gollücke and Ribeiro 2012).

Litchi Fruit (*Litchi chinensis*)

Litchi fruit pericarp (LFP) extract exhibited potential anti-cancer activity against hepato-cellular carcinoma *in vitro* and *in vivo* through inhibition of proliferation and apoptosis induction of cancer cells (Wang *et al.*, 2006a) Wang *et al.* (2006b) demonstrated that litchi fruit extract might have potential anti-cancer activity on both ER positive and negative breast cancers, which could be attributed, in part, to its DNA damage effect, proliferating inhibition and apoptosis induction of cancer cells through up-regulation and down-regulation of multiple genes involved in cell cycle regulation and cell proliferation, apoptosis, signal transduction and transcriptional regulation, motility and invasiveness of cancer cells. ADP-ribosyl transferase (NAD+; poly (ADP-ribose) polymerase)-like 1 (ADPRTL1), Cytochrome P450, subfamily I and Hyaluronan-mediated motility receptor might be the main molecular targets at which LFP water-soluble crude ethanolic extract acted.

The anti-breast cancer activities of epicatechin, proanthocyanidin B2, pro-anthocyanidin B4 and the ethyl acetate fraction was much higher on splenocyte proliferation than that of the reference rutin. Epicatechin and pro-anthocyanidin B2 had lower cyto-toxicities to human breast cancer cell MCF-7 and human embryolic lung fibroblast than paclitaxel (Zhao *et al.*, 2007).

Recent studies have revealed that Litchi pericarp is composed of significant amounts of flavonoids and anthocyanins, including procyanidin B2, B4, epicatechin, cyanidin-3-rutinoside, cyanidin-3-glucoside, quercetin-3-retinoside, quercetin-3-glucoside etc. (Li and Jiang, 2007). These components carry high free radical scavenging properties and could be used as anti-inflammation, anti-oxidation, or anti-cancer agents (Ariga, 2004; Kaur *et al.*, 2009). Therefore it is suggested that flavonoids from litchi fruit pericarp might be potentially useful components for functional foods and/or anti-breast cancer.

In addition to the anti-oxidant activity, litchi fruit pericarp extract displayed a dose- and time-dependent inhibitory effect on human breast cancer, which was attributed, in part, to inhibition of proliferation and induction of apoptosis in cancer cells through up-regulation and down-regulation of multiple genes. Furthermore, various anti-cancer activities were observed for epicatechin, procyanidin B2, procyanidin B4 and the ethyl acetate fraction of LFP tissue extracts. Procyanidin B4 and the ethyl acetate fraction showed a stronger inhibitory effect on HELF than MCF-7 proliferation, while epicatechin and procyanidin B2 have lower cyto-toxicities towards MCF-7 and HELF than paclitaxel (Li and Jiang, 2007). Therefore the authors suggested that flavonoids from LFP might be potentially useful components for functional foods and/or anti-breast cancer.

Pharmacological studies have revealed that Litchi seeds exert anti-hyper-lipidemic, hypoglyceamic, and anti-tumor effects (Chen *et al.*, 2007; Xiong *et al.*, 2008; Xiao *et al.*, 2004). In India, the seeds are powdered as an herbal medicine owing to their astringency, and after oral intake they have the reputation of relieving neuralgic pains (Li and Jiang, 2007). Hsu *et al.* (2012) provided *in vitro* evidence that polyphenol-rich litchi seed ethanol extract serves as a potential chemo-preventive agent for colorectal cancer.

Berries

The anticancer potential of berries has been related, at least in part, to a multitude of bioactive phyto-chemicals that these colorful fruits contain, including polyphenols (flavonoids, proanthocyanidins, ellagitannins, gallotannins, phenolic acids), stilbenoids, lignans, and triterpenoids (Seeram, 2008). This diverse range of phytochemicals with biological properties such as antioxidant, anticancer, anti-neuro-degerative, and anti-inflammatory activities. Six popularly consumed berries–blackberry, black raspberry, blueberry, cranberry, red raspberry and strawberry showed with increasing concentration of berry extract, increasing inhibition of cell proliferation in all of the cell lines (Seeram *et al.*, 2006).

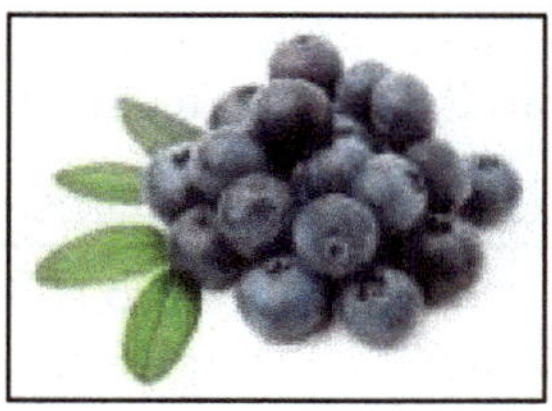

Blue Berry

Duthie (2007) in his review found a strong and convincing evidence that berry extracts and berry phyto-chemicals modulate biomarkers of DNA damage and indicators of malignant transformation *in vitro* and *in vivo*. Data from numerous cell culture and animal models indicate that berry components such as the anthocyanins are potent anti-carcinogenic agents and are protective against genomic instability at several sites in the carcinogenic pathway. Anti-carcinogenic mechanisms include modulation of carcinogen activation and detoxification, decreased DNA binding of the carcinogen, inhibition of oxidative DNA damage, alteration in cell signalling and malignant transformation and inhibition of cell invasiveness and metastasis. But still feels that the evidence in human studies is weak.

Cran Berry (*Vaccinium microcarpon*)

The main phenolic compounds in European, small-fruited cranberries were pro-anthocyanidins comprising 63-71 per cent of the total phenolic content, but anthocyanins, hydroxycinnamic acids, hydroxybenzoic acids, and flavonols were also found. Pro-anthocyanidins are polymeric phenolic compounds consisting mainly of catechin, epicatechin, gallocatechin, and epigallocatechin units. Cranberry phenolic extract inhibited LPS-induced NO production in a dose-dependent manner, but it had no major effect on iNOS of COX-2 expression. At a concentration of 100 μg/ml cranberry phenolic extract inhibited LPS-induced IL-6, IL-1β and TNF-α production. Thus, the phenolics, notably pro-anthocyanidins (oligomers and polymers), in cranberries exert multiple bioactivities that may be exploited in food development (Kylli *et al.*, 2011).

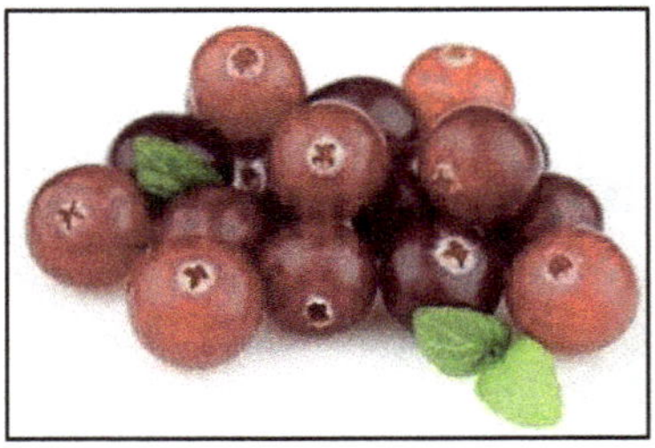

Cran Berry

The enhanced anti-proliferative activity of total polyphenols compared to total cranberry extract and its individual phyto-chemicals suggests synergistic or additive anti-proliferative interactions of the anthocyanins, pro-anthocyanidins, and flavonol glycosides within the cranberry extract (Seeram *et al.*, 2004).

In vitro studies using a variety of tumor models show that polyphenolic extracts from *V. macrocarpon* inhibit the growth and proliferation of breast, colon, prostate, lung, and other tumors, as do flavonols, pro-anthocyanidin oligomers and triterpenoids isolated from the fruit. The phyto-chemicals prevent cardiovascular diseases, various cancers, and infections involving the urinary tract, dental health, and Helicobacter pylori-induced stomach ulcers and cancers (Côté *et al.*, 2010). Possible chemo-preventive mechanisms of action by cranberry phytochemicals include induction of apoptosis in tumor cells, reduced ornithine decarboxylase activity, decreased expression of matrix metallo-proteinases associated with prostate tumor metastasis, and anti-inflammatory activities including inhibition of cyclo-oxygenases. These findings suggest a potential role for cranberry as a dietary chemopreventive and provide direction for future research (Neto, 2007).

Deer Berry (*Vaccinium stamineum*)

Wang *et al.* (2007) found Deer berries to contain potent free radical scavenging activities. Pre-treatment of JB6 P (+) mouse epidermal cells with deer berry fruit extracts produced an inhibition on the activation of activator protein-1 (AP-1) and nuclear factor-kappaB (NF-kappaB) induced by either 12- O-tetra-decanoylphorbol 13-acetate (TPA) or ultraviolet-B (UVB). Deer berry fruit extracts also blocked TPA- or UVB-induced phosphorylation of ERKs and MEK 1/2, two upstream regulators of AP-1 and inhibited proliferation of human leukemia HL-60 cancer cells and human lung epithelial cancer A549 cells and induced apoptosis of HL-60 cells.

Lingon Berry (*Vaccinium vitis-idaea*)

The extract of Lingon berry (also known as red cowberries) suppressed TPA-induced neoplastic transformation of JB6 P(+) cells in a dose-dependent manner. Lingon berry extract also induced the apoptosis of human leukemia HL-60 cells in a dose-independent manner (Wang *et al.*, 2005).

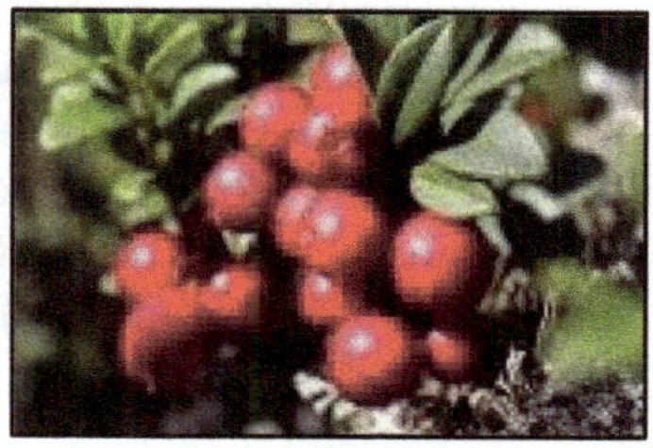

Lingon Berry

Black Raspberry (*Rubus occidentalis*)

The ability of black raspberries to inhibit tumor development may be mediated by impairing signal transduction pathways leading to activation of AP-1 and NF-kappaB. The RU-ME fraction appears to be the major fraction responsible for the inhibitory activity of black raspberries (Huang *et al.*, 2002). In view of the important roles of AP-1 and VEGF in tumor development, one mechanism for the chemo-preventive activity of black raspberries may be inhibition of the PI-3K/Akt/AP-1/VEGF pathway (Huang *et al.*, 2006). Lu *et al.* (2006) showed that pretreatment of mouse epidermal Cl 41 cells with methanol-extracted blackberry fraction RO-ME resulted in a dramatic inhibition of B(a)PDE-induced activation of AP-1 and NF-kappaB, and expression of VEGF and COX-2. The RO-ME fraction appears to be the major fraction responsible for the inhibitory activity of black raspberries.

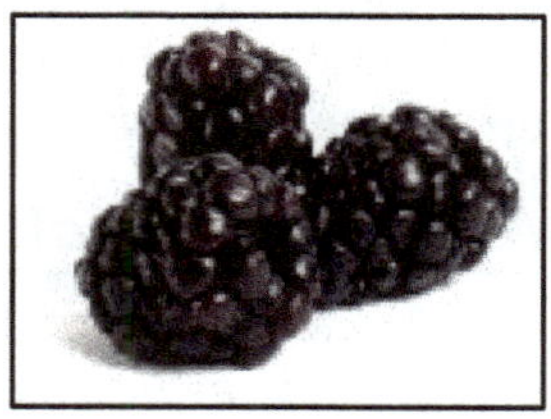

Black Raspberries

Further, Huang *et al.* (2007; 2008a) observed that the inhibition of UV-induced signaling pathways is specific for black raspberries and NF- kappaB. Cyanidin-3-rutinoside, an anthocyanin found in abundance in black raspberries. Black raspberry fractions inhibited the activation of AP-1, NF-kappaB, and nuclear factor of activated T cells (NFAT) by BaPDE as well as their upstream PI-3K/Akt-p70 (S6K) and mitogen-activated protein kinase pathways. In contrast, strawberry fractions inhibited NFAT activation, but did not inhibit the activation of AP-1, NF-kappaB or the PI-3K/Akt-p70 (S6K) and mitogen-activated protein kinase pathways. Consistent with the effects on NFAT activation, tumor necrosis factor-alpha (TNF-alpha) induction by BaPDE was blocked by extract fractions of both black raspberries and strawberries, whereas vascular endothelial growth factor (VEGF) expression, which depends on AP-1 activation, was suppressed only by black raspberry fractions but not strawberry fractions. Li *et al.* (2008) thus demonstrated that black raspberry and strawberry components may target different signaling pathways in exerting their anti-carcinogenic effects.

Black Current (*Ribes nigrum*)

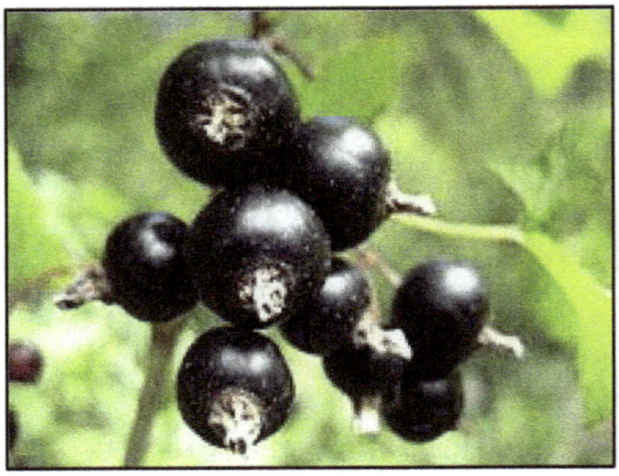

Black Current

Black currant (Raisins) is known to contain high amounts of anthocyanins (250 mg/100 g fresh fruit). Black currant fruits have been used in Asian and European traditional medicine for the treatment of a variety of diseases. Black currant extract has recently been found to be the second most effective amongst nine different berry extracts studied for their free radical scavenging activity.

Constituents present in black currant juice have been found to exert a number of health-promoting effects, including immuno-modulatory, anitimicrobial and anti-inflammatory actions, inhibition of low-density lipoprotein, and reduction of cardiovascular diseases. Bishayee *et al.* (2010) demonstrated that black currant skin containing an anthocyanin-rich fraction inhibits the proliferation of liver cancer cells, possibly due to additive as well as synergistic effects.

Again, Edirisinghe *et al.* (2011) demonstrated that black current concentrates (Ben Gairn and Ben Hope - commercial products) also could activate eNOS via Akt/PI3 kinase pathway *in vitro* in human umbilical vein endothelial cells and that the effect was not dependent on vitamin C.

Amla (*Emblica officinalis gaertn or Phyllanthus emblica*)

Amla, is arguably the most important medicinal plant in the Indian traditional system of medicine, the Ayurveda. Different parts of the plants show anti-diabetic, hypo-lipidemic, anti-bacterial, anti-oxidant, anti-ulcerogenic, hepato-protective, gastro-protective, and chemo-preventive properties (Krishnaveni and Mirunalini, 2010). Baliga and Dsouza (2011) summarized the results of the review and reported that amla and some of its phytochemicals such as gallic acid, ellagic acid, pyrogallol, some nor-sesquiterpenoids, corilagin, geraniin, elaeocarpusin, and pro-delphinidins B_1 and B_2 also possess anti-neoplastic effects. Amla is also reported to possess radio-modulatory, chemo-modulatory, chemo-preventive effects, free radical scavenging, anti-oxidant, anti-inflammatory, anti-mutagenic and immuno-modulatory activities, properties that are efficacious in the treatment and prevention of cancer.

Experimental studies in the past decade have shown that Triphala composed of the three medicinal fruits *Phyllanthus emblica* L. or *Emblica officinalis* Gaertn., *Terminalia chebula* Retz., and *Terminalia belerica* Retz. is useful in the prevention of cancer and that it also possesses anti-neoplastic, radio-protective and chemoprotective effects (Baliga, 2010).

Broccoli (*Brassica oleracea*)

Bioactive chemicals in broccoli include glucosinolates, plant pigments including kaempferol, quercetin, lutein and carotenoids, various vitamins, minerals and amino acids. Cancer prevention is hypothesised to act through various mechanisms including modulation of xenobiotic metabolising enzymes, NF-E2 p45-related factor-2 (Nrf2)-mediated stress-response mechanisms, and protection against genomic instability. Broccoli and broccoli extracts also regulate the progression of cancer through anti-inflammatory effects, effects on signal transduction, epigenetic effects and modulation of the colonic microflora. (Ferguson and Schlothauer, 2012). Broccoli contains isothiocyanates that induce carcinogen-detoxifying enzymes. Glutathione transferase enzymes conjugate isothiocyanates, leading to excretion. Keck and Finley (2006) demonstrated that Se and sulforaphane, alone or as a component of broccoli, may help decrease oxidative stress. They further suggest that Se is the most important element to decrease oxidative stress, but maximizing the Se content of broccoli also may compromise its ability to induce Phase II detoxification proteins. According to Tsai *et al.* (2013) regardless of Se content, the cytotoxicity in HCT116 cells of both high-Se (H-SeB) or low-Se (L-SeB) enzymatic-digested Se-enriched broccoli extracts (SeB) forms appeared to be H2O2-independent, whereas the cytotoxicity in HCT116+Chr.3 of either SeB form appeared to be H2O2-dependent with an increase in anti-oxidative ability for H-SeB.

Broccoli on Lung Cancer

The risk for lung cancer among those in the highest category of total cruciferous vegetable intake was 22 per cent lower in case-control studies and 17 per cent lower in cohort studies compared with those in the lowest category of intake (Lam *et al.*, 2009). Broccoli is a rich source of glucosinolates (Higdon *et al.*, 2007). The anti-carcinogenic properties of cruciferous vegetables may be attributable to isothiocyanates derived specifically from glucosinolates. Several experimental and mechanistic studies support a potential anti-cancer role of isothiocyanates ((Myzak and Dashwood, 2006; Juge *et al.*, 2007). Sulforaphane, an isothiocyanate found in broccoli, is involved in several pathways including induction of detoxifying genes, cell cycle control, and apoptosis; acting as an anti-oxidant (Higdon *et al.*, 2007) and inhibiting histone deacetylase (Myzak *et al.*, 2007).

Broccoli on Prostate Cancer

Epidemiological studies suggest that people who consume more than one portion of cruciferous vegetables per week are at lower risk of both the incidence of prostate cancer and of developing aggressive prostate cancer. Srivastava *et al.* (2003) demonstrated that administration of allyl isothiocyanate inhibits growth of PC-3 xenografts *in vivo* by inducing apoptosis and reducing mitotic activity. Joseph *et al.* (2004) provided evidence that two or more servings per month of cruciferous vegetables may reduce risk of prostate cancer, especially among men with glutathione S-transferase M1-present alleles (Joseph *et al.*, 2004) and are consistent with a role of dietary Isothiocyanates as chemo-preventive agents (Conaway *et al.*, 2002) against prostate cancer. Further, a high intake of broccoli has been found to reduce the risk of aggressive prostate cancer (Kirsh *et al.*, 2007). A protective effect of broccoli was observed when broccoli in combination with the glutathione transferase M1 (GSTM1) null genotype was consumed and to be associated with a lower prevalence of colorectal adenomas because of higher isothiocyanate levels (Lin *et al.*, 1998).

Traka *et al.* (2008) observed that broccoli interacts with GSTM1 genotype to result in complex changes to signalling pathways associated with inflammation and carcinogenesis in the prostate. The authors proposed that these changes may be mediated through the chemical interaction of isothiocyanates with signalling peptides in the plasma. This is the first experimental evidence in humans to support that diets rich in cruciferous vegetables may reduce the risk of prostate cancer and other chronic disease.

Bitter Gourd (*Momordica charantia*)

Several studies have demonstrated that leaf or fruit extracts of *Momordica charantia* (MC) exert antineoplastic effects against various cancers. Phytochemicals in MC that have been documented with cytotoxicity on cancer cells include proteins, triterpenoids, and their glycosides. Ribosome-inactivated proteins and a chemical analogue, MAP30, in MC have been reported to exhibit the cytotoxicity and inhibit the metastasis of the highly metastatic human breast cancer MDA-MB-231 cells and considered to be potential therapeutic agents against breast carcinomas (Lee-Huang *et al.*, 1995; 2000). Fruits of the Thai bitter gourd, strongly enhanced glutathione S-transferase activity and the fruit contain monofunctional phase II enzyme inducers and compounds capable of repressing some monooxygenases, especially those involved in the metabolic activation of chemical carcinogens (Kusamran *et al.*, 1998). Thai bitter gourd fruits but not Chinese bitter gourd may possess chemo-preventive potential. Extracts of MC have been shown to inhibit proliferation of human breast cancer cells by inducing cell cycle arrest and apoptosis (Ray *et al.*, 2010).

Several groups of investigators have reported that treatment of bitter-melon-related products in a number of cancer cell lines induces cell cycle arrest and apoptosis without affecting normal cell growth (Nerurkar and Ray, 2010). Li *et al.* (2012) demonstrated the apoptosis induced by methanol extract of MC (MCME) on human lung adeno-carcinoma CL1-0 cells through caspase- and mitochondria-dependent pathways, which changes of the anti-proapoptotic Bcl-2 and proapoptotic Bax proteins were included.

Methanol extract of *Momordica charantia* (MCME) was evaluated for its cytotoxic activity on four human cancer cell lines, Hone-1 nasopharyngeal carcinoma cells, AGS gastric adeno-carcinoma cells, HCT-116 colorectal carcinoma cells, and CL1-0 lung adeno-carcinoma cells. The findings according to Li *et al.* (2012) pointed to its cytotoxic effects on human cancer cells and exhibited promising anti-cancer activity by triggering apoptosis through the regulation of caspases and mitochondria. Bitter gourd is a very popular vegetable in many Asian countries. MAP30 (a natural component from *M. charantia*, as an anticancer agent against liver cancer) would serve as a novel and relatively safe agent for prophylaxis and treatment of liver cancer (Fang *et al.*, 2012).

Drumstick (*Moringa oleifera*)

The high anti-oxidant/radical scavenging effects observed for different parts of M.oleifera appear to provide justification for their widespread therapeutic use in traditional medicine in different continents. The possibility that this high anti-oxidant/radical scavenging capacity may impact on the cancer chemo-preventive potential of the plant (Atawodi *et al.*, 2010). The anti-neoplastic effects of *M. oleifera* have been evaluated in animal models. Relevant human trials showed that this plant may offer anti-tumor benefits, and could also enhance the sensitivity of tumor cells to ordinary chemotherapy. *M. oleifera* possesses anti-tumor, anti-pyretic, anti-epileptic, anti-inflammatory, anti-ulcer, anti-spasmodic, diuretic, anti-hypertensive, cholesterol-lowering, anti-oxidant, anti-diabetic, and renal- and hepato-protective activities (Paliwal *et al.*, 2011; Anonymous, 2011). The hydro-ethanolic extract of *M. oleifera* reduced the formation of free radicals, enhanced the levels of anti-oxidants in 7, 12-dimethylbenz [a] anthracene induced carcinogenesis rationalizing the ethno-medicinal use of drumstick for the protection against nephro-toxicity induced by chemical carcinogens (Sharma *et al.*, 2012 a;b).

Tulasi (*Ocimum sanctum*)

Ocimum sanctum has been known to possess various beneficial properties including anti-cancer activities. Tulsi arrests cancer if detected at first stage. In laboratory animals, it has been shown to prevent cancer and to protect against radiation. A study from Madras established that hamsters were protected from developing cancer of the mouth by taking holy basil. The seed oil was evaluated for chemo-preventive activity against subcutaneously injected 20-methylcholanthrene induced-fibrosarcoma tumors in the thigh region of Swiss albino mice. Enhanced survival rate and delay in tumor incidence was observed in seed oil supplemented mice. Liver enzymatic (superoxide dismutase, catalase, glutathione-S-transferase), non-enzymatic antioxidants (reduced glutathione) and lipid peroxidation end product, malondialdehyde levels were significantly modulated with oil treatment as compared to untreated 20-methylcholanthrene injected mice. The potential chemo preventive activity of the oil is partly attributable to its antioxidant properties. The chemo - preventive efficacy of seed oil (100-ml/kg) was comparable to that of 80 mg/kg of vitamin E (Prakash *et al.*, 2000). Kim *et al.* (2010) support that Ethanolic extract of *Ocimum sanctum* can be a potent anti-metastatic candidate through inactivation of MMP-9 and enhancement of anti-oxidant enzymes.

Male Wistar rats that were treated with extracts showed low levels of TBARS, ALT, and AST, which clearly indicates the extract had no toxic effects on hepatocytes. Again, there was no significant difference between Ocimum gratissimum and Ocimum canum from Southern Africa except in the levels of vitamins E and C. Thus, George and Chaturvedi (2009) reported that there is a possibility that *O. canum* might be participating through vitamin C and *O. gratissimum* through vitamin E.

At the concentration of 50 μg/kg in the *in vitro* system the flavonoids, orientin and vicenin showed a significantly greater free radical-inhibiting activity. Neither orientin nor vicenin showed any pro-oxidant activity at the concentrations tested. Both compounds inhibited free radical formation in the absence of EDTA. Free radical scavenging appears to be the possible mechanism of radiation protection by these flavonoids (Uma Devi *et al.*, 2000). Thus the results indicated a significant protection by these extracts against ethanol-induced hepato-toxicity ($p<or=0.05$).

Betel Leaves (*Piper betel*)

The mutagenic activity of betel quid and its ingredients using four strains of *S. typhimurium* tester strains was determined. Aqueous extract of betel leaf was not mutagenic in any of the four strains. At the same time, when betel nut extract was fed with betel leaf extract, the lung tumorogenisity induced by the nut reduced from 47 per cent to 38 per cent indicating the protective role of betel leaf. Betel leaf water and acetone extracts reduce the mutagenicity of benzo(a)pyrene and dimethylbenzanthracene. Acetone extract is more potent than water extract in inhibiting mutagenicity of environmental mutagens (Nagabhushan *et al.*, 1987).

Based on the studies on stomach tumor models and mice, betel leaf extract has been proved to be a promising anti-carcinogenic agent in tobacco-induced cancers and also against environmental mutagens. Similarly, it was also observed that the phenolic compound, 'hydroxychavicol (HC)' present in betel leaf suppressed the mutagenic effects of NNK and NNN (N'-nitrosonornicotine) in the test systems of Ames Salmonella/microsome assay and micronucleus test using Swiss male mice thus indicating the role of HC in reducing the risk of oral cancer in betel quid with tobacco chewers (Amonkar *et al.*, 1989).

Chemopreventive efficacy of betel leaf extracts and its constituents on 7, 12-dimethybenz (a) anthrocene induced carcinogenesis and their effect on drug detoxification system in mouse skin showed that there was a significant inhibition in tumor formation of about 85 per cent by betel leaf extract (Azuine *et al.*, 1991). The inhibitory effect of oral administration of betel leaf extract or its constituents - beta-carotene and alpha-tocopherol combined with turmeric was higher than that of individual constituents.

Epidemiological studies have implicated chewing tobacco alone to be more hazardous than chewing tobacco with betel quid. Experimental studies have shown that betel leaf is anti-mutagenic against standard mutagens like benzo[a]pyrene and dimethylbenz[a]anthracene. The tobacco-specific N-nitrosamines (TSNA) are the only carcinogens present in unburnt forms of tobacco, including chewing tobacco. Padma *et al.* (1989 a; b) observed that betel leaf extract suppressed the mutagenic effects of both the nitrosamines to a significant extent.

Purnark, a mixture of extracts of turmeric, betel leaf and catechu, when tested for its chemo-preventive activity against benzo (a) pyrene-induced DNA damage, seemed to give 50-60 per cent protection against BP induced sister chromatid exchange and micronuclei. Betel leaf extract reduced the tumorigenic effects of NNK (nitrosamine 4-(N-nitrosomethylamino)-1-(3-pyridyl)-1-butanone) by 25 per cent and also inhibited the reduction in vitamin A concentration in liver and plasma induced by NNK. Betel leaf thus has protective effect against the mutagenic, carcinogenic and adverse metabolic effects of NNK in mice (Bhide *et al.*, 1991).

It appears that the carcinogenic potential of betel is enhanced by the elevated hormonal profile in pregnant women. There is a need to determine if there is an increased likelihood of developing cancer in betel chewing pregnant women due to increased sensitivity of their lymphocytes to genetic damage compared with non-chewing pregnant women (Ghosh and Ghosh, 1988).

Oils, Butter and Ghee

Dietary fat intake is also associated with incidence of cancer. A strong positive correlation between fat intake and age adjusted incidence and mortality due to breast cancer is evident among women (Wynder *et al.,* 1986). Vegetable oils have been reported to enhance 7,12-dimethylbenz (a) anthracene (DMBA) induced mammary adenocarcinomas more than butter and some other saturated fats in rodents. High intake of unsaturated fatty acids enhances tumour development due to increased synthesis of prostaglandins (Yanagi *et al.,* 1989; Welsch, 1992). Conjugated linoleic acid (CLA) is considered anti-carcinogenic. The CLA content of cow and buffalo ghee prepared by using (a) Desi method, (b) direct cream method without starter, (c) direct cream method with starter, was analyzed. Ghee prepared with desi method was found to contain highest CLA levels and it was higher in buffalo than cow ghee (Aneja and Murthim, 1990). Ghee contains conjugated linoleic acid (CLA) which has been shown unequivocally to inhibit mammary carcinogenesis (Ip *et al.,* 1999).

PPARγ are the key components in regulation of growth and progression of mammary cancer. The expression of PPARγ was significantly more on cow ghee than on soybean oil. In the genesis of breast cancer, evidence suggests that induction of COX-2 and down regulation of PPARγ can be the key components (Badawi and Badr, 2000). Histological analysis showed rapid progression of cancer in soybean oil fed rats than rats fed cow ghee. The expression of cycloxygenase-2(COX-2) was significantly less in cow ghee fed rats compared to those on soybean oil and was associated with decreased tumour incidence. Over expression of COX-2 in rats induces mammary tumours (Liu *et al.,* 2001).

Rani and Kansal (2011) investigated the effect of feeding cow ghee versus soybean oil on DMBA induced mammary cancer and expression of cycloxygenase-2 and perisome proliferators activated receptor-γ (PPARγ) in mammary gland in 21 day old female rats. Animals fed soybean oil had higher tumour incidence (65.4 per cent), tumour weight (6.18g) and tumour volume (6285mm^3) compared to those fed cow ghee (26 per cent, 1.67g, 1925 mm^{3}respectivley). However, further research is essential to understand the regulation of COX-2 and PPARγ apoptotic signaling, cell proliferation and prostaglandin synthesis in response to dietary fat.

Ghee has protective effects against side effects of radiation or chemotherapy. The common side effects of radiation or chemotherapy are loss of appetite, pain, nausea, vomiting, diarrhoea and mucositis which makes eating difficult. Loss of appetite is a cause of concern it results in undesirable weight loss, loss of muscle mass and decreased immunity. Yashtimadhu *(Glycyrrhiza glabra)* Ghrita, a herbal preparation was administered to patients receiving chemotherapy for neck or head malignancies. Application of Yashtinadhu powder with honey and consumption of ghee was effective in prevention and treatment of oral mucositis post radiations (Das *et al.,* 2011).

Whey Protein Concentrate

Animal experiments showed that the concentrates of whey proteins exhibit anti-carcinogenesis and anticancer activity by increasing glutathione (GSH) concentration in relevant tissues, and may have anti-tumor effect on low volume of tumor via stimulation of immunity through the GSH pathway (Bounous, 2000).

Bael (*Aegle marmelos*)

Bael has been used since antiquity for treating various ailments, some of which are now known to be the result of oxidative stress. In studies spanning nearly a decade, it has been observed that bael prevented radiation-induced ill-effects, and the results of these studies indicate that it has the potential to be an effective, nontoxic radio-protective agent (Baliga *et al.*, 2010).

Resveratrol

Resveratrol, a polyphenol is found in grape skins, peanuts, berries and red wine. It has been shown to possess potent growth inhibitory effects against various human cancer cells. Resveratrol has a number of biological effects in a variety of cell culture systems. Resveratrol produces variable anti-tumor effects in different tumor cell lines infact it inhibits all the three major steps of carcinogenesis- initiation, promotion, and progression (Meishiang *et al.*, 1997). Resveratrol has also been shown to have growth-inhibitory activity, and induces apoptotic cell death in a number of human cancer cell lines as well as in animal models of carcinogenesis. In U251 glioma cells, treatment with resveratrol led to growth inhibition, induction of apoptosis and G0/G1-phase cell cycle arrest (Hao *et al.*, 2005). Further, resveratrol inhibited the growth of human skin squamous cell carcinoma A431 xenograft in nude mice. And its mechanism may be associated with the apoptosis of tumor cell through the depression of Survivin (an inhibitor of apoptosis protein), and the activation of caspase-3 (Hao *et al.*, 2013).

Resveratrol dose-dependently reduced the incidence, total number and multiplicity of visible hepatocyte nodules. Mean nodular volume and nodular volume as percentage of liver volume was also inhibited upon resveratrol treatment. Histo-pathological examination of liver tissue confirmed the protective effect of resveratrol. Immuno-histochemical detection of cell proliferation and assay of apoptosis indicated a decrease in cell proliferation and increase of apoptotic cells in the livers of resveratrol-supplemented rats. Resveratrol also induced the expression of pro-apoptotic protein Bax, reduced anti-apoptotic Bcl-2 expression and with a concurrent increase in Bax/Bcl-2 ratio with respect to DENA control thus providing evidence that resveratrol exerts a significant chemo-preventive effect on DENA-initiated hepato-carcinogenesis through inhibition of cell proliferation and induction of apoptosis (Bishayee and Dhir, 2009).

Yin *et al.* (2013) showed that resveratrol effectively inhibited the growth of lung cancer in a dose-dependent manner in nude mice. Dias *et al.* (2013) offered strong pre-clinical evidence for the utilization of dietary stilbenes, particularly 3M-Res, as novel, potent, effective chemo-preventive agents in prostate cancer. In the case of cervical cancer resveratrol treatment induced apoptosis in all cell lines, particularly in CaSki cells, as measured by Annexin-V flow cytometry analysis. There was a decrease in the mitochondrial membrane potential (apoptosis) in HeLa, CaSki, and SiHa cells and an increased lysosomal permeability (autophagy) in C33A, CaLo (HPV18 positive), and HeLa cell lines (García-Zepeda *et al.*, 2013). It is a promising phytomedicine for cancer therapy and further efforts are needed to explore this potential therapeutic strategy.

Anaplastic thyroid carcinoma (ATC) is an extremely aggressive malignancy with undifferentiated features, for which conventional treatments, including radioactive iodine ablation, are usually not effective. Resveratrol inhibited cell growth and enhanced re-differentiation in ATC cells dependent upon the activation of Notch1 signaling. Thus, activation of Notch1 signaling could be a potential therapeutic strategy for ATC patients, and thus warrants further clinical investigation (Yu *et al.*, 2013).

Other Foods

Hui *et al.* (2010) investigated the anticancer effects of an anthocyanin-rich extract from black rice on breast cancer cells *in vitro* and *in vivo*. Oral administration of the extract (100 mg/kg/day) to nude mice bearing MDA-MB-453 cell xenografts significantly suppressed tumor growth and angiogenesis by suppressing the expression of angiogenesis factors MMP-9, MMP-2, and uPA in tumor tissue.

Conclusions

Several studies have provided an insight into the biological activities of various phytochemical constituents of foods and supported a rationale for their use as promising anti-cancer agents. Fruits, especially berries and pomegranate and various cruciferous vegetables such as broccoli were extensively studied and proved to be effective in cancer treatment. However, certain foods such as bael, whey protein concentrate and black rice need to be studied further for their anti-carcinogenic potential. Interestingly, several foods offer relief from the side effects of cancer therapy such as radiation and also counteract the multidrug resistance among cancer patients.

References

Adams LS, Seeram NP, Aggarwal BB, Takada Y, Sand D, *et al.* (2006). Pomegranate juice, total pomegranate ellagitannins, and punicalagin suppress inflammatory cell signaling in colon cancer cells. J. Agric. Food Chem. 54: 930 – 85.

Adhami VM, Khan N, Mukhtar H (2009). Cancer chemoprevention by pomegranate: laboratory and clinical evidence. Nutr. Cancer. 61 (6): 811 - 15.

Afaq F, Malik A, Syed D, Maes D, Matsui MS, *et al.* (2005a). Pomegranate fruit extract modulates UV-B-mediated phosphorylation of mitogen-activated protein kinases and activation of nuclear factor kappa B in normal human epidermal keratinocytes paragraph sign. Photochem. Photobiol, 81: 38 - 45.

Afaq F, Saleem M, Krueger CG, Reed JD, Mukhtar H. (2005b). Anthocyanin- and hydrolyzable tannin-rich pomegranate fruit extract modulates MAPK and NF-kappaB pathways and inhibits skin tumorigenesis in CD-1 mice. Int. J. Cancer. 113: 423 - 33.

Albrecht M, Jiang W, Kumi-Diaka J, Lansky EP, Gommersall LM, Patel A, Mansel RE, Neeman I, Geldof AA, Campbell MJ (2004). Pomegranate extracts potently suppress proliferation, xenograft growth, and invasion of human prostate cancer cells. J. Med. Food. 7 (3): 274 - 83.

Abdullaev FI, Riverón-Negrete L, Caballero-Ortega H, Manuel Hernández J, Pérez-López I, Pereda-Miranda R, *et al.* (2003). Use of *in vitro* assays to assess the potential antigenototoxic and cytotoxic effect of saffron (*Crocus sativus) Toxicol. In vitro.*17: 731 - 36.

Aggarwal S, Ichikawa H, Takada Y, Sandur SK, Shishodia S, Aggarwal BB (2006). Curcumin (diferuloylmethane) down-regulates expression of cell proliferation and antiapoptotic and metastatic gene products through suppression of IkBa kinase and Akt activation. Mol. Pharmacol. 69: 195 - 206.

Alenzi FQ, El-Bolkiny Yel-S, Salem ML (2010). Protective effects of *Nigella sativa* oil and thymoquinone against toxicity induced by the anticancer drug cyclophosphamide. Br J. Biomed. Sci. 67 (1): 20-8.

Ali M, Thomson M, Afzal M (2000). Garlic and onions: their effect on eicosanoid metabolism and its clinical relevance. Prostaglandins Leukot. Essent. Fatty Acids. 62: 55 - 73.

Amin A, Hamza AA, Bajbouj K, Ashraf SS, Daoud S (2011). Saffron: a potential candidate for a novel anticancer drug against hepatocellular carcinoma. Hepatology. 54 (3): 857 - 67.

Amonkar AJ, Padma PR, Bhide SV (1989). Protective effect of hydroxychavicol, a phenolic component of betel leaf, against the tobacco-specific carcinogens. Mutat. Res. 210 (2): 249 - 53.

Anand P, Sundaram C, Jhurani S, Kunnumakkara AB, Aggarwal BB (2008). Curcumin and cancer: an "old-age" disease with an "age-old" solution. Cancer Lett. 267 (1): 133 - 64.

Aneja RP, Murthi TN (1990). Conjugated linoleic acid contents of Indian curds and ghee. Indian J Dairy Sc, 43 (2): 231 - 238.

Anonymous (2011). *Moringa oleifera* Lam. in amelioration of DMBA-induced renal carcinogenesis in Swiss albino mice. J. Biol Med, 3 (2): 27 - 35.

Anter J, de Abreu-Abreu N, Fernández-Bedmar Z, Villatoro-Pulido M, Alonso-Moraga A, Munoz-Serrano A (2011). Targets of red grapes: oxidative damage of DNA and leukaemia cells. Nat. Prod. Commun. 6 (1): 59 - 64.

Aoki H, Takada Y, Kondo S, Sawaya R, Aggarwal BB, Kondo Y (2007). Evidence that curcumin suppresses the growth of malignant gliomas *in vitro* and *in vivo* through induction of autophagy: role of Akt and extracellular signal-regulated kinase signaling pathways. Mol. Pharmacol. 272: 29 - 39.

Arabbi PR, Genovese MI, Lajolo FM (2004). Flavonoids in vegetable foods commonly consumed in Brazil and estimated ingestion by the Brazilian population. J. Agri. Food Chem. 52, 1124 - 31.

Ariga T (2004). The antioxidative function, preventive action on disease and utilization of proanthocyanidins. BioFactors. 21 (1–4): 197 - 201.

Aruna K, Sivaramakrishnan VM (1990). Plant products as protective agents against cancer. Indian J. Exp. Biol. 28 (11): 1008-11.

Aruna K, Sivaramakrishnan VM (1992). Anticarcinogenic effects of some Indian plant products. Food Chem. Toxicol. 30 (11): 953-6.

Asher GN, Spelman K (2013). Clinical utility of curcumin extract. Altern Ther Health Med. 19 (2): 20 - 22.

Atawodi SE, Atawodi JC, Idakwo GA, Pfundstein B, Haubner R, Wurtele G, Bartsch H, Owen RW (2010). Evaluation of the polyphenol content and antioxidant properties of methanol extracts of the leaves, stem, and root barks of Moringa oleiferaLam. J Med Food. 13 (3): 710 - 16.

Azuine MA, Amonkar AJ, Bhide SV (1991). Chemopreventive efficacy of betel leaf extract and its constituents on 7,12-dimethylbenz(a)anthracene induced carcinogenesis and their effect on drug detoxification system in mouse skin. Indian J. Exp. Biol. 29 (4): 346 - 51.

Badawi AF, Badr MZ (2003). Expression of cyclooxygenase-2 and peroxisome proliferator-activated receptor-γ and levels of prostaglandin E2 and 15dexocy Δ12, 14-prostaglandin in human breast cancer and metastasis. Int. J. Cancer. 103: 84-89.

Bakshi HA, Sam S, Feroz A, Ravesh Z, Shah GA, Sharma M (2009). Crocin from Kashmiri saffron (Crocus sativus) induces *in vitro* and *in vivo* xenograft growth inhibition of Dalton's lymphoma (DLA) in mice. Asian Pac. J. Cancer Prev. 10 (5): 887-90.

Baliga MS (2010). Triphala, Ayurvedic formulation for treating and preventing cancer: a review. J. Altern. Complement. Med. 16 (12): 1301 - 308.

Baliga MS, Bhat HP, Pereira MM, Mathias N, Venkatesh P (2010). Radioprotective effects of *Aegle marmelos* (L.) Correa (Bael): a concise review. J Altern Complement Med. 2010 Oct;16(10):1109-16.

Baliga MS, Dsouza JJ (2011). Amla (*Emblica officinalis Gaertn*), a wonder berry in the treatment and prevention of cancer. Eur. J. Cancer. Prev. 20 (3): 225-39.

Banerjee S, Das S (2005). Anti-carcinogenic effects of an aqueous infusion of cloves on skin carcinogenesis. Asian Pac. J. Cancer Prev. 6 (3): 304 308.

Banerjee S, Panda CK, Das S (2006). Clove (*Syzygium aromaticum* L.), a potential chemo-preventive agent for lung cancer. Carcinogenesis. 27 (8): 1645 - 54.

Bardy J, Molassiotis A, Ryder WD, Mais K, Sykes A, Yap B, Lee L, Kaczmarski E, Slevin N (2012). A double-blind, placebo-controlled, randomised trial of active manuka honey and standard oral care for radiation-induced oral mucositis. Br. J. Oral. Maxillofac. Surg. 50 (3): 221 - 26

Bardy J, Slevin NJ, Mais KL, Molassiotis A. (2008). A systematic review of honey uses and its potential value within oncology care. J. Clin. Nurs.17 (19): 2604-23.

Bell C, Hawthorne S (2008). Ellagic acid, pomegranate and prostate cancer – a mini review. J. Pharm. Pharmacol. 60 (2):139 - 44.

Bernatchez PN, Soker S, Sirois MG. (1999). Vascular endothelial growth factors effect on endothelial cell proliferation, migration, and plutelet-activating factor synthesis is FLK-1-1 dependent. J. Biol.Chem. 274: 31047-54.

Bharti AC, Donato N, Aggarwal BB (2003). Curcumin (diferuloylmethane) inhibits constitutive and IL-6-inducible STAT3 phosphorylation in human multiple myeloma cells. J. Immunol. 171: 3863 - 71.

Bhide SV, Padma PR, Amonkar AJ (1991). Antimutagenic and anticarcinogenic effects of betel leaf extract against the tobacco-specific nitrosamine 4-(N-nitrosomethylamino)-1-(3-pyridyl)-1-butanone (NNK). IARC Sci. Publ. (105): 520 - 24.

Bishayee A, Dhir N (2009). Resveratrol-mediated chemoprevention of diethylnitrosamine-initiated hepatocarcinogenesis: inhibition of cell proliferation and induction of apoptosis. Chem. Biol. Interact. 179 (2-3): 131 - 44.

Bishayee A, Háznagy-Radnai E, Mbimba T, Sipos P, Morazzoni P, Darvesh AS, Bhatia D, Hohmann J (2010). Anthocyanin-rich black currant extract suppresses the growth of human hepatocellular carcinoma cells. Nat. Prod. Commun. 5 (10): 1613-8.

Block E (1985). The chemistry of garlic and onions. Sci. Am. 252: 114 - 19.

Bounous G (2000). Whey protein concentrate (WPC) and glutathione modulation in cancer treatment. Anticancer Res. 20 (6C): 4785 - 92.

Brooks JD, Paton VG, Vidanes G (2001). Potent induction of phase 2 enzymes in human prostate cells by sulforaphane. *Cancer. Epidemiol. Biomarkers. Prev.* 10: 949 - 54.

Calaf GM, Echiburú-Chau C, Roy D, Chai Y, Wen G, Balajee AS (2011). Protective role of curcumin in oxidative stress of breast cells. Oncol. Rep. 26 (4): 1029 - 35.

Challier B, Perarnau JM, Viel JF (1998). Garlic, onion and cereal fibre as protective factors for breast cancer: A French case-control study. Eur. J. Epidemiol. 14: 737 - 47.

Chen H, Lv L, Soroka D, Warin RF, Parks TA, Hu Y, Zhu Y, Chen X, Sang S (2012). Metabolism of [6]-shogaol in mice and in cancer cells. Drug. Metab. Dispos. 40 (4): 742 - 53.

Chen H, Soroka DN, Hu Y, Chen X, Sang S (2013). Characterization of thiol-conjugated metabolites of ginger components shogaols in mouse and human urine and modulation of the glutathione levels in cancer cells by [6]-shogaol. Mol. Nutr. Food Res. 57 (3): 447 - 58.

Chen YB, Wu KS, Gu Y, Chen JZ (2007). Research progress in the chemical constituents and pharmacological effects of lychee seeds. Chinese Journal of Infection. 14: 97 - 98.

Citronberg J, Bostick R, Ahearn T, Turgeon DK, Ruffin MT, Djuric Z, Sen A, Brenner DE, Zick SM (2013). Effects of ginger supplementation on cell-cycle biomarkers in the normal-appearing colonic mucosa of patients at increased risk for colorectal cancer: results from a pilot, randomized, and controlled trial. Cancer Prev. Res. (Phila). 6 (4): 271 - 81.

Conaway CC, Yang YM, Chung FL (2002). Isothiocyanates as cancer chemopreventive agents: their biological activities and metabolism in rodents and humans. Curr Drug Metab. 3 (3): 233 - 55

Côté J, Caillet S, Doyon G, Sylvain JF, Lacroix M (2010). Bioactive compounds in cranberries and their biological properties. Crit. Rev. Food Sci. Nutr. 50 (7): 666-79.

Das S (2002). Garlic - A Natural Source of Cancer Preventive Compounds. Asian Pac. J. Cancer Prev. 3 (4): 305 - 311.

Das D, Agarwal SK, Chandola HM (2011). Protective effect of Yashtimadhu (*Glycyrrhiza glabra*) against side effects of radiation/chemotherapy in head and neck malignancies. Ayu. 32 (2): 196-199.

Das I, Chakrabarty RN, Das S (2004). Saffron can prevent chemically induced skin carcinogenesis in Swiss albino mice. Asian Pac. J. Cancer Prev. 5 (1):70-6.

Das KC, Das CK (2002). Curcumin (diferuloylmethane), a singlet oxygen ((1)O(2)) quencher. Biochem. Biophys. Res. Commun. 295: 62 - 66.

Das I, Das S, Saha T (2010). Saffron suppresses oxidative stress in DMBA-induced skin carcinoma: A histopathological study. Acta Histochem. 112 (4): 317-27.

Deschner EE, Ruperto J, Wong G, Newmark HL (1991). Quercetin and rutin as inhibitors of azoxymethanol-induced colonic neoplasia. Carcinogenesis. 12: 1193 - 96.

Dias SJ, Li K, Rimando AM, Dhar S, Mizuno CS, Penman AD, Levenson AS (2013). Trimethoxy-Resveratrol and Piceatannol Administered Orally Suppress and Inhibit Tumor Formation and Growth in Prostate Cancer Xenografts. Prostate. 2013 May 8. doi: 10.1002/pros.22657. [Epub ahead of print].

Dorai T, Cao YC, Dorai B, Buttyan R, Katz AE. (2001). Therapeutic potential of curcumin in human prostate cancer. III. Curcumin inhibits proliferation, induces apoptosis, and inhibits angiogenesis of LNCaP prostate can- cer cells *in vivo*. Prostate. 47(4):293-303.

Dorant E, van den Brandt PA, Goldbohm RA, Sturmans F (1996). Consumption of onions and a reduced risk of stomach carcinoma. Gastroenterology. 110: 12 - 20.

Duncan AM, Merz BE, Xu X, Nagel TC, Phipps WR, Kurzer MS (1999). Soy isoflavones exert modest hormonal effects in premenopausal women. J. Clin. Endocrinol. Metab. 84 (1):192 - 97.

Duthie SJ (2007). Berry phytochemicals, genomic stability and cancer: evidence for chemoprotection at several stages in the carcinogenic process. Mol. Nutr. Food Res. 51 (6):665-74.

Dwivedi V, Shrivastava R, Hussain S, Ganguly C, Bharadwaj M (2011). Comparative anticancer potential of clove (*Syzygium aromaticum*)–an Indian spice–against cancer cell lines of various anatomical origin. Asian Pac. J. Cancer. Prev. 12 (8): 1989 - 93.

Edirisinghe I, Banaszewski K, Cappozzo J, McCarthy D, Burton-Freeman BM (2011). Effect of black currant anthocyanins on the activation of endothelial nitric oxide synthase (eNOS) *in vitro* in human endothelial cells. J. Agric. Food Chem. 59 (16): 8616 - 24.

Escribano J, Alonso GL, Coca-Prados M, Fernandez JA (1996). Crocin, safranal and picrocrocin from saffron (*Crocus sativus* L.) inhibit the growth of human cancer cells *in vitro*. Cancer Lett. 100 (1-2): 23 - 30.

Fang EF, Zhang CZ, Wong JH, Shen JY, Li CH, Ng TB (2012). The MAP30 protein from bitter gourd (*Momordica charantia*) seeds promotes apoptosis in liver cancer cells *in vitro* and *in vivo*. Cancer. Lett. 324 (1): 66 - 74.

Fauzi AN, Norazmi MN, Yaacob NS. (2011) Tualang honey induces apoptosis and disrupts the mitochondrial membrane potential of human breast and cervical cancer cell lines. Food Chem. Toxicol. 49 (4): 871 - 78.

Fenwick GR, Hanley AB (1985). The genus Allium - Part 1. Crit. Rev. Food Sci. Nutr. 22: 199 - 271.

Ferguson LR, Schlothauer RC (2012). The potential role of nutritional genomics tools in validating high health foods for cancer control: broccoli as example. Mol. Nutr. Food Res. 56 (1): 126 - 46.

Ferlay J, Shin HR, Bray F, *et al.* (2010a). Estimates of worldwide burden of cancer in 2008: GLOBOCAN 2008. Int. J. Cancer. 127 (12): 2893 - 917.

Ferlay J, Shin HR, Bray F, *et al.* (2010b). GLOBOCAN 2008 v1.2, Cancer Incidence and Mortality Worldwide: IARC CancerBase No. 10 [Internet]. Lyon, France: International Agency for Research on Cancer, 2010. Available from: http:// globocan.iarc.fr. Accessed May 2011.

Ferrario A, Luna M, Rucker N, Wong S, Gomer CJ (2011). Pro-apoptotic and anti-inflammatory properties of the green tea constituent epigallocatechin gallate increase photodynamic therapy responsiveness. Lasers. Surg. Med. 43 (7): 644 - 50.

Fleischauer AT, Arab L (2001). Garlic and cancer: a critical review of the epidemiologic literature. J. Nutr. 131: 1032S - 40S.

Fleischauer AT, Poole C, Arab L (2000). Garlic consumption and cancer prevention: meta-analyses of colorectal and stomach cancers. Am. J. Clin. Nutr. 72: 1047 - 52.

Fukushima S, Takada N, Hori T, Wanibuchi H (1997). Cancer prevention by organosulfur compounds from garlic and onion. J. Cell. Biochem. Suppl. 27: 100 -105.

Gagandeep, Dhanalakshmi S, Méndiz E, Rao AR, Kale RK (2003). Chemopreventive effects of *Cuminum cyminum* in chemically induced forestomach and uterine cervix tumors in murine model systems. Nutr. Cancer. 47 (2): 171 - 80.

Galeone C, Pelucchi C, Dal Maso L, Negri E, Montella M, Zucchetto A, Talamini R, La Vecchia C (2009). Allium vegetables intake and endometrial cancer risk. Public Health Nutr. 12 (9): 1576 - 79.

Galeone C, Pelucchi C, Levi F, Negri E, Franceschi S, Talamini R, Giacosa A, La Vecchia C (2006). Onion and garlic use and human cancer. Am. J. Clin. Nutr. 84 (5): 1027 - 32.

Galeone C, Pelucchi C, Talamini R, Negri E, Dal Maso L, Montella M, Ramazzotti V, Franceschi S, La Vecchia C (2007). Onion and garlic intake and the odds of benign prostatic hyperplasia. Urology. 70 (4): 672 - 76.

Gao CM, Takezaki T, Ding JH, Li MS, Tajima K (1999). Protective effect of allium vegetables against both esophageal and stomach cancer: a simultaneous case-referent study of a high-epidemic area in Jiangsu Province, China. Jpn. J. Cancer. Res. 90: 614 - 21.

García-Zepeda SP, García-Villa E, Díaz-Chávez J, Hernández-Pando R, Gariglio P (2013). Resveratrol induces cell death in cervical cancer cells through apoptosis and autophagy. Eur. J. Cancer. Prev. 2013 Apr 18. [Epub ahead of print].

George S, Chaturvedi P (2009). A comparative study of the anti-oxidant properties of two different species of *Ocimum* of southern Africa on alcohol-induced oxidative stress. J. Med. Food. 12 (5): 1154 - 58.

Ghashm AA, Othman NH, Khattak MN, Ismail NM, Saini R (2010) Antiproliferative effect of Tualang honey on oral squamous cell carcinoma and osteosarcoma cell lines. BMC Complement Altern Med. 14 (10): 49.

Ghosh PK, Ghosh R (1988). Effect of betel chewing on the frequency of sister chromatid exchanges inpregnant women and women using oral contraceptives. Cancer. Genet. Cytogenet. 32 (2): 211 - 15.

Gollücke AP, Ribeiro DA (2012). Use of grape polyphenols for promoting human health: a review of patents. Recent Pat. Food Nutr. Agric. 4 (1): 26 - 30.

Han SS, Keum YS, Chun SK, Surh YJ. (2002). Suppression of phorbol ester-induced NF-kB activation by capsaicin in cultured human promyelocytic leukemia cells. Arch. Pharma. Res. 25: 475 - 79.

Hanif R, Qiao L, Shiff SJ, Rigas B.(1997) Curcumin, a natural plant phenolic food additive, inhibits cell proliferation and induces cell cycle changes in colon adenocarcinoma cell lines by a prostaglandin-independent pathway. Lab. Clin. Med. 130 (6): 576 - 84.

Hao YQ, Huang WX, Feng HX, Zhang GH, Ning XH, Li HG, Hao CG, Li ZH (2013). [Study of apoptosis related factors regulatory mechanism of resveratrol to human skin squamous cell carcinoma A431 xenograft in nude mice]. Zhonghua. Yi. Xue. Za. Zhi. 93 (6): 464 - 68. [Article in Chinese].

Hao J, Zhang L, Kuo J, Kuo K, G SC, Groc L, Rodriguez AI, Koubi D, Hunter TJ, Corcoran GB, Seidman MD, Levine RA (2005). Resveratrol-induced apoptotic death in human U251 glioma cells. Mol. Cancer Ther. 4: 554 - 61.

Higdon JV, Delage B, Williams DE, Dashwood RH (2007). Cruciferous vegetables and human cancer risk: epidemiologic evidence and mechanistic basis. Pharmacol. Res. 55 (3): 224 - 36.74

Hong MY, Seeram NP, Heber D. (2008). Pomegranate polyphenols down-regulate expression of androgen-synthesizing genes in human prostate cancer cells overexpressing the androgen receptor. J. Nutr. Biochem.19: 848 - 55.

Hora JJ, Maydew ER, Lansky EP, Dwivedi C (2003). Chemopreventive effects of pomegranate seed oil on skin tumor development in CD1 mice. J. Med. Food. 6: 157 - 61.

Hsing AW, Chokkalingam AP, Gao YT, Madigan MP, Deng J, Gridley G, Fraumeni JF Jr. (2002). Allium vegetables and risk of prostate cancer: a population-based study. J. Natl. Cancer. Inst. 94 (21): 1648 - 51.

Hsu CP, Lin CC, Huang CC, Lin YH, Chou JC, Tsia YT, Su JR, Chung YC (2012). Induction of apoptosis and cell cycle arrest in human colorectal carcinoma by Litchi seed extract. J. Biomed. Biotechnol. 2012: 341479.

Hu J, La Vecchia C, Negri E, Chatenoud L, Bosetti C, Jia X, Liu R, Huang G, Bi D, Wang C (1999). Diet and brain cancer in adults. A case control study in northeast China. Int. J. Cancer. 81:20 - 23.

Huang C, Huang Y, Li J, Hu W, Aziz R, Tang MS, Sun N, Cassady J, Stoner GD (2002). Inhibition of benzo(a)pyrene diol-epoxide-induced transactivation of activated protein 1 and nuclear factor kappaB by black raspberry extracts. Cancer. Res. 62 (23): 6857 - 63.

Huang C, Li J, Song L, Zhang D, Tong Q, Ding M, Bowman L, Aziz R, Stoner GD.(2006). Black raspberry extracts inhibit benzo(a)pyrene diol-epoxide-induced activator protein 1 activation and VEGF transcription by targeting the phosphotidyl-inositol 3-kinase/Akt pathway. Cancer Res. 66 (1): 581 - 87.

Huang C, Li J, Song L, Zhang D, Tong Q, Ding M, Bowman L, Aziz R, Stoner GD (2008a). Black raspberry extracts inhibit benzo(a)pyrene diol-epoxide-induced activator protein 1 activation and VEGF transcription by targeting the phosphotidylinositol 3-kinase/Akt pathway. Cancer. Res. 66 (1): 581 - 87.

Huang AC, Lin SY, Su CC, Lin SS, Ho CC, Hsia TC, Chiu TH, Yu CS, Ip SW, Lin TP, Chung JG. (2008b). Effects of curcumin on N-bis(2-hydroxypropyl) nitrosamine (DHPN)-induced lung and liver tumorigenesis in BALB/c mice *in vivo*. *In vivo*. 22 (6): 781 - 85.

Huang C, Zhang D, Li J, Tong Q, Stoner GD (2007). Differential inhibition of UV-induced activation of NF kappa B and AP-1 by extracts from black raspberries, strawberries, and blueberries. Nutr. Cancer. 58 (2): 205 - 212.

Hui C, Bin Y, Xiaoping Y, Long Y, Chunye C, Mantian M, Wenhua L (2010). Anticancer activities of an anthocyanin-rich extract from black rice against breast cancer cells *in vitro* and *in vivo*. Nutr. Cancer. 62 (8): 1128 - 36.

IP C, Banni S, Angioni E, Carta G, McGinley J, Thompson HJ, *et al.* (1999). Conjugated linoleic acid enriched butter fat alters mammary gland morphogenesis and reduces cancer risk in rats. J. Nutr, 129: 2135 - 42.

Jagannathan SK (2011). Can flavonoids from honey alter multidrug resistance? Med. Hypotheses. 76 (4): 535- 37.

Jagannathan SK, Mazumdar A, Mondhe D, Mandal M (2011). Apoptotic effect of eugenol in human colon cancer cell lines. Cell Biol Int. 35(6):607-15.

Jagannathan SK, Mondhe D, Wani ZA, Pal HC, Mandal M. (2010). Effect of honey and eugenol on Ehrlich ascites and solid carcinoma. J. Biomed. Biotechnol. 989163. Epub 2010 Mar 28.

Jeune MA, Kumi-Diaka J, Brown J (2005). Anticancer activities of pomegranate extracts and genistein in human breast cancer cells. J. Med. Food. 8 (4): 469 - 75.

Joseph MA, Moysich KB, Freudenheim JL, Shields PG, Bowman ED, Zhang Y, Marshall JR, Ambrosone CB (2004). Cruciferous vegetables, genetic polymorphisms in glutathione S-transferases M1 and T1, and prostate cancer risk. Nutr. Cancer. 50 (2): 206 - 13.

Juge N, Mithen RF, Traka M. (2007). Molecular basis for chemoprevention by sulforaphane: a comprehensive review. Cell. Mol. Life Sci. 64 (9): 1105–27.

Jurenka JS (2008). Therapeutic applications of pomegranate (*Punica granatum* L.): a review. Altern. Med. Rev. 13 (2): 128-44.

Katiyar SK, Mukhtar H (1997). Tea antioxidants in cancer chemoprevention. J. Cell. Biochem. Suppl. 27: 59-67.

Kaur M, Singh RP, Gu M, Agarwal R, Agarwal C (2006). Grape seed extract inhibits *in vitro* and *in vivo* growth of human colorectal carcinoma cells. Clin. Cancer Res. 12 (20 Pt 1): 6194 - 202.

Kaur M, Agarwal C, Agarwal R (2009a). Anti-cancer and cancer chemopreventive potential of grape seed extract and other grape-based products. J. Nutr. 139 (9): 1806S - 12S.

Kaur M, Velmurugan B, Rajamanickam S, Agarwal R, Agarwal C (2009b). Gallic acid, an active constituent of grape seed extract, exhibits anti-proliferative, pro-apoptotic and anti-tumorigenic effects against prostate carcinoma xenograft growth in nude mice. Pharmaceutical Research. 26 (9): 2133 - 40.

Keck AS, Finley JW (2006). Aqueous extracts of selenium- fertilized broccoli increase selenoprotein activity and inhibit DNA single-strand breaks, but decrease the activity of quinone reductase in Hepa 1c1c7 cells. Food Chem. Toxicol. 44 (5): 695 - 703.

Khan SA (2009). The role of pomegranate (*Punica granatum* L.) in colon cancer. Pak. J. Pharm. Sci. 22 (3): 346 - 48.

Khan GN, Gorin MA, Rosenthal D, Pan Q, Bao LW, Wu ZF, Newman RA, Pawlus AD, Yang P, Lansky EP, Merajver SD (2009). Pomegranate fruit extract impairs invasion and motility in human breast cancer. Integr. Cancer Ther. 8 (3): 242 - 53.

Khan N, Hadi N, Afaq F, Syed DN, Kweon MH, *et al.* (2007). Pomegranate fruit extract inhibits prosurvival pathways in human A549 lung carcinoma cells and tumor growth in athymic nude mice. Carcinogenesis. 28: 163 - 73.

Khanal B, Baliga M, Uppal N (2010). Effect of topical honey on limitation of radiation-induced oral mucositis: an intervention study. Int. J. Oral Maxillofac. Surg. 39 (12): 1181 - 85.

Khanduja KL, Gandhi RK, Pathania V, Syal N (1999). Prevention of N-nitrosodiethylamine-induced lung tumorigenesis by ellagic acid and quercetin in mice. Food Chem. Toxicol. 37: 313 - 18.

Kim HJ, Han MH, Kim GY, Choi YW, Choi YH (2012). Hexane extracts of garlic cloves induce apoptosis through the generation of reactive oxygen species in Hep3B human hepatocarcinoma cells. Oncol. Rep. 28 (5): 1757 - 63.

Kim SC, Magesh V, Jeong SJ, Lee HJ, Ahn KS, Lee HJ, Lee EO, Kim SH, Lee MH, Kim JH, Kim SH (2010). Ethanol extract of *Ocimum sanctum* exerts anti-metastatic activity through inactivation of matrix metalloproteinase-9 and enhancement of anti-oxidant enzymes. Food Chem. Toxicol. 48 (6): 1478 - 82.

Kirsh, VA; Peters U, Mayne ST, Subar AF, Chatterjee N, Johnson CC, Hayes RB (2007). Prospective study of fruit and vegetable intake and risk of prostate cancer. Journal of the National Cancer Institute. 99 (15): 1200 - 209.

Kohno H, Suzuki R, Yasui Y, Hosokawa M, Miyashita K, *et al.* (2004). Pomegranate seed oil rich in conjugated linolenic acid suppresses chemically induced colon carcinogenesis in rats. Cancer Sci. 95: 481 - 86.

Krishnaswamy K, Goud VK, Sesikeran B, Mukundan MA, Krishna TP. (1998) Retardation of experimental tumorigenesis and reduction in DNA adducts by turmeric and curcumin. Nutr. Cancer. 30:163 - 66.

Krishnaveni M, Mirunalini S (2010). Therapeutic potential of *Phyllanthus emblica* (amla): the ayurvedic wonder. Review. J. Basic Clin. Physiol. Pharmacol. 21 (1): 93 - 105.

Kristal AR, Lampe JW (2002). Brassica vegetables and prostate cancer risk: a review of the epidemiological evidence. *Nutr. Cancer.* 42: 1 - 9.

Kumar A, Dhawan S, Hardegen NJ, Aggarwal BB (1998). Curcumin (Diferuloylmethane) inhibition of tumor necrosis factor (TNF)-mediated adhesion of monocytes to endothelial cells by suppression of cell surface expression of adhesion molecules and of nuclear factor-κB activation. Biochem. Pharmacol. 55: 775 - 83.

Kundu JK, Surh YJ. (2009). Molecular basis of chemoprevention with dietary phytochemicals: Redox-regulated transcription factors as relevant targets. Phytochemistry Rev. 8: 333 - 47.

Kunnumakkara AB, Anand P, Aggarwal BB (2008b). Curcumin inhibits proliferation, invasion, angiogenesis and metastasis of different cancers through interaction with multiple cell signaling proteins. Cancer Lett. 269 (2): 199 - 225.

Kunnumakkara AB, Diagaradjane P, Guha S, Deorukhkar A, Shentu S, Aggarwal BB, Krishnan S (2008a). Curcumin sensitizes human colorectal cancer xenografts in nude mice to gamma-radiation by targeting nuclear factor-kappaB-regulated gene products. Clin. Cancer Res. 14 (7): 2128 - 36.

Kunnumakkara AB, Diagaradjane P, Anand P, Harikumar KB, Deorukhkar A, Gelovani J, Guha S, Krishnan S, Aggarwal BB (2009). Curcumin sensitizes human colorectal cancer to capecitabine by modulation of cyclin D1, COX-2, MMP-9, VEGF and CXCR4 expression in an orthotopic mouse model. Int. J. Cancer. 125 (9): 2187 - 97.

Kunnumakkara AB, Guha S, Krishnan S, Diagaradjane P, Gelovani J, Aggarwal BB (2007). Curcumin potentiates antitumor activity of gemcitabine in an orthotopic model of pancreatic cancer through suppression of proliferation, angiogenesis, and inhibition of nuclear factor-kappaB-regulated gene products. Cancer Res. 67 (8): 3853 - 61.

Kusamran WR, Ratanavila A, Tepsuwan A (1998). Effects of neem flowers, Thai and Chinese bitter gourd fruits and sweet basil leaves on hepatic monooxygenases and glutathione S-transferase activities, and *in vitro* metabolic activation of chemical carcinogens in rats. Food Chem. Toxicol. 36 (6): 475 - 84.

Kylli P, Nohynek L, Puupponen-Pimiä R, Westerlund-Wikström B, Leppänen T, Welling J, Moilanen E, Heinonen M (2011). Lingonberry (*Vaccinium vitis-idaea*) and European cranberry (*Vaccinium microcarpon*) proanthocyanidins: isolation, identification, and bioactivities. J. Agric. Food Chem. 59 (7): 3373 - 84.

Lam TK, Gallicchio L, Lindsley K, Shiels M, Hammond E, Tao XG, Chen L, Robinson KA, Caulfield LE, Herman JG, Guallar E, Alberg AJ (2009). Cruciferous vegetable consumption and lung cancer risk: a systematic review. Cancer. Epidemiol. Biomarkers. Prev. 18 (1): 184 - 95.

Lansky EP, Harrison G, Froom P, Jiang WG (2005). Pomegranate (*Punica granatum*) pure chemicals show possible synergistic inhibition of human PC-3 prostate cancer cell invasion across Matrigel. Invest. New Drugs. 23: 121 - 22.

Lazzè MC, Pizzala R, Gutiérrez Pecharromán FJ, Gatòn Garnica P, Antolín Rodríguez JM, Fabris N, Bianchi L (2009). Grape waste extract obtained by supercritical fluid extraction contains bioactive antioxidant molecules and induces antiproliferative effects in human colon adenocarcinoma cells. J. Med. Food. 12 (3): 561 - 68.

Le Bon AM, Siess MH (2000). Organosulfur compounds from Allium and the chemoprevention of cancer. Drug Metabol. Drug Interact. 17 (1-4): 51 - 79.

Lee-Huang S, Huang PL, Chen HC, Huang PL, Bourinbaiar A, Huang HI, Kung HF. (1995). Anti-HIV and anti-tumor activities of recombinant MAP30 from bitter melon. *Gene.* 161 (2): 151 - 56.

Lee-Huang S, Huang PL, Sun Y, Chen HC, Kung HF, Huang PL, Murphy WJ (2000). Inhibition of MDA-MB-231 human breast tumor xenografts and HER2 expression by anti-tumor agents GAP31 and MAP30. *Anti-cancer. Research.* 20 (2): 653 - 59.

Leifert WR, Abeywardena MY (2008). Grape seed and red wine polyphenol extracts inhibit cellular cholesterol uptake, cell proliferation, and 5-lipoxygenase activity. Nutr. Res. 28 (12): 842 - 50.

Li J, Jiang Y (2007). Litchi flavonoids: isolation, identification and biological activity. Molecules. 12 (4): 745 - 58. Review.

Li CJ, Tsang SF, Tsai CH, Tsai HY, Chyuan JH, Hsu HY (2012). *Momordica charantia* extract induces apoptosis in human cancer cells through caspase- and mitochondria-dependent pathways. Evidence-Based Complementary and Alternative Medicine. 2012: 11 pages. 261971.

Li J, Zhang D, Stoner GD, Huang C (2008). Differential effects of black raspberry and strawberry extracts on BaPDE-induced activation of transcription factors and their target genes. Mol. Carcinog. 47 (4): 286 - 94.

Limtrakul P, Anuchapreeda S, Buddhasukh D (2004). Modulation of human multidrug-resistance MDR-1 gene by natural curcuminoids. BMC. Cancer. 4: 13.

Lin HJ, Probst-Hensch NM, Louie AD, Kau IH, Witte JS, Ingles SA, Frankl HD, Lee ER, Haile RW (1998). Glutathione transferase null genotype, broccoli, and lower prevalence of colorectal adenomas. Cancer Epidemiol. Biomarkers Prev. 7 (8): 647 - 52.

Lin JK, Liang YC (2000). Cancer chemoprevention by tea polyphenols. Proc. Natl. Sci. Counc. Repub. China. B. 24 (1): 1 - 13.

Liu RH (2004). Potential synergy of phytochemicals in cancer prevention: mechanism of action. *J. Nutr.* 134: 3479S - 85S.

Liu CH, Chang SH, Narko K, Trifan OC, Wu MT, Smith E *et al.* (2001). Overexpression of cyclooxygenase-2 is sufficient to induce tumerogenesis in transgenic mice. J. Biol. Chem, 276: 18563 - 69.

Liu Y, Whelan RJ, Pattnaik BR, Ludwig K, Subudhi E, Rowland H, Claussen N, Zucker N, Uppal S, Kushner DM, Felder M, Patankar MS, Kapur A (2012). Terpenoids from *Zingiber officinale* (Ginger) induce apoptosis in endometrial cancer cells through the activation of p53. PLoS. One. 7 (12): e53178.

Liu Y, Yadev VR, Aggarwal BB, Nair MG (2010). Inhibitory effects of black pepper (*Piper nigrum*) extracts and compounds on human tumor cell proliferation, cyclooxygenase enzymes, lipid peroxidation and nuclear transcription factor-kappa-B. Nat. Prod. Commun. 5 (8): 1253 - 57.

Lu H, Li J, Zhang D, Stoner GD, Huang C (2006). Molecular mechanisms involved in chemo-prevention of black raspberry extracts: from transcription factors to their target genes. Nutr. Cancer. 54 (1): 69 - 78.

Lu J, Zhang K, Nam S, Anderson RA, Jove R, Wen W. (2010). Novel angiogenesis inhibitory activity in cinnamon extract blocks VEGFR2 kinase and downstream signaling. Carcinogenesis. 31 (3): 481 - 88.

Majdalawieh AF, Carr RI (2010). *In vitro* investigation of the potential immunomodulatory and anti-cancer activities of black pepper (*Piper nigrum*) and cardamom (*Elettaria cardamomum*). J. Med. Food. 13 (2): 371 -81.

Majtan J, Majtanova L, Bohova J, Majtan V (2011). Honeydew honey as a potent antibacterial agent in eradication of multi-drug resistant *Stenotrophomonas maltophilia* isolates from cancer patients. Phytother. Res. 25 (4): 584 - 87.

Malaveille C, Hautefeuille A, Pignatelli B, Talaska G, Vineis P, Bartsch H (1996). Dietary phenolics as anti-mutagens and inhibitory of tobacco related DNA adduction in the urothelium of smokers. Carcinogenesis. 17: 2193 - 200.

Malik A, Afaq F, Sarfaraz S, Adhami VM, Syed DN, Mukhtar H (2005). Pomegranate fruit juice for chemoprevention and chemotherapy of prostate cancer. Proc. Natl. Acad. Sci. USA. 102: 14813 - 18.

Malik A, Mukhtar H (2006). Prostate cancer prevention through pomegranate fruit. Cell. Cycle. 5 (4): 371 - 73.

Manju V, Nalini N (2006). Effect of ginger on bacterial enzymes in 1,2-dimethylhydrazine induced experimental colon carcinogenesis. Eur. J. Cancer Prev. 15 (5): 377 - 83.

Mehta R, Lansky EP (2004). Breast cancer chemopreventive properties of pomegranate (*Punica granatum*) fruit extracts in a mouse mammary organ culture. Eur J Cancer Prev. 13 4): 345 - 48.

Meishiang J, Cai L, Udeani GO, Slowing KV, Thomas CF, Beecher C WW, Fong HHS, Farnsworth NR, Douglas KA, Mehta RG, Moon R C, Pezzuto JM (1997). Cancer chemopreventive activity of resveratrol, a natural product derived from grapes. Science. 275: 218.

Menon LG, Kuttan R, Kuttan G (1999). Anti-metastatic activity of curcumin and catechin. *Cancer Lett.* 141: 159 - 65.

Milner JA (2001). A historical perspective on garlic and cancer. J Nutr 131: 1027S - 31S.

Milner JA (2001). Milner JA (2006). Preclinical perspectives on garlic and cancer. J. Nutr. 136 (3 Suppl): 827S - 831S.

Miroddi M, Calapai F, Calapai G (2011). Potential beneficial effects of garlic in oncohematology. Mini Rev. Med. Chem. 11 (6): 461 - 72.

Mukhopadhyay A, Bueso-Ramos C, Chatterjee D, Pantazis P, Aggarwal BB (2001). Curcumin downregulates cell survival mechanisms in human prostate cancer cell lines. Oncogene. 20: 7597 - 609.

Myzak MC, Dashwood RH (2006). Chemo-protection by sulforaphane: keep one eye beyond Keap1. Cancer Lett. 233 (2): 208 - 18.

Myzak MC, Tong P, Dashwood WM, Dashwood RH, Ho E (2007). Sulforaphane retards the growth of human PC-3 xenografts and inhibits HDAC activity in human subjects. Experimental biology and medicine Maywood, NJ. 232 (2): 227 - 34.

Nagabhushan M, Amonkar AJ, Bhide SV (1987). *In vitro* antimutagenicity of curcumin against environmental mutagens. Food Chem. Toxicol. 25 (7): 545 - 47.

Nagabhushan M, Bhide SV (1992). Curcumin as an inhibitor of cancer. J. Am. Coll. Nutr. 11 (2): 192 - 98.

Nagabhushan M, Nair UJ, Amonkar AJ, D'Souza AV, Bhide SV (1988). Curcumins as inhibitors of nitrosation *in vitro*. Mutat. Res. 202 (1): 163 - 69.

Nalini N, Manju V, Menon VP (2006). Effect of spices on lipid metabolism in 1, 2-dimethylhydrazine-induced rat colon carcinogenesis. J. Med. Food. 9 (2): 237 - 45.

Nalini N, Sabitha K, Viswanathan P, Menon VP (1998). Influence of spices on the bacterial (enzyme) activity in experimental colon cancer. J. Ethnopharmacol. 62 (1): 15 - 24.

Nakamura K, Yasunaga Y, Segawa T, (2002) Curcumin down-regulates AR gene expres- sion and activation in prostate cancer cell lines. Int. J. Oncol. 21 (4): 825 - 30.

Nerurkar P, Ray RB (2010). Bitter melon: antagonist to cancer. Pharm. Res. 27 (6): 1049 - 53.

Neto CC (2007). Cranberry and its phytochemicals: a review of *in vitro* anti-cancer studies. J. Nutr. 137 (1 Suppl): 186S - 193S.

Otsuki N, Dang NH, Kumagai E, Kondo A, Iwata S, Morimoto C (2010). Aqueous extract of *Carica papaya* leaves exhibits anti-tumor activity and immuno-modulatory effects. J. Ethnopharmacol. 127 (3): 760 - 67.

Oyagbemi AA, Saba AB, Azeez OI (2010). Capsaicin: a novel chemopreventive molecule and its underlying molecular mechanisms of action. Indian J. Cancer. 47 (1): 53 - 58.

Pacheco-Palencia LA, Noratto G, Hingorani L, Talcott ST, Mertens-Talcott SU (2008). Protective effects of standardized pomegranate (*Punica granatum* L.) polyphenolic extract in ultraviolet-irradiated human skin fibroblasts. J. Agric. Food Chem. 56: 8434 - 41.

Padma PR, Amonkar AJ, Bhide SV (1989a). Antimutagenic effects of betel leaf extract against the mutagenicity of two tobacco-specific N-nitrosamines. Mutagenesis. 4 (2): 154 - 56.

Padma PR, Lalitha VS, Amonkar AJ, Bhide SV (1989b). Anticarcinogenic effect of betel leaf extract against tobacco carcinogens. Cancer. Lett. 45 (3): 195 - 202.

Pakhale SS, Karibasappa GS, Ramchandani AG, Bhushan B, Sharma A (2007). Scavenging effect of Indian grape polyphenols on 2,2'-diphenyl-1-picrylhydrazyl(DPPH) radical by electron spin resonance spectrometry. Indian J. Exp. Biol. 45 (11): 968 - 73.

Paliwal R, Sharma V, Pracheta, Sharma SH (2011). Hepatoprotective and antioxidant potential of *Moringa oleifera* pods against DMBA-induced hepatocarcinogenesis in male mice. Int. J. Drug Dev. Res. 3 (2): 128 - 38.

Panahi Y, Saadat A, Sahebkar A, Hashemian F, Taghikhani M, Abolhasani E (2012). Effect of ginger on acute and delayed chemotherapy-induced nausea and vomiting: a pilot, randomized, open-label clinical trial. Integr. Cancer. Ther. 11 (3): 04 - 11.

Pantuck AJ, Zomorodian N, Belldegrun AS (2006). Phase-II Study of pomegranate juice for men with prostate cancer and increasing PSA. Curr. Urol. Rep. 7: 7.

Pinto JT, Qiao C, Xing J, Suffoletto BP, Schubert KB, Rivlin RS, et al. (2000). Alterations of prostate biomarker expression and testosterone utilization in human LNCaP prostatic carcinoma cells by garlic-derived S-allylmercaptocysteine. Prostate. 45: 304 - 14.

Plummer SM, Holloway KA, Manson MM, *et al.* (1999). Inhibition of cyclo-oxygenase 2 expression in colon cells by the chemopreventive agent curcumin involves inhibition of NF-κB activation via the NIK/IKK signalling complex. Oncogene. 18: 6013 - 20.

Polasa K, Raghuram TC, Krishna TP, Krishnaswamy K (1992). Effect of turmeric on urinary mutagens in smokers. Mutagenesis. 7 (2):107 - 109.

Potter JD, Steinmetz K (1996). Vegetables, fruit and phyto-estrogens as preventive agents. IARC. Sci. Publ. 139: 61 - 90.

Prakash J, Gupta SK (2000) Chemo-preventive activity of *Ocimum sanctum* seed oil. J. Ethnopharmacol. 72 (1-2): 29 - 34.

Qin B, Panickar KS, Anderson RA (2010). Cinnamon: potential role in the prevention of insulin resistance, metabolic syndrome, and type 2 diabetes. J. Diabetes Sci. Technol. 4 (3): 685 - 93.

Ramchandani AG, Karibasappa GS, Pakhale SS (2008). Antitumor-promoting effects of polyphenolic extracts from seedless and seeded Indian grapes. J. Environ. Pathol. Toxicol. Oncol. 27 (4): 321 - 31.

Rani R, Kansal VK (2011). Study on cow ghee versus 7, 12-dimethylbenz (a) anthracene (DMBA) induced mammary carcinogenesis and expression of cycloxygenase-2 and perisome proliferators activated receptor-γ in rats. Indian J. Med. Res. 133: 497 - 503.

Ranjan D, Chen C, Johnston TD, Jeon H, Nagabhushan M (2004). Curcumin inhibits mitogen stimulated lymphocyte proliferation, NFkappaB activation, and IL-2 signaling. J. Surg. Res. 121 (2): 171 - 77.

Rashad UM, Al-Gezawy SM, El-Gezawy E, Azzaz AN. (2009). Honey as topical prophylaxis against radiochemotherapy-induced mucositis in head and neck cancer. J. Laryngol. Otol. 123 (2): 223 - 28.

Ray RB, Raychoudhuri A, Steele R, Nerurkar P. Bitter melon (*Momordica charantia*) extract inhibits breast cancer cell proliferation by modulating cell cycle regulatory genes and promotes apoptosis. Cancer Research. 70 (5): 1925 - 31.

Rhode J, Fogoros S, Zick S, Wahl H, Griffith KA, Huang J, Liu JR (2007). Ginger inhibits cell growth and modulates angiogenic factors in ovarian cancer cells. BMC Complement. Altern. Med. 7: 44.

Salim EI, Fukushima S (2003). Chemopreventive potential of volatile oil from black cumin (*Nigella sativa* L.) seeds against rat colon carcinogenesis. Nutr. Cancer. 45 (2): 195 - 202.

Samarghandian S, Afshari JT, Davoodi S. (2011).Honey induces apoptosis in renal cell carcinoma. Pharmacogn. Mag. 7 (25): 46 - 52.

Sartippour MR, Seeram NP, Rao JY, Moro A, Harris DM, *et al.* (2008). Ellagitannin-rich pomegranate extract inhibits angiogenesis in prostate cancer *in vitro* and *in vivo*. Int. J. Oncol. 32: 475 - 80.

Seeram NP (2008). Berry fruits for cancer prevention: current status and future prospects. J. Agric. Food Chem. 56 (3): 630 - 35.

Seeram NP, Adams LS, Hardy ML, Heber D (2004). Total cranberry extract versus its phytochemical constituents: anti-proliferative and synergistic effects against human tumor cell lines. J. Agric. Food Chem. 52 (9): 2512 - 17.

Seeram NP, Adams LS, Henning SM, Niu Y, Zhang Y *et al.* (2005). *In vitro* anti-proliferative, apoptotic and antioxidant activities of punicalagin, ellagic acid and a total pomegranate tannin extract are enhanced in combination with other polyphenols as found in pomegranate juice. J. Nutr. Biochem. 16: 360 - 67.

Seeram NP, Adams LS, Zhang Y, Lee R, Sand D, Scheuller HS, Heber D (2006). Blackberry, black raspberry, blueberry, cranberry, red raspberry, and strawberry extracts inhibit growth and stimulate apoptosis of human cancer cells *in vitro*. J. Agric. Food Chem. 54 (25): 9329 - 39.

Seeram NP, Aronson WJ, Zhang Y, Henning SM, Moro A, *et al.* (2007). Pomegranate ellagitannin-derived metabolites inhibit prostate cancer growth and localize to the mouse prostate gland. J. Agric. Food Chem. 55: 7732 - 37.

Sengupta A, Ghosh S, Bhattacharjee S (2004). Allium vegetables in cancer prevention: an overview. Asian Pac, J. Cancer Prev. 5 (3): 237 - 45.

Sethi G, Ahn KS, Chaturvedi MM, Aggarwal BB (2007). Epidermal growth factor (EGF) activates nuclear factor-κB through IκBα kinase-independent but EGF receptor-kinase dependent tyrosine 42 phosphorylation of IκBα. Oncogene. 26: 7324 - 32.

Sharma G, Tyagi AK, Singh RP, Chan DC, Agarwal R (2004). Synergistic anti-cancer effects of grape seed extract and conventional cytotoxic agent doxorubicin against human breast carcinoma cells. Breast Cancer Res. Treat. 85 (1): 1 - 12.

Sharma V, Paliwal R, Janmeda P, Sharma S ((2012a). Renoprotective effects of *Moringa oleifera* pods in 7,12-dimethylbenz [a] anthracene-exposed mice. Journal of Chinese Integrative Medicine. 10 (10): DOI: 10.3736/jcim20121015.

Sharma V, Paliwal R, Janmeda P, Sharma S (2012b). Chemopreventive efficacy of Moringa oleifera pods against 7, 12-dimethylbenz [a] anthracene induced hepatic carcinogenesis in mice. Asian Pac J Cancer Prev. 13 (6): 2563 - 69.

Shen F, Herenyiova M, Weber G (1999). Synergistic down-regulation of signal transduction and cytotoxicity by tiazofurin and quercetin in human ovarian carcinoma cells. Life Sci. 64: 1869 - 76.

Shoma A, Eldars W, Noman N, Saad M, Elzahaf E, Abdalla M, Eldin DS, Zayed D, Shalaby A, Malek HA. (2010). Pentoxifylline and local honey for radiation-induced burn following breast conservative surgery. Curr. Clin. Pharmacol. 5 (4): 251 - 6.

Shukla Y, Singh M (2007). Cancer preventive properties of ginger: a brief review. Food Chem. Toxicol. 45: 683 - 90.

Singh S, Aggarwal BB (1995). Activation of transcription factor NF-k B is suppressed by curcumin (diferuloylmethane) [corrected]. J. Biol. Chem. 270: 24995 - 5000.

Singh M, Singh P, Shukla Y (2012). New strategies in cancer chemoprevention by phytochemicals. Front. Biosci. (Elite Ed). 4: 426 - 52.

Singh SV, Srivastava SK, Choi S, Lew KL, Antosiewicz Xiao D, Zeng Y, Watkins SC, Johnson CS, Trump DL, Lee YJ, Xiao H, Herman-Antosiewicz A (2005). Sulforaphane-induced cell death in human prostate cancer cells is initiated by reactive oxygen species. *J. Biol. Chem.* 280 (20): 19911 - 24.

Singh RP, Tyagi AK, Dhanalakshmi S, Agarwal R, Agarwal C (2004). Grape seed extract inhibits advanced human prostate tumor growth and angiogenesis and upregulates insulin-like growth factor binding protein-3. Int. J. Cancer. 108 (5): 733 - 40.

Srivastava SK, Xiao D, Lew KL, Hershberger P, Kokkinakis DM, Johnson CS, Trump DL, Singh SV (2003). Allyl isothiocyanate, a constituent of cruciferous vegetables, inhibits growth of PC-3 human prostate cancer xenografts *in vivo*. Carcinogenesis. 24 (10): 1665 - 70.

Steinmetz KA, Potter JD (1991). Vegetables, fruit, and cancer. II. Mechanisms. *Cancer Causes Control* 2: 427 - 42.

Surh YJ (2002). Anti-tumor promoting potential of selected spice ingredients with anti-oxidative and anti-inflammatory activities: a short review. Food Chem. Toxicol. 40: 1091 - 97.

Surh YJ, Han SS, Keum YS, Seo HJ, Lee SS (2000). Inhibitory effects of curcumin and capsaicin on phorbol ester-induced activation of eukaryotic transcription factors, NF-kappaB and AP-1. Biofactors. 12 (1-4): 107 - 112.

Surh YJ, Lee SS (1995). Capsaicin, a double-edged sword: Toxicity, metabolism, and chemo-preventive potential. Life Sci. 1845 - 55.

Syed DN, Malik A, Hadi N, Sarfaraz S, Afaq F *et al.* (2006). Photochemopreventive effect of pomegranate fruit extract on UVA-mediated activation of cellular pathways in normal human epidermal keratinocytes. Photochem. Photobiol. 82: 398 - 405.

Szarc vel Szic, K, Ndlovu MN, Haegeman G, Vanden Berghe W (2010). Nature or nurture: let food be your epigenetic medicine in chronic inflammatory disorders. Biochem. Pharmacol. 80: 1816 - 32.

Thoennissen NH, O'Kelly J, Lu D, Iwanski GB, La DT, Abbassi S, Leiter A, Karlan B, Mehta R, Koeffler HP (2010). Capsaicin causes cell-cycle arrest and apoptosis in

ER-positive and -negative breast cancer cells by modulating the EGFR/HER-2 pathway. Oncogene. 29 (2): 285 - 96.

Tomasin R, Gomes-Marcondes MC (2011). Oral administration of Aloe vera and honey reduces Walker tumour growth by decreasing cell proliferation and increasing apoptosis in tumour tissue. Phytother. Res. 25 (4): 619 - 23.

Tomita M, Kawakami H, Uchihara JN, *et al.* (2006). Curcumin (diferuloylmethane) inhibits constitutive active NF-κB, leading to suppression of cell growth of human T-cell leukemia virus type I-infected T-cell lines and primary adult T-cell leukemia cells. Int. J. Cancer. 118: 765 - 72.

Traka M, Gasper AV, Melchini A, Bacon JR, Needs PW, Frost V, Chantry A, Jones AM, Ortori CA, Barrett DA, Ball RY, Mills RD, Mithen RF (2008). Broccoli consumption interacts with GSTM1 to perturb oncogenic signalling pathways in the prostate. PLoS One. 3 (7): e2568.

Tsai CF, Ou BR, Liang YC, Yeh JY (2013). Growth inhibition and antioxidative status induced by selenium-enrichedbroccoli extract and selenocompounds in DNA mismatch repair-deficient human colon cancer cells. Food Chem. 139 (1-4): 267 - 73.

Uma Devi P, Ganasoundari A, Vrinda B, Srinivasan KK, Unnikrishnan MK (2000). Radiation protection by the ocimum flavonoids orientin and vicenin: mechanisms of action. Radiat Res. 154 (4): 455 - 60.

Vainio H, Bianchini F (2003). IARC handbooks of cancer prevention. Fruit and vegetables. IARC Press. Lyon (France). *p.* 376.

Virtanen AL, Matikkala EJ (1976). The isolation of S-methyl L-cysteine sulphoxide and S-n-propyl-L-cysteine from onion (*Allium cepa*) and the antibiotic activity of crushed onion. Acta. Chem. Scand. 13: 1898 - 900.

Wang SY, Feng R, Bowman L, Penhallegon R, Ding M, Lu Y (2005). Anti-oxidant activity in lingonberries (*Vaccinium vitis-idaea* L.) and its inhibitory effect on activator protein-1, nuclear factor-kappaB, and mitogen-activated protein kinases activation. J. Agric. Food. Chem. 53 (8): 3156 - 66.

Wang SY, Feng R, Bowman L, Lu Y, Ballington JR, Ding M (2007). Anti-oxidant activity of *Vaccinium stamineum*: exhibition of anti-cancer capability in human lung and leukemia cells. Planta. Med. 73 (5): 451 - 60.

Wang X, Jiao F, Wang QW, Wang J, Yang K, Hu RR, Liu HC, Wang HY, Wang YS (2012a). Aged black garlic extract induces inhibition of gastric cancer cell growth *in vitro* and *in vivo*. Mol. Med. Report. 5 (1): 66 - 72.

Wang X, Wei Y, Yuan S, Liu G, Zhang YL, Wang W (2006a). Potential anticancer activity of litchi fruit pericarp extract against hepatocellular carcinoma *in vitro* and *in vivo*. Cancer. Lett. 239 (1): 144 - 50.

Wang X, Yuan S, Wang J, Lin P, Liu G, Lu Y, Zhang J, Wang W, Wei Y (2006b). Anti-cancer activity of litchi fruit pericarp extract against human breast cancer *in vitro* and *in vivo*. Toxicol. Appl. Pharmacol. 215 (2): 168 - 78.

Wang Y, Tian WX, Ma XF (2012b). Inhibitory effects of onion (*Allium cepa* L.) extract on proliferation of cancer cells and adipocytes via inhibiting fatty acid synthase. Asian. Pac. J. Cancer. Prev. 13 (11): 5573 - 79.

Welsch CW (1992). Relationship between dietary fat and experimental mammary tumourogenesis: a review and critique. Cancer Res; 52 (Suppl. 7): 2040S - 8S.

Welch C, Wuarin L, Sidell N (1992). Anti-proliferative effect of the garlic compound S-allyl cysteine on human neuroblastoma cells in vitro. Cancer Lett. 63: 211 - 19.

WHO (2008). World Health Organisation. The global burden of disease: 2004 update. 2008. The World Health Organisation. Geneva.

WHO (2012). *Fact sheet - No. 297.*

Wondrak GT, Villeneuve NF, Lamore SD, Bause AS, Jiang T, Zhang DD (2010).

The cinnamon-derived dietary factor cinnamic aldehyde activates the Nrf2-dependent anti-oxidant response in human epithelial colon cells. Molecules. 15 (5): 3338 - 55.

Wynder EL, Rose DP, Cohen LA (1986). Diet and breast cancer in causation and therapy. Cancer. 58: 1804 - 813.

Xiao D, Srivastava SK, Lew KL, Zeng Y, Hershberger P, Johnson CS, Trump DL, Singh SV (2003). Allyl isothiocyanate, a constituent of cruciferous vegetables, inhibits proliferation of human prostate cancer cells by causing G2/M arrest and inducing apoptosis. *Carcinogenesis.* 24: 891 - 97.

Xiao LY, Zhang D, Feng ZM, Chen YW, Zhang H, Lin PY (2004). Studies on the antitumor effect of lychee seeds in mice. Journal of Chinese Medicine. Materials. 27: 517 - 18.

Xiong AH, Shen WJ, Xiao LY, Lv JH (2008). Effect of Semen Litchi containing serum on proliferation and apoptosis of HepG2 cells. Zhongyaocai. 31 (10): 1533 - 36.

Yanagi S, Yamshita M, Sakamoto M, Kumazawa K, Imai S (1989). Comparative effects of butter, margarine, safflower oil and dextrin on mammary tumerogenesis in mice and rates. In Kabara JJ editor. The pharmacological effects of lipids III: The role of lipids in cancer research. Galena, IL. Lauricidin. Inc. pp. 159 - 69.

Yin HT, Tian QZ, Guan L, Zhou Y, Huang XE, Zhang H (2013). *In vitro* and *in vivo* Evaluation of the Antitumor Efficiency of Resveratrol Against Lung Cancer. Asian Pac. J. Cancer Prev. 14 (3): 1703 - 706.

You WC, Zhang L, Gail MH, Ma JL, Chang YS, Blot WJ, Li JY, Zhao CL, Liu WD, Li HQ, Hu YR, Bravo JC, Correa P, Xu GW, Fraumeni JF Jr. (1998). Helicobacter pylori infection, garlic intake and precancerous lesions in a Chinese population at low risk of gastric cancer. Int J Epidemiol 27: 941 - 44.

Yu XM, Jaskula-Sztul R, Ahmed K, Harrison AD, Kunnimalaiyaan M, Chen H (2013). Resveratrol Induces Differentiation Markers Expression in Anaplastic Thyroid Carcinoma via Activation of Notch1 Signaling and Suppresses Cell Growth. Mol. Cancer Ther. 2013 Apr 17. [Epub ahead of print].

Zhao M, Yang B, Wang J, Liu Y, Yu L, Jiang Y (2007). Immuno-modulatory and anticancer activities of flavonoids extracted fromlitchi (*Litchi chinensis* Sonn) pericarp. Int. Immuno-pharmacol. 7 (2): 162 - 66.

Zhu Y, Warin RF, Soroka DN, Chen H, Sang S (2013). Metabolites of ginger component [6]-shogaol remain bioactive in cancer cells and have low toxicity in normal cells: chemical synthesis and biological evaluation. PLoS One. 8 (1): e54677.

Chapter 4

Anti-Cognitive-Impairment Foods

Cognition is a group of mental processes that include attention, memory, comprehension, learning, reasoning, solving problems, thinking, concentration, planning, organization and decision making. Age related decline in cognition and memory to some extent is normal, but sometimes it can signal problems.

Memory is one of the most complex functions of the brain and involves multiple neural pathways and neuro-transmitter systems. Depression has become a universal problem, with lack of motivation and lassitude as major symptoms. Cure of cognitive disorders such as amnesia, attention deficit and Alzheimer's disease is still a nightmare in the field of medicine. Nootropic agents such as piracetam, aniracetam and choline esterase inhibitors like Donepezil are being used to improve memory, mood and behavior, but the resulting side effects associated with these agents have made their use limited. Several environmental factors including diet influence the growth, development and functioning of brain. Over the past 40 years, several lines of investigation have shown that the chemistry and function of both the developing and the mature brain are influenced by diet. Coultrap *et al.* (2008) provided evidence that dietary alterations later in life may prevent or postpone the cognitive declines associated with ageing.

Protein, energy (Winick, 1976), iron (Felt and Lozoff, 1996; Lozoff *et al.*, 1991), essential fatty acids (polyunsaturated fatty acids) and folate are some of the dietary factors that were found to impact the brain (Bättig and Welzl, 1993). Examples are the effect of folate deficiency on neural tube development during early gestation, the influence of essential fatty acid deficiency during gestation and postnatal life on the development of visual function in infants, and the effects of tryptophan or tyrosine intake (alone or as a constituent of dietary protein) on the production of the brain neuro-transmitters derived from them (serotonin and the catecholamines, respectively). Chronic deficiencies of certain minerals such as zinc, iron, magnesium and iodine, and insufficient dietary intake of long-chain polyunsaturated fatty acids may have a significant impact on the development and severity of the symptoms of attention deficit hyper-activity disorder (ADHD) in children (Konikowska *et al.*, 2012).

In the past few decades, it has become clear that many other constituents of the diet, apart from macro and micronutrients influence brain function. *E.g.* Caffeine contained in coffee, tea, chocolate, and soft drinks is a mild stimulant that may improve mental alertness and performance. γ-Amino-butyric acid (GABA) is found in many foods such as tomatoes, unpolished rice, chocolate, tea, fermented foods and fish. Though it has been recognized as a functional food, very few studies have been conducted on the relevance of GABA to learning behavior, object recognition, memory or working memory (Menzies *et al.*, 2007). Thus, some foods or food constituents were found to possess biochemical effects whereas others, functional and behavioral effects.

Essential Fatty Acids

It is well known that the two essential fatty acids, linoleic and alpha linolenic are most important for brain function. *n*-3 PUFAs influence cognition during ageing. These are the prime structural components of brain cell membranes and are also an important part of the enzymes within cell membranes that transport valuable nutrients in and out of the cells.

The Eskimos who eat a lot of fish have a lower incidence of degenerative diseases of the central nervous system, such as multiple sclerosis. Omega-3 polyunsaturated fatty acids (*n*-3 PUFAs) are one diet-related factor suggested to influence cognitive decline during ageing. The *n*-3 long-chain (LC) PUFAs eicosa-pentaenoic acid (EPA) and docosa-hexaenoic acid (DHA) are crucial to brain development and normal brain functioning (Neuringer *et al.*, 1988). DHA concentration in the brain decreases with age in humans (Soderberg *et al.*, 1991).

After birth the DHA content of the brain in formula fed infants was below that of breastfed infants as the breast milk contains DHA (Makrides *et al.*, 1994). Thus, presence of DHA in the diet could directly influence DHA accretion in the brain. But hydrogenated or partially hydrogenated fat hinder the brain's work. High-fat foods not only clog the arteries, but damage brain function.

DHA is particularly important to brain functioning due to its influence on neural membrane properties, which modulate cell signaling (Uauy and Dangour, 2006). Infants with low amounts of dietary DHA have reduced brain development and diminished visual acuity. The increased intelligence and academic performance of breastfed infants has been attributed in part to the increased DHA content of human milk. Experimental animals whose diets are low in DHA have been found to have smaller brains and delayed central nervous system development. Some children with poor school performance because of ADD (Attention Deficiency Disorder) have been shown to have insufficient essential fatty acids in their diet. The underlying biochemical mechanisms are poorly understood. Improvements in mild memory complaints with 900 mg of DHA were reported by Yurko-Mauro *et al.* (2010). Positive effects were observed on Verbal Recognition Memory and significant decreases in resting heart rate with DHA indicating improved learning and episodic memory functions and cardiovascular benefits in age-related cognitive decline (Yurko-Mauro, 2010).

Cognitive deficits are ameliorated and memory performance is improved by DHA supplementation (Moriguchi and Salem, 2003; Chung *et al.*, 2008, Sugimoto *et al.*, 2002). DHA and EPA levels, either individually or in combination, have been associated with better cognitive function in normal older adults (Whalley *et al.*, 2004; 2008, Whalley *et al.*, 2008) or reduced risk of cognitive decline (Heude *et al.*, 2003), substantial inhibition of Aβ fibrillation (Hashimoto and Hossain, 2011) and lower risk of developing dementia (Schaefer *et al.*, 2006). Ueda *et al.* (2011) showed that the senescence-accelerated mice given a high poly-unsaturated fatty acid diet had higher brain concentrations of poly-unsaturated fatty acid, better memory and greater longevity. Apart from improving memory, the reaction time of memory also improved in healthy, young adults on supplementation with DHA, whose habitual diets were low in the same (Stonehouse *et al.*, 2013). The long-term dietary ω3 PUFA supplementation positively impacts the anxiety and cognitive performances in the adult mouse lemur and may improve the same in humans also (Vinot *et al.*, 2011). Increasing n-3 PUFA (DHA and EPA) intakes may reduce depressive symptoms and the risk of progressing to dementia in older people with mild cognitive impairment (Sinn *et al.*, 2012).

Some clinical evidence suggests that an ARA:DHA ratio greater than 1:1 is associated with improved cognitive outcomes (Hoffman *et al.*, 2009). Combined supplementation of DHA with iron improved verbal and nonverbal learning and memory, particularly in children with anemia (Baumgartner *et al.*, 2012), and DHA and phytonutrient lutein showed cognitive benefits in older adults (Johnson *et al.*, 2008).

Amino Acids and Neurotransmitters

Tryptophan is the precursor to the neuro-transmitter serotonin. Numerous studies showed that the availability of this amino acid to brain neurons directly influences the rate at which it is converted to a neuro-transmitter (Fernstrom, 1983). Administering either the amino acid itself (Ashcroft *et al.*, 1965) or meals that raise tryptophan availability to serotonergic neurons (Fernstrom and Wurtman, 1971; Fernstrom and Fernstrom, 1995) rapidly stimulated serotonin production and enhanced serotonin release in neurons (Sharp *et al.*, 1992) thus producing changes in brain function. In humans, administration of oral tryptophan can modify sleep and mood via its actions to stimulate neuronal serotonin production and release (Borbely and Youmbi–Balderer, 1987; Young and Gauthier, 1981). The radial arm maze and the passive avoidance tests on animals showed that the increase in brain 5 Hydroxy-tryptamine metabolism following long term tryptophan administration may be involved in enhancement of memory (Khaliq *et al.*, 2006). While single oral administration of tryptophan was not effective in memory enhancement, repeated intake significantly enhanced memory functions of rats as evidenced by the decreased latency time to reach the hidden platform in Water Maze test (Khaliq *et al.*, 2007). Older adults with mild cognitive impairment showed significant improvements in several measures of cognitive function when supplemented with an oily emulsion of DHA-phospholipids containing melatonin and tryptophan for 12 weeks, compared with the placebo (Rondanelli *et al.*, 2012). In a double-blind study for 14 days, S-Adenosyl **Methionine** (SAMe) supplementation was found to result in significant improvements in depressive symptoms compared to 22 per cent of the Imipramine treated patients (Bell *et al.*, 1988).

Tyrosine is the precursor to the catecholamine neurotransmitters dopamine, norepinephrine and epinephrine. Analogous to the ability of tryptophan to stimulate serotonin production, elevating tyrosine concentrations in brain catecholamine neurons, particularly dopamine and norepinephrine neurons, can stimulate transmitter production. Tyrosine administration appears to improve cognition and performance (Banderet and Lieberman, 1989) in soldiers under stressful conditions. Further work is required before the usefulness of tyrosine is established or accepted. Mahoney *et al.* (2007) and O'Brien *et al.* (2007a and b) demonstrated that cold exposure degrades cognitive performance and supplementation with tyrosine alleviates working memory decrements.

B Complex Vitamins and Neurotransmitters

B vitamins appear to slow cognitive and clinical decline in people with mild cognitive impairment, in particular in those with elevated homocysteine (de Jager *et al.*, 2012). In a multivariate analysis, Moorthy *et al.* (2012) showed an association between low plasma vitamin B-12 concentrations and poor Mini-Mental Status Exam (MMSE) scores and higher depression scores; and between low vitamin B-6 concentrations and low MMSE, attention span and executive function. Walker *et al.* (2012) reported that long-term daily supplementation of folic acid and vitamin B-12 promotes performance on immediate and delayed memory but not processing speed among community-dwelling older adults with elevated psychological distress.

Choline is the precursor to another neuro-transmitter acetylcholine. Neuronal choline concentrations can be altered by dietary choline intake, in the form of either free choline or phosphatidyl-choline (lecithin) (Cohen and Wurtman, *et al.*, 1976; Hirsch and Wurtman, 1978). Oral choline and phosphatidyl-choline have found some application in brain functions involving cholinergic neurons. Choline and lecithin have also been studied as potential memory enhancers, on the basis of the notion that acetylcholine neurons in the hippocampus play an important role in memory and that enhancing transmitter production might improve memory. Supplementing the maternal diet with additional choline (approximately 4.5 times the amount in normal rodent chow) dramatically improved the performance of the adult trisomic offspring in a Radial Arm Water Maze task and partially normalized adult hippocampal neurogenesis thus contributing functionally to their improved spatial cognition (Velazquez *et al.*, 2013).

Folic Acid and Brain Development

During the past decade, clinical observation has strongly linked folic acid to brain development. The incidence of neural tube defects (*e.g.* spina bifida) is notably higher in children of women who are folate deficient during pregnancy and can be reduced by folic acid supplementation during pregnancy; ideally, supplementation should begin before conception (Rosenberg, 1992). The clearest demonstration of this relation derives from a study by the Medical Research Council (MRC) Vitamin Study Research Group, which conducted a randomized, double-blind trial involving folate supplementation of women before conception (MRC, 1991). Folate deficiency, by impeding DNA, protein, or lipid synthesis, could conceivably influence neuronal and glial growth and proliferation during critical points in neural tube development, leading in some cases to induce neural tube defects. Hence, initiating supplementation before conception is important because the fundamental construction of the CNS occurs during the first trimester; a time when many women are unaware that they are pregnant.

Various biochemical actions of folate might be involved in the functioning of brain. 1. Maintaining adequate methionine pools for the synthesis of *S*-adenosylmethionine (Bottiglieri, 1994), 2. As a cofactor in methylation reactions in catecholamine synthesis and metabolism (Turner, 1977). 3. Maintenance of adequate amounts of tetrahydro-biopterin (Hamon *et al.*, 1986), and 4. A key cofactor in the synthesis of serotonin and the catecholamine neuro-transmitters (Turner, 1977). These neurotransmitters are important in maintaining normal affective state (mood). Folate supplementation (15 mg/d) for 6 months showed improvements in the depressed and schizophrenic patients treated with standard pharmacotherapy (Godfrey *et al.*, 1990). Intake of folic acid has been linked to other psychiatric conditions as well as to deficits in learning and memory, particularly in the elderly (Wahlin *et al.*, 1996; Riggs *et al.*, 1996; Joyal, 1993). Shooshtari *et al.* (2012) showed that folic acid may improve both short- and long-term memories, dose dependently, although it affects motor balance at lower dose. Coenzyme Q10 and folic acid have also been shown to possess therapeutic and preventive effects on cognitive impairments in Alzheimer's disease The mechanism of effects of folic acid on cognition and motor coordination is yet to be understood.

Iodine and Brain Development

Iodine deficiency results in a global loss of 10-15 intellectual quotient points at a population level, and constitutes the world's greatest single cause of preventable brain damage and mental retardation (Delange, 2000). Iodine is a key nutrient in the fetal development process, especially with respect to the brain. The associated disturbances due to maternal thyroxine deficiency range from increased neonatal morbidity and mortality and severe mental dysfunction, to hyperactivity, attention disorders and a substantial decrease of IQ of an irreversible nature in the progeny. Young children are particularly at risk because the brain still needs iodine for its development during the first two years of life. Iodine deficiency affects the thyroid function and the mental development, and is the main cause of brain damage in childhood. In addition, iodine deficiency in children is responsible for disorders in physical and cognitive development and hypothyroidism.

There is much anecdotal evidence coming from long-standing observations in Europe supported by recent reports from China and India, indicating that iodine-deficient village populations suffer from general lethargy, poor work performance and defective school performance in children. These effects are due to hypothyroidism, particularly cerebral hypothyroidism (Hetzel, 2000). Recently, Liu *et al.* (2013) reported that the spatial learning and memory ability of 40-day-old marginal iodine-deficient rats had a downward trend compared with the normal control group. Free thyroxine levels significantly decreased after pregnancy in rats with marginal iodine deficiency, affecting the expression of related proteins in the brain of offspring. As a consequence, iodine deficiency is the leading preventable cause of impaired mental function in the world, affecting as many as 2 billion people (35.2 per cent of the entire population) (Puig-Domingo and Vila, 2013). A child's performance at school is affected by Impaired cognitive and motor development. It is because of these adverse effects on brain development that the 58th World Health Assembly passed a resolution to urge a renewed effort from the international community, including WHO and UNICEF, to address iodine deficiency in the 54 countries most affected.

Iodine supplementation given to school-age children improved performance on tests of intellectual functioning. Randomized controlled trials showed that iodine supplementation in iodine-deficient mothers before pregnancy or during early pregnancy improved the motor and cognitive performance of their offspring (Pharoah and Connolly, 1987; Cao *et al.*, 1994; Connolly *et al.*, 1979). Zimmerman *et al.* (2006) reported that iodine repletion with 400 mg I (as oral iodized oil) to moderately iodine-deficient school children in rural south eastern Albania improved information processing, fine motor skills, and visual problem solving abilities. Gordon *et al.* (2009) also conducted a similar randomized placebo controlled double blind trial on mildly iodine-deficient children and demonstrated improved perceptual reasoning through 4 subtests from the Wechsler Intelligence Scale for Children by supplying 150μg for 28 weeks. Iodine supplementation improved perceptual reasoning in mildly iodine-deficient children. Selenium deficiency superimposed by iodine deficiency partly prevents the neurological damage (Delange, 2000). Iodine prophylaxis given before or during pregnancy has resulted in improved cognitive functioning in offspring in Ecuador.

Iron

Iron deficiency affects cognitive functions, specifically short-term memory, attention and visual motor coordination in anaemic children as compared to normal healthy children (Hamid *et al.*, 2010). Bandhu *et al.* (2011) demonstrated that the hematological status is associated with some effects on cognition.

Iron is a co-factor of tyrosine hydroxylase which is a critical enzyme in dopamine synthesis. Dopamine has been implicated in the patho-physiology of ADHD. Large-scale cross-sectional field study suggested that lower ferritin level might be associated with parent-reported hyperactivity after controlling for important confounding factors (Oner *et al.*, 2012). Those teens who don't get enough iron do poorly in school. Children and adults who are deficient, suffer from decreased attention spans. Treatment of the school children with iron sulfate for 12 months improved the scores and time required in a visual attention test. Also there was a favorable change in the scores obtained by one the subtests of the Wechsler Intelligence Scale for Children (WISC) Test (Vega Franco *et al.*, 1994).

Iron therapy resulted in significant improvements in Mental Development Index which was associated with improvement in attention span and cooperativeness among 15 months old young children (Walter *et al.*, 1983). Similarly, in pregnant women aged 14-24 years also iron supplementation significantly improved short-term memory and attention span (Groner *et al.*, 1986). In a recent longitudinal study, multiple micronutrient supplementation but not iron and folic acid supplementation alone to pregnant under-nourished or anemic women has been found to improve the motor and cognitive abilities of their children up to 3.5 years later, particularly both motor function and visual attention/spatial ability (Prado *et al.*, 2012).

Water

Adequate hydration is essential for human homeostasis and survival, including maintenance of brain function. Since the brain is 80 per cent water it is imperative that the brain is kept hydrated. Even a slight dehydration in the brain can raise the stress hormone in a person affecting clarity of thought. Just 2 per cent dehydration impairs performance in tasks that require attention, psychomotor, and immediate memory skills, as well as assessment of the subjective state (Adan, 2012).

Other Nutrients in Brain Function

Inositol may improve symptoms of depression and mood disorders. Inositol and choline also assist in neurotransmitter function. These nerve impulses help with memory capacity. Supplementation of 12 g/day of inositol resulted in positive therapeutic improvements similar to common anti-depressant drugs, but without untoward side effects (Levine *et al.*, 1995). Zinc is important for growth and maturation of the brain, and is especially related to behavior. Sandstead (2012) found that subclinical zinc deficiency changes brain function. Simultaneous treatment with a broad mixture of other micronutrients and/or an adequate omnivorous diet appeared to enhance the efficacy of zinc. Dietary supplementation after traumatic brain injury, but not zinc injection, significantly improved ($P < 0.05$) cognitive behavior as measured by the Morris water maze test (Cope *et al.*, 2012). Further, zinc-supplemented offspring showed reversal of neuronal morphologic changes in the learning and memory ability (Yu *et al.*, 2013). Phosphatidylcholine found in soy lecithin readily gets converted to acetylcholine. Oral co-intake with 1,2-dilynoleoyl-sn-glycero-3-phosphocholine (DLPhtCho) (50 mg) and 1-palmitoyl-2-oleoyl-sn-glycero-3-phosphocholine (POPhtCho) (45 mg) once after breakfast everyday raised the Mini Mental State Examination score to over 20, corresponding to normal cognitive functions, throughout 5 months after intake, and the increase in the score was significantly greater than that for oral intake with DLPhtCho (100 mg/day) alone or POPhtCho (90 mg/kg) alone (Nagata *et al.*, 2011).

Anti-oxidants in Brain Function

The free radical theory of ageing predicts that reactive oxygen species are involved in the decline in cognitive function associated with ageing. Bickford *et al.* (1999; 2000) reported that diets supplemented with nutritional sources of anti-oxidants, either spinach, strawberries or blueberries, reverse age-induced decline in beta-adrenergic receptor function in cerebellar Purkinje neurons. They have shown that age-related deficits in motor learning and memory can be reversed with anti-oxidant foods. Similar observations were made by Gemma *et al.* (2002) as they found spirulina, with high Oxygen Radical Absorbance Capacity (ORAC) to reverse and apple (a food with intermediate ORAC) to have an intermediate effect and cucumber (low ORAC) to have no effect on cerebellar beta-adrenergic receptor physiology, indicating that the reversal of impaired beta-adrenergic receptor function might be related to the ORAC dose.

Foods and Brain

Traditionally food is believed to influence the cognitive abilities. Various foods were attributed a role in brain function *e.g.* Ladies finger is given the title "Maths vegetable", Too much of sweet and/or Curds from buffalo milk consumption was considered to dull the brain and Vallarai (brahmi) was said to improve memory. Interestingly several of these beliefs were scientifically proved later. In addition, several foods that play a role in cognitive function of brain have also been researched extensively and documented.

Fish

The brain is made up of 60 per cent fat. Consuming foods rich in omega-3 fatty acids keeps cell membranes flexible and maximizes their ability to allow important nutrients get into the brain. Fatty fish and marine omega-3 consumption were associated with a reduced risk, while cholesterol and saturated fat with an increased risk of impaired cognitive function in the middle-aged population (Kalmijn *et al.*, 2004). According to Kesse-Guyot (2011) cognitive complaints, an early indicator of cognitive decline, are less frequent among the elderly who have a high long-chain n-3 fatty acid intake. A consistent finding across studies is that higher intake of fish is related to less cognitive decline (van Gelder *et al.*, 2007; Kalmijn *et al.*, 1997a; 1997b; Morris *et al.*, 2005) and incidence of dementia (Kalmijn *et al.*, 1997 a; Barberger-Gateau *et al.*, 2002; Morris *et al.*, 2003) in prospective studies, and associated with better cognitive performance in non-clinical samples (Kalmijn *et al.*, 2004; Morris *et al.*, 2005; Nurk *et al.*, 2007; Dangour *et al.*, 2009), in cross-sectional analyses. Oily fish (eg. mackerel, herring, trout), are the major dietary sources of EPA and DHA. Morris *et al.* (2003), Kalmijn *et al.* (2004); van Gelder *et al.* (2007) found significant positive relationship between cognitive outcomes and dietary intake levels of *n*-3 LC PUFAs.

Vinot *et al.* (2011) observed that ω3-supplemented animals exhibited not only lower anxiety level (significant reduction in spontaneous loco-motor activity by 31 per cent,($p<0.001$), compared to control animals, but also better performances in a reference spatial memory task (80 per cent of successful trials vs. 35 per cent in controls, $p<0.05$). Thus they showed that the long-term dietary ω3 PUFA supplementation positively impacts the anxiety and cognitive performances in adult mouse lemur. Hence, supplementation of human food with ω3 fatty acids may represent a valuable dietary strategy to improve behavioral and cognitive functions. *Yellow fin Tuna, a* cold-water fish, is a rich source of omega-3 fatty acids as well as the B vitamin niacin, which protects the brain against Alzheimer's disease.

Supplementation with 1 or 2 g of fish oil brought out significant increase in oxy-hemoglobin and hemoglobin indicating increased cerebral blood flow during the cognitive tasks as compared to placebo (Jackson *et al.*, 2012). According to Denny

Joseph and Muralidhara (2012) the prophylactic protection offered by fish oil may be due to its ability to enhance GSH levels, anti-oxidant potential that offset protein oxidation and specific modulatory effects on brain mitochondria.

Fruits and Vegetables

Recent studies suggest that consumption of diets rich in anti-oxidants and anti-inflammatory components such as those found in fruits, nuts, vegetables, spices, or even reduced caloric intake, may lower age-related cognitive declines, risk of dementia (Loef and Walach, 2012) and the risk of developing neuro-degenerative disease (Joseph *et al.*, 2009; Letenneur *et al.*, 2007). Blueberries, strawberries, prunes, kiwi, dark leafy greens like spinach and many others provide benefits as per ADA and foods rich in vitamin E such as dark green vegetables, nuts, olive oil, and other foods prevent brain cell damage and also lower the risk of Alzheimer's disease. According to Ye *et al.* (2012) variety, more than total quantity of fruit and vegetable intake may offer cognitive protection in middle-aged and older adults.

Many studies have been conducted on anti-oxidants for their effectiveness in reducing the deleterious effects of brain ageing and behavior. Phytochemicals found in fruits and vegetables (Youdim and Joseph, 2001), anti-oxidant vitamins such as vitamins A, C, E; bioflavonoids such as flavones, tannins, and anthocyanins (Cantuti-Castelvetri *et al.*, 2000) and essential fatty acids (Youdim *et al.*, 2000) have been implicated in preventing the onset of age-related deficits in cognitive behavior and Morris water maze performance (Joseph *et al.*, 1998).

Phytochemicals such as flavanoids and anthocyanins can cross the blood brain barrier and protect brain from degenerative damage (Casadesus *et al.*, 2004; Kalt *et al.*, 2008). The anti-oxidant rich fruits and vegetables are strawberries, cranberries, spinach, raspberries, brussel sprouts, plums, broccoli, oranges, red grapes, red bell pepper, cherries and kiwis. Several studies proved that dietary supplementation with fruit or vegetable extracts high in anti-oxidants (eg, blueberry or spinach extracts) might decrease the vulnerability to oxidative stress that occurs in ageing thus improving motor and cognitive behavior and prevent age related neuro-degenerative diseases (Josheph *et al.*, 1999; 2004; 2005; 1998; Youdim *et al.*, 2000; Casadesus *et al.*, 2004; Shukitt-Hale *et al.*, 2008; Lau *et al.*, 2007). They also found that in addition to anti-oxidant and anti-inflammatory activities, their ability to increase cellular signaling and neuronal communication might be involved in the beneficial effects of these extracts.

Berries on Brain Function

The polyphenolic compounds contained in berries have been shown to cross the blood brain barrier and localize in various brain regions important for learning and memory. Talavéra *et al.* (2005) confirmed this in their research that showed increased total anthocyanin content in the brain on anthocyanin enriched diet (blackberry anthocyanins and peonidin 3-*O*-glucoside).

Plant polyphenols appear to have direct actions on signaling pathways involved in stress protection in neurons. This view further supports the potential for effective nutritional interventions to attenuate brain ageing, neuro-degeneration, and functional declines (Joseph *et al.*, 2009). Blueberry (*Vaccinium ashei*) and blackberry (*Rubus fruticosus/Rubus ulmifolius*) contain anti-oxidant anthocyanins and thus are especially good for the brain. Blueberries have the highest anti-oxidant capacities among fruits and vegetables (Elks *et al.*, 2011; Krikorian *et al.*, 2010). Blueberries also reverse age-related declines in neuronal signal transduction as well as cognitive and motor deficits (Malin *et al.*, 2011).

Supplementation with the blueberry extract concentrated in polyphenols to adult mice showed significant cognitive enhancement. The higher anti-oxidant potential inhibits AChE activity (Papandreou *et al.*, 2009) and increases hippocampal plasticity Lau *et al.* (2005 and 2007) and Casadesus *et al.* (2004). Higher intake of flavonoids, particularly from berries, appears to reduce rates of cognitive decline in older adults (Devore *et al.*, 2012).

The measurement of anthocyanins and flavanols in the brain following blueberry supplementation may indicate that changes in spatial working memory in aged animals are linked to the effects of flavonoids on the extracellular signal-related kinase - cAMP-response element-binding protein - brain-derived neurotrophic factor pathway (Williams *et al.*, 2008; Joseph *et al.*, 2009; Rendeiro *et al.*, 2012; 2013). The beneficial effects of blueberry extract, according to Brewer *et al.* (2010), may involve transient stress signaling and oxyradical production protection that may translate into improved cognition (Andres-Lacueva *et al.*, 2005), reversed cognitive declines in object recognition (Goyarzu *et al.*, 2004) and reduced number of neuro-degenerative processes in the brain of aged animals (Galli *et al.*, 2006).

A non-significant trend was noted by Crews *et al.* (2005) on a subjective, self-report questionnaire where twice as many participants in the cranberry group rated their overall abilities to remember by treatment end as "improved" compared to placebo controls. Blueberry, cranberry, strawberry, and blackberry significantly attenuated age-related motor and cognitive deficits and reversed neuronal and behavioral (cognitive) function in aged rats (Joseph *et al.*, 1999; Shukitt-Hale *et al.*, 2005; 2006a; 2006b; 2009).

Vepsäläinen *et al.* (2013) found that anthocyanin-rich bilberry and blackcurrant diets also favorably modulated the processing of amyloid precursor protein and alleviated behavioral abnormalities in a mouse model of Alzheimer's disease.

Ramirez *et al.* (2005) showed that lyophilised berries (blueberry, bilberry) significantly enhanced short-term memory, but not long-term memory in the inhibitory avoidance task, and induced an increase in the number of crossings in the first exposure to the open field. However, treated rats did not present any improvement of memory retention in open field habituation. In contrast, Barros *et al.* (2006) showed that the administration of a lyophilized extract of blue berries significantly enhanced long-term memory in the inhibitory avoidance task, induced an increase in the number of crossings during open-field habituation and had an anxiolytic effect in the elevated plus-maze task. Moreover, the extract reduced oxidative DNA damage in brain tissue *in vitro* suggesting that supplementation with *Vaccinium ashei* berries to mice improves performance on memory tasks and has a protective effect on DNA damage, possibly due to the anti-oxidant activity of polyphenols, including anthocyanins.

However, Joseph *et al.* (1999) opined that anti-oxidant activity alone cannot predict the potency of these compounds against certain disorders affected by ageing suggesting that berry fruit polyphenols may possess a multiplicity of actions aside from anti-oxidant activity. Other possible mechanisms for the berry fruit's positive effects include: direct effects on signaling to enhance neuronal communication (Joseph *et al.*, 2003), the ability to buffer against excess calcium (Joseph *et al.*, 2004), enhancement of neuro-protective stress shock proteins (Galli *et al.*, 2006), and reduction of stress signals such as nuclear factor κ B (NF-κB) (Goyarzu *et al.*, 2004).

Grape Seeds (*Vitis vinifera*)

Sreemantulu *et al.* (2005) provided scientific support for the anti-stress (adaptogenic), anti-oxidant and nootropic activities of grape seed extract and substantiated the traditional claims for the usage of grapes and grape seeds in stress induced disorders. Intake of pro-anthocyanidin from grape seed extract in moderately low quantity was found to be effective in up-regulating the anti-oxidant defense mechanism by attenuating lipid peroxidation and protein oxidation. Changes in the cholinergic system, however, indicated an increase in the acetyl choline concentration with a moderate reduction in acetylcholine esterase activity, suggesting that pro-anthocyanidin has a potent role in enhancing cognition in older rats. Balu *et al.* (2005; 2006) revealed that grape seed extract has inhibiting effect on the accumulation of age-related oxidative DNA damages in spinal cord and in various brain regions such as cerebral cortex, striatum and hippocampus. Liu *et al.* (2011) and Wang *et al.* (2008) observed Grape seed polyphenolic extract to inhibit Aβ oligomerization *in vitro* and attenuate cognitive impairment and AD-related neuropathology in the brains of transgenic mice. Ashadevi *et al.* (2011) demonstrated it to be a neuroprotectant in the hippocampus and a preventive agent in cognitive loss with ageing.

Amla (*Emblica officinalis*)

Amla churna, an Ayurvedic preparation, (50, 100, and 200 mg/kg, p.o.) produced a dose-dependent improvement in memory scores of young and aged rats. Furthermore, it reversed the amnesia induced by scopolamine (0.4 mg/kg, i.p.) and diazepam (1 mg/kg, i.p.) (Vasudevan and Parle, 2007a). The churna may prove to be a useful remedy for the management of Alzheimer's disease on account of its multifarious beneficial effects such as, memory improving property, cholesterol lowering property and anti-cholinesterase activity (Vasudevan and Parle, 2007b) and thus may be useful for the treament of cognitive impairments induced by cholinergic dysfunction (Golechha *et al.*, 2012).

Litchi (*Litchi chinensis*)

Oligomerised litchi fruit-derived polyphenol (OLFP, also called Oligonol has been reported to attenuate early cognitive impairment in male senescence-accelerated mice, and diminish stress of the endoplasmic reticulum in neuronal cells (Sakurai *et al.*, 2013).

Mulberry (*Morus nigra*)

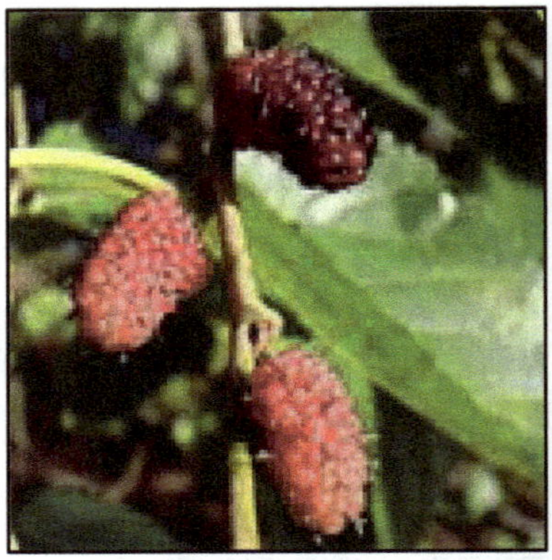

Mulberry

The berries being a rich source of Zeaxanthin, Lutein, Resveratrol - another polyphenol flavonoid, along with Iron, ß carotene, Vitamin K and B complex vitamins are potential natural cognitive enhancers and neuroprotectants. It was found that anthocyanin in mulberry fruit, could protect against cerebral ischemia (Shin *et al.*, 2006). Kaewkaen *et al.* (2012) observed that mulberry fruit extract enhanced memory and the effect might be partly associated with the increased cholinergic function and its neuroprotective effect, and partly via the decreased oxidative stress in hippocampus.

Olives

De Nicoló *et al.* (2013) showed that olive polyphenols may increase the levels of nerve growth factor and brain-derived neurotrophic factor in crucial areas of the limbic system and olfactory bulbs. These factors play a key role in learning and memory processes, and in the proliferation and migration of endogenous progenitor cells present in the rodent brain.

Walnut (*Juglans regia*)

Walnuts contain a number of potentially neuro-protective compounds like vitamin E, folate, melatonin, several anti-oxidative polyphenols. Walnuts are well known for their high levels of PUFAs, specifically the ω-6 fatty acid linoleic acid (LA) and the ω-3 fatty acid α-linolenic acid (ALA). LA and ALA can either exist as membrane components or can be metabolized via the arachidonic acid cascade to generate numerous lipid messengers including prostaglandins, eicosapentaenoic acid (EPA), and docosahaenoic acid (DHA). High-anti-oxidant foods such as berries, concord grapes, and walnuts may increase "health span" and enhance cognitive and motor function in ageing (Joseph *et al.*, 2009). Though no significant increases were detected for mood, non-verbal reasoning or memory on the walnut-supplemented diet in young healthy normal adults, inferential verbal reasoning increased significantly by 11 2 per cent (Pribis *et al.*, 2011).

A significant improvement in learning and memory of walnut treated rats compared to controls was observed. Analysis of brain monoamines exhibited enhanced serotonergic levels in rat brain fed walnuts suggesting that walnut may exert its hypophagic and nootropic actions via an enhancement of brain 5-HT metabolism (Haider *et al.*, 2011). Recently, Poulose *et al.* (2013) demonstrated the effectiveness of a walnut-supplemented diet in activating the autophagy function in brain beyond its traditionally known anti-oxidant and anti-inflammatory benefits. Willis *et al.* (2009) reported that the 2 per cent walnut diet improved performance on rod walking, while the 6 per cent walnut diet improved performance on the medium plank walk; the higher dose of the 9 per cent walnut diet did not improve psychomotor performance and on the large plank actually impaired performance. All of the walnut diets improved working memory in the Morris water maze and showed that moderate dietary walnut supplementation can improve cognitive and motor performance in aged rats.

Walnut extract induced a decrease in tumor necrosis-alpha production, internalization of the lipo-polysaccharide receptor and toll-like receptor 4. The anti-inflammatory effects of walnut were dependent on functional activation of phospholipase D2. Thus Willis *et al.* (2010) were the first ones to describe the anti-inflammatory effects of walnuts in microglia, which could lead to nutritional interventions in the prevention and treatment of neuro-degeneration. Shabani *et al.* (2012) observed walnut consumption to improve memory and motor abilities in cisplatin treated rats. Cisplatin increased latency of response to nociception, and walnut reversed this effect of cisplatin.

Mango (*Mangifera indica*)

Chronic treatment (7 days) of the ethanolic extract of *Mangifera indica* fruit and vitamin C significantly ($p < 0.05$) reversed the ageing and scopolamine induced memory deficits as judged by the step down passive avoidance task and elevated plus-maze task in mice (Kumar *et al.*, 2009).

Soya (*Glycine max*)

Kritz-Silverstein *et al.* (2003) reported that soya isoflavone supplementation has a favorable effect on cognitive function, particularly verbal memory, in postmenopausal women. Thorp *et al.* (2009) found soya isoflavone supplementation in healthy males enhanced cognitive processes which appear to be dependent on oestrogen activation. Although data from humans, cultures, and animal models show soy isoflavones to have a positive effect on brain function, Lee *et al.* (2005) who found it to be difficult to elucidate the mechanism of action on cognitive function and the nervous system, suggested two putative pathways: (1) an estrogen receptor-mediated pathway and (2) inhibition of tyrosine kinase, in particular by genistein. Soya derived phosphatidylserine has been shown to have beneficial effects on cognitive functions. Phosphatidylserine containing omega-3 fatty acids significantly improved immediate verbal recall in the treatment group compared to the placebo group and cognitive performance in non-demented elderly with memory complaints (Vakhapova *et al.*, 2010).

The investigation by Ding *et al.* (2011, 2013a) showed that soya isoflavone reduced the cytokine cascade and inflammatory response induced by Aβ1-42 which could result in the improvement of spatial learning and memory in the rats. Its mechanism might be associated with the protection of synaptic plasticity by improving the synaptic structure and regulating the synaptic related proteins. Soya isoflavone could alleviate the oxidative damage and maintain the redox imbalance in brain mitochondria damaged by Aβ1-42. This might result from regulation of the Nrf2/HO-1 pathway (Ding *et al.*, 2013b).

Saffron (*Crocus sativus*)

Saffron's active constituent is crocin (crocetin di-gentiobiose ester). Ghadrdoost *et al.* (2011) found crocin significantly decreased plasma levels of corticosterone, as measured after the end of stress. Their observations indicate that saffron and its active constituent crocin can prevent the impairment of learning and memory as well as the oxidative stress damage to the hippocampus induced by chronic stress thus, proving that saffron may be useful in pharmacological alleviation of cognitive deficits. Abe and Saito (2000) found saffron extract to improve ethanol-induced impairments of learning behaviors, prevent hippocampal long-term potentiation, and a form of activity-dependent synaptic plasticity that may underly learning and memory. This effect of saffron extract is attributed to crocin but not crocetin. Crocin and daunorubicin inhibits neuronal cell death induced by both internal and external apoptotic stimuli (Soeda *et al.*, 2001).

Turmeric (C*urcuma longa*)

Recent evidence suggests that curcumin, an active principle of turmeric, has potential for neuro-protective efficacy as it activates a key enzyme that protects the brain against oxidation which is thought to be a major factor responsible for neuro-degenerative disorders in ageing like Alzheimer's disease (Li and Wang, 2009). Curcumin protects retinal neurons and micro-vessels against I/R injury. The beneficial effects of curcumin on neurovascular degeneration may occur through its inhibitory effects on injury-induced activation of NF-κB and STAT3, and on over-expression of MCP-1. Curcumin may therefore serve as a promising candidate for retinal ischemic diseases (Wang *et al.*, 2011).

Curcumin possesses multiple desirable characteristics required for a neuro-protective drug such as anti-inflammatory, anti-oxidant, and anti-protein-aggregate activities (Cole *et al.*, 2003; Ringman *et al.*, 2005). Rathore *et al.* (2008) reported that pre-treatment with curcuma oil, isolated from powdered rhizomes of *C. longa*, and significantly reduced the levels of mitochondrial membrane potential, reactive oxygen species, peroxy-nitrite levels, caspase-3 activities leading to delayed neuronal death. Further; there is attenuation of delayed neuronal death via a caspase-dependent pathway. This illustrates the neuroprotective activity of the oil against cerebral ischemia.

Evidence for an impact on ageing brain has been recently produced in rats, where chronic curcumin treatment was shown to result in reduced lipid peroxidation, accumulation of the pigment lipofuscin and to increase the anti-oxidant defense enzymes glutathione peroxidase and superoxide dismutase as well as sodium potassium ATPase, which normally decline (Bala *et al.*, 2006). Curcumin dose dependently improved cerebral blood flow in streptozotocin treated mice together with amelioration of memory impairment both in preventive and therapeutic manner (Awashti *et al.*, 2010). Curcumin has at least 10 known neuroprotective actions and many of these might be realized *in vivo*. Indeed, accumulating cell culture and animal model data show that dietary curcumin is a strong candidate for use in the prevention or treatment of major disabling age-related neuro-degenerative diseases like

Alzheimer's, Parkinson's, and stroke. Promising results have already led to ongoing pilot clinical trials (Cole *et al.*, 2007).

Cumin Seeds (*Cuminum cyminum*)

Koppula and Choi, (2011) found the cognition, as determined by the acquisition, retention, and recovery in rats, to be dose-dependent and provided scientific support for the anti-stress, anti-oxidant, and memory-enhancing activities of cumin extract. They also substantiated that the traditional use of cumin seeds as a culinary spice in foods is beneficial.

Black Cumin Seeds (*Nigella sativa*)

Experimental evidences have demonstrated that *Nigella sativa* seed (NS) has positive modulation effects on aged rats with memory impairments. These seeds prevent hippocampal pyramidal cell loss and enhance consolidation of recall capability of stored information and spatial memory in rats. Bin Sayeed *et al.* (2013) demonstrated the role of NS in enhancing memory, attention and cognition. Therefore, further investigations are needed on black cumin seed as a potential food supplement for preventing or delaying the progress of Alzheimer disease.

Onion (*Allium cepa*)

Shri and Singh (2008) demonstrated that the pretreatment with methanolic extract of outer scales (100 mg/kg and 200 mg/kg) and edible portions (100 mg/kg and 200 mg/kg) of onion bulb markedly reduced cerebral infarct size and attenuated impairment in short-term memory and motor coordination along with a marked decrease in mitochondrial TBARS. Hwang *et al.* (2009) also proved the neuro-protective effects of onion extract and its major component, quercetin, on ischemic damage in the gerbil hippocampus - related to memory function. On the basis of this observation, the authors suggest that repeated administration of onion extract and quercetin can protect against neuronal damage from transient cerebral ischemia.

Nishimura *et al.* (2006) demonstrated that 2-n-propyl trisulfide present in onion ameliorated memory impairment in SAMP8 mouse by its anti-oxidant effect.

Garlic (*Allium sativum*)

Aged garlic extract (AGE) supplementation to senescence-accelerated-prone mouse 8 (SAMP8) from 2 months of age markedly improved the learning deficits of SAMP8 in the Morris water maze test and prevented the decrease in survival ratio (Moriguchi *et al.*, 1994; 1996; 1997). Chronic ingestion of AGE prevented this shrinkage in the frontal cerebrum and kept the brain size at the control level indicating that AGE has an anti-ageing effect on the senescence-accelerated Mouse (Nishiyama *et al.*, 1997). S-allylcysteine, a major thioallyl compound present in aged garlic extract was found to be responsible for significant attenuation of the memory deficit and age-related changes of senescence-accelerated mice (Nishiyama *et al.*, 2001). Feeding of aged garlic extract prevented deterioration of hippocampal based memory tasks in mice, suggesting that aged garlic extract has a potential for preventing progression of Alzheimer's disease (Chauhan and Sandoval, 2007; Borek, 2006).

Haider *et al.* (2008) observed a significant improvement in memory function in garlic-treated rats in the passive avoidance test. Moreover, increased brain 5-hydroxytryptamine levels were associated with improved cognitive performance.

Ginger (*Zingiber officinale*)

According to Arabian folklore, ginger has been claimed to improve memory and has also been traditionally used as an ingredient for cognitive enhancement. Cognitive function and neurons density in hippocampus of rats receiving ginger rhizome extract were improved while the brain infarct volume was decreased. The cognitive enhancing effect and neuro-protective effect occurred partly via the anti-oxidant activity of the extract (Wattanathorn *et al.*, 2011). Ginger extract at doses of 400 and 800mg once daily for 2 months tested on working memory and cognitive function using computerized battery tests and the auditory oddball paradigm of event-related potentials at three different time periods of middle-aged healthy women significantly decreased P300 latencies, increased N100 and P300 amplitudes, and exhibited enhanced working memory (Saenghong *et al.*, 2012).

Curry Leaves (*Murraya koenigii*)

Dementia is a syndrome of gradual onset and continuous decline of higher cognitive functioning. It is a common disorder in older persons and has become more prevalent today. Significant improvement in memory scores of young and aged mice fed curry leaves (20 and 30 mg/kg, p.o.) was demonstrated by Vasudevan and Parle (2009) and Mani *et al.* (2012). The alkaloidal extract of curry leaves improved the level of protective antioxidants such as glutathione peroxidase, reduced glutathione, glutathione reductase, superoxide dismutase and catalase in brain homogenate at higher doses (20 and 40mg/kg, p.o.). Moreover, a dose dependent decline was noted in lipid peroxidation and the nitric oxide assay at all doses (10, 20 and 40mg/kg, p.o.). Interestingly, significant progress was noted with the supplementation of curry leaves by an improvement of the acetylcholine levels and a reduction in the acetylcholinesterase activity in aged mouse brain. In addition, a significant elevation of serum albumin, alkaline phosphatase, alanine transaminase, aspartate transaminase and total protein as well as a decline in creatinine, total cholesterol, urea nitrogen and glucose levels with curry leaves also ameliorated the hepatic and renal functions in normal ageing process. Thus Mani *et al.* (2012; 2013) showed the possible utility of Murraya koenigii leaves in neuro-protection against neurodegenerative disorders such as Alzheimer's disease.

Noni (*Morinda citrifolia*)

Noni is widely used for different illnesses including disorders of central nervous system. Recently, Noni has been reported to prevent amyloid beta induced memory impairment in mice. Ethanolic extract of Noni fruits and its chloroform and ethyl acetate fractions significantly improved memory and cerebral blood flow. However, butanol fraction had no effect. Further, increased oxidative stress and AChE activity following scopolamine was significantly attenuated in a dose dependent inhibition *in vitro* by ethanolic extract of Noni and its fractions (Pachauri *et al.*, 2012).

Wolf Berries (*Lycium barbarum*)

It has been shown that pre-treatment using extracts of *Lycium barbarum* containing mostly polysaccharides (LBP) could protect the cultured primary cortical neurons from β-amyloid peptide neurotoxicity (Yu *et al.*, 2005). Yang *et al.* (2012) showed a seven-day oral pre-treatment with LBP, to effectively improve neurological deficits, decrease infarct size and cerebral edema as well as protect the brain from blood brain barrier disruption, aquaporin-4 up-regulation, and glial activation. LBP may be used as a prophylactic neuroprotectant in patients at high risk for ischemic stroke. Ho *et al.* (2010) also demonstrated that LBP exerted neuro-protective effects on cortical neurons exposed to plasma homocystine and thus has the potential to be a disease modifying agent for the prevention of AD.

Brahmi (*Bacopa monnieri*)

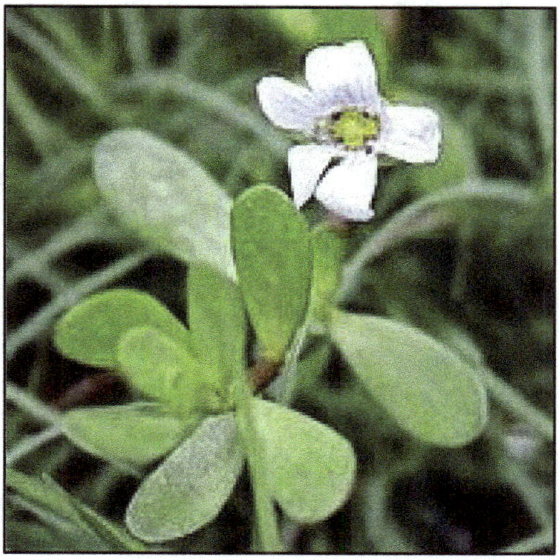

Bacopa monnieri

An Australian survey showed brahmi to be one of the most popular aids for memory among 60–64-year-old consumers (Jorm *et al.*, 2004). Laboratory studies on rats indicate that extracts of the plant improve memory capacity (Morgan and Stevens, 2010). Some studies in mice suggest that ingestion of *Bacopa* for a 12 week period can significantly improve cognitive ability by accelerating the rate of learning and enhancing memory (Prakash and Sirsi, 1962; Singh and Dhawan, 1997; Stough *et al.*, 2001; 2008; Roodenrys *et al.*, 2002). Memory-enhancing effects of brahmi have been attributed to saponins (bacosides, bacopasides, or bacopasaponins). Bacopasaponin constituents have been shown to facilitate mental retention in avoidance response in rats (Singh *et al.*, 1988).

Bacopasaponin have also been shown to reverse amnesic effects of neurotoxin, scopolamine, phenytoin, electroshock, and immobilization stress (Bhattacharya *et al.*, 2001; Kishore and Singh, 2005; Vohora *et al.*, 2000) and diazepam-induced amnesia in the Morris water maze test (Saraf *et al.*, 2008).

In some trials, though the extract did not restore or enhance memory formation, it did improve retention (Roodenrys *et al.*, 2002; Nathan *et al.*, 2004). Aged human subjects treated with standardized brahmi extract of 300 mg/day orally for 12 weeks confirmed it as a potential and safe cognitive performance enhancer (Calabrese *et al.*, 2008). In 98 healthy older people over 55 years of age *Bacopa* significantly improved memory acquisition and retention (Morgan and Stevens, 2010). A recent systematic review found some evidence to suggest that *Bacopa* improves memory free recall, but there was a lack of evidence for enhancement of other cognitive abilities (Pase *et al.*, 2012).

Treatment with brahmi reduced beta-amyloid levels in the brain of an Alzheimer's disease doubly transgenic mouse model of rapid amyloid deposition (PSAPP mice) suggesting brahmi to be therapeutically useful for the treatment of cognitive impairment, thus supporting its possible anti-Alzheimer's properties (Dhanasekaran *et al.*, 2007; Holcomb *et al.*, 2006).

Apart from these, co-administration of *Bacopa* extract during aluminium treatment significantly prevented the aluminium-induced decrease in SOD activity as well as the increased oxidative damage to lipids and proteins. Protective effect was also observed at microscopic level. These observations showed that Bacopa's neuro-protective effects were comparable to those of l-deprenyl at both biochemical and microscopic levels (Jyoti and Sharma, 2006). Several observations have strongly implicated that *Bacopa monniera* has potential to protect brain from oxidative damage resulting from aluminium toxicity (Jyoti *et al.*, 2007) and MeHg-induced neurotoxicity (Sumathi *et al.*, 2012) in rat.

Mandukaparni (*Centella asiatica*)

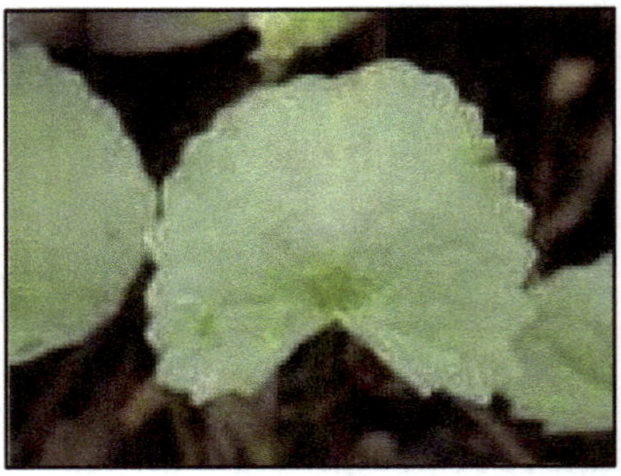

Mandukaparni

Centella asiatica (CA) is a common medicinal plant used in the ayurvedic system of medicine to treat various ailments and as a memory enhancer. Ashwagandha, Brahmi, Vacha, and Shank Pushpi at the right proportions are found to work in combination to prevent mental restlessness and agitation.

The *Medhya rasayana* are a group of medicines in Ayurveda known to act on the nervous system have been claimed to improve mental ability (Sharma, 1992). These drugs contain mainly extracts from plants such as *Centella asiatica*, *Acorus calamus*, jatamansi and *Bacopa monnieri.* Brahmi is a great herb for the brain. But without Ashwagandha, Brahmi has a different effect and is not as helpful.

CA grows in wet places throughout India. It is used in Ayurvedic preparations either as whole plants or as leaves in the fresh or extract form (Sharma, 1992). It is also used as a tonic for promoing brain growth and improving memory (Anbuganapathi, 1995). In addition, the plant is used in children with learning difficulties to improve general mental ability and in people suffering from cognitive disorders (Sivarajan, 1994; Rajagopalan, 1995; Shah, 1992; Appa Rao *et al.*, 1973.; Joshi and Parle, 2006). Fresh leaf juice (extract) of CA has been claimed to improve learning and memory in different clinical studies (Sivarajan, 1994; Dash *et al.*, 1996; Rajagopalan, 1995; Shah, 1992; Appa Rao *et al.*, 1973; Satyavati *et al.*,1976). Administration of fresh leaf extracts of CA during the growth spurt (neonatal) period facilitates dendritic growth in the hippocampal CA3 neurons. Increased dendritic arborization may be the neuronal basis (Rao, 2006), for the improved learning and memory reported earlier (Rao *et al.*, 2005). Brahmi rasayana (BR) significantly improved learning and memory in young mice and reversed the amnesia induced by both scopolamine (0.4 mg kg(-1) i.p.) and natural ageing. BR significantly decreased whole brain acetyl cholinesterase activity.

BR might prove to be a useful memory restorative agent in the treatment of dementia seen in elderly (Joshi and Parle, 2006).

Shinomol and Muralidhara (2008a) observed that CA has the propensity to modulate both endogenous and neuro-toxicant induced oxidative impairments in the brain and may be effectively employed as a neuroprotective adjuvant to abrogate oxidative stress *in vivo*. and (Shinomol and Muralidhara, 2008b; 2010) opined that it may be wholly or in part related to the enhancement of glutathione, thiols and antioxidant machinery in the brain regions of prepubertal mice. Dhanasekaran *et al.* (2009) reported that CA can impact the amyloid cascade altering amyloid beta pathology in the brains of PSAPP mice and modulating components of the oxidative stress response that has been implicated in the neuro-degenerative changes in Alzheimer's disease.

Okra (*Abelmoschus esculentus*)

Quercetin, rutin and okra extract treatments reversed cognitive deficits, including impaired dentate gyrus cell proliferation, and protected against morphological changes in the CA3 region in dexamethasone-treated mice (Tongjaroenbuangam *et al.*, 2011).

Buck Wheat (*Fagopyrum esculentum*)

Pu *et al.* (2004) observed that Buckwheat polyphenol (BWP) ameliorate spatial memory impairment by inhibiting glutamate release and the delayed generation of NO(x)(-) in rats subjected to repeated cerebral ischemia.

Kokum (*Garcinia indica*)

Garcinol, a naturally occurring Histone acetyl-transferase inhibitor derived from the rind of Kokum fruit (Balasubramanyam *et al.*, 2004) regulates chromatin function and hence useful in the treatment of newly acquired or recently reactivated traumatic memories (Maddox *et al.*, 2013).

Coffee

The larger improvement of performance in fatigued subjects confirms that caffeine is a mild stimulant. Caffeine has also been reported to prevent cognitive decline in healthy subjects but the results of the studies are heterogeneous, some finding no age-related effect while others reported effects only in one sex and mainly in the oldest population. In conclusion, it appears that caffeine cannot be considered a;pure' cognitive enhancer. Its indirect action on arousal, mood and concentration contributes in large part to its cognitive enhancing properties (Nehlig, 2010). The cognitive and mood effects of caffeine are well documented. Caffeine, in a dose-dependent manner, mitigated many adverse effects of exposure to multiple stressors. Caffeine (200 and 300 mg) significantly improved visual vigilance, choice reaction time, repeated acquisition, self-reported fatigue and sleepiness with the greatest effects on tests of vigilance, reaction time, and alertness. Even in the most adverse circumstances, moderate doses of caffeine can improve cognitive function, including vigilance, learning, memory, and mood state (Lieberman *et al.*, 2002; Brice and Smith, 2002).

Besides improving cognitive function, chronic coffee consumption modulated the endogenous anti-oxidant system in the brain. Therefore, chronic coffee ingestion, through the protection of the anti-oxidant system, may play an important role in preventing age-associated decline in the cognitive function (Abreu *et al.*, 2011). Caffeine intake was found to be related to moderately better cognitive maintenance over 5 years in older women with vascular disorders (Vercambre *et al.*, 2013).

Aged rats supplemented with a 0.55 per cent coffee diet, equivalent to ten cups of coffee, performed better in psychomotor testing (rotarod) and in a working memory task (Morris water maze) compared to aged rats fed a control diet. A diet with 0.55 per cent coffee appeared to be optimal. The 0.165 per cent coffee-supplemented group (three cups) showed some improvement in reference memory performance in the Morris water maze. In a subsequent study, the effects of caffeine alone did not account for the performance improvements, showing that the neuroprotective benefits of coffee are not due to caffeine alone, but rather to other bioactive compounds in coffee (Shukitt-Hale *et al.*, 2013). The findings of Jang *et al.* (2013) also suggested that caffeine-free decaffeinated coffee may prevent memory impairment in human through the inhibition of NF-κB activation and subsequent TNF-α production.

Smith (2013) observed that caffeine interacted with extraversion in the predicted direction for serial recall and running memory tasks. Caffeine improved simple reaction time and the speed of encoding of new information, effects which were not modified by extraversion thus implying possible biological mechanisms underlying effects of caffeine on cognitive performance.

Wheat Germ

Wheat germ is a powerful brain food because it is rich in vitamin E and selenium (both very potent anti-oxidant nutrients), as well as choline and magnesium.

The development of biotech drugs such as peptides and proteins that act in the central nervous system has been significantly impeded by the difficulty of delivering them across the blood-brain barrier. Improvements in spatial memory in ethylcholine aziridium-treated rats were observed following intranasal administration of 25 microg/kg and 12.5 microg/kg of vasoactive intestinal peptide loaded by unmodified nano-particles and wheat germ-agglutinin-modified nano-particles, respectively. Distribution profiles of wheat germ agglutinin-conjugated nanoparticles in the nasal cavity presented their higher affinity to the olfactory mucosa than to the respiratory mucosa. Inhibition experiment with specific sugars suggested that the interaction between the nasal mucosa and the wheat germ agglutinin-functionalized nanoparticles were due to the immobilization of carbohydrate-binding pockets on the surface of the nano-particles. The results clearly indicated wheat germ agglutinin-modified nano-particles might serve as promising carriers especially for biotech drugs such as peptides and proteins (Gao *et al.*, 2007).

Conclusions

Most of the studies have concentrated on age-related cognition and memory. Berries, Garlic, Ginger, Turmeric, Soya etc., appear to be memory boosters as well as anti-ageing foods. It is interesting to note that Mulberry fruit improves cognition. But further research is needed to elucidate the possible active ingredient. Studies on Ladies finger, Kokum, Noni, Cumin seeds, Walnuts, *Mangifera indica* etc. are very scanty but seem to be worth researching upon. Mental fatigue and stress being the root cause of lack of memory in many cases, anti-stress foods or relaxants such as coffee and tea seem to be good choice. But, the upper limits may be worked out to avoid untoward effects of overdose. Thus, Foods for Nerves need further exploration.

References

Abe K, Saito H (2000). Effects of saffron extract and its constituent crocin on learning behaviour and long-term potentiation. Phytother. Res. 14 (3): 149 - 52.

Abreu RV, Silva-Oliveira EM, Moraes MF, Pereira GS, Moraes-Santos T (2011). Chronic coffee and caffeine ingestion effects on the cognitive function and anti-oxidant system of rat brains. Pharmacol. Biochem. Behav. 99 (4): 659 - 64.

Adan A (2012). Cognitive performance and dehydration. J. Am. Coll. Nutr. 31 (2): 71 - 78.

Anbuganapathi, GA (1995). Synergetic effect of vallarai and brahmi on learning ability of albino mice and school children. Paper presented at the International Seminar on Recent Trends in Pharmaceutical Sciences; Ootacamund. February. pp. 18 - 20.

Andres-Lacueva C, Shukitt-Hale B, Galli RL, Jauregui O, Lamuela-Raventos RM, Joseph JA (2005). Anthocyanins in aged blueberry-fed rats are found centrally and may enhance memory. Nutr. Neurosci. 8: 111 - 20.

Appa Rao MVR, Srinivasan K, Rao KT (1973). The effect of mandookaparni (*Centella asiatica*) on the general mental ability (medhya) of mentally retarded children. *J. Res. Indian Med.* **8**: 9 - 16.

Ashadevi S, Sagar Chandrasekar BK, Manjula KR, Ishii N (2011). Grape seed proanthocyanidin lowers brain oxidative stress in adult and middle-aged rats. Exp. Gerontol. 46 (11): 958 - 64.

Ashcroft GW, Eccleston D, Crawford TBB. (1965). 5-Hydroxyindole metabolism in rat brain: a study of intermediate metabolism using the technique of tryptophan loading-I. J. Neurochem. 12: 483 - 92.

Awasthi H, Tota S, Hanif K, Nath C, Shukla R (2010). Protective effect of curcumin against intra-cerebral streptozotocin induced impairment in memory and cerebral blood flow. Life Sci. 86 (3-4): 87 - 94.

Bala K, Tripathy BC, Sharma D (2006). Neuroprotective and anti-ageing effects of curcumin in aged rat brain regions. Biogerontology. 7 (2): 81 - 89.

Balasubramanyam K, Altaf M, Varier RA, Swaminathan V, Ravindran A, *et al.* (2004). Polyisoprenylated benzophenone, garcinol, a natural histone acetyltransferase inhibitor, represses chromatin transcription and alters global gene expression. J. Biol. Chem. 279: 33716 - 26.

Balu M, Sangeetha P, Haripriya D, Panneerselvam C (2005).Rejuvenation of antioxidant system in central nervous system of aged rats by grape seed extract. Neurosci. Lett. 383 (3): 295 - 300.

Balu M, Sangeetha P, Murali G, Panneerselvam C (2006). Modulatory role of grape seed extract on age-related oxidative DNA damage in central nervous system of rats. Brain Res. Bull. 68 (6): 469 - 73.

Banderet LE, Lieberman HR (1989). Treatment with tyrosine, a neuro-transmitter precursor, reduces environmental stress in humans. Brain. Res. Bull. 22: 759 - 62.

Bandhu R, Shankar N, Tandon OP, Madan N (2011). Event related potentials in anemic school–going girls of age group 8 to 10 years. Indian J. Physiol. Pharmacol. 55 (3): 234 - 40.

Barberger-Gateau P, Letenneur L, Deschamps V, Peres K, Dartigues J-F, Renaud S. (2002). Fish, meat, and risk of dementia: cohort study. B.M.J. 325 (7370): 932 - 33.

Barros D, Amaral OB, Izquierdo I, Geracitano L, do Carmo Bassols Raseira M, Henriques AT, Ramirez MR (2006). Behavioral and genoprotective effects of Vaccinium berries intake in mice. Pharmacol. Biochem. Behav. 84 (2): 229 - 34.

Bättig K, Welzl H (1993). Psychopharmacological profile of caffeine. In: Garattini S, ed. Caffeine, coffee and health. Raven Press. New York. pp. 213 - 53.

Baumgartner J, Smuts CM, Malan L, Kvalsvig J, van Stuijvenberg ME, Hurrell RF, Zimmermann MB (2012). Effects of iron and n-3 fatty acid supplementation, alone and in combination, on cognition in school children: a randomized, double-blind, placebo-controlled intervention in South Africa. Am. J. Clin. Nutr. 96 (6): 1327 - 38.

Bell KM, Plon L, Bunney WE, Jr., Potkin SG (1988). S-adenosylmethionine treatment of depression: a controlled clinical trial. *American Journal of Psychiatry.* 145 (9): 1110 - 14.

Bhattacharya SK, Kumar A, Ghosal S (2001). Effect of *Bacopa monniera* on animal models of Alzheimer's disease and perturbed central cholinergic markers of cognition in rats. In: Mori A, editor; Satoh T, editor. Molecular Aspects of Asian Medicines. PJD Publications. Westbury, NY.

Bickford PC, Shukitt-Hale B, Joseph J (1999). Effects of ageing on cerebellar noradrenergic function and motor learning: nutritional interventions. Mech. Ageing Dev. 111 (2-3): 141 - 54.

Bickford PC, Gould T, Briederick L, Chadman K, Pollock A, Young D, Shukitt-Hale B, Joseph J (2000). Antioxidant-rich diets improve cerebellar

Bin Sayeed MS, Asaduzzaman M, Morshed H, Hossain MM, Kadir MF, Rahman MR (2013). The effect of Nigella sativa Linn. seed on memory, attention and cognition in healthy human volunteers. J. Ethnopharmacol. 2013 May 21. [Epub ahead of print].

Borbély A, Youmbi-Balderer G (1987). Effects of tryptophan on human sleep. Interdisciplinary Top. Gerontol. 22: 111 - 27.

Borek C (2006). Garlic reduces dementia and heart-disease risk. J. Nutr. 136 (3 Suppl): 810S - 812S.

Bottiglieri T, Hyland K, Reynolds EH (1994). The clinical potential of ademetionine (*S*-adenosyl-methionine) in neurological disorders. Drugs. 48: 137 - 52.

Brewer GJ, Torricelli JR, Lindsey AL, Kunz EZ, Neuman A, Fisher DR, Joseph JA (2010). Age-related toxicity of amyloid-beta associated with increased pERK and pCREB in primary hippocampal neurons: reversal by blueberry extract. J. Nutr. Biochem. 21 (10): 991 - 98.

Brice CF, Smith AP (2002). Effects of caffeine on mood and performance: a study of realistic consumption. Psychopharmacology (Berl). 164 (2): 188 - 92.

Calabrese C, Gregory WL, Leo M, Kraemer D, Bone K, Oken B (2008). Effects of a standardized Bacopa monnieri extract on cognitive performance, anxiety, and depression in the elderly: a randomized, double-blind, placebo-controlled trial. J. Altern. Complement. Med. 14 (6): 707 - 713.

Cantuti-Castelvetri I, Shukitt-Hale B, Joseph JA (2000). Neuro-behavioral aspects of anti-oxidants in ageing. Int. J. Dev. Neurosci. 18: 367 - 81.

Cao XY, Jiang XM, Dou ZH, Rakeman MA, Zhang ML, O'Donnell K, Ma T, Amette K, DeLong N, DeLong GR (1994). Timing of vulnerability of the brain to iodine deficiency in endemic cretinism. N. Engl. J. Med. 331: 1739 - 44.

Casadesus G, Shukitt-Hale B, Stellwagen HM, Zhu X, Lee HG, Smith MA, Joseph JA (2004). Modulation of hippocampal plasticity and cognitive behavior by short-term blueberry supplementation in aged rats. Nutr. Neurosci. 7 (5-6): 309 - 16.

Chauhan NB, Sandoval J (2007). Amelioration of early cognitive deficits by aged garlic extract in Alzheimer's transgenic mice. Phytother. Res. 21 (7): 629 - 40.

Chung WL, Chen JJ, Su HM (2008). Fish oil supplementation of control and (n-3) fatty acid-deficient male rats enhances reference and working memory performance and increases brain regional docosahexaenoic acid levels. J. Nutr. 138 (6): 1165 - 71.

Cohen EL, Wurtman RJ (1976). Brain acetylcholine: control by dietary choline. Science. 191: 561 - 62.

Cole GM, Teter B, Frautschy SA (2007). Neuroprotective effects of curcumin. Adv. Exp. Med. Biol. 595: 197 - 212.

Cole GM, Yang F, Lim GP, Cummings JL, Masterman DL, Frautschy SA (2003). A rationale for curcuminoids for the prevention or treatment of Alzheimer's disease. Curr. Med. Chem-Immun. Endoc. and Metab. Agents. 3: 15 - 25.

Connolly KJ, Pharoah PO, Hetzel BS (1979). Fetal iodine deficiency and motor performance during childhood. Lancet. 2: 1149 - 51.

Cope EC, Morris DR, Scrimgeour AG, Levenson CW (2012). Use of zinc as a treatment for traumatic brain injury in the rat: effects on cognitive and behavioral outcomes. Neurorehabil. Neural. Repair. 26 (7): 907 - 913.

Coultrap SJ, Bickford PC, Browning MD (2008). Blueberry-enriched diet ameliorates age-related declines in NMDA receptor-dependent LTP. Age (Dordr). 30 (4): 263 - 72.

Crews WD Jr, Harrison DW, Griffin ML, Addison K, Yount AM, Giovenco MA, Hazell J (2005). A double-blinded, placebo-controlled, randomized trial of the neuro-psychologic efficacy of cranberry juice in a sample of cognitively intact older adults: pilot study findings. J. Altern. Complement. Med. 11 (2): 305 - 309.

Dangour A, Allen E, Elbourne D, Fletcher A, Richards M, Uauy R (2009). Fish consumption and cognitive function among older people in the UK: Baseline data from the OPAL study. The Journal of Nutrition, Health and Ageing. 13 (3): 198 - 202.

Dash PK, Mistry IU, Rao AR, Patel KS (1996). Role of medhya rasayana in school children. *Ayu.* **12**: 15. De Nicoló S, Tarani L, Ceccanti M, Maldini M, Natella F, Vania A, Chaldakov GN, Fiore M (2013). Effects of olive polyphenols administration on nerve growth factor and brain-derived neurotrophic factor in the mouse brain. Nutrition. 29 (4): 681 - 87.

de Jager CA, Oulhaj A, Jacoby R, Refsum H, Smith AD (2012). Cognitive and clinical outcomes of homocysteine-lowering B-vitamin treatment in mild cognitive impairment: a randomized controlled trial. Int. J. Geriatr. Psychiatry. 27 (6): 592 - 600.

De Nicoló S, Tarani L, Ceccanti M, Maldini M, Natella F, Vania A, Chaldakov GN, Fiore M (2013). Effects of olive polyphenols administration on nerve growth factor and brain-derived neurotrophic factor in the mouse brain. Nutrition. 29 (4): 681 - 87.

Delange F (2000). The role of iodine in brain development. Proc. Nutr. Soc. 59 (1): 75 - 79.

Denny Joseph KM, Muralidhara M (2012). Fish oil prophylaxis attenuates rotenone-induced oxidative impairments and mitochondrial dysfunctions in rat brain. Food Chem. Toxicol. 50 (5): 1529 - 37.

Devore EE, Kang JH, Breteler MM, Grodstein F (2012). Dietary intakes of berries and flavonoids in relation to cognitive decline. Ann Neurol. 72 (1): 135 - 43.

Dhanasekaran M, Holcomb LA, Hitt AR, Tharakan B, Porter JW, Young KA, Manyam BV (2009). *Centella asiatica* extract selectively decreases amyloid beta levels in hippocampus of Alzheimer's disease animal model. Phytother. Res. 23 (1): 14 - 19.

Dhanasekaran M. Tharakan B. Holcomb LA, *et al.* (2007). Neuroprotective mechanisms of ayurvedic antidementia botanical *Bacopa monniera*. Phytother. Res. 21: 965 - 69.

Ding BJ, Ma WW, He LL, Zhou X, Yuan LH, Yu HL, Feng JF, Xiao R (2011). Soybean isoflavone alleviates β-amyloid 1-42 induced inflammatory response to improve learning and memory ability by down regulation of Toll-like receptor 4 expression and nuclear factor-κB activity in rats. Int. J. Dev. Neurosci. 29 (5): 537 - 42.

Ding J, Xi YD, Zhang DD, Zhao X, Liu JM, Li CQ, Han J, Xiao R (2013a). Soybean isoflavone ameliorates β-amyloid 1-42-Induced learning and memory deficit in rats by protecting synaptic structure and function. Synapse. 2013 Jun 14. doi: 10.1002/syn.21692. [Epub ahead of print].

Ding J, Yu HL, Ma WW, Xi YD, Zhao X, Yuan LH, Feng JF, Xiao R (2013b). Soy isoflavone attenuates brain mitochondrial oxidative stress induced by beta-amyloid peptides 1-42 injection in lateral cerebral ventricle. J. Neurosci. Res. 91 (4): 562 - 67.

Elks CM, Reed SD, Mariappan N, Shukitt-Hale B, Joseph JA, Ingram DK, Francis J (2011). A blueberry-enriched diet attenuates nephropathy in a rat model of hypertension via reduction in oxidative stress. PLoS One. 6 (9): e24028.

Felt BT, Lozoff B (1996). Brain iron and behavior of rats are not normalized by treatment of iron deficiency anemia during early development. J, Nutr. 126: 693 - 701.

Fernstrom JD, Wurtman RJ (1971). Brain serotonin content: increase following ingestion of carbohydrate diet. Science. 174: 1023 - 25.

Fernstrom JD (1983). Role of precursor availability in control of monoamine biosynthesis in brain. Physiol. Rev. 63: 484 - 546.

Fernstrom MH, Fernstrom JD (1995). Brain tryptophan concentrations and serotonin synthesis remain responsive to food consumption after the ingestion of sequential meals. Am. J. Clin. Nutr. 61: 312 - 19.

Galli RL, Bielinski DF, Szprengiel A, Shukitt-Hale B, Joseph JA (2006) Blueberry supplemented diet reverses age-related decline in hippocampal HSP70 neuro-protection. Neurobiol. Ageing 27: 344 - 50.

Gao X, Wu B, Zhang Q, Chen J, Zhu J, Zhang W, Rong Z, Chen H, Jiang X (2007). Brain delivery of vasoactive intestinal peptide enhanced with the nanoparticles conjugated with wheat germ agglutinin following intranasal administration. J. Control. Release. 121 (3): 156 - 67.

Gemma C, Mesches MH, Sepesi B, Choo K, Holmes DB, Bickford PC (2002). Diets enriched in foods with high antioxidant activity reverse age-induced decreases in cerebellar beta-adrenergic function and increases in pro-inflammatory cytokines. J. Neurosci. 22 (14): 6114 - 20.

Ghadrdoost B, Vafaei AA, Rashidy-Pour A, Hajisoltani R, Bandegi AR, Motamedi F, Haghighi S, Sameni HR, Pahlvan S (2011). Protective effects of saffron extract and its active constituent crocin against oxidative stress and spatial learning and memory deficits induced by chronic stress in rats. Eur. J. Pharmacol. 667 (1-3): 222 - 29.

Godfrey PS, Toone BK, Carney MW, Flynn TG, Bottiglieri T, Laundy M, Chanarin I, Reynolds EH (1990). Enhancement of recovery from psychiatric illness by methylfolate. Lancet. 336: 392 - 95.

Golechha M, Bhatia J, Arya DS (2012). Studies on effects of *Emblica officinalis* (Amla) on oxidative stress and cholinergic function in scopolamine induced amnesia in mice. J. Environ. Biol. 33 (1): 95 - 100.

Gordon RC, Rose MC, Skeaff SA, Gray AR, Morgan KM, Ruffman T (2009). Iodine supplementation improves cognition in mildly iodine-deficient children. Am. J. Clin. Nutr. 90 (5): 1264 - 71.

Goyarzu P, Malin DH, Lau FC, Taglialatela G, Moon WD, Jennings R, Moy E, Moy D, Lippold S, Shukitt-Hale B, Joseph JA (2004). Blueberry supplemented diet: effects on object recognition memory and nuclear factor-kappa B levels in aged rats. Nutr. Neurosci. 7: 75 - 83.

Groner JA, Holtzman NA, Charney E, Mellits ED (1986). A randomized trial of oral iron on tests of short-term memory and attention span in young pregnant women. J. Adolesc. Health. Care. 7 (1): 44 - 48.

Haider S, Batool Z, Tabassum S, Perveen T, Saleem S, Naqvi F, Javed H, Haleem DJ (2011). Effects of walnuts (*Juglans regia*) on learning and memory functions. Plant. Foods. Hum. Nutr. 66 (4): 335 - 40.

Haider S, Naz N, Khaliq S, Perveen T, Haleem DJ (2008). Repeated administration of fresh garlic increases memory retention in rats. J. Med. Food. 11 (4): 675 - 79.

Hamid Jan JM Jr, Amal KM, Rohani A, Norimah AK (2010). Association of Iron Deficiency with or without Anaemia and Cognitive Functions among Primary School Children in Malaysia. Malays J Nutr. 16 (2): 261 - 70.

Hamon CG, Blair JA, Barford PA (1986). The effect of tetrahydrofolate on tetrahydrobiopterin metabolism. J. Ment. Defic. Res. 30: 179 - 83.

Hashimoto M, Hossain S (2011). Neuroprotective and ameliorative actions of polyunsaturated fatty acids against neuronal diseases: beneficial effect of docosahexaenoic acid on cognitive decline in Alzheimer's disease. J. Pharmacol. Sci. 116 (2): 150 - 62.

Hetzel BS (2000). Iodine and Neuropsychological Development. *Journal of Nutrition.* Supplement. 130: 493S - 495S.

Heude B, Ducimetière P, Berr C; EVA Study (2003). Cognitive decline and fatty acid composition of erythrocyte membranes–The EVA Study. Am. J. Clin. Nutr. 77 (4): 803 - 808.

Hirsch MJ, Wurtman RJ (1978). Lecithin consumption elevates acetylcholine concentrations in rat brain and adrenal gland. Science. 202: 223 - 25.

Ho YS, Yu MS, Yang XF, So KF, Yuen WH, Chang RC (2010). Neuroprotective effects of polysaccharides from wolfberry, the fruits of *Lycium barbarum,* against homocysteine-induced toxicity in rat cortical neurons. J. Alzheimers. Dis. 19 (3): 813 - 27.

Hoffman DR, Boettcher JA, Diersen-Schade DA (2009). Toward optimizing vision and cognition in term infants by dietary docosahexaenoic and arachidonic acid supplementation: a review of randomized controlled trials. Prostaglandins. Leukot. Essent. Fatty Acids. 81 (2-3): 151 - 58.

Holcomb LA, Dhanasekaran M, Hitt AR, Young KA, Riggs M, Manyam BV (2006). *Bacopa monniera* extract reduces amyloid levels in PSAPP mice. J. Alzheimers. Dis. 9 (3): 243 - 51.

Hwang IK, Lee CH, Yoo KY, Choi JH, Park OK, Lim SS, Kang IJ, Kwon DY, Park J, Yi JS, Bae YS, Won MH (2009). Neuroprotective effects of onion extract and quercetin against ischemic neuronal damage in the gerbil hippocampus. J. Med. Food. 12 (5): 990 - 95.

Jackson PA, Reay JL, Scholey AB, Kennedy DO (2012). Docosahexaenoic acid-rich fish oil modulates the cerebral hemodynamic response to cognitive tasks in healthy young adults. Biol. Psychol. 89 (1): 183 - 90.

Jang YJ, Kim J, Shim J, Kim CY, Jang JH, Lee KW, Lee HJ (2013). Decaffeinated coffee prevents scopolamine-induced memory impairment in rats. Behav. Brain. Res. 245: 113 - 19.

Johnson EJ, McDonald K, Caldarella SM, Chung HY, Troen AM, Snodderly DM (2008). Cognitive findings of an exploratory trial of docosahexaenoic acid and lutein supplementation in older women. Nutr. Neurosci. 11 (2): 75 - 83.

Jorm AF, Rodgers B, Christensen H (2004). Use of medications to enhance memory in a large community sample of 60-64 year olds. Int. Psychogeriatr. 16: 209 - 217.

Joseph J, Cole G, Head E, Ingram D (2009). Nutrition, Brain Ageing, and Neurodegeneration. The Journal of Neuroscience. 29 (41): 12795 - 801.

Joseph JA, Denisova NA, Arendash G, Gordon M, Diamond D, Shukitt-Hale B, Morgan D (2003). Blueberry supplementation enhances signaling and prevents behavioral deficits in an Alzheimer disease model. Nutr. Neurosci. 6: 153 - 62.

Joseph JA, Fisher DR, Carey AN (2004) Fruit extracts antagonize Abeta- or DA-induced deficits in Ca^{2+} flux in M1-transfected COS-7 cells. J. Alzheimers. Dis. 6:403 - 411.

Joseph JA, Shukitt-Hale B, Casadesus G (2005). Reversing the deleterious effects of ageing on neuronal communication and behavior: beneficial properties of fruit polyphenolic compounds. American Journal of Clinical Nutrition. 81 (1): 313S - 6S.

Joseph JA, Shukitt-Hale B, Denisova NA, Bielinski D, Martin A, McEwen JJ, Bickford PC (1999). Reversals of age-related declines in neuronal signal transduction, cognitive, and motor behavioral deficits with blueberry, spinach, or strawberry dietary supplementation. J. Neurosci. 19: 8114 - 21.

Joseph JA, Shukitt-Hale B, Denisova NA, Prior RL, Cao G, Martin A, Taglialatela G, Bickford PC (1998). Long-term dietary strawberry, spinach or vitamin E supplementation retards the onset of age-related neuronal signal-transduction and cognitive behavioral deficits. J. Neurosci. 18: 8047 - 55.

Joseph JA, Shukitt-Hale B, Willis LM (2009). Grape juice, berries, and walnuts affect brain ageing and behavior. J. Nutr. 139 (9): 1813S - 7S.

Joshi H and Parle M (2006). *Brahmi rasayana* improves learning and memory in mice. *Evid. Based Complement. Alternat. Med.* **3 (1)**: 79 - 85.

Joyal CC, Lalonde R, Vikis-Freibergs V, Botez MI (1993). Are age-related behavioral disorders improved by folate administration? Exp. Ageing Res. 19: 367 - 76.

Jyoti A, Sethi P, Sharma D (2007). *Bacopa monniera* prevents from aluminium neurotoxicity in the cerebral cortex of rat brain. J. Ethnopharmacol. 111 (1): 56 - 62.

Jyoti A, Sharma D (2006). Neuro-protective role of *Bacopa monniera* extract against aluminium-induced oxidative stress in the hippocampus of rat brain. Neurotoxicology. 27 (4): 451 - 57.

Kaewkaen P, Tong-Un T, Wattanathorn J, Muchimapura S, Kaewrueng W, Wongcharoenwanakit S (2012). Mulberry Fruit Extract Protects against Memory Impairment and Hippocampal Damage in Animal Model of Vascular Dementia. Evid. Based Complement. Alternat. Med. 2012: 263520.

Kalmijn S, Feskens EJM, Launer LJ, Kromhout D (1997a). Polyunsaturated Fatty Acids, Antioxidants, and Cognitive Function in Very Old Men. Am. J. Epidemiol. 145 (1): 33 - 41.

Kalmijn S, Launer LJ, Ott A, Witteman JC, Hofman A, Breteler MM (1997b). Dietary fat intake and the risk of incident dementia in the Rotterdam Study. Ann. Neurol. 42 (5): 776 - 82.

Kalmijn S, van Boxtel MPJ, Ocke M, Verschuren WMM, Kromhout D, Launer LJ. (2004). Dietary intake of fatty acids and fish in relation to cognitive performance at middle age. Neurology. 62 (2): 275 - 80.

Kalt W, Blumberg JB, McDonald JE, Vinqvist-Tymchuk MR, Fillore SA, Graf BA, O'Leary JM, Milbury PE (2008). Identification of anthocyanins in the liver, eye, and brain of blueberry-fed pigs. J. Agric. Food Chem. 56: 705 - 12.

Kesse-Guyot E, Péneau S, Ferry M, Jeandel C, Hercberg S, Galan P; SU.VI.MAX 2 Research Group. (2011). Thirteen-year prospective study between fish consumption, long-chain n-3 fatty acids intakes and cognitive function. J. Nutr. Health. Ageing. 15 (2): 115 - 20.

Khaliq S, Haider S, Ahmed SP, Perveen T, Haleem DJ (2006). Relationship of brain tryptophan and serotonin in improving cognitive performance in rats. Pak. J. Pharm. Sci. 19 (1): 11 - 15.

Khaliq S, Haider S, Haleem DJ (2007). Comparative effects of single dose and repeated oral tryptophan administration on indoleamine synthesis and memory functions in rats. Pak. J. Pharm. Sci. 20 (1): 71 - 76.

Kishore K, Singh M (2005). Effect of bacosides, alcoholic extract of *Bacopa monniera* Linn. (brahmi), on experimental amnesia in mice. Indian J. Exp. Biol. 43: 640 - 45.

Konikowska K, Regulska-Ilow B, Rózanska D (2012). The influence of components of diet on the symptoms of ADHD in children. Rocz. Panstw. Zakl. Hig. 63 (2): 127 - 34.

Koppula S, Choi DK (2011). *Cuminum cyminum* extract attenuates scopolamine-induced memory loss and stress-induced urinary biochemical changes in rats: a noninvasive biochemical approach. Pharm. Biol. 49 (7): 702 - 708.

Krikorian R, Shidler MD, Nash TA, Kalt W, Vinqvist-Tymchuk MR, Shukitt-Hale B, Joseph JA (2010). Blueberry supplementation improves memory in older adults. J. Agric. Food Chem. 58 (7): 3996 - 4000.

Kritz-Silverstein D, Von Mühlen D, Barrett-Connor E, Bressel MA (2003). Isoflavones and cognitive function in older women: the soy and post-menopausal health in ageing (SOPHIA) Study. Menopause. 10 (3): 196 - 202.

Kumar S, Maheshwari KK, Singh V (2009). Effects of *Mangifera indica* fruit extract on cognitive deficits in mice. J. Environ. Biol. 30 (4): 563 - 66.

Lau FC, Shukitt-Hale B, Joseph JA (2005). The beneficial effects of fruit polyphenols on brain ageing. Neurobiol. Ageing. 26 Suppl.1: 128 - 32.

Lau FC, Shukitt-Hale B, Joseph JA (2007). Nutritional intervention in brain ageing: reducing the effects of inflammation and oxidative stress. Subcell. Biochem. 42: 299 - 318.

Lee YB, Lee HJ, Sohn HS (2005). Soy isoflavones and cognitive function. J. Nutr. Biochem. 16 (11): 641 - 49.

Letenneur L, Proust-Lima C, Le Gouge A, Dartigues JG, Barberger-Gateau P (2007). Flavonoid intake and cognitive decline over a 10-year period. Am. J. Epidemiol. 165: 1364 - 71.

Levine J, Barak Y, Gonzalves M, Szor H, Elizur A, Kofman O, Belmaker RH (1995). Double-blind, controlled trial of inositol treatment of depression. *American Journal of Psychiatry*. 152 (5): 792 - 94.

Li Y, Wang P (2009). Neuroprotective effects of curcumin. Zhongguo. Zhong. Yao. Za. Zhi. 34 (24): 3173 - 75.[Article in Chinese].

Lieberman HR, Tharion WJ, Shukitt-Hale B, Speckman KL, Tulley R (2002). Effects of caffeine, sleep loss, and stress on cognitive performance and mood during U.S. Navy SEAL training. Sea-Air-Land. Psychopharmacology. (Berl). 164 (3): 250 - 61.

Liu P, Kemper LJ, Wang J, Zahs KR, Ashe KH, Pasinetti GM (2011). Grape seed polyphenolic extract specifically decreases aβ*56 in the brains of Tg2576 mice. J. Alzheimers. Dis. 26 (4): 657 - 66.

Liu Y, Zhang L, Li J, Shan Z, Teng W (2013). Maternal marginal iodine deficiency affects the expression of relative proteins during brain development in rat offspring. J. Endocrinol. 217 (1): 21 - 29.

Loef M, Walach H (2012). Fruit, vegetables and prevention of cognitive decline or dementia: a systematic review of cohort studies. J. Nutr. Health Ageing. 16 (7): 626 - 30.

Lozoff B, Jimenez E, Wolf AW (1991). Long-term developmental outcome of infants with iron deficiency. N. Engl. J. Med. 325: 687 - 94.

Maddox SA, Watts CS, Doyère V, Schafe GE (2013). A naturally-occurring histone acetyltransferase inhibitor derived from *Garcinia indica* impairs newly acquired and reactivated fear memories. PLoS One. 8 (1): e54463.

Mahoney CR, Castellani J, Kramer FM, Young A, Lieberman HR (2007). Tyrosine supplementation mitigates working memory decrements during cold exposure. Physiol. Behav. 92 (4): 575 - 82.

Makrides M, Neumann MA, Byard RW, Simmer K, Gibson RA (1994). Fatty acid composition of brain, retina, and erythrocytes in breast- and formula-fed infants. Am. J. Clin. Nutr. 60: 189 - 94.

Malin DH, Lee DR, Goyarzu P, Chang YH, Ennis LJ, Beckett E, Shukitt-Hale B, Joseph JA (2011). Short-term blueberry-enriched diet prevents and reverses object recognition memory loss in ageing rats. Nutrition. 27 (3): 338 - 42.

Mani V, Ramasamy K, Ahmad A, Parle M, Shah SA, Majeed AB (2012). Protective effects of total alkaloidal extract from *Murraya koenigii* leaves on experimentally induced dementia. Food Chem. Toxicol. 50 (3-4): 1036 - 44.

Mani V, Ramasamy K, Ahmad A, Wahab SN, Jaafar SM, Kek TL, Salleh MZ, Majeed AB (2013). Effects of the total alkaloidal extract of *Murraya koenigii* leaf on oxidative stress and cholinergic transmission in aged mice. Phytother. Res. 27 (1): 46 - 53.

Menzies L, Ooi C, Kamath S, Suckling J, McKenna P, Fletcher P, Bullmore E, Stephenson C (2007). Effects of gamma-aminobutyric acid-modulating drugs on working memory and brain function in patients with schizophrenia. Arch. Gen. Psychiatry. 64 (2): 156 - 67.

Moorthy D, Peter I, Scott TM, Parnell LD, Lai CQ, Crott JW, Ordovás JM, Selhub J, Griffith J, Rosenberg IH, Tucker KL, Troen AM (2012). Status of vitamins B_{12} and B_6 but not of folate, homocysteine, and the methylenetetrahydrofolate reductase C677T polymorphism are associated with impaired cognition and depression in adults. J. Nutr. 142 (8): 1554 - 60.

Morgan A, Stevens J (2010). Does *Bacopa monnieri* improve memory performance in older persons? Results of a randomized, placebo-controlled, double-blind trial. Journal of Alternative and Complementary Medicine. 16 (7): 753 - 59.

Moriguchi T, Saito H, Nishiyama N (1996). Aged garlic extract prolongs longevity and improves spatial memory deficit in senescence-accelerated mouse. Biol. Pharm. Bull. 19 (2): 305 - 307.

Moriguchi T, Saito H, Nishiyama N (1997). Anti-ageing effect of aged garlic extract in the inbred brain atrophy mouse model. Clin. Exp. Pharmacol. Physiol. 24 (3-4): 235 - 42.

Moriguchi T, Salem N Jr. (2003). Recovery of brain docosahexaenoate leads to recovery of spatial task performance. J. Neurochem. 87 (2): 297 - 309.

Moriguchi T, Takashina K, Chu PJ, Saito H, Nishiyama N (1994). Prolongation of life span and improved learning in the senescence accelerated mouse produced by aged garlic extract. Biol. Pharm. Bull. 17 (12): 1589 - 94.

Morris MC, Evans DA, Bienias JL, Tangney CC, Bennett DA, Wilson RS, Aggarwal N, Schneider JA (2003). Consumption of Fish and n-3 Fatty Acids and Risk of Incident Alzheimer Disease. Archives of neurology. 60 (7): 940 - 46.

Morris MC, Evans DA, Tangney CC, Bienias JL, Wilson RS (2005). Fish consumption and cognitive decline with age in a large community study. Archives of neurology. 62 (12): 1849 - 53.

MRC (1991). Vitamin Study Research Group. Prevention of neural tube defects: results of the Medical Research Council Vitamin Study. Lancet. 338: 131 - 37.

Nagata T, Yaguchi T, Nishizaki T (2011). DL- and PO-phosphatidylcholines as a promising learning and memory enhancer. Lipids. Health. Dis. 28: 10: 25.

Nathan PJ, Tanner S, Lloyd J, Harrison B, Curran L, Oliver C, Stough C (2004). Effects of a combined extract of *Ginkgo biloba* and *Bacopa monniera* on cognitive function in healthy humans. Human Psychopharmacology. 19 (2): 91 - 96.

Nehlig, A (2010). Is caffeine a cognitive enhancer? J. Alzheimers. Dis. 20. Suppl. 1: S85 - 94.

Neuringer M, Anderson GJ, Connor WE (1988). The essentiality of n-3 fatty acids for the development and function of the retina and brain. Annu. Rev. Nutr. 8: 517 - 41.

Nishimura H, Higuchi O, Tateshita K, Tomobe K, Okuma Y, Nomura Y (2006). Antioxidative activity and ameliorative effects of memory impairment of sulfur-containing compounds in *Allium* species. Biofactors. 26 (2): 135 - 46.

Nishiyama N, Moriguchi T, Morihara N, Saito H (2001). Ameliorative effect of S-allylcysteine, a major thioallyl constituent in aged garlic extract, on learning deficits in senescence-accelerated mice. J. Nutr. 131 (3s): 1093S - 5S.

Nishiyama N, Moriguchi T, Saito H (1997). Beneficial effects of aged garlic extract on learning and memory impairment in the senescence-accelerated mouse. Exp. Gerontol. 32 (1-2): 149 - 60.

Nurk E, Drevon CA, Refsum H, Solvoll K, Vollset SE, Nygard O, Nygaard HA, Engedal K, Tell GS, Smith AD. (2007). Cognitive performance among the elderly and dietary fish intake: the Hordaland Health Study. Am. J. Clin. Nutr. 86 (5): 1470 - 78.

O'Brien C, Mahoney C, Tharion WJ, Sils IV, Castellani JW (2007a). Dietary tyrosine benefits cognitive and psychomotor performance during body cooling. Physiol. Behav. 90 (2-3): 301 - 307.

O'Brien C, Tharion WJ, Sils IV, Castellani JW (2007b). Cognitive, psychomotor, and physical performance in cold air after cooling by exercise in cold water. Aviat. Space. Environ. Med. 78 (6): 568 - 73.

Oner P, Oner O, Azik FM, Cop E, Munir KM (2012). Ferritin and hyperactivity ratings in attention deficit hyperactivity disorder. Pediatr. Int. 54 (5): 688 - 92.

Pachauri SD, Tota S, Khandelwal K, Verma PR, Nath C, Hanif K, Shukla R, Saxena JK, Dwivedi AK (2012). Protective effect of fruits of *Morinda citrifolia* L. on scopolamine induced memory impairment in mice: a behavioral, biochemical and cerebral blood flow study. J. Ethnopharmacol. 139 (1): 34 - 41.

Papandreou MA, Dimakopoulou A, Linardaki ZI, Cordopatis P, Klimis-Zacas D, Margarity M, Lamari FN (2009). Effect of a polyphenol-rich wild blueberry extract on cognitive performance of mice, brain antioxidant markers and acetylcholinesterase activity. Behav. Brain Res. 198 (2): 352 - 58.

Pase MP, Kean J, Sarris J, Neale C, Scholey AB, Stough C (2012). The cognitive-enhancing effects of *Bacopa monnieri*: a systematic review of randomized, controlled human clinical trials. Journal of alternative and complementary medicine. 18 (7): 647 - 52.

Pharoah PO, Connolly KJ (1987). A controlled trial of iodinated oil for the prevention of endemic cretinism: a long-term follow-up. Int. J. Epidemiol. 16: 68 - 73.

Poulose SM, Bielinski DF, Shukitt-Hale B (2013). Walnut diet reduces accumulation of polyubiquitinated proteins and inflammation in the brain of aged rats. J. Nutr. Biochem. 24 (5): 912 - 19.

Prado EL, Alcock KJ, Muadz H, Ullman MT, Shankar AH; SUMMIT Study Group (2012). Maternal multiple micronutrient supplements and child cognition: a randomized trial in Indonesia. Pediatrics. 130 (3): e536 - 46.

Prakash JC, Sirsi M (1962). Comparative study of the effects of Brahmi and chlorpromazine on motor learning in rats. J. Sci. Ins. Res. 21: 93 - 96.

Pribis P, Bailey RN, Russell AA, Kilsby MA, Hernandez M, Craig WJ, Grajales T, Shavlik DJ, Sabatè J (2011). Effects of walnut consumption on cognitive performance in young adults. Br. J. Nutr. 19: 1 - 9.

Pu F, Mishima K, Egashira N, Iwasaki K, Kaneko T, Uchida T, Irie K, Ishibashi D, Fujii H, Kosuna K, Fujiwara M (2004). Protective effect of buckwheat polyphenols against long-lasting impairment of spatial memory associated with hippocampal neuronal damage in rats subjected to repeated cerebral ischemia. J. Pharmacol. Sci. 94 (4): 393 - 402.

Puig-Domingo M, Vila L (2013). The implications of iodine and its supplementation during pregnancy in fetal brain development. Curr. Clin. Pharmacol. 8 (2): 97 - 109.

Rajagopalan, V (1995), Effect of Ayushman-8 in manasa mandata (mental retardation). Paper presented at the Seminar on Research in Ayurveda and Siddha; New Delhi. CCRAS. pp. 20–2.

Ramirez MR, Izquierdo I, do Carmo Bassols Raseira M, Zuanazzi JA, Barros D, Henriques AT (2005). Effect of lyophilised Vaccinium berries on memory, anxiety and locomotion in adult rats. Pharmacol. Res. 52 (6): 457 - 62.

Rao MKG, Rao Muddanna S, Rao Gurumadhva S. (2005), *Centella asiatica* (Linn.) induced behavioural changes during growth spurt period in neonatal rats. *Neuroanatomy*. **4**: 18 - 23.

Rao, MKG, Rao M, Rao SG, (2006). *Centella asiatica* (L.) leaf extract treatment during the growth spurt period enhances hippocampal CA3 neuronal dendritic arborization in rats. Evid. Based Complement. Alternat. Med. 3 (3): 349 - 57.

Rathore P, Dohare P, Varma S, Ray A, Sharma U, Jagannathan NR, Ray M (2008). Curcuma oil: reduces early accumulation of oxidative product and is anti-apoptogenic in transient focal ischemia in rat brain. Neurochem. Res. 33: 1672 - 82.

Rendeiro C, Vauzour D, Kean RJ, Butler LT, Rattray M, Spencer JP, Williams CM (2012). Blueberry supplementation induces spatial memory improvements and region-specific regulation of hippocampal BDNF mRNA expression in young rats. Psychopharmacology. (Berl). 223 (3): 319 - 30.

Rendeiro C, Vauzour D, Rattray M, Waffo-Téguo P, Mérillon JM, Butler LT, Williams CM, Spencer JP (2013). Dietary levels of pure flavonoids improve spatial memory performance and increase hippocampal brain-derived neurotrophic factor. PLoS One. 8 (5): e63535.

Riggs KM, Spiro A, Tucker K, Rush D (1996). Relations of vitamin B_{12}, vitamin B_6, folate, and homocysteine to cognitive performance in the Normative Ageing Study. Am. J. Clin. Nutr. 63: 306 - 14.

Ringman JM, Frautschy SA, Cole GM, Masterman DL, Cummings JL (2005). A potential role of the curry spice curcumin in Alzheimer's disease. Curr. Alzheimers. Res. 2: 131 - 36.

Rondanelli M, Opizzi A, Faliva M, Mozzoni M, Antoniello N, Cazzola R, Savarè R, Cerutti R, Grossi E, Cestaro B (2012). Effects of a diet integration with an oily emulsion of DHA-phospholipids containing melatonin and tryptophan in elderly patients suffering from mild cognitive impairment. Nutr. Neurosci. 15 (2): 46 - 54.

Roodenrys S, Booth D, Bulzomi S, Phipps A, Micallef C, Smoker J (2002). Chronic effects of Brahmi (*Bacopa monnieri*) on human memory. Neuropsychopharmacology. 27 (2): 279 - 81.

Rosenberg IH (1992). Folic acid and neural tube defects: time for action? N Engl J Med 327: 1875 - 77.

Saenghong N, Wattanathorn J, Muchimapura S, Tongun T, Piyavhatkul N, Banchonglikitkul C, Kajsongkram T (2012). Zingiber officinale Improves Cognitive Function of the Middle-Aged Healthy Women. Evid. Based Complement. Alternat. Med. 2012: 383062.

Sakurai T, Kitadate K, Nishioka H, Fujii H, Ogasawara J, Kizaki T, Sato S, Fujiwara T, Akagawa K, Izawa T, Ohno H (2013). Oligomerised lychee fruit-derived polyphenol attenuates cognitive impairment in senescence-accelerated mice and endoplasmic reticulum stress in neuronal cells. Br. J. Nutr. 28: 1-10.

Sandstead HH (2012). Subclinical zinc deficiency impairs human brain function. J. Trace. Elem. Med. Biol. 26 (2-3): 70 - 73.

Saraf K, Prabhakar S, Pandhi P, Anand A (2008). *Bacopa monniera* ameliorates amnesic effects of diazepam qualifying behavioral-molecular partitioning. Neuroscience 155 (2): 476 - 84.

Satyavati, GV, Gupta, AK, Tandon, N. (1976). *Medicinal Plants of India.* 1st edition. Indian Council of Medical Research. New Delhi.

Schaefer EJ, Bongard V, Beiser AS, Lamon-Fava S, Robins SJ, Au R, Tucker KL, Kyle DJ, Wilson PW, Wolf PA (2006). Plasma phosphatidylcholine docosahexaenoic acid content and risk ofdementia and Alzheimer disease: the Framingham Heart Study. Arch. Neurol. 63 (11): 1545 - 50.

Shabani M, Nazeri M, Parsania S, Razavinasab M, Zangiabadi N, Esmaeilpour K, Abareghi F (2012). Walnut consumption protects rats against cisplatin-induced neurotoxicity. Neurotoxicology. 33 (5): 1314 - 21.

Shah LP (1992). An open clinical trial of mentat in hyperkinetic children. *Probe.* **31**: 125 - 29.

Sharma, PV (1992). *Dravyaguna Vignana.* 13th edition. Chaukhamba Publications. Vishwa Bharati Academy. New Delhi. India. pp. 3 - 5.

Sharp T, Bramwell SR, Grahame-Smith DG (1992). Effect of acute administration of L-tryptophan on the release of 5-HT in rat hippocampus in relation to serotoninergic neuronal activity: an *in vivo* micro-dialysis study. Life Sci. 50: 1215 - 23.

Shin WH, Park SJ, Kim EJ (2006). Protective effect of anthocyanins in middle cerebral artery occlusion and reperfusion model of cerebral ischemia in rats. *Life Sciences.* 79 (2):130 - 37.

Shinomol and Muralidhara (2008 a). Effect of *Centella asiatica* leaf powder on oxidative markers in brain regions of prepubertal mice *in vivo* and its *in vitro* efficacy to ameliorate 3-NPA-induced oxidative stress in mitochondria. Phytomedicine. 15 (11): 971 - 84.

Shinomol and Muralidhara (2008 b). Prophylactic neuroprotective property of *Centella asiatica* against 3-nitropropionic acid induced oxidative stress and mitochondrial dysfunctions in brain regions of prepubertal mice. Neurotoxicology. 29 (6): 948-57.

Shinomol GK, Ravikumar H, Muralidhara (2010). Prophylaxis with *Centella asiatica* confers protection to prepubertal mice against 3-nitropropionic-acid-induced oxidative stress in brain. Phytother. Res. 24 (6): 885 - 92.

Shooshtari MK, Moazedi AA, Parham GA (2012). Memory and motor coordination improvement by folic acid supplementation in healthy adult male rats. Iran. J. Basic. Med. Sci. 15 (6): 1173 - 79.

Shri R, Singh B.K. (2008). Neuroprotective effect of methanolic extracts of *Allium cepa* on ischemia and reperfusion-induced cerebral injury. Fitoterapia. 79 (2): 86 - 96.

Shukitt-Hale B, Carey A, Simon L, Mark DA, Joseph JA (2006a). The effects of Concord grape juice on cognitive and motor deficits in ageing. Nutrition. 22: 295 - 302.

Shukitt-Hale B, Cheng V, Bielinski D, Carey AN, Lau FC, Seeram NP, Heber D, Joseph JA (2006b). Differential brain regional specificity to blueberry and strawberry polyphenols in improved motor and cognitive function in aged rats. Soc. Neurosci. Abstr. 32: 81 - 15.

Shukitt-Hale B, Cheng V, Joseph JA (2009). Effects of blackberries on motor and cognitive function in aged rats. Nutr. Neurosci. 12: 135 - 40.

Shukitt-Hale B, Galli R, Meterko V, Carey A, Bielinski D, McGhie T, Joseph JA (2005) Dietary supplementation with fruit polyphenolics ameliorates age-related deficits in behavior and neuronal markers of inflammation and oxidative stress. AGE. 27: 49 - 57.

Shukitt-Hale B, Lau FC, Joseph JA (2008). Berry fruit supplementation and the ageing brain. J. Agric. Food Chem. 56 (3): 636 - 41.

Shukitt-Hale B, Miller MG, Chu YF, Lyle BJ, Joseph JA (2013). Coffee, but not caffeine, has positive effects on cognition and psychomotor behavior in ageing. Age (Dordr). 2013 Jan 24 [Epub ahead of print].

Singh HK, Dhawan BN (1997). Neuro-psychopharmacological effects of the ayurvedic nootropic *Bacopa monniera* Linn. (Brahmi). Indian J. Pharmacol. 29: 359 - 65.

Singh HK, Rastogi RP, Sriman RC, Dhawan BN (1988). Effect of bacoside A and B on avoidance response in rats. Phytother. Res. 2: 70 - 75.

Sinn N, Milte CM, Street SJ, Buckley JD, Coates AM, Petkov J, Howe PR (2012). Effects of n-3 fatty acids, EPA v. DHA, on depressive symptoms, quality of life, memory and executive function in older adults with mild cognitive impairment: a 6-month randomised controlled trial. Br. J. Nutr. 107 (11): 1682 - 93.

Sivarajan, VV (1994). *Ayurvedic Drugs and Their Plant Sources.* Indira Balachandran. Oxford and IBH Publishing Company. New Delhi. India. p. 97. 289, 290.

Smith AP (2013). Caffeine, extraversion and working memory. J Psychopharmacol. 27 (1): 71 - 76.

Soderberg M, Edlund C, Kristensson K, Dallner G (1991). Fatty-acid composition of brain phospholipids in ageing and in Alzheimers-disease. Lipids. 26 (6): 421 - 25.

Soeda S, Ochiai T, Paopong L, Tanaka H, Shoyama Y, Shimeno H (2001). Crocin suppresses tumor necrosis factor-alpha-induced cell death of neuronally differentiated PC-12 cells. Life Sci. 69 (24): 2887 - 98.

Sreemantula S, Nammi S, Kolanukonda R, Koppula S, Boini KM (2005). Adaptogenic and nootropic activities of aqueous extract of *Vitis vinifera* (grape seed): an experimental study in rat model. BMC Complement. Altern. Med. 5: 1.

Stonehouse W, Conlon CA, Podd J, Hill SR, Minihane AM, Haskell C, Kennedy D (2013). DHA supplementation improved both memory and reaction time in healthy young adults: a randomized controlled trial. Am. J. Clin. Nutr. 97 (5): 1134 - 43.

Stough C, Downey LA, Lloyd J, Silber B, Redman S, Hutchison C, Wesnes K, Nathan PJ (2008). Examining the nootropic effects of a special extract of *Bacopa monniera* on human cognitive functioning: 90 day double-blind placebo-controlled randomized trial. Phytotherapy Research. 22: 1629 - 34.

Stough C, Lloyd J, Clarke J, Downey L, Hutchison C, Rodgers T, Nathan P (2001). The chronic effects of an extract of *Bacopa monnieri* (Brahmi) on cognitive function in healthy human subjects. Psychopharmacology 156 (4): 481 - 84.

Sugimoto Y, Taga C, Nishiga M, Fujiwara M, Konishi F, Tanaka K, Kamei C (2002). Effect of docosahexaenoic acid-fortified *Chlorella vulgaris* strain CK22 on the radial maze performance in aged mice. Biol. Pharm. Bull. 25 (8): 1090 - 92.

Sumathi T, Shobana C, Christinal J, Anusha C (2012). Protective effect of *Bacopa monniera* on methyl mercury-induced oxidative stress in cerebellum of rats. Cell. Mol. Neurobiol. 32 (6): 979 - 87.

Talavéra S, Felgines C, Texier O, Besson C, Gil-Izquierdo A, Lamaison JL, Rémésy C (2005). Anthocyanin metabolism in rats and their distribution to digestive area, kidney, and brain. J. Agric. Food Chem. 53 (10): 3902 - 908.

Thorp AA, Sinn N, Buckley JD, Coates AM, Howe PR (2009). Soya isoflavone supplementation enhances spatial working memory in men. Br. J. Nutr. 102 (9): 1348 - 54.

Tongjaroenbuangam W, Ruksee N, Chantiratikul P, Pakdeenarong N, Kongbuntad W, Govitrapong P (2011). Neuro-protective effects of quercetin, rutin and okra (*Abelmoschus esculentus* Linn.) in dexamethasone-treated mice. Neurochem. Int. 59 (5): 677 - 85.

Turner AJ (1977). Commentary: the roles of folate and pteridine derivatives in neurotransmitter metabolism. Biochem. Pharmacol. 26: 1009 - 14.

Uauy R, Dangour AD (2006). Nutrition in brain development and ageing: Role of essential fatty acids. Nutrition Reviews. 64 (5): S24 - S33.

Ueda Y, Wang MF, Irei AV, Sarukura N, Sakai T, Hsu TF (2011). Effect of dietary lipids on longevity and memory in the SAMP8 mice. J. Nutr. Sci.Vitaminol. (Tokyo). 57 (1): 36 - 41.

Vakhapova V, Cohen T, Richter Y, Herzog Y, Korczyn AD (2010). Phosphatidylserine containing omega-3 fatty acids may improve memory abilities in non-demented elderly with memory complaints: a double-blind placebo-controlled trial. Dement. Geriatr. Cogn. Disord. 29 (5): 467 - 74.

Van Gelder BM, Tijhuis M, Kalmijn S, Kromhout D (2007). Fish consumption, n-3 fatty acids, and subsequent 5-y cognitive decline in elderly men: the Zutphen Elderly Study. pp. 1142 - 47.

Vasudevan M, Parle M (2007a). Memory enhancing activity of Anwala churna (*Emblica officinalis* Gaertn.): an Ayurvedic preparation. Physiol. Behav. 91 (1): 46 - 54.

Vasudevan M, Parle M (2007b). Effect of Anwala churna (*Emblica officinalis* Gaertn): an ayurvedic preparation on memory deficit rats. Yakugaku. Zasshi. 127 (10): 1701 - 77.

Vasudevan M, Parle M (2009). Antiamnesic potential of *Murraya koenigii* leaves. Phytother. Res. 23 (3): 308 - 316.

Vega Franco L, Robles Martínez B, Mejía AM (1994). Effect of iron deficiency on attention capacity among school children. Gac Med Mex. 1994 Mar-Apr;130(2):67-71. [Article in Spanish].

Velazquez R, Ash JA, Powers BE, Kelley CM, Strawderman M, Luscher ZI, Ginsberg SD, Mufson EJ, Strupp BJ (2013). Maternal choline supplementation improves spatial learning and adult hippocampal neurogenesis in the Ts65Dn mouse model of Down syndrome. Neurobiol. Dis. 58C: 92 - 101.

Vepsäläinen S, Koivisto H, Pekkarinen E, Mäkinen P, Dobson G, McDougall GJ, Stewart D, Haapasalo A, Karjalainen RO, Tanila H, Hiltunen M (2013). Anthocyanin-enriched bilberry and blackcurrant extracts modulate amyloid precursor protein processing and alleviate behavioral abnormalities in the APP/PS1 mouse model of Alzheimer's disease. J. Nutr. Biochem. 24 (1): 360 - 70.

Vercambre MN, Berr C, Ritchie K, Kang JH (2013). Caffeine and cognitive decline in elderly women at high vascular risk. J. Alzheimers. Dis. 35 (2): 413 - 21.

Vinot N, Jouin M, Lhomme-Duchadeuil A, Guesnet P, Alessandri JM, Aujard F, Pifferi F (2011). Omega-3 fatty acids from fish oil lower anxiety improve cognitive functions and reduce spontaneous locomotor activity in a non-human primate. PLoS. One. 6 (6): e20491.

Vohora D, Pal SN, Pillai KK (2000). Protection from phenytoin-induced cognitive deficit by *Bacopa monniera*, a reputed Indian nootropic plant. J. Ethnopharmacol. 71: 383 - 90.

Wahlin A, Hill RD, Winblad B, Backman L. (1996). Effects of serum vitamin B12 and folate status on episodic memory performance in very old age: a population-based study. Psychol. Ageing. 11: 487 - 96.

Walker JG, Batterham PJ, Mackinnon AJ, Jorm AF, Hickie I, Fenech M, Kljakovic M, Crisp D, Christensen H (2012). Oral folic acid and vitamin B_{12} supplementation to prevent cognitive decline in community-dwelling older adults with depressive symptoms–the Beyond Ageing Project: a randomized controlled trial. Am. J. Clin. Nutr. 95 (1): 194 - 203.

Walter T, Kovalskys J, Stekel A (1983). Effect of mild iron deficiency on infant mental development scores. J. Pediatr. 102 (4): 519 - 22.

Wang J, Ho L, Zhao W, Ono K, Rosensweig C, Chen L, Humala N, Teplow DB, Pasinetti GM (2008). Grape-derived polyphenolics prevent Abeta oligomerization and attenuate cognitive deterioration in a mouse model of Alzheimer's disease. J. Neurosci. 28 (25): 6388 - 92.

Wang L, Li C, Guo H, Kern TS, Huang K, Zheng L (2011). Curcumin inhibits neuronal and vascular degeneration in retina after ischemia and reperfusion injury. PLoS. One. 6 (8): e23194.

Wattanathorn J, Jittiwat J, Tongun T, Muchimapura S, Ingkaninan K (2011). *Zingiber officinale* Mitigates Brain Damage and Improves Memory Impairment in Focal Cerebral Ischemic Rat. Evid. Based Complement. Alternat. Med. 2011: 429505.

Whalley LJ, Deary IJ, Starr JM, Wahle KW, Rance KA, Bourne VJ, Fox HC (2008). n-3 Fatty acid erythrocyte membrane content, APOE varepsilon4, and cognitive variation: an observational follow-up study in late adulthood. Am. J. Clin. Nutr. 87 (2): 449 - 54.

Whalley LJ, Fox HC, Wahle KW, Starr JM, Deary IJ (2004). Cognitive ageing, childhood intelligence, and the use of food supplements: possible involvement of n-3 fatty acids. Am. J. Clin. Nutr. 80 (6): 1650 - 57.

Williams CM, El Mohsen MA, Vauzour D, Rendeiro C, Butler LT, Ellis JA, Whiteman M, Spencer JP (2008). Blueberry-induced changes in spatial working memory correlate with changes in hippocampal CREB phosphorylation and brain-derived neurotrophic factor (BDNF) levels. Free Radic. Biol. Med. 45 (3): 295 - 305.

Willis LM, Bielinski DF, Fisher DR, Matthan NR, Joseph JA (2010). Walnut extract inhibits LPS-induced activation of BV-2 microglia via internalization of TLR4: possible involvement of phospholipase D2. Inflammation. 33 (5): 325 - 33.

Willis LM, Shukitt-Hale B, Cheng V, Joseph JA (2009). Dose-dependent effects of walnuts on motor and cognitive function in aged rats. Br. J. Nutr. 101: 1140 - 44.

Winick M (1976). Malnutrition and brain development. Oxford University Press. New York.

Yang D, Li SY, Yeung CM, Chang RC, So KF, Wong D, Lo AC (2012). *Lycium barbarum* extracts protect the brain from blood-brain barrier disruption and cerebral edema in experimental stroke. PLoS. One. 7 (3): e33596.

Ye X, Bhupathiraju SN, Tucker KL (2012). Variety in fruit and vegetable intake and cognitive function in middle-aged and older Puerto Rican adults. Br. J. Nutr. 2012 May 1:1-8. [Epub ahead of print].

Youdim KA, Joseph JA (2001). A possible emerging role of phytochemicals in improving age-related neurological dysfunctions: a multiplicity of effects. Free Radic. Biol. Med. 30: 583 - 94.

Youdim KA, Martin A, Joseph JA (2000). Essential fatty acids and the brain: possible health implications. Int. J. Dev. Neurosci. 18: 383 - 99.

Young SN, Gauthier S (1981). Tryptophan availability and the control of 5-hydroxy-tryptamine and tryptamine synthesis in human CNS. Adv. Exp. Med. Biol. 133: 221 - 30.

Yu MS, Leung SK, Lai SW, Che CM, Zee SY, So KF, Yuen WH, Chang RC (2005). Neuroprotective effects of anti-ageing oriental medicine *Lycium barbarum* against beta-amyloid peptide neurotoxicity. Exp. Gerontol. 40: 716 - 27.

Yu X, Jin L, Zhang X, Yu X (2013). Effects of maternal mild zinc deficiency and zinc supplementation in offspring on spatial memory and hippocampal neuronal ultra-structural changes. Nutrition. 29 (2): 457 - 61.

Yurko-Mauro K (2010). Cognitive and cardiovascular benefits of docosahexaenoic acid in ageing and cognitive decline. Curr. Alzheimer. Res. 7 (3): 190 - 96.

Yurko-Mauro K, McCarthy D, Rom D, Nelson EB, Ryan AS, Blackwell A, Salem N Jr, Stedman M; MIDAS (2010). Beneficial effects of docosahexaenoic acid on cognition in age-related cognitive decline. Alzheimers Dement. 6 (6): 456 - 64.

Zimmermann MB, Connolly K, Bozo M, Bridson J, Rohner F, Grimci L (2006). Iodine supplementation improves cognition in iodine-deficient school children in Albania: a randomized, controlled, double-blind study. Am. J. Clin. Nutr. 83 (1): 108 - 14.

Chapter 5
Anti-Diabetic Foods

Globally, the prevalence of chronic, non-communicable diseases is increasing at an alarming rate and diabetes is one of them. Uncontrolled diabetes can lead to a lot of complications like coronary artery disease, cerebrovascular disease, peripheral vascular disease, retinopathy, nephropathy and neuropathy and may result in morbidity and/or mortality (Haque *et al.*, 2011). Despite the introduction of hypoglycaemic agents from natural and synthetic sources, diabetes and its secondary complications continue to be a major medical problem to people (Ravi *et al.*, 2005). It has been estimated that up to one-third of patients with diabetes mellitus use some form of complementary and alternative medicine.

There is the wider appeal of 'natural' dietary adjuncts as functional foods through which patients can gain added benefits to the management of their disease (Swanston-Flatt *et al.*, 1991). The lack of such adjuncts to combat hyperglycaemia and its accompanying complications presents an opening to revisit traditional anti-diabetic plants (Gray and Flatt, 1997). As illustrated by Gray and Flatt (1998a), there is a need for gathering scientific validation for the use of certain traditional anti-diabetic plants, and this has encouraged botanical exploration in the quest for new anti-diabetic drugs. The World Health Organization has listed 21,000 plants, which are used for medicinal purposes around the world. Among these 2500 species are in India, out of which 150 species are used commercially on a fairly large scale. India is the largest producer of medicinal herbs and is called as botanical garden of the world (Seth and Sharma, 2004). WHO (1980) has pointed out that prevention of diabetes and its complications is not only a major challenge for the future, but also essential to attain health for all. Hence, in recent years, considerable attention is accorded towards identification of plants with anti-diabetic ability and a number of them have shown varying degrees of hypoglycemic or anti-hyperglycemic activity (Ayyanar *et al.*, 2008).

According to Aggarwal (2010), curcumin directly interacts with adipocytes, pancreatic cells, hepatic stellate cells, macrophages, and muscle cells. There, it suppresses the pro-inflammatory transcription factors nuclear factor-kappa B, signal transducer and activators of transcription-3, and Wnt/beta-catenin, and it activates peroxisome proliferator-activated receptor-gamma and Nrf2 cell-signaling pathways, thus leading to the downregulation of adipokines, including tumor necrosis factor (Chan, 1995) interleukin-6, resistin, leptin, and monocyte chemotactic protein-1, and the upregulation of adiponectin and other gene products. These curcumin-induced alterations reverse insulin resistance, hyperglycemia, hyperlipidemia, and other symptoms linked to obesity. Shehzad *et al.* (2011) thus recommended that these results enable translation of curcumin to the clinical practice for the treatment and prevention of obesity-related chronic diseases.

A few vegetables that are commonly consumed in India have been claimed to possess anti-diabetic potency. Extensive work has been carried out in this regard on bitter gourd (*Momordica charantia*), and ivy gourd (*Coccinia indica*), cabbage (*Brassica oleracia*), green leafy vegetables, beans and tubers both in experimental animals and human diabetic subjects. A limited number of studies on other vegetables such as cabbage (*Brassica oleracia*), green leafy vegetables, beans and tubers have shown hypo-glycaemic effect in both experimental animals and humans. (Platel and Srinivasan, 1997).

Several other plants, *M. charantia, Eugenia jambolana, Mucuna pruriens, T. cordifolia, T. foenum graecum, O. sanctum, P. marsupium, Murraya koeingii* and *Brassica juncea* have shown varying degrees of hypoglyceamic (Grover *et al.*, 2002). Yadav *et al.* (2010) reported that the ethanol extract of *E. jambolana* seeds, water extract of *M. charantia* fruits, ethanol extract of *G. sylvestre* leaves, and water extract of fenugreek seeds have higher hypoglyceamic potential and may be used as complementary medicine to treat the diabetic population by significantly reducing the dosage of standard drugs.

Spices such as garlic (*Allium sativum*), onion (*Allium cepa*), and turmeric (*Curcuma longa*) have been confirmed to possess anti-diabetic potential, cumin seeds (*Cuminum cyminum*), ginger (*Zingiber officinale*), mustard (*Brassica nigra*), and coriander (*Coriandrum sativum*) have also been reported to be hypoglyceamic (Srinivasan, 2005).

Use of medicinal plants is common in Jordanian traditional medicinal system for the treatment of diabetes. The anti-oxidant activity of these plant extracts and their potential role in radical scavenging agreed with their potential use by Jordanian population as traditional anti-diabetic agents (Al-Mustafa and Al-Thunibat (2008). Yeh *et al.* (2003) through a review of well designed randomized controlled trials on anti-diabetic herbs, found the best evidence for efficacy of *Coccinia indica* and American ginseng. Other supplements with positive preliminary results include *Gymnema sylvestre, Aloe vera* and *Momordica charantia*.

Based on a large number of chemical and pharmacological research work, numerous antidiabetic bioactive compounds have been found in Chinese medicinal plants (Li *et al.*, 2004). Pharmacological and clinical evaluations by Jia *et al.* (2003) indicated that the Chinese anti-diabetic drug formulas such as polysaccharide containing drugs restore the functions of pancreatic tissues and cause an increase in insulin output by the functional beta cells, while other ingredients enhance the microcirculation, increase the availability of insulin and facilitate the metabolism in insulin-dependent processes. These drugs had a mild, but significant blood glucose lowering effect and that the long-term use of these agents may be advantageous over chemical drugs in alleviating some of the chronic diseases and complications caused by diabetes. Additionally, the use of these natural agents in conjunction with conventional drug treatments, such as a chemical agent or insulin, permits decreases the dose requirement of the drug and/or frequency of administration and thereby alleviates the side effects most commonly observed. *S. cumini* exerts a dual effect resembling that of a combination of mechanism of action of sulfonylurea and biguanides and may exhibit its hypoglyceamic action through stimulation of surviving β cells of islets.

The hypoglyceamic effect is claimed to be mediated through an insulin secretagogic effect or through an influence on enzymes involved in glucose metabolism. Several traditional anti-diabetic plant materials which are components of a normal diet do indeed exert anti-diabetic activity by improving various parameters of glucose metabolism for which, mushrooms, bitter gourd, and fenugreek seeds are good examples (Day *et al.*, 1989; Swanston-Flatt *et al.*, 1989; 1990; Gray and Flatt, 1998 1998b; Subbulakshmi and Naik, 2001). Mitra (2007) found a composite of Tulsi (*Ocimum sanctum*) leaves, Amla (*Emblica officinalis*), Bitter Gourd (*Momordica charantia*), Gurmur (*Gymnema sylvestre*) leaves and Jamun (*Syzygium cumini*) fruit and its seed fed to mild diabetic patients to be effective not only in changing the blood bio-chemical parameters but also the overall picture of Insulin resistance.

Nutritional and Non-nutritional Anti-diabetic Agents

Most plants exhibit their anti-diabetic effect probably through their fiber, nutrient or phytchemical content. Mineral deficiencies are common in diabetes and can exacerbate insulin resistance. Several of these minerals are co-factors for signaling intermediaries of insulin action and key enzymes of glucose metabolism. Plants rich in minerals have also been shown to benefit glycemic control in diabetic patients, for example manganese in Lucerne and chromium in brewer's yeast (Day, 1990). Vitamins such as vitamins E and C along with various phytochemicals prevent oxidative stress induced complications and comorbidities whereas dietary fibre aids in the management of blood sugar.

Naturally-occurring compounds that have been shown to improve insulin sensitivity include Chromium (Cr) and polyphenols found in cinnamon (*Cinnamomon cassia*). These compounds also have similar effects on insulin signalling and glucose control. Not all studies on both supplemental Cr and cinnamon have reported beneficial effects and the responses are related to the duration of the study, form of Cr or cinnamon used and the extent of obesity and glucose intolerance of the subjects (Anderson, 2008).

Again, supplementation of a combination of three novel supplements (niacin-bound chromium, Maitake mushroom and (-)-hydroxycitric acid from *Garcinia cambogia*) resulted in a lower systolic blood pressure and maintenance of body weight as compared to control animals. From these observations, Talpur *et al.* (2003) concluded that elderly diabetics and even ageing individuals might benefit from a similar regimen.

Several plants have provided entirely new hypoglycemic compounds such as castanospermine in Castanospermum australe and neomyrtillin in bilberry (Day, 1990). Unfortunately, many of these compounds are alkaloids, flavonoids and glycosides which do not lend themselves readily to pharmaceutical development (Day, 1995). It is also likely that traditional anti-diabetic plants are sources of agents which can benefit the co-morbid conditions of dyslipidaemia, hypertension or atherosclerosis; *e.g.* the lipid lowering properties of garlic. Complications of diabetes may also be targeted by anti-diabetic plants; for example evening primrose oil, a source of γ-linolenic acid, has been shown to benefit nerve conduction disorders in diabetes.

Anti-oxidants in Diabetes

Oxidative stress is an important aspect of glucose toxicity in pancreatic β-cells. Flavonoids have been shown to exert a variety of biological effects including antioxidant, anti-inammatory, and anti-cancer effects in different cell types (Chowdhury *et al.*, 2002; Bahia *et al.*, 2008). In particular, flavonoids have been shown to have potent anti-diabetic and anti-oxidant activity in experimental diabetic animal models (Kamalakkannan and Prince, 2006).

Diets rich in flavanols reverse vascular dysfunction in diabetes, highlighting therapeutic potentials in cardiovascular disease (Balzer. *et al.*, 2008). A single ingestion of flavanol-containing cocoa was dose-dependently associated with significant acute increases in circulating flavanols and a 30-day, thrice-daily consumption of flavanol-containing cocoa increased baseline flow-mediated dilation of the brachial artery by 30 per cent.

Yamagata *et al.* (2011) observed that apigenin inhibited high glucose levels and tumor necrosis factor-α (TNF-α)-induced adhesion molecule levels in human endothelial cells. Suh *et al.* (2012) demonstrated that flavonoid apigenin protected pancreatic β-cells from 2-deoxy-D-ribose (dRib)-induced oxidative cell damage. The anti-oxidants, N-acetyl-L-cysteine and alpha lipoic acid also prevented both dRib-induced oxidative damage and activation of transcriptional factors, nuclear factor-κB and activator protein. It has been reported that apigenin has the potential to regulate disease-induced thyroid dysfunction and lipid peroxidation too, apart from regulating blood glucose level (Panda and Kar, 2007).

Kuhad and Chopra (2008) emphasized the involvement of oxidative stress and inflammation in the development of cognitive impairment in diabetic animals and confirmed the therapeutic potential of sesamol (3, 4-methylenedioxyphenol), a phenolic antioxidant and anti-inflammatory molecule, in diabetes-associated cognitive decline. Kuhad *et al.* (2008) further demonstrated that chronic treatment with lycopene (1, 2 and 4 mg/kg; p.o.) significantly and dose dependently attenuated cognitive deficit, increased acetyl-cholinesterase activity, oxidative-nitrosative stress and inflammation in diabetic rats. Chronic treatment with curcumin (60 mg/kg; p.o.)

significantly attenuated cognitive deficit, cholinergic dysfunction, oxidative stress and inflammation in diabetic rats. Kuhad and Chopra (2007) emphasized the involvement of cholinergic dysfunction, oxidative stress and inflammation in the development of cognitive impairment in diabetic animals and pointed towards the potential of curcumin as an adjuvant therapy to conventional anti-hyperglycemic regimens for the prevention and treatment of diabetic encephalopathy.

Quercetin, a bioflavonoid widely distributed in the plants is reported to be a potent anti-diabetic, anti-oxidant, acetylcholinesterase (AChE) inhibitor, and memory enhancer. Bhutada *et al.* (2010) found that the treatment with quercetin (5-20 mg/kg, p.o., twice daily for 30 days) in streptozotocin-induced diabetic rats prevented the changes in blood glucose, body weight, and performance in Morris water and elevated plus maze tasks.

Berberine, an isoquinoline alkaloid is reported to exhibit anti-diabetic and anti-oxidant effect, inhibit AChE, and increase GLP release. Bhutada *et al.* (2011) demonstrated that treatment with berberine prevents the changes in oxidative stress and ChE activity, and consequently memory impairment in diabetic rats.

Bittergourd also improved the anti-oxidant status, indicated by low levels of thiobarbituric acid-reactive substances and normal levels of reduced glutathione. However, rats reverted to diabetic conditions and were found to be under oxidative stress after termination of treatment (Chaturvedi and George, 2010).

Anti-diabetic Foods

Fenugreek (*Trigonella foenum graecum*)

Consumption of fenugreek seeds has been a traditional dietary advice to diabetics for the control of blood glucose level. Available data suggest that though several anti-diabetic plants of Iran need further study, the best evidence in glycaemic control was found in *Citrullus colocynthus, Ipomoea betatas, Silybum marianum* and *Trigonella foenum graecum* (Shojaii *et al.*, 2011).

The action of fenugreek in lowering blood glucose levels is almost comparable to the effect of insulin. In a majority of patients, a mild improvement in clinical symptoms such as polydipsia and polyuria were observed along with a reduction in anti-diabetic drug doses. Extensive research provided the scientific basis for the mechanim of anti-diabetic action of fenugreek seeds. The gel forming characters of fenugreek fiber reduces gastric emptying, glucose absorption and the insulin response. The soluble dietary fiber (SDF) fraction of fenugreek seeds exerts anti-diabetic effects mediated through inhibition of carbohydrate digestion and absorption, and enhancement of peripheral insulin action (Hannan *et al.*, 2007). Ali *et al.* (1995) had confirmed the involvement of the major constituent of SDF fraction, a galactomannan in the hypo-glycaemic effect. Besides SDF, a novel amino acid 4-hydroxyleucine present in fenugreek seeds was found to increase glucose stimulated insulin release by isolated islet cells in both rats and humans (Sauvaire *et al.*, 1998).

In addition to decreasing blood glucose level, administration of fenugreek seeds also normalized creatinine kinase activity in heart, skeletal muscle and liver of diabetic rats besides reducing hepatic and renal glucose-6-phosphatase, and fructose 1, 6-biphosphatase activity (Gupta *et al.*, 1999). Fenugreek extract lowered kidney/body weight ratio, blood glucose, blood lipid levels and improved hemorheological properties in experimental diabetic rats following repeated treatment for 6 weeks (Xue *et al.*, 2007). The extract exhibited hypo-lipidemic action in addition to hypo-glycaemic effects in the streptozotocin-induced diabetic rats (Ahmed *et al.*, 2001). Fenugreek also showed anti-oxidant potential to protect the organs such as liver and pancreas against the oxidative damage induced by diabetes, apart from controlling the blood glucose levels (Sankar *et al.*, 2012).

The hypoglyceamic response of fenugreek seemed to be dose dependent. Animal studies proved that an oral administration of 2 and 8 g/kg of fenugreek plant extract produced dose dependent decrease in the blood glucose levels in both normal as well as diabetic rats (Khosla *et al.*, 1995) and appropriate dose of fenugreek administration has been proposed for diabetic patients. Incorporating around 25g fenugreek seeds in the daily diet can serve as an effective supportive therapy in the management of diabetes. Not only a significant reduction in blood glucose but also a significant reduction in cholesterol, triglycerides and urinary sugar levels was observed on consumption of fenugreek (Raghuram, 1996).

The most effective dose recognized was 1 g/kg body weight but that is still lower than the standard anti-diabetic drug. No acute or delayed toxicity was observed with ethanol extract of methi seed when it was administered orally at a high dose level of 3 g/kg body weight, which is higher than effective anti-hyperglycemic dose (Mowla *et al.*, 2009). Interestingly, addition of fenugreek to vanadium significantly removed the toxicity of vanadium when used to reduce blood glucose levels (Baquer *et al.*, 2011).

Bitter Gourd/Bitter Melon/Karela (*Momordica charantia*)

Bitter gourd is a vegetable indigenous to South America and Asia, used in native medicines of Asia and Africa, Oriental and Latin American countries. It is believed to be anti-dotal, anti-pyretic tonic, appetizing, stomachic, anti-bilious and laxative. It has been widely studied for its beneficial effects on blood glucose levels. Bitter gourd has been found to show anti-hyperglycemic activities when administered in experimental rats (Singh *et al.*, 2008; Malik *et al.*, 2011; Clouatre *et al.*, 2011; Choudhary *et al.*, 2012; Sitasawad *et al.*, 2000; Ahmed *et al.*, 2001; Sekar *et al.*, 2005; Virdi *et al.*, 2003).

The hypoglyceamic efficacy in an aqueous extract of seeds of two varieties, namely a country and a hybrid variety of *M. charantia* clearly proved the anti-diabetic properties. Both the varieties showed safe and significant hypoglyceamic effects which were more pronounced in country variety compared to hybrid variety (Sekar and Subramanian, 2005a). The extract exerted rapid protective effects against lipid peroxidation by scavenging of free radicals thereby reducing the risk of diabetic complications (Sekar and Subramanian, 2005b). Metabolic and hypoglyceamic effects of bitter gourd extracts have been demonstrated in cell culture, animal, and human studies. (Krawinkel and Keding, 2006).

Active Components

Bitter gourd contains bitter glycosides, saponins, alkaloids, reducing sugars, phenolics, oils, free acids, polypeptides, sterols, 17-amino acids including methionine and a crystalline product named p-insulin. It is reported to have hypoglyceamic activity in addition to being anti-haemorrhoidal, astringent, stomachic, emmenagogic, hepatic stimulant, anthelminthic and blood purifier.

Bitter gourd also contains charantin, vicine, and polypeptide-p, (anti-diabetic components) as well as other unspecific bioactive components such as anti-oxidants. Keller *et al.* (2011) discovered that a saponin-rich fraction isolated from *M. charantia*, stimulate insulin secretion in an *in vitro*, static incubation assay. 11β-Hydroxysteroid dehydrogenase type 1 (11β-HSD1) catalyzes the intracellular regeneration of active cortisol from inert cortisone in key metabolic tissues, thus regulating ligand access to glucocorticoid receptors.

Out of the three anti-diabetic compounds namely, charantin, momordenol and momordicilin from bitter gourd, momordicilin was found to show minimum binding energy and thus found to be the most active compound in the respective target site (Hazarika *et al.*, 2012).

Effect on Carbohydrate and Lipid Metabolism

Bitter melon can suppress the visceral fat accumulation and inhibit adipocyte hypertrophy, which may be associated with marked down-regulated expressions of lipogenic genes in the adipose (Huang *et al.*, 2008).

According to Chaturvedi (2012) the effects of bitter gourd including transport of glucose in the cells, transport of fatty acids in the mitochondria, modulation of insulin secretion, and elevation of levels of uncoupling proteins in adipose and skeletal muscles are similar to those of AMP-activated protein kinase (AMPK) and thyroxine. Therefore it is proposed that effects of bitter gourd on carbohydrate and fat metabolism are through thyroxine and AMPK.

There is strong evidence that increased adipose 11β-HSD1 activity may be an important aetiological factor in the current obesity and diabetes type 2 epidemics. Blum *et al.* (2012) showed that bitter gourd extract capsules contain at least one ingredient with selective 11β-HSD1 inhibitory activity thus providing an interesting additional explanation for the well-documented anti-diabetic and hypoglyceamic effects of bitter gourd.

The methanol extract of bitter gourd normalised blood glucose level, reduced triglyceride and LDL levels and increased HDL level in diabetic rats fed a high-fat and a low-carbohydrate diet (Chaturvedi *et al.*, 2004). However, the animals reverted to a diabetic state once the extract was discontinued (Chaturvedi, 2005).

Bittergourd consumption along with high fat diet ameliorates the negative influence of dietary fat on the body composition. Rats fed on the High fat + Bitter Melon (HF +BM) diet gained less weight and had less visceral fat than those fed the HF diet ($P < 0.05$). The addition of BM did not change apparent fat absorption. BM supplementation to the HF diet improved insulin resistance, lowered serum insulin and leptin but raised serum free fatty acid concentration ($P < 0.05$). Chen *et al.* (2003) showed for the first time that BM reduces adiposity in rats fed a HF diet. BM appears to have multiple influences on glucose and lipid metabolism that strongly counteract the untoward effects of a high fat diet.

Shih *et al.* (2009) demonstrated that bitter melon was effective in ameliorating the fructose diet-induced hyper-glycemia, hyper-leptinemia, hyper-insulinemia, and hyper-triglyceridemia as well as in decreasing the levels of free fatty acid. Bitter melon reversed fructose diet-induced hypo-adiponectinemia, which provides a therapeutic advantage to insulin resistance in improving insulin sensitivity. Additionally, bitter melon decreased the weights of epididymal and retroperitoneal white adipose tissue. Furthermore, they demonstrated that bitter melon significantly increased the mRNA expression and protein of glucose transporter 4 (GLUT4) in skeletal muscle.

Again, Roffey *et al.* (2007) reported that water-soluble component(s) in bitter gourd enhanced the glucose uptake at sub-optimal concentrations of insulin in 3T3-L1 adipocytes, which was accompanied by and might be the result of increased adiponectin secretion from the 3T3-L1 adipocytes. The mechanism of action of the extract in alloxan-induced diabetic rats seemed to be enhancing insulin secretion by the islets of Langerhans, reducing glycogenesis in liver tissue, enhancing peripheral glucose utilisation and increasing serum protein levels. Further, the treatment restored the altered histological architecture of the islets of Langerhans. Hence, the biochemical, pharmacological and histo-pathological profiles of bitter gourd clearly indicate its potential anti-diabetic activity and other beneficial effects in amelioration of diabetes associated complications including hyper-lipidemia and obesity (Fernandes *et al.*, 2007).

Mechanism of Action

Singh and Gupta (2007) observed the presence of small scattered islets among the acinar tissue when experimental diabetic animals were administered the acetone extract of bitter gourd fruit powder. These small scattered islets were suggestive of the neo formation of islets from pre-existing islet cells, which if proved by further studies will be beneficial for diabetic population. Alleviation of pancreatic damage and an increase in the number of beta cells in neonatal diabetic rats fed with bitter gourd fruit extract was observed by Abdollahi *et al.* (2011). The islet size, total beta cell area and number of β-cells almost doubled in the diabetic rats treated with bitter gourd extract as compared to the untreated diabetic rats, and the extract-treated diabetic rat beta cells were found to be abundant with insulin granules (Hafizur *et al.*, 2011). Experiment conducted on rats (Leatherdale *et al.*, 1981; Day, 1990; Chaturvedi *et al.*, 2004; Zheng *et al.*, 2005) and maturity onset diabetic patients (Welihinda *et al.*, 1986), showed that bitter gourd improved glucose tolerance without any significant increase in serum insulin response, along with protective effect on development of diabetes induced cataract.

Singh *et al.* (2008) further observed that the blood glucose once lowered by the treatment with bitter gourd fruit extract remained static even after discontinuation of the extract for 15 days and the blood sugar never fell below normal values even with a high dose of this extract. Kumar *et al.* (2009) demonstrated the significance of Glut-4, PPAR gamma and PI3K up-regulation by bitter gourd in augmenting the glucose uptake and homeostasis. According to Sitasawad *et al.* (2000) feeding the aqueous juice of bittergourd fruit resulted in reduction of STZ-induced hyper-glycemia in mice. It also markedly reduced the STZ-induced lipid peroxidation in pancreas of mice, RIN cells and islets. Further, it reduced the STZ-induced apoptosis in RIN cells indicating the mode of protection of bittergourd juice on RIN cells, islets and pancreatic beta-cells.

Mode of Ingestion

Sitasawad *et al.* (2000) confirmed hypoglycemic effect of BF juice and provides sufficient documentation to define its role and action for its potential and promising use in treating diabetes.In non-insulin dependent diabetic patients (Ahmad *et al.*, 1999) the juice of bitter gourd produced significant reduction in fasting as well as post prandial blood sugars after an oral glucose tolerance test. Cummings *et al.* (2004) found the fruit juice to act like insulin to exert its hypo-glycaemic effect and stimulate amino acid uptake into skeletal muscle cells just like insulin. Significant improvement in fasting blood glucose, serum insulin, β-cell number and function was observed with administration of bitter gourd extract to the diabetic rat model (Hafizur *et al.*, 2011).

In a human study, Baldwa and his team, as early as 1977, administered insulin like compound obtained from the bitter gourd fruit and tissue culture. This compound was homologous to animal insulin and showed consistent hypoglyceamic effect on diabetic subjects. It showed the onset of action within 30-60 min and the peak effect of six hours after the administration of the dose without any hyper-sensitivity reaction among the subjects. Time course experiments performed in rat adipocytes by Yibchok-anun (2006) revealed that *M. charantia* protein extract significantly increased glucose uptake after 4 and 6 h of incubation. Thus, the *M. charantia* protein extract, a slow acting chemical, exerted both insulin secretagogue and insulinomimetic activities to lower blood glucose concentrations *in vivo*.

Extracts of fruit pulp, seed, leaves and whole plant was shown to have hypoglyceamic effect in various animal models. Polypeptide p, isolated from fruit, seeds and tissues of bitter gourd showed significant hypoglyceamic effect when administered subcutaneously to langurs and humans (Khanna *et al.*, 1981). 200 mg/kg ethanolic extract showed an anti-hyperglycemic effect in normal and STZ diabetic rats. This may be because of inhibition of glucose-6-phosphatase besides fructose-1, 6-biphosphatase in the liver and stimulation of hepatic glucose-6-phosphate dehydrogenase activities (Shibib *et al.*, 1993).

Dried bitter gourd powder at 10 per cent level in the diet in streptozotocin induced diabetic rats brought down the fasting blood glucose level by about 30 per cent. In addition, bitter gourd supplementation alleviated the rise in water consumption, urine volume and urine sugar during diabetes by about 30 per cent as compared to the controls. Renal hyper-trophy was higher in diabetic controls and bitter gourd supplementation partially, but effectively prevented it by 38 per cent. Increased glomerular filtration rate in diabetes was significantly reduced by 27 per cent in the experimental group (Shetty *et al.*, 2005a; b).

Transdermal patches made up of bitter gourd extract showed improvement in blood glucose parameters of experimental rats without any incidence of skin irritation or reaction (Bhujbal *et al.*, 2011).

Synergistic Effect

A combination of extracts of bitter gourd and fenugreek when administered to alloxan induced diabetes rats for 30 days showed improvement in the fasting blood sugars along with protection of the heart, kidneys and liver tissue against oxidative stress (Tripathi and Chandra, 2009; 2010).

β-Glucan purified from oats (OG) and bitter melon (MC), water extracts have shown favorable effects on diabetes and its complications. In variable compositions (OG:MC = 1:1, 1:2, 1:4, 1:6, 1:8, 1:10, 2:1, 4:1, 6:1, 8:1, 10:1) the extracts were administered orally once a day for 28 days following 7 days post streptozotocin (STZ) dosing. The changes of hyperglycaemia, diabetic nephropathy, hepatopathy, and hyper-lipemia observed as the result of STZ-induced diabetes were dramatically decreased in the OG and MC single-dosing group, and all composition groups. Among variable compositions, the OG:MC 1:2 mixed group showed the most synergic effects (Kim *et al.*, 2012).

The ethanol extract of *E. jambolana* seeds, water extract of *M. charantia* fruits, ethanol extract of *G. sylvestre* leaves, and water extract of fenugreek seeds have higher hypoglyceamic and anti-hyperglyceamic potential and may be used as complementary medicine to treat the diabetic population by significantly reducing the dosage of standard drug (Yadav *et al.*, 2010).

Comparison with Hypoglyceamic Drugs

Diabetes mellitus is associated with an increase in sialic acid concentration along with other complications. Comparison of serum sialic acid concentration of patients, following bitter melon and rosiglitazone treatment revealed no significant difference but it was shown that bitter melon could be more effective in the management of diabetes and its related complications as compared to rosiglitazone (Inayat-ur-Rahman *et al.*, 2009).

The seed varieties of bittergourd were more effective than the glibenclamide, a known synthetic drug in normalizing the impaired oxidative stress in streptozotocin induced-diabetic rats (Sekar and Subramanian, 2005 c).

Bitter melon fruit aqueous extract reduced the blood glucose level similar to glibenclamide and increased the serum insulin level in the treated diabetic rats. The fruit extract alleviated pancreatic damage and increased the number of β-cells in the diabetic treated rats suggesting that oral feeding of the fruit extract may have a significant role in the renewal of pancreatic β-cells in the diabetic control group rats (Abdollahi *et al.*, 2011).

Bitter melon may have additive effects when taken with other glucose-lowering agents (Basch *et al.*, 2003). Yadav *et al.* (2005) found that the fruit extract and sodium orthovanadate, a well-known insulin mimetic and an anti-diabetic compound exhibited hypo-lipidemic as well as hypoglyceamic effect in diabetic rats and their effect was pronounced when administered in combination. Bitter melon significantly reduced fructosamine levels from baseline among patients with type 2 diabetes who received 2,000 mg/day. However, the hypoglyacemic effect of bitter melon was less than metformin (1,000 mg/day) (Fuangchan *et al.*, 2011). Huang *et al.* (2008) showed that Bitter melon can reduce insulin resistance as effective as the anti-diabetic drug thiazolidinedione.

In spite of the fact that numerous pre-clinical studies have documented the anti-diabetic and hypo-glycaemic effects of bitter gourd through various postulated mechanisms, Leung *et al.* (2009) called for better-designed clinical trials to further elucidate its possible therapeutic effects.

Safety

Bitter gourd has the potential to become a component of the diet or a dietary supplement for diabetic and pre-diabetic patients. According to Virdi *et al.* (2003) the aqueous extract powder of fresh unripe whole fruits did not show any signs of nephro-toxicity and hepato-toxicity as judged by histological and biochemical parameters. Thus the aqueous extract powder of *M. charantia* appears to be a safe alternative to reduce blood glucose.

Malik *et al.* (2011) also reported that bitter gourd has potent neuro-protective activity against global cerebral ischemia-reperfusion induced neuronal injury and consequent neurological deficits in diabetic mice. Snee *et al.* (2011) suggested that incorporating variety of foods along with bittergourd in commonly consumed recipes can mask bitter taste of bitter melon. Furthermore, providing positive health information can elicit a change in the intent to consume bitter melon-containing dishes despite mixed palatability results.

Jamun (*Eugenia jambolana*)

Jamun commonly known as Jambolan or Black Plum is found throughout the plains. Jamun was one of the significant anti-diabetic plants and it has long been reported for its use in many pharmacological conditions mainly diabetes. During the last four decades, numerous folk medicine and scientific reports on the anti-diabetic effects of this plant have been cited in the literature. Clinical and experimental studies suggest that, different parts of the plant especially fruits, seeds and stem bark possess promising activity against diabetes mellitus (Mukherjee *et al.*, 2006). The folkloric practice was consumption of juice extracted from the jamun leaf mixed with honey or cow's milk, or fresh fruits consumed twice a day orally after food for 3 months. Jamun seed extract (JSEt) has also been shown to possess hypo-glycaemic action. The decrease in thiobarbituric acid reactive substances (TBARS) and increase in reduced glutathione (GSH), superoxide dismutase (SOD) and catalase (CAT) clearly showed the anti-oxidant property of the JSEt. The effect of JSEt was most prominently seen in the case of animals given 5.0 g/kg body weight. JSEt was more effective than glibenclamide (Prince *et al.*, 1998).

Anti-hyperglyceamic effect of aqueous and alcoholic extract as well as lyophilized powder shows reduction in blood glucose level (Sheela and Augusti, 1992). The hypoglyceamic activity of jamun pulp extract in streptozotocin induced diabetic mice was seen within 30 min of administration while the seed of the same fruit required 24 h. The oral administration of the extract resulted in increased serum insulin levels in diabetic rats. Insulin secretion was found to be stimulated on incubation of plant extract with isolated islets of Langerhans from normal as well as diabetic animals. These extracts also inhibited insulinase activity from liver and kidney (Acherekar *et al.*, 1991) thus delaying the inactivation of insulin in the body. The elevated levels of cholesterol, phospholipids, triglycerides and free fatty acids were restored to near normal by jamun kernel or glibenclamide treatment in streptozotocin induced diabetic rats. Ravi *et al.* (2004a; 2004b; 2005) concluded that Jamun kernel possesses hypo-lipidemic effect, which may be due to the presence of flavonoids, saponins, glycosides and triterpenoids in the extract. Thus the efficacy of *Eugenia jambolana* seed kernel in the amelioration of diabetes may be attributed to its hypoglyceamic property along with its anti-oxidant potential of the seed kernel which also compared well with glibenclamide, a standard hypoglyceamic drug. Ravi *et al.* (2004 c) confirmed that the inorganic constituents play a important role in the antidiabetic nature of jamun seeds.

The ethanolic extract of dried jamun seed kernel (200 mg/kg) showed anti-hyperglyceamic effect on 10th day of its administration. There was a decrease in cholesterol level with little or no effect on triglycerides level. Interestingly, the extract was not only effective in reversing the increased propensity to ulceration in diabetic rats but also decreased the acid-pepsin output better than glibenclamide. Hence, Chaturvedi *et al.* (2009a) observed the ulcer protective effect of jamun was due to its antidiabetic and gastric antisecretory effects. Because of its both anti-hyperglyceamic and mucosal defensive actions, it could be a better choice for treating gastric ulcers co-occurring with diabetes (Chaturvedi *et al.* (2009b). Sridhar *et al.* (2005) also observed the anti-diabetic effect of jamun seed powder with an oral dose of 500 mg/kg. Subacute toxicity studies with a single administration of 2.5 and 5.0 g/kg seed powder showed no mortality or abnormality.

Garlic (*Allium sativum*) in Diabetes

Garlic has been used safely since ancient times as both food and medicine in human populations for several clinical conditions. Its usaga as a hypo-lipidemic agent is more popular. But, garlic also plays a beneficial role in diabetes. Several mechanisms were elucidated to explain the role of garlic in diabetes. Garlic was thought to increase hepatic metabolism, insulin release from pancreatic beta cells and/or exhibit insulin sparing effect (Bever and Zahnd 1979). Aqueous homogenate of garlic (10 ml/kg/day) administered orally to sucrose fed rabbits (10 g/kg/day in water for two months) significantly increased hepatic glycogen and free amino acid content, decreased fasting blood glucose, and triglyceride levels in serum in comparison to sucrose controls (Zacharias *et al.*, 1980). Allicin, a sulfur-containing compound is responsible for the pungent odour of garlic and it has been shown to have significant hypoglyceamic activity (Sheela and Augusti, 1992). S-allyl cystein sulfoxide (SACS), the precursor of allicin and garlic oil controlled lipid peroxidation better than glibenclamide and insulin. It also improved diabetic cmplications. SACS also stimulated *in vitro* insulin secretion from beta cells isolated from normal rats (Augusti and Sheela, 1996). Garlic was able to reduce blood glucose significantly compared with the control group (Jelodar *et al.*, 2005) thus further reiterating the benefit of garlic in diabetes.

In addition to fresh garlic, fermented form of the spice was also found to exhibit several therapeutic benefits. Yeast (Saccharomyces cerevisiae)-fermented aged black garlic (FBG) exhibited potent anti-oxidative effects. Jung *et al.* (2011b) suggested that the bioactivities of black garlic can be improved by yeast fermentation as FBG showed favourable hepato-protective, nephro-protective, hypo-lipidemic, and anti-obesity effects compared with the control, but no hypoglyceamic effects.

Fermented Garlic also prevented the risk factors of CVD among diabetics. Regular and prolonged use of therapeutic amounts of aged garlic extracts lowered blood homocysteine levels and showed prevention of some complications of diabetes mellitus. Padiya *et al.* (2011) observed significant ($p < 0.05$) reduction in body weight gain and serum glycated hemoglobin levels in fructose fed rats after garlic administration.

The anti-oxidant property of garlic is an added advantage to diabetics in the prevention of metabolic syndrome. Administration of raw garlic homogenate normalized both hepatic TBARS and GSH levels and thus concluded that raw garlic homogenate is effective in improving insulin sensitivity while attenuating metabolic syndrome and oxidative stress in fructose-fed rats. El-Demerdash *et al.* (2005) reported a cumulative effect of garlic and onion juices on oxidative stress and hyperglyceamia, and consequently they also alleviated liver and renal damage caused by alloxan-induced diabetes.

Consumption of garlic along with hypoglyceamic medications was proved to potentiate the action of the drug while contributing its own benefits. According to Ashraf *et al.* (2011) garlic is a good supplement in the management of patients with diabetes and hyper-lipidemia as combination of garlic (300 mg) tablet with typical anti-diabetic medicine (Metformin 500 mg) has shown to improve glyceamic control. In addition, (Ashraf *et al.*, 2005; 2011) there was a considerable decrease in mean total cholesterol and triglycerides and a significant increase in HDL cholesterol as compared to placebo group (Metformin 500 mg alone).

Onion (*Allium cepa*)

There are a few sporadic studies on onion as a hypoglycemic agent. An oral dose of 50 g of onion juice significantly controlled post-prandial glucose levels in diabetic patients (Mathew and Augusti, 1975). *A. cepa* and *A. sativum* possess a high level of anti-oxidant activity, which is attributed to the flavonoids and organosulphur compounds and have been demonstrated to possess anti-diabetic potential (Bhanot and Shri, 2010). But Islam *et al.* (2008) observd that a high fat diet impaired the anti-diabetic effect of freeze dried onion powder in diabetic rat model.

Administration of a sulfur containing amino acid from *Allium cepa*, S-methyl cysteine sulphoxide (SMCS) (200 mg/kg for 45 days) to alloxan induced diabetic rats significantly controlled blood glucose as well as lipids in serum and tissues and normalized the activities of enzymes involved in glucose metabolism, liver hexokinase, glucose 6-phosphatase and HMG Co A reductase (Roman-Ramos, 1995; Kumari *et al.*, 1995). The hypo-glycaemic and hypo-lipidaemic actions of *A. cepa* were associated with anti-oxidant activity, since superoxide dismutase activities decreased while lipid hydroperoxide and lipoperoxide concentrations did not increase in diabetic rats treated with *A. cepa* (Campos *et al.*, 2003).

Onion peel extract (OPE) improved glucose response and insulin resistance associated with type 2 diabetes by alleviating metabolic dysregulation of free fatty acids, suppressing oxidative stress, up-regulating glucose uptake at peripheral tissues, and/or down-regulating inflammatory gene expression in liver. Moreover, in most cases, OPE showed greater potency than pure quercetin equivalent providing a basis for the use of onion peel to improve insulin insensitivity in type 2 diabetes (Jung *et al.*, 2011a).

Barley in Diabetes

The ancient Hindu physician, Charaka had identified barley as a low glyceamic dietary substitute for diabetic patients around 2800 years ago. He also advocated different invigorating agents like honey, triphala and vinegar for use with barley-based diet and drink. Barley and its various products have been reported to possess preventive and therapeutic anti-diabetic properties, both in experimental animals and clinical studies.

Naismith *et al.* (1991) reported that barley reduced blood glucose level, water consumption and weight loss. Mahdi *et al.* (1994) observed that substitution of barley for sucrose reduced the elevated plasma concentration of 7-S collagen and of laminin P2, peptide fragments that retain antigenicity of the parent proteins. It is suggested that the beneficial property of barley is due to its high content of chromium. Malted barley extract alleviated many of the symptoms of diabetes in genetically obese mice and thus can be a good supplement for normalization of blood glucose levels in humans (Hong and Maeng, 2004). Li *et al.* (2003a) demonstrated that barley enabled glycemic control and improved glucose tolerance compared with rice or alpha-corn starch. Barley diet significantly improved the area under the plasma glucose concentration time curves, lowered the fasting plasma glucose and glycosylated hemoglobin levels, and decreased plasma total cholesterol, triglycerides and free fatty acid levels (Li *et al.*, 2003b).

Reports are available with barley administration on low glyceamic index and high insulinemic index (Shukla *et al.*, 1991), significant improvement in glycemic and insulinemic indices (Liljeberg *et al.*, 1996), improvement in glyceamic response and insulinemic response, reduced dependence on oral hypoglycemic drugs (Pick *et al.*, 1998) and improvement in impaired carbohydrate and lipid metabolism (Urooj *et al.*, 1998). However, no significant change in total cholesterol, HDL- cholesterol, triglycerides or in fasting and postprandial blood glucose level was also observed by Keogh, (2003). This lack of effect may be, at least in part, a consequence of structural changes in β-glucan that result from the commercial processing of the barley into a highly enriched β-glucan product or from the freezing, storage, or baking of the product during the intervention period. Reduction in postprandial glycemic peak with better insulin response, glycemic and insulinemic response (Poppitt *et al.*, 2007) and overall metabolic improvement in patients (Hinata *et al.*, 2007) were also noticed. The therapeutic benefits of barley made it suitable for its selection as a dietary substitute and inclusion of other fortifying agents in barley based diet and drink (Tiwari, 2008).

Cinnamon (*Cinnamomum tamala/Clitoria ternatea*)

Cinnamon has a long history as an anti-diabetic spice. The available *in vitro* and animal *in vivo* evidence suggests that cinnamon has anti-inflammatory, anitimicrobial, anti-oxidant, anti-tumor, cholesterol-lowering, and immuno-modulatory effects. In addition, Sharma and Majumdar (1990) found cinnamon to inhibit b-galactocidase and a-glucocidase. *In vitro* studies have demonstrated that cinnamon may act as an insulin mimetic, to potentiate insulin activity or to stimulate cellular glucose metabolism.

However, Vanschoonbeek *et al.* (2006) found that cinnamon supplementation (1.5 g/d) did not improve whole-body insulin sensitivity or oral glucose tolerance. On reviewing the available studies on cinnamon, Kirkham *et al.* (2009) also could not draw definite conclusions regarding the use of cinnamon as an antidiabetic agent due to limited number of well controlled studies. But they confirmed its potential to reduce postprandial blood glucose levels. Pham *et al.* (2007) and Mang *et al.* (2006) also reported that cinnamon has a possible modest effect in lowering plasma glucose levels in patients with poorly controlled type 2 diabetes. However, they suggested that clinicians should refrain themselves from recommending cinnamon supplementation in place of the proven standard of treatment.

But, animal studies have demonstrated strong dose dependent hypoglyceamic properties of cinnamon (Gruenwald *et al.*, 2010).Supplementation with 2g of cinnamon daily for 12 weeks resulted not only in a significant reduction in fasting plasma glucose (FPG), but also in waist circumference and body mass index (BMI) compared to baseline in the cinnamon group. The mean HbA1c was significantly decreased in the cinnamon group (8.22 per cent to 7.86 per cent) compared with placebo group (8.55 per cent to 8.68 per cent). However, the changes were not significant when compared to placebo group. There were no significant differences in total cholesterol, triglycerides, HDL and LDL cholesterol either between or within the groups. Mean systolic and diastolic blood pressures were also significantly reduced after 12 weeks in the cinnamon group compared with the placebo group (Akilen *et al.*, 2010).

Addition of cinnamon to the High fat/High fructose (HF/HF) diet increased the glucose infusion rates to those of the control rats. HF/HF+Cinnamon group (CN) prevented a reduction in pancreas weight induced by the HF/HF diet. This deleterious effect of mesenteric white fat accumulation observed in HF/HF rats was also alleviated when cinnamon was added to the diet thus suggesting that CN alters body composition in association with improved insulin sensitivity in animals fed a high fat/high fructose diet to induce insulin resistance (Couturier *et al.*, 2010). The study by Kim and Chaung (2010) also showed that cinnamon extract significantly increases insulin sensitivity, reduces serum, and hepatic lipids, and improves hyperglyceamia and hyperlipidemia possibly by regulating the PPAR-medicated glucose and lipid metabolism. Cinnamon intake, either as a whole or as cinnamon extract, results in a statistically significant reduction in Fasting Blood Glucose (FBG) (-0.49±0.2 mmol/L; n=8, P=.025); and intake of cinnamon extract alone also lowered FBG (-0.48 mmol/L±0.17; n=5, P=.008) (Davis and Yokoyama, 2011).

Curry Leaves (*Murraya koenigii*)

Curry leaves significantly altered the hepatic glycogen metabolism through enzyme modulation *i.e.* decreased hepatic gluconeogenesis and glycogenolysis by decreasing the activity of glycogen phosphorylase and gluconeogenic enzymes, and increased glycogenesis due to increased activity of glycogen synthetase (Khan *et al.*, 1995). Similar results were also observed later by Yadav *et al.* (2002) with different doses of curry leaves (5 per cent, 10 per cent and 15 per cent) fed to normal rats for 7 d as well as mild diabetic and moderate diabetic rats for 5 weeks. Results showed significant hypoglyceamic and anti-hyperglyceamic effects in diabetic rats.

Aqueous extract of curry leaves lowered blood glucose level in normal as well as in diabetic rabbits (Kesari *et al.*, 2005) Aqueous as well as methanol extracts of the leaves showed significant reduction ($P<0.05$) in blood glucose levels of diabetic rats as compared to diabetic control rats. Plasma insulin was also significantly high on 43rd and 58th days of treatment suggesting that the hypoglyceamic effect may be mediated through stimulating insulin synthesis and/or secretion from the beta cells of pancreatic islets of Langerhans (Vinuthan *et al.*, 2004; Lawal *et al.*, 2008).

Similarly, Arulselvan and Subramanian (2007) demonstrated the anti-oxidant and pancreatic β-cell protective effect of *M. koenigii.* The extract of *M. koenigii* reverted the increased levels of glucose, glycosylated hemoglobin, insulin, thiobarbituric acid reactive substances (TBARS) to normalcy while improving the enzymatic and non-enzymatic anti-oxidant concentrations. In addition, curry leaf administration showed nephroprotective activity in diabetic rats as the aqueous extract of leaves produced a significant dose-dependant decrease in serum urea and creatinine levels, and a marked increase in the levels of plasma anti-oxidant capacity. Histological studies of the kidneys of these animals showed comparable tissue regeneration by the aqueous extract (Yankuzo *et al.*, 2011) thus, scientifically supporting the traditional belief of using the leaves of *Murraya koenigii* as adjuvant, in the treatment of pain disorders related to renal impairments among diabetics.

Curry leaves also exhibited anti-inflammatory effect in diabetic mice. A reduction in interleukin-2, 4 and 10, tumor necrosis factor-α expression and the reduction of apoptosis in pancreatic cells revealed the anti-inflammatory response (Paul *et al.*, 2011).

The hypoglycemic effect of curry leaves was not found to be affected by processing. Freeze dried curry leaves lowered blood glucose level and improved glucose tolerance in normal and diabetic rats on oral administration (Chatterji *et al.*, 2010).

Honey on Diabetes

Charaka Samhita (Shastri *et al.*, 1962) emphasized that honey should also be taken along with various food preparations made up of barley. Animal experiments (Akhtar and Khan, 1989) and observations made in normal human volunteers, type-I diabetic patients (Samanta *et al.*, 1985) type-II diabetic patients (Al-Wailli, 2004), and in young adults with impaired glucose tolerance (Agrawal *et al.*, 2007) showed that honey attenuates postprandial hyperglyceamic response and hence may serve as a suitable sugar substitute for diabetics.

White Beans (*Phaseolus vulgaris*)

White bean pods are among the most widely used traditional remedies against diabetes mellitus. Venkateswaran and Pari (2002) found oral administration of Phaseolus vulgaris pod extract (200 mg/kg body weight) for 45 days to result in a significant reduction in thiobarbituric acid reactive substances and hydroperoxides. The extract also causes a significant increase in reduced glutathione, superoxide dismutase, catalase, glutathione peroxidase and glutathione-S-transferase in the liver and kidneys of rats with streptozotocin-induced diabetes. Apart from significant reduction in the elevated blood glucose, serum triglycerides, free fatty acids, phospholipids, total cholesterol, very-low-density lipoprotein cholesterol, and low-density lipoprotein cholesterol the extract also caused a significant decrease in plasma thiobarbituric acid-reactive substances (TBARS), hydroperoxides, vitamin E, and ceruloplasmin. The decreased serum levels of high-density lipoprotein cholesterol, anti-atherogenic index (AAI), plasma insulin, vitamin C, and glutathione in the diabetic rats were also reversed toward normalization (Venkateswaran *et al.*, 2002). The administration of Phaseolus vulgaris pods (PPEt) to diabetic animals normalized blood glucose and resulted in a marked improvement of altered carbohydrate metabolic enzymes during diabetes (Pari and Venkateswaran, 2003). The effect at 200 mg/kg of body weight was better than that of glibenclamide (Pari and Venkateswaran, 2004). Because of their fiber content and an alpha-amylase inhibitory effect, beans might be more useful as food components in preventing or ameliorating type 2 diabetes (Helmstädter, 2010; Barrett and Udani, 2011).

Green Tea (*Cassia auriculata*)

Tannins from the seed powder, decoction of flower buds of mature tea tree have been reported to be helpful. Sabu *et al.* (2002) found the aqueous extract of green tea polyphenols (GTP) to inhibit lipid peroxidation (LP), scavenge hydroxyl and superoxide radicals *in vitro*. The observations of Latha and Pari (2003) showed that the aqueous extract of Cassia auriculata possesses an anti-hyperglycemic effect and suggest that enhanced gluconeogenesis during diabetes is shifted towards normal and that the extract enhances the utilization of glucose through increased glycolysis. The effect of the extract was more prominent than that of glibenclamide. *Cassia auriculata* flower extract (CFEt), at doses of 0.15, 0.30 and 0.45 g/kg body weight for 30 days, suppressed the elevated blood glucose and lipid levels in diabetic rats (Pari and Latha, 2002). Apart from significant reduction in fasting blood glucose and glycosylated haemoglobin in both mild and severe diabetic rats, serum lipid levels were reversed towards normal in both the groups of rats (Gupta *et al.*, 2009a). Phytochemical screening of CLEt revealed the presence of alkaloids, flavonoids, saponins, tannins and cardiac glycosides with anti-hyperglyceamic and anti-oxidant properties suggesting the extract's protective role against diabetic complications (Gupta *et al.*, 2009 b).

Banana (*Musa sapientum*)

Musa sapientum ('Ney Poovan') commonly known as 'banana' is mainly used in Indian folk medicine for the treatment of diabetes mellitus. Oral administration of 0.15, 0.20 and 0.25 g/kg of chloroform extract of the *Musa sapientum* flowers (MSFEt) for 30 days resulted in a significant reduction in blood glucose, glycosylated haemoglobin and an increase in total hemoglobin, but in the case of 0.25 g/kg dose, the effect was highly significant. It also prevented weight loss (Pari and Umamaheswari, 1999; 2000).

Amla (*E. officinalis*) and Diabetes

Amla works by stimulating pancreas in diabetics. Though *E. officinalis* have been reported to possess beneficial anti- diabetic properties by various mechanisms, the homogeneous hypoglyceamic activity could be achieved only by the use of triphala Methanolic extract (75 per cent) of *Terminalia chebula, Terminalia belerica, Emblica officinalis* and their combination named 'Triphala' (equal proportion of above three plant extracts) are being used extensively in Indian system of medicine (Sabu and Kuttan, 2002). Oral administration of the extracts (100 mg/kg body weight) reduced the blood sugar level in normal and in alloxan (120 mg/kg) diabetic rats significantly within 4 h. Continued, daily administration of the drug produced a sustained effect.

Bilva Bael Fruit/Bengal Quince, Bel or Bilva (*Aegle marmelos*)

Aegle marmelos extract effectively reduced the oxidative stress induced by alloxan and produced a reduction in blood sugar (Sabu and Kuttan, 2004). Kesari *et al.* (2006) showed that the aqueous extract of bel seed (250 mg/kg) reduced the fasting blood glucose by 61 per cent and urine sugar by 75 per cent from their pretreatment levels. It brought about fall in the level of total cholesterol (TC) by 25 per cent with increase of 33 per cent in high density lipoprotein (HDL) and decrease of 54 and 46 per cent in low density lipoprotein (LDL) and triglyceride (TG), respectively in diabetic rats.

The histopathological study by Kamalakkannan and Prince (2005) on the bel fruit extract treated groups showed improved functional state of the pancreatic ss-cells and partially reversed the damage caused by streptozotocin to the pancreatic islets. The extract of A. marmelos modulates the activity of enzymic and nonenzymic antioxidants and enhances the defense against reactive oxygen species-generated damage in diabetic rats (Narendhirakannan and Subramanian, 2010). Abraham *et al.* (2010) demonstrated that the pyridoxine treatment alone and in combination with insulin and A. marmelose had a role in the regulation of insulin synthesis and release, normalizing diabetic related oxidative stress and neuro-degeneration affecting the motor ability of an individual by serotonergic receptors through 5-HT (2A) function.

Bhatti *et al.* (2011) showed that the ethanol extract of bel leaves attenuated the severity of the condition and improved the myocardium in the early stages of alloxan-induced diabetic cardiomyopathy at a dose of 200 mg kg(-1). Sharma *et al.* (2011) reported that the protective effect of fruit aqueous extract in type 2 diabetic rats is due to the preservation of β-cell function and insulin-sensitivity through increased PPARγ expression.

Methanol extract of the bark of *Aegle marmelos* at 200 and 400 mg/kg showed significant reduction in blood glucose level by 19.14 per cent and 47.32 per cent, respectively in diabetic rats. It also significantly increased insulin level, and produced similar effects on other biochemical parameters. Histological studies showed the regenerative effect on the β-cells of diabetic rats. Immuno-histochemical observations in the extract treated diabetic rats showed increased insulin-immunoreactive β-cells (Gandhi *et al.*, 2012).

Gurmar (*Gymnema sylvestre*)

The Hindi word Gur-mar, Madhunaashini in Sanskrit, Chakkarakolli in Malayalam, Podapatri in Telugu, literally means sugar destroyer. Extracts of this plant are widely used in Australian, Japanese, Vietnamese and Indian folk medicine. Gymnema preparations have a profound action on the modulation of taste, particularly suppressing sweet taste sensations. It is used in the treatment of diabetes mellitus and in food additives against obesity and caries. Anti-allergic, antiviral, lipid lowering and other effects are also reported (Porchezhian and Dobriyal, 2003). The EtOH/H_2O extracts of the leaves of gurmar were shown to be able to inhibit glucose absorption in rats (Zhu *et al.*, 2008). Supplementation of the diet with *G.sylvestre* reduced polyphagia, fatigue, blood glucose (fasting and post-prandial), and glycated hemoglobin and there was a favorable shift in lipid profiles and in other clinico-biochemical tests (Kumar *et al.*, 2010).

Gupta (1983) Gupta and Variyar (1964), Khare *et al.* (1983), Baskaran *et al.* (1990), Murakami *et al.* (1996) and Kinghorn *et al.* (2001) reported that Gymnema saponins I-II and gymnemic acids I-IX present in *G.sylvestre* neutralize excess sugar in diabetics. The administration of Inula racemosa and *G. sylvestre* extracts in combination proved to be more effective than the individual extracts. These effects were comparable to a standard corticosteroid-inhibiting drug, ketoconazole (Gholap and Kar, 2003). Daisy *et al.* (2009) reported that the dihydroxy gymnemic triacetate, the compound from *G. sylvestre*, possessed hypoglycemic and hypolipidemic activity in long-term treatment. Ahmed *et al.* (2010) found the gymnemic acid of leaf and callus extracts were responsible for the significant increase in the regeneration of β-cells in treated rats, when compared with the standard diabetic rats. All these studies confirm that *G.sylvestre* could be used as a drug for treating diabetes.

According to the authors, these extracts may not prove to be effective in thyroid hormone mediated type II diabetes but for corticosteroid induced diabetes mellitus (Gholap and Kar, 2004). According to Al-Romaiyan (2010; 2012) *G.sylvestre* stimulates insulin secretion from mouse and human islets *in vitro*, at least in part as a consequence of Ca (2+) influx and protein kinase activation. Feeding *G. sylvestre* extract to the diabetic rats decreased the activity of glutathione peroxidase in cytosolic liver and glutamate pyruvate transaminase in serum to normal levels (Kang *et al.*, 2012).

Aloe vera

Aloe vera gel, the leaf pulp or mucilage, aloe latex, commonly referred to as aloe juice is a bitter yellow exudate from the pericyclic tubules just beneath the outer skin of the leaves. Extracts of aloe gum effectively increases glucose tolerance in both normal and diabetic rats (Al-Awadi *et al.*, 1987). Single as well as chronic doses of bitter principle of the same plant also showed hypoglyceamic effect in diabetic rats. This action of *Aloe vera* and its bitter principle is through stimulation of synthesis and/or release of insulin from pancreatic beta cells. Noel *et al.* (1997) have also reported aloe vera to be hypoglyceamic. Oral administration of ethanolic extract of *Aloe vera* at a concentration of 300 mg/kg

(-1) body weight for 21 days resulted in a significant reduction in fasting blood glucose, thiobarbituric acid reactive substances, hydroperoxides and alpha-tocopherol and significant improvement in ascorbic acid, reduced glutathione and insulin in the plasma of diabetic rats. Interestingly, the ethanolic extract of *Aloe vera* appeared to be more effective than glibenclamide in controlling oxidative stress (Rajasekaran *et al.*, 2005a). Treatment with the extract also resulted in a significant increase in reduced glutathione, superoxide dismutase, catalase, glutathione peroxidase and glutathione-S-transferase in the liver and kidney of diabetic rats. These results clearly showed the anti-oxidant property of *Aloe vera* gel extract (Rajasekaran *et al.*, 2005b). The increased levels of lipid peroxidation and hydroperoxides in tissues of diabetic rats were reverted back to near normal levels after the treatment with gel extract.

Oral administration of *Aloe vera* gel extract at a dose of 300 mg/kg body weight per day to STZ-induced diabetic rats for a period of 21 days resulted in a significant reduction in fasting blood glucose, hepatic transaminases (aspartate aminotransferase and alanine aminotransferase), plasma and tissue (liver and kidney) cholesterol, triglycerides, free fatty acids and phospholipids and a significant improvement in plasma insulin. The decreased plasma levels of high-density lipoprotein-cholesterol and increased plasma levels of low-density lipoprotein-cholesterol and very low-density lipoprotein-cholesterol in diabetic rats were restored to near normal levels following treatment with the extract. The altered fatty acid composition in the liver and kidney of diabetic rats was also restored following treatment with the extract (Rajasekaran *et al.*, 2006).

Colocasia (*Colocasia esculenta*)

Colocasia commonly known as 'Alu and dasheen' is widely used in traditional system of medicine for the treatment of diabetes mellitus. Kumawat *et al.* (2010) reported that 400 mg/kg of ethanolic extract of colocasia leaves showed anti-hyperglycaemic activity in alloxan induced diabetic rats.

Soya (*Glycine max*)

Cederroth *et al.* (2008) reported that mice fed with soy-rich diet have improved adipose and glucose metabolism. According to yhem activation of the AMPK pathway by dietary soy is likely involved and may mediate the beneficial effects of dietary soy in peripheral tissues. Hence they suggested that dietary soy could prove useful to prevent obesity and associated disorders.

McCue *et al.* (2005) reported that sprouting and dietary fungal bioprocessing of soybean improved the anti-diabetic potential of soybean extracts, potentially through modulation of the phenolic profile of the extract, and further suggested that enzyme inhibitory activity may be linked to phenolic anti-oxidant mobilization during spouting and/or bio-processing.

Cranberry (*Vaccinium oxycoccos/Oxycoccus palustris*)

The enhanced functionality in terms of high alpha-glucosidase and alpha-amylase inhibitory activities of Cranberry indicated the potential for diabetes management, and the high ACE-I inhibitory activity indicated its potential for hypertension management (Apostolidis *et al.*, 2006).

Tulasi/holy basil (*Ocimum sanctum*)

Since ancient times, Tulasi is known for its medicinal properties. The aqueous extract of leaves of *Ocimum sanctum* showed the significant reduction in blood sugar level in both normal and alloxan induced diabetic rats (Vats *et al.*, 2002). Significant reduction in fasting blood glucose, uronic acid, total amino acid, total cholesterol, triglyceride and total lipid indicated the hypoglyceamic and hypo-lipidemic effects of tulsi in diabetic rats (Rai *et al.*, 1997). Oral administration of plant extract (200 mg/kg) for 30 days led to decrease in the plasma glucose level by approximately 9.06 and 26.4 per cent on 15 and 30 days of the experiment respectively. Renal glycogen content increased 10 fold while skeletal muscle and hepatic glycogen levels decreased by 68 and 75 per cent respectively in diabetic rats as compared to control (Vats *et al.*, 2004).

Neem (*Azadirachta indica*)

Siddiqui (1942) found the active principle in neem to be the bitter principles nimbin, nimbinin, nimbidin. Siddiqui (1942), Murthy *et al.* (1978), Pillai and Santhakumari (1981) have all reported that neem leaf juice, bark and flowers to lower the blood glucose in diabetics. Hydroalcoholic extracts of this plant was found to show anti-hyperglycemic activity in streptozotocin treated rats and this effect is because of increase in glucose uptake and glycogen deposition in isolated rat hemi diaphragm.

Conclusions

Diabetes and its complications are worldwide metabolic disorders. The current researchers are focusing on the plant foods and herbs to attenuate the same. Bitter gourd, fenugreek seeds, cinnamon, barley, garlic and aloe vera have been studied extensively confirming their anti-diabetic properties. Numerous herbs are found to be effective in diabetes. Since, it is out of scope of this book, information on herbs has not been included in it.

References

Abdollahi M, Zuki AB, Goh YM, Rezaeizadeh A, Noordin MM (2011). Effects of *Momordica charantia* on pancreatic histopathological changes associated with streptozotocin-induced diabetes in neonatal rats. Histol. Histopathol. 26 (1): 13 - 21.

Abraham PM, Paul J, Paulose CS (2010). Down regulation of cerebellar serotonergic receptors in streptozotocin induced diabetic rats: Effect of pyridoxine and *Aegle marmelose*. Brain Res. Bull. 82 (1-2): 87 - 94.

Acherekar S., Kaklij G.S., Kelkar S.M. (1991). Hypoglyceamic activity of *Eugenia jambolana* and *ficus bengalensis*: mechanism of action. *In vivo*. 5: 143 - 147.

Aggarwal BB (2010). Targeting inflammation-induced obesity and metabolic diseases by curcumin and other nutraceuticals. Annu. Rev. Nutr. 30: 173 - 99.

Agrawal OP, Pachauri A, Yadav H, Urmila J, Goswamy HM, Chapperwal A, Bisen PS, Prasad GB (2007). Subjects with impaired glucose tolerance exhibit a high degree of tolerance to honey. J. Med. Food, 10: 473 - 78.

Ahmad N, Hassan MR, Halder H, Bennoor KS (1999). Effect of *Momordica charantia* (Karolla) extracts on fasting and postprandial serum glucose levels in NIDDM patients. Bangladesh Med. Res. Counc. Bull. 25 (1): 11 - 13.

Ahmed AB, Rao AS, Rao MV (2010). *In vitro* callus and *in vivo* leaf extract of *Gymnema sylvestre* stimulate β-cells regeneration and anti-diabetic activity in Wistar rats. Phytomedicine. 17 (13): 1033 - 39.

Ahmed I, Lakhani MS, Gillett M, John A, Raza H (2001). Hypo-triglyceridemic and hypocholesterolemic effects of anti-diabetic *Momordica charantia* (karela) fruit extract in streptozotocin-induced diabetic rats. Diabetes Res. Clin. Pract. 51 (3): 155 - 61.

Akhtar MS, and Khan MS (1989). Glycemic response to three different honeys given to normal and alloxan diabetic rabbits. J. Pak. Med. Assoc. 39: 107 - 113.

Akilen R, Tsiami A, Devendra D, Robinson N (2010). Glycated hemoglobin and blood pressure-lowering effect of cinnamon in multi-ethnic Type 2 diabetic patients in the UK: a randomized, placebo-controlled, double-blind clinical trial. Diabet. Med. 27 (10): 1159 - 67.

Al-Awadi FM, Gumaa KA (1987). Studies on the activity of individual plants of an anti-diabetic plant mixture. Acta. Diabetol. Lat. 24 (1): 37 - 41.

Al-Mustafa AH, Al-Thunibat OY (2008). Anti-oxidant activity of some Jordanian medicinal plants used traditionally for treatment of diabetes. Pak. J. Biol. Sci. 11 (3): 351 - 58.

Al-Romaiyan A, Liu B, Asare-Anane H, Maity CR, Chatterjee SK, Koley N, Biswas T, Chatterji AK, Huang GC, Amiel SA, Persaud SJ, Jones PM (2010). A novel *Gymnema sylvestre* extract stimulates insulin secretion from human islets *in vivo* and *in vitro*. Phytother. Res. 24 (9): 1370 - 76.

Al-Romaiyan A, Liu B, Docherty R, Huang GC, Amiel S, Persaud SJ, Jones PM (2012). Investigation of intracellular signalling cascades mediating stimulatory effect of a *Gymnema sylvestre* extract on insulin secretion from isolated mouse and human islets of Langerhans. Diabetes Obes. Metab. 6; 9999 (9999). [Epub ahead of print].

Ali L, Azad Khan AK, Hassan Z, Mosihuzzaman M, Nahar N, Nasreen T, Nur-e-Alam M, Rokeya B (1995). Characterization of the hypoglyceamic effects of *Trigonella foenum graecum* seed. Planta. Med. 61 (4): 358 - 60.

Al-Wailli NS (2004). Natural honey lowers plasma glucose, C-reactive protein, homocysteine and blood lipids in healthy, diabetic and hyper-lipidemic subjects: Comparison with dextrose and sucrose. J. Med. Food, 7, 100 - 107.

Anderson RA (2008). Chromium and polyphenols from cinnamon improve insulin sensitivity. Proc. Nutr. Soc. 67 (1): 48 - 53.

Apostolidis E, Kwon YI, Shetty K (2006). Potential of cranberry-based herbal synergies for diabetes and hypertension management. Asia Pac. J. Clin. Nutr. 15 (3): 433 - 41.

Arulselvan P, Subramanian SP (2007). Beneficial effects of *Murraya koenigii* leaves on antioxidant defense system and ultra structural changes of pancreatic β-cells in experimental diabetes in rats [J]. Chem. Biol. Interact. 165 (2) : 155 - 64.

Ashraf R, Aamir K, Shaikh AR, Ahmed T (2005). Effects of garlic on dyslipidemia in patients with type 2 diabetes mellitus. J. Ayub. Med. Coll. Abbottabad. 17 (3): 60 - 64.

Ashraf R, Khan RA, Ashraf I (2011). Garlic (*Allium sativum*) supplementation with standard anti-diabetic agent provides better diabetic control in type 2 diabetes patients. Pak. J. Pharm. Sci. 24 (4): 565 - 70.

Augusti KT, Sheela CG (1996). Antiperoxide effect of S-allyl cysteine sulfoxide, an insulin secretagogue in diabetic rats. Experientia. 52: 115 - 120.

Ayyanar M, Sankarasivaraman K and Ignacimuthu S (2008). Traditional Herbal Medicines Used for the Treatment of Diabetes among Two Major Tribal Groups in South Tamil Nadu, India. Ethnobotanical Leaflets. 12: 276 - 80.

Bahia PK, Rattray M, Williams RJ (2008). Dietary flavonoid (-)epicatechin stimulates phosphatidylinositol 3-kinase-dependent anti-oxidant response element activity and up-regulates glutathione in cortical astrocytes. J. Neurochem. 106 (5): 2194 - 204.

Baldwa VS, Bhandari CM, Pangaria A, Goyal RK (1977). Clinical trial in patients with diabetes mellitus of an insulin-like compound obtained from plant source. Ups. J. Med. Sci. 82 (1): 39 - 41.

Balzer J, Rassaf T, Heiss C, Kleinbongard P, Lauer T, Merx M, Heussen N, Gross HB, Keen CL, Schroeter H, Kelm M (2008). Sustained benefits in vascular function through flavanol-containing cocoa in medicated diabetic patients a double-masked, randomized, controlled trial. J. Am. Coll. Cardiol. 51 (22): 2141 - 49.

Baquer NZ, Kumar P, Taha A, Kale RK, Cowsik SM, McLean P (2011). Metabolic and molecular action of *Trigonella foenum-graecum* (fenugreek) and trace metals in experimental diabetic tissues. J. Biosci. 36 (2): 383 - 96.

Barrett ML, Udani JK (2011). A proprietary alpha-amylase inhibitor from white bean (*Phaseolus vulgaris*): a review of clinical studies on weight loss and glycemic control. Nutr. J. 10: 24.

Basch E, Gabardi S, Ulbricht C (2003). Bitter melon (*Momordica charantia*): a review of efficacy and safety. Am. J. Health Syst. Pharm. 60 (4): 356 - 59.

Bever BO, Zahnd GR (1979). Plants with oral hypoglyceamic action. Quart. J. Crude Drug Res. 17: 139 - 146.

Baskaran K, Kizar AB, Shanmugasundaram, Radha K, Shanmugsundaram ERB (1990). Anti-diabetic effect of a leaf extract from *Gymnema sylvestre* in NIDDM patients. J. Ethnopharmacol. 30: 296 - 305.

Bhanot A, Shri R (2010). A comparative profile of methanol extracts of *Allium cepa* and *Allium sativum* in diabetic neuropathy in mice. Pharmacognosy. Res. 2 (6): 374 - 84.

Bhatti R, Sharma S, Singh J, Ishar MP (2011). Ameliorative effect of *Aegle marmelos* leaf extract on early stage alloxan-induced diabetic cardiomyopathy in rats. Pharm. Biol. 49 (11): 1137 - 43.

Bhujbal SS, Hadawale SS, Kulkarni PA, Bidkar JS, Thatte VA, Providencia CA, Yeola RR (2011). A novel herbal formulation in the management of diabetes. Int. J. Pharm. Investig. 1 (4): 222 - 26.

Bhutada P, Mundhada Y, Bansod K, Bhutada C, Tawari S, Dixit P, Mundhada D (2010). Ameliorative effect of quercetin on memory dysfunction in streptozotocin-induced diabetic rats. Neurobiol. Learn. Mem. 94 (3): 293 - 302.

Bhutada P, Mundhada Y, Bansod K, Tawari S, Patil S, Dixit P, Umathe S, Mundhada D (2011). Protection of cholinergic and anti-oxidant system contributes to the effect of berberine ameliorating memory dysfunction in rat model of streptozotocin-induced diabetes. Behav. Brain. Res. 220 (1): 30 - 41.

Blum A, Loerz C, Martin HJ, Staab-Weijnitz CA, Maser E (2012). *Momordica charantia* extract, a herbal remedy for type 2 diabetes, contains a specific 11 β-hydroxysteroid dehydrogenase type 1 inhibitor. J. Steroid. Biochem. Mol. Biol. 128 (1-2): 51 - 55.

Campos KE, Diniz YS, Cataneo AC, Faine LA, Alves MJ, Novelli EL (2003). Hypoglyceamic and antioxidant effects of onion, *Allium cepa*: dietary onion addition, antioxidant activity and hypoglyceamic effects on diabetic rats. Int. J. Food Sci. Nutr. 54 (3): 241 - 46.

Cederroth CR, Vinciguerra M, Gjinovci A, Kühne F, Klein M, Cederroth M, Caille D, Suter M, Neumann D, James RW, Doerge DR, Wallimann T, Meda P, Foti M, Rohner-Jeanrenaud F, Vassalli JD, Nef S (2008). Dietary phytoestrogens activate AMP-activated protein kinase with improvement in lipid and glucose metabolism. Diabetes. 57 (5): 1176 - 85.

Chan MM (1995). Inhibition of tumor necrosis factor by curcumin, a phytochemical. Biochem. Pharmacol. 49 (11): 1551 - 56.

Chatterji S, Singh RK, Shukla S, Yadav DK, Watal G (2010). Glyceamic effect of freeze dried *Murraya koenigii* – an evidence based study [J]. Int. J. Pharma. Bio. Sci. 1(2): 1 - 9.

Chaturvedi P (2005). Role of Momordica charantia in maintaining the normal levels of lipids and glucose in diabetic rats fed a high-fat and low-carbohydrate diet. Br. J. Biomed. Sci. 62 (3): 124 - 26.

Chaturvedi P (2012). Antidiabetic potentials of *Momordica charantia:* multiple mechanisms behind the effects. J. Med. Food. 15 (2): 101 - 107.

Chaturvedi A, Bhawani G, Agarwal PK, Goel S, Singh A, Goel RK (2009a). Antidiabetic and antiulcer effects of extract of *Eugenia jambolana* seed in mild diabetic rats: study on gastric mucosal offensive acid-pepsin secretion. Indian J. Physiol. Pharmacol. 53 (2): 137 - 46.

Chaturvedi A, Bhawani G, Agarwal PK, Goel S, Singh A, Goel RK (2009b). Ulcer healing properties of ethanolic extract of *Eugenia jambolana* seed in diabetic rats: study on gastric mucosal defensive factors. Indian J. Physiol.Pharmacol. 53 (1): 16 - 24.

Chaturvedi P, George S, Milinganyo M, Tripathi YB (2004). Effect of *Momordica charantia* on lipid profile and oral glucose tolerance in diabetic rats. Phytother. Res. 18 (11): 954 - 56.

Chaturvedi P, George S (2010). *Momordica charantia* maintains normal glucose levels and lipid profiles and prevents oxidative stress in diabetic rats subjected to chronic sucrose load. J. Med. Food. 13 (3): 520 - 27.

Chen Q, Chan LL, Li ET (2003). Bitter melon (*Momordica charantia*) reduces adiposity, lowers serum insulin and normalizes glucose tolerance in rats fed a high fat diet. J. Nutr. 133 (4): 1088 - 93.

Choudhary SK, Chhabra G, Sharma D, Vashishta A, Ohri S, Dixit A (2012). Comprehensive evaluation of anti-hyperglyceamic activity of fractionated *Momordica charantia* Seed Extract in Alloxan-Induced Diabetic Rats. Evid. Based Complement. Alternat. Med. 2012: 293650.

Chowdhury AR, Sharma S, Mandal S, Goswami A, Mukhopadhyay S, Majumder HK (2002). Luteolin, an emerging anti-cancer flavonoid, poisons eukaryotic DNA topoisomerase I. Biochem J. 366 (Pt 2): 653 - 61.

Clouatre DL, Rao SN, Preuss HG (2011). Bitter melon extracts in diabetic and normal rats favorably influence blood glucose and blood pressure regulation. J. Med. Food. 14 (12): 1496 - 504.

Couturier K, Batandier C, Awada M, Hininger-Favier I, Canini F, Anderson RA, Leverve X, Roussel AM (2010). Cinnamon improves insulin sensitivity and alters the body composition in an animal model of the metabolic syndrome. Arch. Biochem. Biophys. 501 (1): 158 - 61.

Cummings E, Hundal HS, Wackerhage H, Hope M, Belle M, Adeghate E, Singh J (2004). *Momordica charantia* fruit juice stimulates glucose and amino acid uptakes in L6 myotubes. Mol. Cell. Biochem. 261 (1-2): 99 - 104.

Daisy P, Eliza J, Mohamed Farook KA (2009). A novel dihydroxy gymnemic triacetate isolated from *Gymnema sylvestre* possessing normoglycemic and hypolipidemic activity on STZ-induced diabetic rats. J. Ethnopharmacol. 126 (2): 339 - 44.

Davis PA, Yokoyama W (2011). Cinnamon intake lowers fasting blood glucose: meta-analysis. J. Med. Food. 14 (9): 884 - 89.

Day C (1990). Hypoglyceamic compounds from plants. In New Anti-diabetic Drugs. CJ Bailey and PR Flatt, editors. Smith-Gordon. London: pp. 267 - 78.

Day C (1995). Hypoglyceamic plant compounds. Practical. Diabetes. 2: 269 - 71.

Day C, Cartwright T, Provost J and Bailey CJ (1989). Hypo-glycaemic effect of *Momordica charantia* extracts. Planta. Medica. 56: 426 - 29.

El-Demerdash FM, Yousef MI, El-Naga NI (2005). Biochemical study on the hypoglyceamic effects of onion and garlic in alloxan-induced diabetic rats. Food Chem. Toxicol. 43 (1): 57 - 63.

Fernandes NP, Lagishetty CV, Panda VS, Naik SR (2007). An experimental evaluation of the anti-diabetic and anti-lipidemic properties of a standardized *Momordica charantia* fruit extract. BMC. Complement. Altern. Med. 7: 29.

Fuangchan A, Sonthisombat P, Seubnukarn T, Chanouan R, Chotchaisuwat P, Sirigulsatien V, Ingkaninan K, Plianbangchang P, Haines ST (2011). Hypoglyceamic effect of bitter melon compared with metformin in newly diagnosed type 2 diabetes patients. J. Ethnopharmacol. 134 (2): 422 - 28.

Gandhi GR, Ignacimuthu S, Paulraj MG (2012). Hypoglyceamic and β-cells regenerative effects of *Aegle marmelos* (L.) Corr. bark extract in streptozotocin-induced diabetic rats. Food Chem. Toxicol. 50 (5): 1667 - 74.

Gholap S, Kar A (2003). Effects of Inula racemosa root and *Gymnema sylvestre* leaf extracts in the regulation of corticosteroid induced diabetes mellitus: involvement of thyroid hormones. Pharmazie 58 (6): 413 - 15.

Gholap S, Kar A (2004). Hypo-glycaemic effects of some plant extracts are possibly mediated through inhibition in corticosteroid concentration. Pharmazie. 59 (11): 876 - 78.

Gray AM and Flatt PR (1997). Nature's own pharmacy: the diabetes perspective. Proceedings of the Nutrition Society. 56: 507 - 517.

Gray AM and Flatt PR (1998a). Actions of the traditional anti-diabetic plant *Agrimony eupatoria* (agrimony): effects of hyperglycaemia, cellular glucose metabolism and insulin secretion. British Journal of Nutrition. 80: 109 - 114.

Gray AM and Flatt PR (1998b). Insulin-releasing and insulin-like activity of *Agaricus campestris* (mushroom). Journal of Endocrinology. 157 (2): 259 - 66.

Grover JK, Yadav S, Vats V (2002). Medicinal plants of India with anti-diabetic potential. J. Ethnopharmacol. 81 (1): 81 - 100.

Gruenwald J, Freder J, Armbruester N (2010). Cinnamon and health. Crit. Rev. Food Sci. Nutr. 50 (9): 822 - 34.

Gupta SS (1983). Effect of *Gymnema sylvestre* and *Pterocarpus marsupium* on glucose tolerance in albino rats. Ind. J. Med.Res. 7: 501.

Gupta D, Raju J, Baquer NZ (1999). Modulation of some gluconeogenic enzyme activities in diabetic rat liver and kidney: effect of anti-diabetic compounds. Indian J. Expt. Biol. 37: 196 - 99.

Gupta S, Sharma SB, Bansal SK, Prabhu KM (2009 a). Anti-hyperglyceamic and hypolipidemic activity of aqueous extract of *Cassia auriculata* L. leaves in experimental diabetes. J. Ethnopharmacol. 123 (3): 499 - 503.

Gupta S, Sharma SB, Prabhu KM, Bansal SK (2009 b). Protective role of *Cassia auriculata* leaf extract on hyperglyceamia-induced oxidative stress and its safety evaluation. Indian J. Biochem. Biophys. 46 (5): 371 - 77.

Gupta SS, Variyar MC (1964). Experimental studies on pituitary diabetes, Part IV, effect of *Gymnena sylvestre* and *Coccinia indica* W and A against hypoglyceamic response of somatotropis and corticotrophin hormones. Ind. J. Med. Res. 52: 200 - 204.

Hafizur RM, Kabir N, Chishti S (2011). Modulation of pancreatic β-cells in neonatally streptozotocin-induced type 2 diabetic rats by the ethanolic extract of *Momordica charantia* fruit pulp. Nat. Prod. Res. 25 (4): 353 - 67.

Hannan JM, Ali L, Rokeya B, Khaleque J, Akhter M, Flatt PR, Abdel-Wahab YH (2007). Soluble dietary fibre fraction of *Trigonella foenum-graecum* (fenugreek) seed improves glucose homeostasis in animal models of type 1 and type 2 diabetes by delaying carbohydrate digestion and absorption, and enhancing insulin action. Br. J. Nutr. 97 (3): 514 - 21.

Haque N, Salma U, Nurunnabi TR, Uddin MJ, Jahangir MF, Islam SM, Kamruzzaman M (2011). Management of type 2 diabetes mellitus by lifestyle, diet and medicinal plants. Pak. J. Biol. Sci. 14 (1): 13 - 24.

Hazarika R, Parida P, Neog B, Yadav RN (2012). Binding Energy calculation of GSK-3 protein of Human against some anti-diabetic compounds of *Momordica charantia* Linn. (Bitter melon). Bioinformation. 8 (6): 251 - 54.

Helmstädter A (2010). Beans and diabetes: *Phaseolus vulgaris* preparations as antihyperglycemic agents. J. Med. Food. 13 (2): 251 - 54.

Hinata M, Ono M, Midorokawa S and Nakanishi K (2007). Metabolic improvements of male prisoners with type 2 diabetes in Fukushima prison, Japan. Diab. Res. Clin. Pract. 77: 327 - 32.

Hong H and Maeng JW (2004). Effects of malted barley extracts and banana extract on blood glucose levels in genetically diabetic mice. J. Med. Food, 7: 487 - 90.

Huang HL, Hong YW, Wong YH, Chen YN, Chyuan JH, Huang CJ, Chao PM (2008). Bitter melon (*Momordica charantia* L.) inhibits adipocyte hypertrophy and down regulates lipogenic gene expression in adipose tissue of diet-induced obese rats. Br. J. Nutr. 99 (2): 230 - 39.

Inayat-ur-Rahman, Malik SA, Bashir M, Khan R, Iqbal M (2009). Serum sialic acid changes in non-insulin-dependant diabetes mellitus (NIDDM) patients following bitter melon (*Momordica charantia*) and rosiglitazone (Avandia) treatment. Phytomedicine. 16 (5): 401 – 405.

Islam MS, Choi H, Loots du T (2008). Effects of dietary onion (*Allium cepa* L.) in a high-fat diet streptozotocin-induced diabetes rodent model. Ann Nutr. Metab. 53 (1): 6 - 12.

Jelodar GA, Maleki M, Motadayen MH, Sirus S (2005). Effect of fenugreek, onion and garlic on blood glucose and histopathology of pancreas of alloxan-induced diabetic rats. Indian J. Med. Sci. 59 (2): 64 - 69.

Jia W, Gao W, Tang L (2003). Antidiabetic herbal drugs officially approved in China. Phytother. Res. 17 (10): 1127 - 34.

Jung JY, Lim Y, Moon MS, Kim JY, Kwon O (2011a). Onion peel extracts ameliorate hyperglyceamia and insulin resistance in high fat diet/streptozotocin-induced diabetic rats. Nutr. Metab. (Lond). 8 (1): 18.

Jung YM, Lee SH, Lee DS, You MJ, Chung IK, Cheon WH, Kwon YS, Lee YJ, Ku SK (2011b). Fermented garlic protects diabetic, obese mice when fed a high-fat diet y antioxidant effects. Nutr. Res. 31 (5): 387 - 96.

Kamalakkannan N, Prince PS (2005). The effect of *Aegle marmelos* fruit extract in streptozotocin diabetes: a histopathological study. J. Herb. Pharmacother. 5 (3): 87 - 96.

Kamalakkannan N, Prince PS (2006). Anti-hyperglyceamic and anti-oxidant effect of rutin, a polyphenolic flavonoid, in streptozotocin-induced diabetic wistar rats. Basic Clin. Pharmacol. Toxicol. 98 (1): 97 - 103.

Kang MH, Lee MS, Choi MK, Min KS, Shibamoto T (2012). Hypoglyceamic activity of *Gymnema sylvestre* extracts on oxidative stress and antioxidant status in diabetic rats. J. Agric. Food Chem. 60 (10): 2517 - 24.

Keller AC, Ma J, Kavalier A, He K, Brillantes AM, Kennelly EJ (2011). Saponins from the traditional medicinal plant *Momordica charantia* stimulate insulin secretion *in vitro*. Phytomedicine. 19 (1): 32 - 37.

Keogh GF, Cooper GJ, Mulvev TB, McArdle BH, Coles GD, Monro JA and Poppitt SD (2003). Randomized controlled crossover study of the effect of a highly beta-glucan enriched barley on cardiovascular disease risk factors in mildly hyper-cholesterolemic men. Am. J. Clin. Nutr. 78: 711 - 18.

Kesari AN, Gupta RK, Singh SK, Diwakar S, Watal G (2006). Hypoglyceamic and anti-hyperglycemic activity of *Aegle marmelos* seed extract in normal and diabetic rats. J. Ethnopharmacol. 107 (3): 374 - 79.

Kesari AN, Gupta RK, Watal G (2005). Hypoglycemic effects of *Murraya koenigii* on normal and alloxan-diabetic rabbits [J]. J. Ethnopharmacol, 97 (2): 247 - 51.

Khan BA, Abraham A, Leelamma S (1995). Hypoglyceamic action of *Murraya koenigii* (curry leaf) and *Brassica juncea* (mustard): mechanism of action [J]. Indian J. Biochem. Biophys. 32 (2): 106 - 108.

Khanna P, Jain SC, Panagariya A, Dixit VP (1981). Hypoglyceamic activity of polypeptide- p from a plant source. J. Nat. Prod. 44: 648 - 55.

Khare AK, Tondon RN, Tewari JP (1983). Hypoglyceamic activity of an indigenous drug: *Gymnema sylvestre* in normal and diabetic persons. Ind. J. Physiol. Pharmacol. 27 (3): 257 - 58.

Khosla P, Gupta DD, Nagpal RK (1995). Effect of *Trigonella foenum graecum* (fenugreek) on blood glucose in normal and diabetic rats. Indian J. Physiol. Pharmacol. 39: 173 - 74.

Kim SH, Choung SY (2010). Anti-hyperglycemic and anti-hyperlipidemic action of *Cinnamoum Cassiae* (Cinnamon bark) extract in C57BL/Ks db/db mice. Arch. Pharm. Res. 33 (2): 325 - 33.

Kim JW, Cho HR, Moon SB, Kim KY, Ku S (2012). Synergic effects of bitter melon and β-Glucan composition on STZ-induced rat diabetes and its complications. J Microbiol. Biotechnol. 22 (1): 147–55.

Kinghorn, A. Douglas; Compadre, César M. (2001). Less common high-potency sweeteners". In Nabors, Lyn O'Brien. Alternative Sweeteners. CRC Press. pp. 209 - 33. ISBN 978-0-8247-0437-7.

Kirkham S, Akilen R, Sharma S, Tsiami A (2009). The potential of cinnamon to reduce blood glucose levels in patients with type 2 diabetes and insulin resistance. Diabetes. Obes. Metab. 11 (12): 1100 - 113.

Krawinkel MB, Keding GB (2006). Bitter gourd (*Momordica charantia*): A dietary approach to hyperglycemia. Nutr. Rev. 64 (7 Pt 1): 331 - 37.

Kuhad A, Chopra K (2007). Curcumin attenuates diabetic encephalopathy in rats: behavioral and biochemical evidences. Eur. J. Pharmacol. 576 (1-3): 34 - 42.

Kuhad A, Chopra K (2008). Effect of sesamol on diabetes-associated cognitive decline in rats. Exp. Brain. Res. 185 (3): 411 - 20.

Kuhad A, Sethi R, Chopra K (2008). Lycopene attenuates diabetes-associated cognitive decline in rats. Life Sci. 83 (3-4): 128 - 34.

Kumar R, Balaji S, Uma TS, Sehgal PK (2009). Fruit extracts of *Momordica charantia* potentiate glucose uptake and up-regulate Glut-4, PPAR gamma and PI3K. J. Ethnopharmacol. 126 (3): 533 - 37.

Kumar SN, Mani UV, Mani I (2010). An open label study on the supplementation of *Gymnema sylvestre* in type 2 diabetics. J Diet Suppl. 7 (3): 273 - 82.

Kumari K, Mathew BC, Augusti KT. (1995). Antidiabetic and hypolipidaemic effects of S-methyl cysteine sulfoxide, isolated from *Allium cepa* Linn. Ind. J. Biochem. Biophys. 32: 49 - 54.

Kumawat NS, Chaudhari SP, Wani NS, Deshmukh TA, Patil VR (2010). Antidiabetic activity of ethanol extract of *Colocasia esculenta* leaves in alloxan induced diabetic rats. International Journal of Pharm. Tech. Research. 2 (2): 1246 – 49.

Latha M, Pari L (2003). Antihyperglyceamic effect of *Cassia auriculata* in experimental diabetes and its effects on key metabolic enzymes involved in carbohydrate metabolism. Clin. Exp. Pharmacol. Physiol. 30 (1-2): 38 - 43.

Lawal HA, Atiku MK, Khelpai DG, Wannang NN (2008). Hypoglyceamic and hypolipidaemic effect of aqueous leaf extract of *Murraya koenigii* in normal and alloxan-diabetic rats [J]. Niger. J. Physiol. Sci, 23 (1-2): 37 - 40.

Leatherdale BA, Panesar RK, Singh G, Atkins TW, Bailey CJ, Bignell AH (1981). Improvement in glucose tolerance due to *Momordica charantia* (karela). Br. Med. J. (Clin. Res. Ed.). 282 (6279): 1823 - 24.

Leung L, Birtwhistle R, Kotecha J, Hannah S, Cuthbertson S (2009). Anti-diabetic and hypoglyceamic effects of *Momordica charantia* (bitter melon): a mini review. Br. J. Nutr. 102 (12): 1703 - 708.

Li J, Jia W, Kaneko T, Qin LQ and Sato A (2004). Effects of fiber intake on the blood pressure, lipids and heart rate in Goto Kakizaki rats. Nutrition. 20, 1003 - 1007.

Li J, Kaneko, T, Qin LQ, Jia W, Wang Y and Sato A (2003 a). Long term effects of high dietary fiber intake on glucose tolerance, and lipid metabolism in GK rats: Comparison among barley, rice and corn starch. Metabolism, 52, 1206 - 210.

Li J, Kaneko T, Wang Y, Qin LQ and Sato A (2003 b). Effect of dietary fiber on the glucose tolerance in spontaneously diabetic rats – Comparison among barley, rice and corn starch. Nippon. Eiseigaku. Zasshi. 58: 281 - 86.

Liljeberg HG, Granfeldt YE and Bjorck IM (1996). Products based on a high fiber-based barley genotype, but not common barley or oats lower postprandial glucose and insulin response in healthy humans. J. Nutr. 126: 458 - 66.

Mahdi GS, Naismith DJ, Price, RG, Taylor SA, Risteli J and Risteli L. (1994). Modulating influence of barley on the altered metabolism of glucose and of basement membranes in diabetic rat. Ann. Nutr. Metab. 38: 61 - 67.

Malik ZA, Singh M, Sharma PL (2011). Neuroprotective effect of *Momordica charantia* in global cerebral ischemia and reperfusion induced neuronal damage in diabetic mice. J. Ethnopharmacol. 133 (2): 729 - 34.

Mang B, Wolters M, Schmitt B, Kelb K, Lichtinghagen R, Stichtenoth DO, Hahn A (2006). Effects of a cinnamon extract on plasma glucose, HbA, and serum lipids in diabetes mellitus type 2. Eur. J. Clin. Invest. 36 (5): 340 - 44.

Mathew PT, Augusti KT. (1975). Hyp-glycemic effects of onion, *Allium cepa* Linn. on diabetes mellitus- a preliminary report. Ind. J. Physiol. Pharmacol. 19: 213 - 17.

McCue P, Kwon YI, Shetty K (2005). Anti-diabetic and anti-hypertensive potential of sprouted and solid-state bioprocessed soybean. Asia Pac. J. Clin. Nutr. 14 (2): 145 - 52.

Mitra A (2007). Effrcts of a composite of Tulsi leaves, Amla, Bitter Gourd, Gurmar leaves, Jamun fruit and seed in Type 2 Diabetic Patients. Journal of Clinical and Diagnostic Research. 1: 511 - 20.

Mowla A, Alauddin M, Rahman MA, Ahmed K. (2009) Anti-hyperglyceamic effect of *Trigonella foenum-graecum* (fenugreek) seed extract in alloxan-induced diabetic rats and its use in diabetes mellitus: a brief qualitative phytochemical and acute toxicity test on the extract. Afr. J. Tradit. Complement. Altern. Med. 6 (3): 255 - 61.

Mukherjee PK, Maiti K, Mukherjee K, Houghton PJ, (2006). Leads from Indian medicinal plants with hypoglyceamic potentials. Journal of Ethnopharmacol. 106: 1– 28.

Murakami N, Murakami T, Kadoya M, Matsuda H, Yamahara J, Yoshikawa M (1996). New hypoglyceamic constituents in 'gymnemic acid' from *Gymnema sylvestrae*. Chem. Pharma. Bull. Tokyo. 44 (2): 469 - 71.

Murthy KR, Rao KN, Rao DK, Murthy LBG (1978). A preliminary study on hypoglyceamic and anti-hyperglycemic effects of *azadirachta indica*. Ind. J. Pharmacol. 10: 247.

Naismith DJ, Mahdi, GS, and Shakir NN (1991). Therapeutic value of barley in the management of diabetes. Ann. Nutr. Metab. 35: 61 - 64.

Narendhirakannan RT, Subramanian S (2010). Biochemical evaluation of the protective effect of *Aegle marmelos* (L.), Corr. leaf extract on tissue anti-oxidant defense system and histological changes of pancreatic beta-cells in streptozotocin-induced diabetic rats. Drug. Chem. Toxicol. 33 (2): 120 - 30.

Noel PH, Pugh JA, Larne AC, Marsh G (1997). The use of traditional plant medicines for NIDDM in South Texas. Phytotherapy Res. 11 (7): 512 - 17.

Padiya R, Khatua TN, Bagul PK, Kuncha M, Banerjee SK (2011). Garlic improves insulin sensitivity and associated metabolic syndromes in fructose fed rats. Nutr. Metab. (Lond). 27: 8: 53.

Panda S, Kar A (2007). Apigenin (4',5,7-trihydroxyflavone) regulates hyper-glycaemia, thyroid dysfunction and lipid peroxidation in alloxan-induced diabetic mice. J. Pharm. Pharmacol. 59 (11): 1543 - 48.

Pari L, Latha M (2002). Effect of *Cassia auriculata* flowers on blood sugar levels, serum and tissue lipids in streptozotocin diabetic rats. Singapore Med. J. 43 (12): 617 - 21.

Pari L, Umamaheswari JU (1999). Hypoglyceamic effect of *Musa sapientum* L. in alloxan-induced diabetic rats. J. Ethnopharmacol. 68 (1-3): 321 - 25.

Pari L, Umamaheswari J. (2000) Antihyperglyceamic activity of *Musa sapientum* flowers: effect on lipid peroxidation in alloxan diabetic rats. Phytother. Res. 14 (2): 136 - 38.

Pari L, Venkateswaran S (2003). Effect of an aqueous extract of *Phaseolus vulgaris* on the properties of tail tendon collagen of rats with streptozotocin-induced diabetes. Braz. J. Med. Biol. Res. 36 (7) 861 - 70.

Pari L, Venkateswaran S (2004). Protective role of *Phaseolus vulgaris* on changes in the fatty acid composition in experimental diabetes. J. Med. Food. 7 (2): 204 - 209.

Paul S, Bandyopadhyay TK, Bhattacharyya A (2011). Immuno-modulatory effect of leaf extract of *Murraya koenigii* in diabetic mice. Immuno-pharmacol Immuno-toxicol. 2011 Mar 14.

Pham AQ, Kourlas H, Pham DQ (2007). Cinnamon supplementation in patients with type 2 diabetes mellitus. Pharmaco-therapy. 27 (4): 595 - 99.

Pick, M. E., Hawrysh, Z. J., Gee, M. I. and Toth, E (1998). Barley bread products improve glycemic control of type 2 subjects. Int. J. Food Sci. Nutr. 49: 71 - 78.

Pillai NR, Santhakumari G (1981). Hypoglyceamic activity of *Melia azadirachta* Linn. (neem). Ind. J. Med. Res. 74: 931 - 33.

Platel K, Srinivasan K (1997). Plant foods in the management of diabetes mellitus: vegetables as potential hypoglycaemic agents. Nahrung. 41 (2): 68 - 74.

Poppitt SD, van Drunen JD, McGill AT, Mulvey TB, Leahy FE (2007). Supplementation of a high-carbohydrate breakfast with barley beta-glucan improves postprandial glycaemic response for meals but not beverages. Asia Pac. J. Clin. Nutr. 16 (1): 16 - 24.

Porchezhian E, Dobriyal RM (2003). An overview on the advances of *Gymnema sylvestre*: chemistry, pharmacology and patents.

Prince PS, Menon VP, Pari L (1998). Hypoglyceamicactivity of *Syzigium cumini* seeds: effect on lipid peroxidation in alloxan diabetic rats. J. Ethnopharmacol. 61 (1): 1 - 7.

Raghuram TC (1996). Diet and Diabetes Mellitus. In: Textbook of Human Nutrition. ed by Bamji M, Pralhad Rao N, Vinodini Reddy. New Delhi, Oxford and IBH. pp. 333 - 345.

Rai V, Iyer U, Mani UV. (1997) Effect of Tulasi (*Ocimum sanctum*) leaf powder supplementation on blood sugar levels, serum lipids and tissue lipid in diabetic rats. Plant Food for Human Nutrition. 50: 9 - 16.

Rajasekaran S, Ravi K, Sivagnanam K, Subramanian S (2006). Beneficial effects of *Aloe vera* leaf gel extract on lipid profile status in rats with streptozotocin diabetes. Clin. Exp. Pharmacol. Physiol. 33 (3): 232 - 37.

Rajasekaran S, Sivagnanam K, Subramanian S (2005a). Anti-oxidant effect of *Aloe vera* gel extract in streptozotocin-induced diabetes in rats. Pharmacol. Rep. 57 (1): 90 - 96.

Rajasekaran S, Sivagnanam K, Subramanian S (2005b). Modulatory effects of *Aloe vera* leaf gel extract on oxidative stress in rats treated with streptozotocin. J. Pharm. Pharmacol. 57 (2): 241 - 46.

Ravi KP, Ramachandran B, Subramanian S (2004a). Protective effect of *Eugenia jambolana* seed kernel on tissue antioxidants in streptozotocin-induced diabetic rats. Biol. Pharm. Bull. 27 (8): 1212 - 17.

Ravi KP, Rajasekaran S, Subramanian S (2005). Anti-hyperlipidemic effect of *Eugenia jambolana* seed kernel on streptozotocin induced diabetes in rats. Food and Chemical Toxicology. 43 (9): 1433 - 39.

Ravi K, Sekar DS, Subramanian S (2004c). Hypoglyceamic activity of inorganic constituents in *Eugenia jambolana* seed on streptozotocin-induced diabetes in rats. Biol. Trace. Elem. Res. 99 (1-3): 145 - 55.

Ravi K, Sivagnanam K, Subramanian S (2004b). Anti-diabetic activity of *Eugenia jambolana* seed kernels on streptozotocin-induced diabetic rats. J. Med. Food. 7 (2): 187 - 91.

Roffey BW, Atwal AS, Johns T, Kubow S (2007). Water extracts from *Momordica charantia* increase glucose uptake and adiponectin secretion in 3T3-L1 adipose cells. J. Ethnopharmacol. 112 (1): 77 - 84.

Roman-Ramos R, Flores-Saenz JL, Alaricon-Aguilar FJ (1995). Anti-hyperglyceamic effect of some edible plants. J. Ethnopharmacol. 48: 25 - 32.

Sabu MC, Kuttan R (2002). Anti-diabetic activity of medicinal plants and its relationship with their anti-oxidant property. J. Ethnopharmacol. 81 (2): 155 - 60.

Sabu MC, Kuttan R (2004). Anti-diabetic activity of *Aegle marmelos* and its relationship with its anti-oxidant properties. Indian J. Physiol. Pharmacol. 48 (1): 81 - 88.

Sabu MC, Smitha K, Kuttan R (2002). Anti-diabetic activity of green tea polyphenols and their role in reducing oxidative stress in experimental diabetes. J. Ethnopharmacol. 83 (1-2): 109 - 16.

Samanta A, Burden AC, and Jones GR (1985). Plasma glucose response to glucose and honey in patients with diabetes mellitus: An analysis of glycaemic and peak incremental indices. Diab. Med. 2: 371 - 73.

Sankar P, Subhashree S, Sudharani S (2012). Effect of *Trigonella foenum-graecum* seed powder on the anti-oxidant levels of high fat diet and low dose streptozotocin induced type II diabetic rats. Eur Rev Med Pharmacol Sci. 16. Suppl. 3: 10 - 17.

Sauvaire Y, Petit P, Broca C, Manteghetti M, Baissac Y, Fernandez-Alvarez J, Gross R, Roy M, Leconte A, Gomis R, Ribes G (1998). 4-hydroxyisoleucine: a novel amino acid potentiator of insulin secretion. Diabetes. 47: 206 - 210.

Sekar DS, Sivagnanam K, Subramanian S (2005). Anti-diabetic activity of *Momordica charantia* seeds on streptozotocin induced diabetic rats. Pharmazie. 60 (5): 383 - 87.

Sekar SD, Subramanian S (2005a). Beneficial effects of *Momordica charantia* seeds in the treatment of STZ-induced diabetes in experimental rats. Biol. Pharm. Bull. 28 (6): 978 - 83.

Sekar SD, Subramanian S (2005b). Anti-oxidant properties of *Momordica charantia* (bitter gourd) seeds on Streptozotocin induced diabetic rats. Asia. Pac. J. Clin. Nutr. 14 (2): 153 - 58.

Sekar SD, Subramanian S (2005c). Antioxidant properties of Momordica Charantia (bitter gourd) seeds on Streptozotocin induced diabetic rats. Asia. Pac. J. Clin. Nutr. 14 (2): 153 -58.

Seth SD, Sharma B (2004). Medicinal plants of India. I.J.M.R.120: 9 - 11.

Sharma AK, Bharti S, Goyal S, Arora S, Nepal S, Kishore K, Joshi S, Kumari S, Arya DS (2011). Upregulation of PPARγ by *Aegle marmelos* ameliorates insulin resistance and β-cell dysfunction in high fat diet fed-streptozotocin induced type 2 diabetic rats. Phytother. Res. 25 (10): 1457 - 65.

Sharma AK, Mujumdar M (1990). Some observations on the effect of *Clitoria ternata* Linn.On changes in serum sugar level and small intestinal mucosal carbohydrate activities in alloxan diabetes. Calcutta. Med. J. 87 (11-12): 168 - 71.

Shastri R *et al.* (eds). (1962). Charaka Samhita of Agnivesha, Vidyabhavan Ayurveda Granthamal 32 Part II. Chaukhambha Vidya Bhawan, Varanasi. pp. 236 - 42.

Sheela CG, Augusti KT (1992). Anti-diabetic effects of S-allyl cysteine sulphoxide isolated from garlic *Allium sativum* Linn. Indian J. Exp. Biol. 30: 523 - 526.

Shehzad A, Ha T, Subhan F, Lee YS (2011). New mechanisms and the anti-inflammatory role of curcumin in obesity and obesity-related metabolic diseases. Eur. J. Nutr. 50 (3): 151 - 61.

Shetty AK, Kumar GS, Sambaiah K, Salimath PV (2005a). Effect of bitter gourd (*Momordica charantia*) on glycaemic status in streptozotocin induced diabetic rats. Plant Foods Hum. Nutr. 60 (3): 109 - 112.

Shetty AK, Kumar GS, Salimath PV (2005b). Bitter gourd (*Momordica charantia*) modulates activities of intestinal and renal disaccharidases in streptozotocin-induced diabetic rats. Mol. Nutr. Food Res. 49 (8): 791 - 96.

Shibib BA, Khan LA, Rahman R (1993). Hypoglyceamic activity of *Coccinia indica* and *Momordica charantia* in diabetic rats: depression of the hepatic gluconeogenic enzymes glucose-6-phosphatase and fructose-1, 6-biphosphatase and elevation of liver and red-cell shunt enzyme glucose-6-phosphate dehydrogenase. Biochem. J. 292: 267–270.

Shih CC, Lin CH, Lin WL, Wu JB (2009). *Momordica charantia* extract on insulin resistance and the skeletal muscle GLUT4 protein in fructose-fed rats. J. Ethnopharmacol. 123 (1): 82 - 90.

Shojaii A, Hashem Dabaghian F, Goushegir A, Abdollahi Fard M (2011). Anti-diabetic plants of Iran. Acta. Med. Iran. 49 (10): 637 - 42.

Shukla K, Narain JP, Puri P, Gupta A, Bijlani L, Mahapatra SC, Karmakar MG (1991). Glycemic response to maize, bajra and barley. Indian J. Physiol. Pharmacol. 35: 249 - 254.

Siddiqui S (1942). A note on the isolation of three new bitter principles from the neem oil. Current Sc. 11: 278.

Singh N, Gupta M (2007). Regeneration of beta cells in islets of Langerhans of pancreas of alloxan diabetic rats by acetone extract of *Momordica charantia* (Linn.) (bitter gourd) fruits. Indian J. Exp. Biol. 45 (12): 1055 - 62.

Singh N, Gupta M, Sirohi P, Varsha (2008). Effects of alcoholic extract of *Momordica charantia* (Linn.) whole fruit powder on the pancreatic islets of alloxan diabetic albino rats. J. Environ. Biol. 29 (1): 101 - 106.

Sitasawad SL, Shewade Y, Bhonde R (2000). Role of bittergourd fruit juice in stz-induced diabetic state *in vivo* and *in vitro*. J. Ethnopharmacol. 73 (1-2): 71 - 79.

Snee LS, Nerurkar VR, Dooley DA, Efird JT, Shovic AC, Nerurkar PV (2011). Strategies to improve palatability and increase consumption intentions for *Momordica charantia* (bitter melon): a vegetable commonly used for diabetes management. Nutr. J. 10: 78.

Sridhar SB, Sheetal UD, Pai MR, Shastri MS (2005). Preclinical evaluation of the antidiabetic effect of *Eugenia jambolana* seed powder in streptozotocin-diabetic rats. Braz. J. Med. Biol. Res. 38 (3): 463 - 68.

Srinivasan K (2005). Plant foods in the management of diabetes mellitus: spices as beneficial antidiabetic food adjuncts. Int. J. Food Sci. Nutr. 56 (6): 399 - 414.

Subbulakshmi G, Naik M (2001). Indigenous foods in the treatment of Diabetes Mellitus. Bombay Hospital Journal. 43 (4): 548 – 61.

Suh KS, Oh S, Woo JT, Kim SW, Kim JW, Kim YS, Chon S (2012). Apigenin attenuates 2-deoxy-D-ribose-induced oxidative cell damage in HIT-T15 pancreatic β-cells. Biol. Pharm. Bull. 35 (1): 121 - 26.

Swanston-Flatt SK, Day C, Bailey CJ and Flatt PR (1990). Traditional plant treatments for diabetes: studies in normal and streptozotocin diabetic mice. Diabetologia 33: 462 - 64.

Swanston-Flatt SK, Day C, Flatt PR, Gould BJ, Bailey CJ (1989). Glycaemic effects of traditional European plant treatments for diabetes. Studies in normal and streptozotocin diabetic mice. Diabetes Research. 10: 69 - 73.

Swanston-Flatt SK, Flatt PR, Day C, Bailey CJ (1991). Traditional dietary adjuncts for the treatment of diabetes mellitus. Proceedings of the Nutrition Society.50: 641 - 51.

Talpur N, Echard BW, Yasmin T, Bagchi D, Preuss HG (2003). Effects of niacin-bound chromium, Maitake mushroom fraction SX and (-)-hydroxycitric acid on the metabolic syndrome in aged diabetic Zucker fatty rats. Mol. Cell. Biochem. 252 (1-2): 369 - 77.

Tiwari AK (2008). Invigorated barley in diabetes. Current Science. 95 (1): 25 - 29.

Tripathi UN, Chandra D (2009). The plant extracts of *Momordica charantia* and *Trigonella foenum-graecum* have anti-oxidant and anti-hyperglyceamic properties for cardiac tissue during diabetes mellitus. Oxid. Med. Cell. Longev. 2 (5): 290 - 96.

Tripathi UN, Chandra D (2010). Anti-hyperglycemic and anti-oxidative effect of aqueous extract of *Momordica charantia* pulp and *Trigonella foenum graecum* seed in alloxan-induced diabetic rats. Indian J. Biochem. Biophys. 47 (4): 227 - 33.

Urooj A, Vinutha, S R., Puttaraj S, Leelavathy K and Haridas Rao P (1998). Effect of barley incorporation in bread on its quality and glyceamic responses in diabetics. Int. J. Food Sci. Nutr., 49, 265 - 70.

Vanschoonbeek K, Thomassen BJ, Senden JM, Wodzig WK, van Loon LJ (2006). Cinnamon supplementation does not improve glyceamic control in postmenopausal type 2 diabetes patients. J. Nutr. 136 (4): 977 - 80.

Vats V, Grover JK., Rathi SS (2002). Evaluation of anti-hyperglyceamic and hypoglycemic effect of *Trigonella foenum-graecum* Linn, *Ocimum sanctum* Linn. and *Pterocarpus marsupium* Linn in normal and alloxanized diabetic rats. J. Ethnopharmacol. 79: 95 - 100.

Vats V, Yadav SP. Grover JK (2004). Ethanolic extract of *Ocimum sanctum* leaves partially attenuates streptozotocin induced alteration in glycogen content and carbohydrate metabolism in rats. J. Ethnopharmacol. 90: 155 - 60.

Venkateswaran S, Pari L (2002). Anti-oxidant effect of *Phaseolus vulgaris* in streptozotocin-induced diabetic rats. Asia Pac. J. Clin. Nutr. 11 (3): 206 - 209.

Venkateswaran S, Pari L, Saravanan G (2002). Effect of *Phaseolus vulgaris* on circulatory anti-oxidants and lipids in rats with streptozotocin-induced diabetes. J. Med. Food. 5 (2): 97 - 103.

Vinuthan MK, Girish Kumar V, Ravindra JP, Jayaprakash, Narayana K 2004). Effect of extracts of *Murraya koenigii* leaves on the levels of blood glucose and plasma insulin in alloxan-induced diabetic rats [J]. Indian J. Physiol. Pharmacol, 48 (3): 348 - 52.

Virdi J, Sivakami S, Shahani S, Suthar AC, Banavalikar MM, Biyani MK (2003). Anti-hyperglycemic effects of three extracts from *Momordica charantia*. J. Ethnopharmacol. 88 (1): 107 - 111.

Welihinda J, Karunanayake EH, Sheriff MH, Jayasinghe KS (1986). Effect of *Momordica charantia* on the glucose tolerance in maturity onset diabetes. J. Ethnopharmacol. 17 (3): 277 - 82.

World Health Organization (1980). Second Report of the WHO Expert Committee on Diabetes Mellitus. Technical Report Series 646, p 66. Geneva: World Health Organization.

Xue WL, Li XS, Zhang J, Liu YH, Wang ZL, Zhang RJ (2007). Effect of *Trigonella foenum-graecum* (fenugreek) extract on blood glucose, blood lipid and hemorheological properties in streptozotocin-induced diabetic rats. Asia Pac J Clin Nutr. 16. Suppl.1: 422 - 26.

Yadav M, Lavania A, Tomar R, Prasad GB, Jain S, Yadav H.(2010). Complementary and comparative study on hypoglycemic and antihyperglycemic activity of various extracts of *Eugenia jambolana* seed, *Momordica charantia* fruits, *Gymnema sylvestre*, and *Trigonella foenum graecum* seeds in rats. Appl. Biochem. Biotechnol. 160 (8): 2388 - 400.

Yadav UC, Moorthy K, Baquer NZ (2005). Combined treatment of sodium orthovanadate and *Momordica charantia* fruit extract prevents alterations in lipid profile and lipogenic enzymes in alloxan diabetic rats. Mol. Cell. Biochem. 268 (1-2): 111 - 20.

Yadav S, Vats V, Dhunnoo Y, Grover JK (2002). Hypoglycemic and antihyperglyceamic activity of *Murraya koenigii* leaves in diabetic rats[J]. J Ethnopharmacol, 82 (2-3) : 111 - 16.

Yamagata K, Miyashita A, Chino M, Matsufuji H (2011). Apigenin inhibits tumor necrosis factor alpha plus high glucose-induced LOX-1 expression in human endothelial cells. Microvasc. Res. 81 (1): 60 - 67.

Yankuzo H, Ahmed QU, Santosa RI, Akter SF, Talib NA (2011). Beneficial effect of the leaves of *Murraya koenigii* (Linn.) Spreng (Rutaceae) on diabetes-induced renal damage *in vivo* [J]. J Ethnopharmacol. 135 (1): 88 -94.

Yeh GY, Eisenberg DM, Kaptchuk TJ, Phillips RS (2003). Systematic review of herbs and dietary supplements for glyceamic control in diabetes. Diabetes Care. 26 (4): 277 - 94.

Yibchok-anun S, Adisakwattana S, Yao CY, Sangvanich P, Roengsumran S, Hsu WH (2006). Slow acting protein extract from fruit pulp of *Momordica charantia* with insulin secretagogue and insulinomimetic activities. Biol. Pharm. Bull. 29 (6): 1126 - 31.

Zacharias NT, Sebastian KL, Philip B, Augusti KT (1980). Hypoglyceamic and hypolipidaemic effects of garlic in sucrose fed rabbits. Ind. J. Physiol. Pharmacol. 24: 151 - 54.

Zheng ZX, Teng JY, Liu JY, Qiu JH, Ouyang H, Xue C (2005). [The hypoglycemic effects of crude polysaccharides extract from *Momordica charantia* in mice]. Wei. Sheng. Yan. Jiu. 34 (3): 361 - 63. [Article in Chinese].

Zhu XM, Xie P, Di YT, Peng SL, Ding LS, Wang MK (2008). Two new triterpenoid saponins from *Gymnema sylvestre*. J. Integr. Plant. Biol. 50 (5): 589 - 92.

Chapter 6

Anti-Fertility Foods

Overpopulation is becoming a global problem causing a drain on economic, social and natural resources. Several measures have been employed especially by the developing and underdeveloped countries to control population growth. Control of fertility with hormonal preparations containing estrogen and progesterone has been proved to be effective. The safety of long term use of these contraceptives, however, is controversial. To this effect, World Health Organization has given much attention in the search for safe, affordable and socially acceptable alternatives.

The literature survey by Maurya *et al.* (2004) showed that approximately 318 different plants are in traditional/folkloric use worldwide for controlling fertility, of which 227 plants are of Indian origin. So far, 74 plants have been screened for their anti-fertility potential, 48 of them have been found to be effective. Active principles of about 15 plants have been identified during the period under review. If such potentially effective plant foods are proved to be useful, their ready availability from natural sources can nevertheless give them a definite advantage over the synthetic options (Bingel and Fong, 1988).

The search for a relatively cheap, widely available, acceptable and effective contraceptive of plant origin that is equally non-invasive in administration, non-hormonal in action, non-toxic and relatively long-acting has lead to a number of animal trials in the interest of population control. Current efforts in India to develop a male contraceptive are mainly directed towards (i) development of anti-spermatogenic agents to suppress sperm production, (ii) prevention of sperm maturation, (iii) prevention of sperm transport through vas deferens or rendering these sperm infertile and (iv) prevention of sperm deposition. Research work in the field of prevention of sperm transport through vas deferens has made significant advances.

Vaginal contraception, the oldest method of fertility regulation that remained virtually forgotten for a few decades has recently come under focal review due to an increase in STDs and HIV infections worldwide. Gupta, (2005) reviewed the situation and commented that today it is being considered very strongly that a conceptual microbicidal spermicide can tender protection against pregnancy as well as STDs (including AIDS), simultaneously. A strong detergent like nonoxynol-9 (N-9) has been used as a spermicide in many local contraceptive preparations and studies have shown that it also exhibits significant microbicidal activity in vitro. However, recent clinical trials have shown that detergent spermicides do not provide any protection against STDs and AIDS but may in fact even promote their transmission. This has largely been attributed to their surfactant nature that irritates the vagina and kills the normal vaginal flora making it more susceptible to STD infections. An urgent need for a suitable non-detergent spermicide has thus emerged to replace N-9 among local contraceptive preparations. Incorporating the active ingredient from the fruit pericarp of *Sapindus mukorossi* has been suggested (Gupta, 2005).

Self-induced abortion seems to occur with tea infusions of hot spices like oregano, cinnamon or oregano mixed with chocolate (Misago and Fonseca, 1999). Taking ginger, clove and combination of ergot, gin and vinegar is also common to induce bleeding and effect abortion. In Nigeria women consumed potash mixed with lime juice, thrice a day for 3 days to terminate a month old conception, but for pregnancies older than a month cactus juice with fresh egg is used. To effect abortion after 2 months of pregnancy, a stronger solution of potash, lime juice, washing blue with a generous helping of gin is used. In India raw papaya, cooked banana stem, pineapple and mango are supposed to interfere with pregnancy. Indian women are known to have jaggery with omum (ajwain) along with generous doses of ghee with the belief that the heat giving effect of the mixture would cause stomach cramps and disturb conception (Mankekar, 1973).

Many of the abortifacients were traditionally used either as coating of abortion sticks to be inserted in the cervix, or as gastrointestinal irritants. The Task Force on Plants for Fertility Regulation set up by the World Health Organization identified approximately thirty plants demonstrating anti-implantational properties. None of these have reached the stage of clinical evaluation (Chaudhury, 2001). However, three plants from India have shown promise in their use in female contraception *i.e. Hibiscus rosa-sinensis* (Tewari, 1974); *Vicoa indica* (Chaudhury, 1985) and *Embelia ribes* (Joshi *et al.*, 1977). The combination of *Embelia ribes*, Borax and *Piper longum* has been tried in phase-I clinical trials at three centers in the country and the results were encouraging (Chaudhury, 2001).

Kamboj (1988) reviewed 103 plant species from India that have been tested for anti-implantation activity. 40 plants were found to have the effect. 23 plants were tested in rodents for abortifacient activity, and all but 2 were active in 50 per cent or more. Farnsworth *et al.* (1975) reported that Vinblastine, demecolene, and podophyllotoxin possess known cyto-toxic and anti-fertility properties. Naturally occurring plant sources such as steroid estrogens, estrogenic isoflavins, coumestans, and cyto-toxic agents show anti-fertility properties. Later Farnsworth and Waller, (1982) reviewed the researches on plant-derived agents that prevent sperm production if taken orally by the male, or incapacitate or kill sperm on contact if used vaginally by the female. Of 1600 Indian plants tested, 90 showed positive semen coagulating properties.

The practice of traditional medicine for the control of fertility in most parts of the world is based on the uses of plant medicines for many years. The fact that herbal medicines have been employed for such a long time does not guarantee their efficacy and safety.

Many of the anti-fertility compounds identified in plants to date perturb spermatogenesis by causing testicular dysfunction. The roots of *Aristolochia indica* and *Plumbago zeylanica*; the leaves of *Azadirachta indica*, *Catharanthus roseus*, *Vinca rosea* and *Ocimum sanctum*; the flowers of *Hibiscus rosa-sinensis* and *Malvaviscus conzatii*; the seeds of *C. papaya* and *Vitex negundo*; and the fruit of *Momordica charantia* have been identified as candidates for male fertility regulation (Manivannan et al, 2009). In contradiction to a number of other essential oils, fennel and anise oils and to a very slight extent eucalyptus oil too have definite oestrogenic activities (Zondek and Bergmann, 1938).

A few reports have suggested that some dietary factors might be related to semen quality. Mínguez-Alarcón *et al.* (2012) found a positive association between dietary intakes of cryptoxanthin, vitamin C, lycopene and β-carotene and total motile sperm count while vitamin C alone on semen volume too. Higher intake of fruits and vegetables, dark green vegetables, skim milk, poultry and sea food was associated with a lower risk of asthenozoospermia (reduced sperm motility) (Eslamian *et al.*, 2012) and semen quality (Gaskins *et al.*, 2012a).

Anti-fertility Food Components

Saturated Fat and Infertility

Animal studies have shown that dietary fats affect male fertility (Blesbois *et al.*, 2004; Estienne *et al.*, 2008; Stoffel *et al.*, 2008; Bongalhardo *et al.*, 2009; Roqueta-Rivera *et al.*, 2010). Human and animal studies have also correlated a specific fatty acid composition of sperm with semen quality (Zalata *et al.*, 1998; Conquer *et al.*, 1999; Gulaya *et al.*, 2001; Aksoy *et al.*, 2006; Tavilani *et al.*, 2006, 2007; Safarinejad *et al.*, 2010).

In their preliminary cross-sectional study Attaman *et al.* (2012) found high intake of saturated fats was negatively related to sperm concentration whereas higher intake of omega-3 fats was positively related to sperm morphology. Jensen *et al.* (2013) found a significant dose-response association between high intake of saturated fat and lower sperm concentration & total sperm count in men. Men in the highest quartile of saturated fat intake had a 38 per cent lower sperm concentration and a 41 per cent lower total sperm count than did men in the lowest quartile. They reason it out as the changes in diet over the past decades implying that reduction in saturated fat intake may be beneficial for both general and reproductive health.

Trans unsaturated fats may increase the risk of ovulatory infertility when consumed instead of carbohydrates or unsaturated fats commonly found in nonhydrogenated vegetable oils. Each 2 per cent increase in the intake of energy from trans unsaturated fats, as opposed to that from carbohydrates, was associated with a 73 per cent greater risk of ovulatory infertility after adjustment for known and suspected risk factors for this condition [relative risk (RR) = 1.73; 95 per cent]. Obtaining 2 per cent of energy intake from trans fats rather than from n-6 polyunsaturated fats was associated with a similar increase in the risk of ovulatory infertility (RR = 1.79; 95 per cent). In addition, obtaining 2 per cent of energy from trans fats rather than from monounsaturated fats was associated with a more than doubled risk of ovulatory infertility (RR = 2.31; 95 per cent) (Chavarro *et al.*, 2007a).

Recently, high frequency of subnormal human sperm counts is reported. It has been suggested that environmental estrogens could be responsible for the putative secular decline in sperm counts. Dairy foods contain large amounts of estrogens. While some studies have suggested dairy as a possible contributing factor for decreased semen quality, no consistent reports are seen across studies. Afeiche *et al.* (2013) found that intake of full-fat dairy was inversely related to sperm motility and morphology. These associations were driven primarily by intake of cheese and were independent of overall dietary patterns. Chavarro *et al.* (2007b) followed the pre-menopausal women without a history of infertility who attempted a pregnancy or became pregnant during an 8-year period. They found that high intake of low-fat dairy foods to increase the risk of anovulatory infertility whereas intake of high-fat dairy foods to decrease this risk.

Folate

Folate is necessary for the synthesis of DNA, transfer RNA, and the amino acids cysteine and methionine. Thus, it plays an important role in human reproduction (Ebisch *et al.*, 2007). In animals, folic acid supplementation increased ovulation rates (and subsequently litter sizes) in pigs (Matte *et al.*, 1984) while folic acid deficiency decreased ovulation in rats (Willmott *et al.*, 1968). Previous human studies documented higher pregnancy rates among users of micronutrient supplements either with (Westphal *et al.*, 2004) or without (Czeizel *et al.*, 1996) fertility disorders. Further, regular use of multivitamins was associated with a decreased risk of ovulatory infertility with B vitamins, in particular folic acid, explaining some of this association (Chavarro *et al.*, 2008; Gaskins *et al.*, 2012b).

Acrylamide

The presence of acrylamide has been reported in a variety of human foods including heat-processed starchy foods such as potato chips and bread. Kermani-Alghoraishi *et al.* (2010) reported that acrylamide, decreased sperm vitality and displayed abnormal sperm parameters in progressive motility and total motility through effects on membrane integrity.

Anti-fertility Foods

Papaya (*Carica papaya* Linn.)

The traditional use of papaya to treat many diseases, especially skin conditions and its prohibition for consumption during pregnancy is well known.

Gopalakrishnan and Rajasekharasetty (1978) observed that unripe fruits of papaya interrupt estrous cycle and induce abortions. The abortifacient property seems to decrease as the fruit becomes stale or ripe. Exogenous progesterone counteracts partially the adverse effects on pregnancy and the surviving foeti are without any distinct malformations. Adebiyi *et al.* (2002) suggested that normal consumption of ripe papaya during pregnancy may not pose any significant risk. However, the unripe or semi-ripe papaya (which contains high concentration of the latex that produces marked uterine contractions) could be unsafe in pregnancy. The fruit, seed and latex of papaya have emmenagogic, abortifacient and oxytocic activity (Casey, 1960, Saha *et al.*, 1961). It was also reported to be uterotonic due to the presence of 5 hydroxy tryptamine (Paton, 1968; Barlow and Khan, 1959). No anti-fertility effect was observed in the case of papaya seeds at a dose of 100-500 mg per kg body wt (Bodhankar *et al.*, 1974) and petroleum ether extract of raw papaya pulp at a dose of 100 mg per kg body wt. However, the raw pulp exhibited anti-implantation activity in the petroleum ether extract at 500 mg per kg body wt and the alcoholic extract at 100-500 mg per kg body wt and also abortifacient activity in the alcoholic extract at 500 mg/kg body wt (Garg and Garg, 1970).

The seeds of *Carica papaya* have been well recognized to possess compounds that putatively control fertility. Adebiyi *et al.* (2003) conclude that at high concentration, *Carica papaya L.* seeds extracted with 80 per cent ethanol are capable of causing irreversible uterine tocolysis probably due to the damageing effect of isothiocyanate (its chief phytochemical) on the myometrium.

A preclinical, short-term evaluation through a series of experiments using various extraction procedures of the seeds of *C. papaya* revealed spermatogenic arrest, leading to azoospermia or total inhibition of sperm motility in rats, rabbits and langur monkeys (Lohiya *et al.*, 1994a; 1999a; 1999b; 2000; 2005; 2006; 2008). *Carica papaya* seed extract may selectively act on the developing germ cells, possibly through Sertoli cells, leading to azoospermia. The inhibitory effect of benzene chromatographic fraction of the chloroform extract could be due to its effect on sperm motility (Lohiya *et al.*, 2002; Manivannan *et al.*, 2004). Sperm motility is inhibited by benzene chromatographic fraction of the chloroform extract of *papaya* seed in langur monkey (Lohiya, *et al.*, 2008). The suppression of spermatogenesis by water extract of papaya seed has been reported. It was suggested that this is possibly mediated through the loss of cell processes by Sertoli cells (Uche-Nwachi *et al.*, 2001). Methanol sub fraction is safe for long-term treatment and the mechanism of contraception is shown by its effect on spermatid differentiation in the testis, possibly mediated by the Sertoli cell factors (Manivannan *et al.*, 2009).

Investigations by Oderinde *et al.* (2002) lead to the clear conclusion that low dose aqueous crude extract of *Carica papaya* (Linn) seeds does not adversely affect prenatal development. The altered toxicological profile indicates that the abortifacient property is a high dose side effect. The results indicate that *Carica papaya* toxicity can adversely affect the foetus. Kusemiju *et al.* (2002) suggest that the aqueous extracts of *Carica papaya* bark is safe and could serve as an effective male contraceptive in animals as they observed complete loss of fertility which was attributed to decline in sperm motility and alteration in their morphology. Uche-Nwachi *et al.* (2011) concluded from their study that the water extract of papaya seed suppresses the activities of steroidogenic enzymes in the testis of Sprague Dawley rats, and that this may contribute to reversible suppression of spermatogenesis, a property that gives a possible male contraceptive potent.

Pathak *et al.* (2000) observed total suppression of cauda epididymal sperm motility to coincide with a decrease in sperm count, viability and an increase in per cent abnormal spermatozoa during 60-150 days observation period. Chloroform extract of the seeds of *Carica papaya* exerts anti-fertility effects in rats without adverse toxicity and that the effects may be directly rendered on the spermatozoa.

Udoh *et al.* (2005) observed that the papaya extract interfered with the pituitary - gonadal axis to influence male reproductive functions, which confirmed its anti-fertility property. The testes of rats treated with papaya extract at 50 and 200 mg/kg revealed gradual degeneration of germ cells, Sertoli cells and Leydig cells as well as germinal epithelium. Ripe papaya extract fed group of mice experienced embryonic resorption while this effect was observed in none of the mice given green papaya extract. The differences in the protein bands of the two stages of ripening of papaya may have contributed to the difference in abortive effects of green and ripe papaya (Anuar *et al.*, 2008).

Neem (*Azadirachta indica*)

Numerous investigators have reported that neem leaves, bark, seeds and oils possess antifertility properties in male and female rats (Riar *et al.*, 1991; Jacobson, 1995; Dhaliwal *et al.*, 1998; Kasturi *et al.*, 2002; Upadhyay *et al.*, 1990; 1992; Shakti *et al.*, 1990; Sadre *et al.*, 1983). Several reports cited in literature on the antifertility effect of *Neem* showed anti-implantation or abortifacient effect in rodents if administered early from day 2 to 7 postcoitum (Talwar *et al.*, 1997; Mukherjee *et al.*, 1999; Juneja *et al.*, 1994). Also praneem (purified *Neem* extract) given orally from day 8 to 10 postcoitum resulted in complete resorption of embryos (Mukherjee and Talwar, 1996).

A new vaginal contraceptive, NIM-76 was developed from neem oil having antimicrobial activity against Escherichia coli, *K. pneumoniae* and *C. albicans* (SaiRam *et al.*, 2002). The contraceptive property of neem oil has been reported (Upadhyay *et al.*, 1994). The neem seed oil, leaf extracts and NIM-76 act as powerful spermicide and significantly inhibited spermatogenesis, decreased sperm motility, count and cessation of fertility. These conditions were reversed by the withdrawal of neem products 4-6 weeks later (Sadre *et al*, 1983). Ogbuewu *et al.* (2009) reported no significant reduction *in libido* of rabbit bucks fed graded levels of neem leaf meal based diets.

Neem seed oil possesses anti-implantation and abortifacient properties. Sinha *et al.* (1984) found spermatozoa of human and Rhesus monkey were immotile and die within 30 min of contact with neem seed oil in an intra-vaginal dose of 1.0 mL. Vaginal biopsy revealed no side effect, while radio-isotope studies indicate non-absorption in the vagina and non anti-ovulatory (Sinha *et al.*, 1984). These findings enabled neem oil formulation 'sensal' use in India as powerful contraceptive (Ogbuewu *et al.*, 2009). Dallaqua *et al.* (2012) also reported that both neem seed oil and azadirachtin impaired intrauterine development of fetus and altered anti-oxidant/oxidative status during pregnancy in rats.

The leaf extracts of neem showed 100 per cent immobilization and mortality of human spermatozoa at a 3 mg dose within 20 seconds (Khan and Awasthy, 2003; Khillare and Shrivastav, 2003). Treatment of mice with neem leaf extract (aqueous) caused adverse effects on sperm motility, acrosomal morphology and number of spermatozoa (Mishra and Singh, 2005). Neem leaf extract has spermatotoxic effect (Ogbuewu *et al.*, 2009).

Ogbuewu *et al.* (2009) and Mohan *et al.* (1997) reported significant reduction in semen volume, sperm count, higher incidence of morphological abnormalities of spermatozoa, fertilizing ability of rabbit bucks fed neem leaf meal based diets and hatchability of eggs on birds fed neem kernel cakes.

The active fraction was identified to be a mixture of six components, which comprises of saturated, mono and di-unsaturated free fatty acids and their methyl esters. The anti-fertility activity with the active fraction was reversible in nature. There was no systemic toxic effect following the administration of the active fraction. Garg *et al.* (1998) for the first time proposed that an active fraction from neem seeds, responsible for long term and reversible blocking of fertility after a single intrauterine administration with high efficacy. The spermicidal activity of NIM-76 was confirmed using a fluorescent staining technique. NIM-76 was found to affect the motility of the sperm in a dose-dependent manner. Supplementation of pentoxifylline, which is known to enhance the motility of the sperm, could not prevent the spermicidal action of NIM-76 locking of fertility after a single intrauterine administration with high efficacy. The capability of NIM-76 to selectively kill sperm without affecting normal cells makes it a highly desirable potential vaginal contraceptive agent (Sharma *et al.*, 1996).

Juneja *et al.* (1996) confirmed that the postcoital intrauterine treatment of neem oil during preimplantation period causes fertility block in mouse by lowering the epidermal growth factor receptor localization in the luminal and glandular epithelium, by causing massive leukocytes infiltration into the uteri, by degenerating the early embryos, and by causing the post-implantation embryonic resorptions in the uteri. Kaushik and Upadhyay (1995) showed that the mode of antifertility action of intrauterine neem treatment (IUNT) is not because of uterine unresponsiveness to the ovarian hormones but is due to impairment of embryo development thus confirming their earlier observations. They also showed that the anti-fertility effect of IUNT is at the pre-implantation stage, localized and without any adverse or toxic effect on the fetal development in the contralateral uterine horn of the unilaterally treated rats. Upadhyay *et al.* (1994) demonstrated further that an IUNT can be used for long-term, reversible contraception, without any apparent side effects, and that the method could provide an alternate to currently used intrauterine contraceptive devices (IUCD).

Neem oil, extracted from the seeds of *Azadirachta indica* has also been found by Bardhan *et al.* (1991) to act as a good spermicidal agent. Pre and post coital application of the oil intra vaginally prevented pregnancy in rhesus monkey. Neem oil at subcutaneous doses up to 0.3 ml/rat did not possess any estrogenic, anti-estrogenic or progestational activity and appeared not to interfere with the action of progesterone.

Thus, Prakash *et al.* (1988) expects that neem oil would elicit less side effects than the steroidal contraceptives, since the post-coital contraceptive effect of neem oil seems to be non-hormonal.

Khillare and Shrivastav (2003) studied the neem leaf also on the spermicidal activity and found the minimum effective spermicidal concentrations for tender and old neem leaf extracts were 2.91 +/- 0.669 mg/million sperm and 2.75 +/- 0.754 mg/million sperm, respectively. With an increase in concentration, there is a linear decrease in percentage motility, becoming zero at a 3-mg dose within 20s.

Garg *et al.* (1994) identified a potent spermicide free from side effects by combination strategy. The positive synergistic effect in the spermicidal activity of the components - purified neem seeds extract (Praneem), reetha saponins and quinine hydrochloride indicates reduced concentrations of each to achieve effective spermicidal activity (0.39 per cent neem oil, 0.015 per cent reetha saponins, and 0.0012 per cent quinine hydrochloride). Reetha saponin contains considerable oleanolic acid or hederagenin, which have a mild detergent effect, inactivating sperm. Quinine chloride strengthens spermicidal activity and antimicrobial activity. Neem extract induces local cell-mediated immunity. Contraceptive developers can formulate the combination of these 3 components either as a cream or pessary.

The treatment with aqueous leaf extract of neem had adverse effects on motility, morphology, and number of spermatozoa in the cauda epididymidis, level of fructose in the seminal vesicle, and on litter size. After 42 days of withdrawal of the treatment, the alterations induced in the reproductive organs recovered to control levels (Mishra and Singh, 2005). The polar and non-polar fractions of *A. indica* and *M. azedarach* (mountain variety) seed extracts significantly reduced the number of normal follicles in rats, with maximum reduction occurring with 6 mg polar fraction of *Azadirachta* extract. This is consistent with its use in folk medicine as an anti-conceptional agent (Roop *et al.*, 2005).

Administration of alcoholic extract of Neem flower disrupted the estrous cycle in Sprague-Dawley rats and caused a partial block in ovulation and thus has the potential of being developed into a female contraceptive (Gbotolorun *et al.*, 2008). There are differences in the observations which could be attributed to the fact that there is variability in *Neem* with respect to azadirachtin content (Sidhu *et al.*, 2003).

A polyherbal pessary formulated with purified ingredients from neem (*Azadirachta indica*) leaves, *Sapindus mukerossi* (pericarp of fruit) and *Mentha citrata* oil showed spermicidal action on human sperm *in vitro* and *in vivo*. When applied in the vagina before mating, it prevented rabbits from conceiving (Raghuvanshi *et al.*, 2001).

Garlic (*Allium sativum*)

Garlic bulbs have been reported to have abortifacient (Casey 1960) and emmenagogic properties (Saha *et al.*, 1961; Khory and Katrak, 1999; Wealth of India 1972, Warrier *et al.*, 1994; Husain *et al.*, 1992). It has been reported that garlic powder (Dixit and Joshi, 1982) or crude garlic preparations (Hammami *et al.*, 2008) impaired testicular and male reproductive tract functions. Moreover, garlic metabolites such as diallyl trisulfide have been reported to have spermicidal effects (Chakrabarti *et al.*,

2003; Qian *et al.*, 1986). The mechanisms of garlic action on male reproduction function, and particularly on spermatogenesis, however, remain unknown. Crude garlic consumption for one month reduced testosterone secretion and altered spermatogenesis at 10 per cent, 15 per cent and 30 per cent doses (Hammami *et al.*, 2008). Hammami *et al.* (2009) showed that feeding with crude fresh crushed garlic has inhibitory effects on Leydig steroidogenic enzyme expression and Sertoli cell markers. These alterations might induce germ cell death (spermatocytes and spermatids) via an apoptotic process. According to Abdelmalik (2011), the testicular apoptosis with disruption in spermatogenesis following chronic crude garlic consumption could be correlated with two possible theories: being an anti-hyper-cholesterolemic agent, it might inhibit steroidogenesis resulting in a decrease in testosterone level and being one of the famous phytoestrogens it possibly has direct estrogen-like actions on adult male rat testes.

Hammami and El May (2012) have shown that garlic impairs testicular functions and has spermicidal effect on spermatozoa. The seminiferous tubules of rats treated with garlic fractions [one soluble in water (aqueous solution obtained by grinding and centrifugation) and the other one precipitated by ethanol (alcoholic precipitate obtained by precipitation of the aqueous solution)] showed an increased number of tubules deprived of spermatozoa. Hammami *et al.* (2013) reported through histological and molecular studies that one or several substances, soluble in water and precipitated by alcohol, impaired spermatogenesis.

Cumin Seeds (*Cuminum cyminum*)

Animals treated with methanol extract of cumin seeds showed a marked reduction in sperm density in the cauda epididymis and testes, and sperm motility in the cauda epididymis. Reduction in fertility was 69.0 per cent and 76.0 per cent in 100 and 200 mg/rat/day dose levels, respectively. The circulatory hormones were also reduced significantly. Testicular biochemical analysis of protein, sialic acid, glycogen, ascorbic acid and fructose indicated a marked decline, whereas testicular cholesterol content was significantly increased, which showed altered biochemistry of the reproductive organs. Thus, Gupta *et al.* (2011) confirmed that *C. cyminum* treatment resulted in the inhibition of spermatogenesis and fertility without producing apparent toxic effects. Abortifacient effect seems to be due to the presence of coumingine (Abdo and Al–Kafaw, 1969).

Fenugreek Seeds (*Trigonella foenum graecum*)

Setty *et al.* (1976) reported that a 2 per cent concentration of the saponin fraction of fenugreek showed *in vitro* spermicidal action against rat and human semen. Literature also demonstrated that on feeding diets containing 30 per cent fenugreek seeds, a decrease in the testis weight, histopathological damage to the seminiferous tubules and interstitial tissues; and a decrease in the plasma concentration of the androgen hormone and sperm concentrations was observed in male rabbits and histo-pathologically evident proliferative changes of the endometrial glands and also a significant increase in the circulating plasma progesterone concentrations at 10 and 20 days of gestation in female rabbits. Reduction of both fetal and placental weights at 20 days of gestation, and of the litter size indicated a significant reduction of developing fetuses in the female rabits (Kassem *et al.*, 2006). Supplementation with fenugreek seed extract to female albino wistar rats reduced uterine weights along with the levels of FSH, LH, progesterone and estrogen. These results confirmed the traditional belief on the antiestrogenic activity of fenugreek seeds (Amin and Subhadra, 2008)

Lemon (*Citrus limonum*)

Citrus-limonum is native of North West region of India. The petroleum ether, alcoholic and aqueous extracts of *Citrus-limonum* (lemon) seeds were investigated for anti-fertility effect in female albino mice. The alcoholic extract showed significant anti-fertility effect as compared to petroleum ether and aqueous extracts. The fraction of ethyl-acetate (12-25 fractions) showed most encourageing anti-fertility activity. In the second part of the study, the alcoholic extract and its ethyl-acetate fraction (12-25 fractions) were observed to exhibit anti-zygotic action. Withdrawal of the test drug resulted in complete restoration of fertility. Thus the ethyl-acetate fraction (12-25 fractions) of alcoholic extract of lemon seeds exerted reversible anti-fertility effect in female mice by virtue of its anti-zygotic action (Kulkarni *et al.*, 2005).

Salawu *et al.* (2010) found a significant (P = 0.001) reduction in the number of ova shed in rats administered undiluted lime juice also in comparison with the control animals. Ovulation was partially blocked, as shown by the reduced number of ova observed in the oviducts from the rats given undiluted lime juice (5.10 ±2.37) in comparison with the control rats (12.70 ± 1.14).

Drumstick (*Moringa oleifera*)

Sethi *et al.* (1988) observed 100 per cent abortifacient activity with the plant extract of *Moringa oleifera* and none of the parameters of anti-fertility activity could be detected. The aqueous extract of *M. oleifera* when administered to pregnant rats, no deciduoma was observed on 5th day of pregnancy and the luminal epithelium remained unstimulated. The lumen was enlarged and the uterus was non-oedematous. It has been concluded that the administration of aqueous extract of *M. oleifera* to pregnant rats could not stimulate the uterus which remained non-receptive throughout the period of treatment, and therefore, the fertilized eggs may not be welcomed by the unprepared uterus (Prakash *et al.*, 1987). Administration of the extract in ovariectomized rats stimulated the uterine histo-architecture as revealed by increases in the height of luminal epithelium, well developed glands, loose stroma and rich vascularity. The cervix showed metaplastic changes in the epithelium with marked keratinization. In the vagina, cornification was very prominent, rugae increased and stroma was loose. Conjoint administration of the extract with estradiol showed a synergistic action, and an inhibition was observed when administered conjointly with progesterone (Shukla *et al.*, 1989). Shukla *et al.* (1988a) concluded from his investigation that the anti-fertility effect of the *Moringa oleifera* root extract appears to be due to multiple attributes. Biochemical observations supplemented with the histological findings have been correlated with the anti-implantation action of the aqueous extract in the light of its hormonal properties (Shukla *et al.*, 1988b).

Pineapple (*Ananas comosus*)

The pineapple juice is believed to be an anti-fertility fruit in Malaya (Casey, 1960). Pineapple exhibited 60 per cent anti-implantation activity at a concentration of 50 ml/kg in rats (Bhaduri *et al.*, 1968). The ethanol and petroleum ether extracts of the fruit also yielded similar results in the past. The fruit, fruit juice and leaf have been reported to be abortifacient and emmenagogic (Casey, 1960; Saha *et al.*, 1961) while the leaf and fruit has been reported to be uterotonic due to the presence of 5 hydroxy tryptamine (Paton, 1968; Barlow and Khan, 1959). Resorptive activity at 100mg/kg body wt. has been reported on consumption of pineapple fruit by Prakash *et al.* (1978) but no anti-fertility effect at 100-200mg/kg body wt. (Prakash and Mathur, 1976) was observed with the unripe fruit. Reports in the past suggest that pineapple has exhibited estrogenic activity (Feurt and Fox, 1955). Singh *et al.* (1985) implied that a compound; 5-stigmastene-3β, 7α-diol isolated from pineapple leaves induced anti-fertility effect in mice. The juice from unripe fruits demonstrated encourageing anti-implantation activity showing 40 per cent of implants only.

Pomegranate

The pericarp of pomegranate at 3g and 9g per day for 4 weeks resulted in infertile matings in rats and guinea pigs respectively (Gujaral *et al.*, 1960) but no antifertility effect was observed in the fruit at a dose 200 mg/kg body wt (Prakash and Mathur, 1976). The fruit peel, however, demonstrated a high incidence of pseudo pregnancies (Gujaral *et al.*, 1960). Besides the root and bark of pomegranate being abortifacient and emmenagogic (Watt and Breyer-Brandwijk 1962), the fruit pulp also has been reported to be uterotonic (Dhawan and Saxena, 1958).

Soya Beans (*Glycine max*)

Cederroth *et al.* (2010a) reviewed the evidence regarding the potential detrimental effects of soy and phyto-oestrogens on male reproductive function and fertility in humans and animals. There are some indications that phyto-oestrogens, alone or in combination with other endocrine disruptors, may alter reproductive hormones, spermatogenesis, sperm capacitation and fertility and therefore feeding infants on soy-based formula, should be avoided (Cederroth *et al.*, 2010a). Review of the studies on the influence of dietary soy and phytoestrogens on testicular and reproductive functions showed that long-term exposure to dietary soy and phytoestrogens may affect male reproductive function resulting in a small decrease in sperm count and fertility (Cederroth *et al.*, 2010b).

Grape Fruit (*Citrus sinensis/Citrus paradise*)

Fingerová *et al.* (2003) that grapefruit juice may increase bioavailability of orally administered estradiol and progesterone. The response varies markedly between individuals. This observation may be of some importance also for users of OC and HRT.

Garden Cress Seeds (*Lepidium sativum*)

The garden cress seed oil has been reported to have variable proportion of benzyl isothiocyanate, benzyl cyanide, lignoceric and behenic acid, and posses estrogenic activity on immature rats, as 3-4 drops of the oil in the diet, demonstrated consistently better development, higher weights of ovaries and several hemorrhagic follicles in the ovaries (Sahasrabuddhe and De, 1943). Studies conducted in 1976 reported that the seeds did not exhibit any anti-fertility effect at a dose of 150 - 200mg/kg body wt. (Prakash *et al.*, 1978; Prakash and Mathur, 1976). But the seeds have been reported to have abortifacient activity (Casey, 1960; Saha *et al.*, 1961; Warrier *et al.*, 1994; Malhi and Trivedi 1972; Hussain *et al.*, 1992), spasmolytic activity, galactogogic and emmenagogic activity (Warrier *et al.*, 1994; Wealth of India, 1972).

Later in 1984, between the β sitosterol and glucotropaeolin (Wealth of India, 1972; Kirtikar and Basu, 1984) present in garden cress seeds, the β sitosterol has been reported to have anti implantation activity at a dose of 100-150 mg/kg in rats. Probably due to this, garden cress seed oil was suggested as an effective postcoital contraceptive (Singh *et al.*, 1984).

Mustard Seeds (*Brassica juncea*)

Mustard seeds extracted in water is drunk with a belief that they have abortifacient properties (Casey, 1960) and mustard is an anti-fertility plant (Malhi and Trivedi, 1972).

Mustard hip baths were used in fever, uterine derangement, amenorrhea and dysmenorrhea (Khory and Katrak, 1999). These effects of mustard could be due to the various compounds present in it like signirin, enzyme myrosin, sinapine sulphocyanide, lecithin, glucosinoles, allyl isothiocyanate (Wealth of India, 1972; Asolkar *et al.*, 1992; Khory and Katrak, 1999; Kirtikar and Basu, 1984).

Betel Leaves (*Piper betel* Linn.)

It is believed among the rural population in South India that betel leaf consumption after delivery delays conception. The extract was found to reduce fertility to 0 per cent within 60 days. Suppression of cauda epididymal sperm count and motility ($p < 0.05$) was observed. The contraceptive effect of the extract of leaf-stalk of *Piper betle* Linn. was found to be mainly on the maturation process of spermatozoa in epididymides without influencing hystemic hormonal profiles. Withdrawal of the extract restored all altered parameters including organ weights and fertility after 60 days (Sarkar *et al.*, 2000; Dhar *et al.*, 1992).

Ginger (*Zingiber officinale*)

Farnsworth and colleagues (1975) also reported ginger to have abortifacient qualities, but the active constituent responsible for this was not identified. Dose and time-dependent decreases in motility accompanied by concomitant decrease in grading 3 and 4 were noticed in human semen samples treated with methanolic extract of ginger. Accordingly Jorsaraei *et al.* (2008) concluded that ginger can induce the toxic effects on sperm parameters.

Black/Long Pepper (*Piper longum, Piper nigrum*)

Piperine effectively inhibited implantation, produced abortion and delayed labor when it was given from day 2 through 5, day 8 through 12 and day 15 until labor, respectively. Piyachaturawat *et al.* (1982) from their observations suggested that the anti-fertility activity of piperine did not operate through any hormonal actions or uterotonic activity. Daware *et al.* (2000) showed that piperine interferes with several crucial reproductive events in a mammalian model.

Coriander Seeds (*Coriandrum sativum*)

The aqueous extract of fresh coriander seeds produced a significant decrease in serum progesterone levels on day-5 of pregnancy which may be responsible for the anti-implantation effect observed by Al-Said *et al.* (1987).

Turmeric (*Curcuma longa* L)

C. longa treatment causes reversible suppression of spermatogenesis and fertility, thereby suggesting the potential of this plant in the regulation of male fertility (Mishra and Singh, 2009). Incubation of sperm with curcumin caused a concentration-dependent decrease in sperm forward motility, capacitation/acrosome reaction, and murine fertilization *in vitro*. At higher concentrations, there was a complete block of sperm motility and function within 5-15 min. Administration of curcumin, especially intravaginally, caused a significant ($P<0.001$) reduction in fertility. The antifertility effect of curcumin was reversible. This is the first study to report the inhibitory effect of curcumin on sperm function, fertilization, and fertility. The findings suggest that curcumin may constitute a double-edged sword to block conception, infection, and cancer, thus providing an ideal contraceptive (Naz, 2011).

Betel Nut

The betelnut commonly consumed in rural and tribal areas, besides being abortifacient and emmenagogic (Casey, 1960; Saha *et al.*, 1961) has been reported to show uterotonic activity due to the presence of the active constituent arecoline or the tannin content (Saha and Kashinathan, 1961). The petroleum ether, ethanol, water extracts of betelnut have showed anti-implantation activity at 500mg/kg in rats (Garg and Garg, 1970) while the water extract of this plant was ineffective at 0.05 – 0.2 ml twice a day in mice (Matsui *et al.*, 1967).

Peas

An interesting observation about *Pisum sativum*, 'peas' is that when contributing to 20 per cent of the diet, it decreased litter production and when contributing to 30 per cent of diet, it abolished litter production in rats only during the first 10 days of pregnancy (Sanyal, 1956). The active compound responsible for this action 'm Xylohydroquinone' isolated from pea oil was experimentally found to reduce pregnancy rates in Indian women (Sanyal, 1960) and earlier showed similar effects in the Tibetan population, where the staple diet consists of corn and peas (Sanyal, 1956).

Dates

Dates have also been reported in literature to be used as aphrodisiacs (Khory and Katrak, 1999; Husain *et al.*, 1992). The date seed has been reported to demonstrate the presence of ergosterol and estrone. The non saponifiable fraction of fatty oil from dried date pollen showed the presence of estrogenic substances and has also exhibited gonadotrophic activity on immature rats (Wealth of India, 1972; Hussain *et al.*, 1992).

Coconut

In Java, nut milk is used for contraception purpose (Asolkar *et al.*, 1992). Coconut has also been reported to have abortifacient effect (Casey, 1960) while its dried kernel has been considered to be an aphrodisiac (Khory and Katrak, 1999).

Cowpeas (*Vigna unguiculata*)

Histological studies showed severe degenerative changes in the testis and the presence of multinucleated giant cells in the epididymis of the cowpea fed group, that did not have fertile matings. It is proposed that cowpeas may contain some factors that could have antifertility effects, although the nature of such factors was not known (Umapathy, 1993).

Non-Conventional Foods

Brahmi (*Cintella asiatica*)

In Brahmi-treated males fertility was notably suppressed. The alterations caused in the above reproductive end points by the plant extract were reversible, and by 56 days of treatment withdrawal, the parameters recovered to control levels. Thus Singh and Singh (2009) found Brahmi treatment to cause reversible suppression of spermatogenesis and fertility, without producing apparent toxic effects.

Cotton Seed

The anti-fertility effect of the cottonseed oil, gossypol, had been first observed in China, where it was administered orally to over 40,000 healthy males, with an effectiveness of 99 per cent (Tso and Lee, 1982). The authors of this study found gossypol to be a vaginal contraceptive with an added advantage of vaginal lubricating quality. They also found gossypol to cause total immobilization of spermatozoa in male seminal fluid. Kalla and Vasudev (1980) observed that treatment with gossypol depletes production of adenosine triphosphate in the sperms and thus their metabolism does not proceed normally, rendering them immotile. It appears that the high vulnerability of the testis–to gossypol and the uncoupling of oxidative phosphorylation in the respiratory chain of mitochondria of germ cells may be the mechanism responsible for infertility induction. In an attempt to mitigate the gastric side effects of gossypol, one group of clinicians adopted enteric-coated tablets for the clinical trial. They found that both the anti- fertiltiy effect and the systemic side effects of these tablets were much less than those of ordinary tablets. On the contrary, Zatuchni and Osborn (1981) reported that around 4000 Chinese men used gossypol contraceptive pill for at least 6 months, and some for more than 4 years. The efficacy rate of the pill was 99.89 per cent. Infertility was produced by cotton seed flour diets even with a low concentration of gossypol (defatted cottonseed flour); this effect was reversible at least after 6 weeks of gossypol-containing diets, even in the groups fed diets with a high gossypol concentration (Sotelo *et al.*, 1982). Male fertility returned

(Penningroth, 1984) by 3 months after discontinuation of the pill, and there were no apparent serious side effects on the babies borne by the wives of the men who had stopped using gossypol. Thus, gossypol was proved to be an effective anti-spermatogenic agent for certain susceptible animals and humans, and represents the only reasonable approach to reach the stage of large scale clinical testing (Qian and Wang, 1984). Porat (1990) who surveyed the research on gossypol is uncertain if infertility induced by gossypol is reversible or not.

Gossypol seems to disrupt estrous cycles, pregnancy, and early embryo development in females of all non-ruminant species studied. Probable mechanisms include an endocrine effect on the ovary as well as a cytotoxic effect on the uterus or embryo. The female ruminant seems to be relatively insensitive to the anti-fertility effect of gossypol; however, *in vitro* data indicate some inhibition of embryonic development and ovarian steroidogenesis. The anti-fertility effect of gossypol has been studied most in males of nonruminant species. The effects of gossypol in the male are both dose- and time-dependent. At effective doses, gossypol causes males to be infertile because of sperm immotility and depressed sperm counts. Extensive damage to the germinal epithelium has been shown in both rams and bulls fed diets containing gossypol (Randel *et al.*, 1992).

According to Porat (1990) the most common toxic side effect of cotton seed consumption is hypo-kalemia, which is severe enough to cause temporary paralysis in 1 per cent of 8806 volunteers in a study conducted in China. Whether potassium loss can be reversed by supplementation, or by taking potassium-sparing diuretics, has been questioned. Similarly, the extent and permanence of renal damage presumed responsible for potassium loss is uncertain.

Yet, the extensive investigations on formal animal toxicology and on the recovery of fertility in men after withdrawl of gossypol treatment led to the decision by the Special Programme of Research, Development and Research Training in Human Reproduction at the World Health Organization, that gossypol would not be acceptable as an antifertility drug (Waites *et al.*, 1998). Roychoudhury *et al.* (2009) confirmed the dose and time dependent alterations of rabbit spermatozoa motility parameters by gossypol and also indicated that a higher immobilizing potential of unfiltered gossypol in comparison to filtered one in rabbits.

Castor Bean (*Ricinus communis*)

The protein contents of castor bean extract, separated by polyacrylamide gel electrophoresis, revealed the presence of several protein bands, ricin toxin being a major constituent of the extract. Both castor bean extract (CBE) and ricin A-chain (RAC) administered intraperitoneally on days 5-9 of pregnancy, exhibited a pronounced decrease in maternal body weight gain and in death of all fetuses. A significant ($p < 0.01$) decrease of implantation sites resulted after rabbits were treated with RAC on the first 6 consecutive days of pregnancy indicating that CBE and RAC possess potent effects on implantation and ovulation in rabbits (Salhab *et al.*, 1999). The seed extract possesses an anti-fertility effect in female guinea pigs, which might be extrapolated in human beings. These findings might support the accredited claim of its traditional use to avoid unwanted pregnancies (Makonnen *et al.*, 1999).

The ether extracts of castorbean seed possessed antifertility activity and contraceptive efficacy in female and male rodents and the *in vitro* study showed significant inhibitory activity in the primary cultured rat decidual stromal cells. Zhang *et al.* (2007) presumed that gamma-sitosterol may be the main component contributing to inhibit the viability of decidual stromal cells. Nithya *et al.* (2012) also confirmed that 50 per cent ethanolic extract of the root of *Ricinus communis* possesses reversible anti-fertility effect. According to them, a 62-kDa protein (Rp) from this extract is responsible for the anti-fertility effects. They also showed that the protein Rp possesses spermicidal activity *in vitro* and its effects are similar to that of nonoxynol 9.

The Anti-fertility Effect of Selected Foods

Food	*Effect*
Mint leaves	Anti-implantation activity at 100-500mg/kg body wt (Bodhankar *et al.*, 1974).
Bitter gourd	Antifertility due to cytotoxic constituents like cucurbitacins (Belkin and Fitzgerald, 1952).
Asafoetida	Prevented conception for a year when followed in a specific regimen with other plant extracts (Das, 1966).Reinvestigation of the anti-fertility effect suggested by Farnsworth *et al.*, 1975).
Pepper	Abortifacient (Malhi and Trivedi, 1972; Casey, 1960; Saha *et al.*, 1961).

Amin and Subhadra (2008)

Bael (*Aegle marmelos*)

The leaf extract of bael (bilvapatra) suppresses fertility in male rats (Chauhan *et al.*, 2007; Chauhan and Agarwal, 2009). Complete recovery of fertility was observed following the withdrawal of drug. Absence of any deleterious effect on the vital organs points to the safe use of the extract.

Ajwain

Omum seeds have also been shown to have emmenagogic activity (Saha *et al.*, 1961). The active component responsible for this effect remains unidentified. It could include the omum oil containing petroselenic acid, thymol, carvacrol, α and β pinene, camphene, myrcene, D-3-carene, limonene, γ terpinene, r cymene, phenol glucoside–2 -methyl 3 glucosyloxy 5 isopropyl phenol (Hussain *et al.*, 1992) or any other yet undiscovered compound.

Tulasi (*Ocimum sanctum*)

Tulasi leaves showed encourageing results when tested for anti-fertilizing, anti-zygotic, blasto-cystotoxic, anti-implantation, and early abortifacient activity (Vohora *et al.*, 1969).

Conclusions

There is an urgent need for research to develop new contraceptive modalities especially for men and also for women and to make existing methods more safe, affordable and acceptable. Though many plants not mentioned in classic literature were found to be active according to Kamboj (1988), a lot more work has been done in the last 2 decades; but still it seems more focus is needed on all Indian plants for anti-implantation, anti-fertility effects under strict WHO guidelines in order to control the population especially in India and improve the health of the nation. However, experimental studies are required to confirm the association between dietary fat intake and fertility among men and women. Most of the work focused on herbals and some foods like dates, coconut etc. are quite earlier ones and there is a scarcity of recent reports.

References

Abdelmalik SW (2011). Histological and ultra-structural changes in the adult male albino rat testes following chronic crude garlic consumption. Ann. Anat. 193 (2): 134 - 41.

Abdo MS, Al–Kafaw AA (1969). In: Planta Med 17:14. In: Farnsworth NR, Bingel AS, Cordell GA, Crane FA, Fong HS (1975). Potential value of plants as sources of new anti-fertility agents –I. J. Pharm. Sci. 64 (4): 535 - 98.

Adebiyi A, Adaikan PG, Prasad RN (2002). Papaya (*Carica papaya*) consumption is unsafe in pregnancy: fact or fable? Scientific evaluation of a common belief in some parts of Asia using a rat model. Br. J. Nutr. 88 (2): 199 - 203.

Adebiyi A, Ganesan Adaikan P, Prasad RN (2003). Tocolytic and toxic activity of papaya seed extract on isolated rat uterus. Life Sci. 74 (5): 581 - 92.

Afeiche M, Williams PL, Mendiola J, Gaskins AJ, Jørgensen N, Swan SH, Chavarro JE (2013). Dairy food intake in relation to semen quality and reproductive hormone levels among physically active young men. Hum. Reprod. 28 (8): 2265 - 75.

Aksoy Y, Aksoy H, Altinkaynak K, Aydin HR, Ozkan A (2006). Sperm fatty acid composition in subfertile men. Prostaglandins Leukot. Essent. Fatty Acids. 75 (2): 75 - 79.

Al-Said MS, Al-Khamis KI, Islam MW, Parmar NS, Tariq M, Ageel AM (1987). Post-coital anti-fertility activity of the seeds of *Coriandrum sativum* in rats. J. Ethnopharmacol. 21 (2): 165 - 73.

Amin JA and Subhadra, M (2008). Phytosteroids and phenolic compounds in spices and spice mixes, PhD thesis (unpublished data). College of Home Science, Nirmala Niketan, Mumbai.

Anuar NS, Zahari SS, Taib IA, Rahman MT (2008). Effect of green and ripe *Carica papaya* epicarp extracts on wound healing and during pregnancy. Food Chem. Toxicol. 46 (7): 2384 - 89.

Asolkar LV, Kakkar KK, Chakre OJ (1992). Glossary of Indian medicinal plants with active principles. CSIR Publication, New Delhi. 2nd suppl. part –I, A-K.

Attaman JA, Toth TL, Furtado J, Campos H, Hauser R, Chavarro JE (2012). Dietary fat and semen quality among men attending a fertility clinic. Hum. Reprod. 27 (5): 1466 - 74.

Bardhan J, Riar SS, Sawhney RC, Kain AK, Thomas P, Ilavazhagan G (1991). Neem oil - a fertility controlling agent in rhesus monkey. Indian J. Physiol. Pharmacol. 35 (4): 278 - 80.

Barlow RB, Khan I (1959). Actions of some analogues of tryptamine on the isolated rat uterus and on the isolated rat fundus strip preparations. Br. J. Pharmacol. Chemother. 14 (1): 99 - 107.

Belkin M, Fitzgerald DB (1952). J Nat Cancer Inst 13:607 in Farnsworth NR, Bingel AS, Cordell GA, Crane FA, Fong HS (1975). Potential value of plants as sources of new anti-fertility agents – II. J. Pharm. Sci. 64 (5): 717 - 54.

Bhaduri H, Ghose CR, Bose AN, Moza BK, Basu UP (1968). Indian J. Exp. Biol. 6:.252. In: Farnsworth NR, Bingel AS, Cordell GA, Crane FA, Fong HS (1975). Potential value of plants as sources of new anti-fertility agents - I. J. Pharm. Sci. 64 (4): 535 – 98.

Bingel AS, Fong HH (1988). Potential fertility regulating plants In: Economical and Medicinal Plant Research. Wagner H, Hikino H, Farnsworth NR (eds). Academic Press. London. Chapter. 4. vol 2. pp 96 - 115.

Blesbois E, Douard V, Germain M, Boniface P, Pellet F (2004). Effects of n-3 polyunsaturated dietary supplementation on the reproductive capacity of male turkeys. Theriogenology. 61: 537 - 49.

Bongalhardo DC, Leeson S, Buhr MM (2009). Dietary lipids differentially affect membranes from different areas of rooster sperm. Poult. Sci. 88 (5): 1060 - 69.

Bodhankar SL, Garg SK, Mathur VS (1974). Antifertility screening of plants. Part IX. Effect of five indigenous plants on early pregnancy in female albino rats. Indian J. Med. Res. 62 (6): 831 - 37.

Casey RC (1960). Indian J Med Sci 14:590. In: Farnsworth NR, Bingel AS, Cordell GA, Crane FA, Fong HS (1975). Potential value of plants as sources of new anti-fertility agents - I. J. Pharm. Sci. 64 (4): 535 - 98.

Cederroth CR, Auger J, Zimmermann C, Eustache F, Nef S (2010a). Soy, phyto-oestrogens and male reproductive function: a review. Int. J. Androl. 33 (2): 304 - 16.

Cederroth CR, Zimmermann C, Beny JL, Schaad O, Combepine C, Descombes P, Doerge DR, Pralong FP, Vassalli JD, Nef S (2010b). Potential detrimental effects of a phytoestrogen-rich diet on male fertility in mice. Mol. Cell. Endocrinol. 321 (2):152 - 60.

Chakrabarti K, Pal S, Bhattacharyya AK (2003). Sperm immobilization activity of *Allium sativum* L. and other plant extracts. Asian J. Androl. 5: 131 - 35.

Chaudhury RR (1985) Plant Contraceptives: Translating folklore into scientific application. In: Advances in maternal and child health. (eds) DB Jelliffe and EFP Jelliffe (Oxford: Oxford University Press) vol. 5. p. 58.

Chaudhury RR (2001). Traditional methods of fertility regulation. In: Current status in fertility regulation - Indigenous and modern approaches (eds) SR Chaudhury, CM Gupta and VP Kamboj (Lucknow: CDRI) pp XI–XXI.

Chauhan A, Agarwal M (2009). Assessment of the contraceptive efficacy of the aqueous extract of *Aegle marmelos Corr*. leaves in male albino rats. Hum Fertil (Camb). 12 (2): 107 - 118.

Chauhan A, Agarwal M, Kushwaha S, Mutreja A (2007). Suppression of fertility in male albino rats following the administration of 50 per cent ethanolic extract of *Aegle marmelos*. Contraception. 76 (6): 474 - 81.

Chavarro JE, Rich-Edwards JW, Rosner BA, Willett WC (2007a). Dietary fatty acid intakes and the risk of ovulatory infertility. Am. J. Clin. Nutr. 85 (1): 231 - 37.

Chavarro JE, Rich-Edwards JW, Rosner BA, Willett WC (2007b). Diet and lifestyle in the prevention of ovulatory disorder infertility. Obstet. Gynecol. 110 (5): 1050 - 58.

Chavarro JE, Rich-Edwards JW, Rosner BA, Willett WC (2008). Use of multivitamins, intake of B vitamins, and risk of ovulatory infertility. Fertil. Steril. 89 (3): 668 - 76.

Conquer JA, Martin JB, Tummon I, Watson L, Tekpetey F (1999). Fatty acid analysis of blood serum, seminal plasma, and spermatozoa of normozoospermic vs. asthenozoospermic males. Lipids. 34 (8): 793 - 99.

Czeizel AE, Metneki J, Dudas I (1996). The effect of preconceptional multivitamin supplementation on fertility. Int. J. Vitam. Nutr. Res. 66: 55 - 58.

Dallaqua B, Saito FH, Rodrigues T, Calderon IM, Rudge MV, Herrera E, Damasceno DC (2012). Treatment with *Azadirachta indica* in diabetic pregnant rats: negative effects on maternal outcome. J. Ethnopharmacol. 143 (3): 805 - 11.

Das PC (1966). Chem Abstr 64,19328h in Farnsworth NR, Bingel AS, Cordell GA, Crane FA, Fong HS (1975). Potential value of plants as sources of new anti-fertility agents - I. J. Pharm. Sci. 64 (4): 535 - 98.

Daware MB, Mujumdar AM, Ghaskadbi S (2000). Reproductive toxicity of piperine in Swiss albino mice. Planta. Med. 66 (3): 231 - 36.

Dhaliwal PK, Roop JK & Guraya SS (1998). Anti-fertility activity of neem-seed oil in cyclic female rats. In: Dhaliwal GS, Randhawa NS, Arora A & Dhawan AK. (Eds). Ecological Agriculture and Sustainable Development. Vol. 2. Indian Ecological Society and Centre for Research in Rural and Industrial Development, Chandigarh, India, 340 - 46.

Dhar JD, Setty BS, Lakshmi V, Bhakuni DS (1992). Post-coital anti-fertility activity of the marine plant, *Achrostichum aureum* L. in rat. Indian J. Med. Res. 96: 150 - 52.

Dhawan BN, Saxena PN (1958). Evaluation of some indigenous drugs for stimulant effect on rat uterus: a preliminary report. Indian J. Med. Res. 46 (6): 808 - 811.

Dixit VP, Joshi S (1982). Effects of chronic administration of garlic (*Allium sativum* Linn) on testicular function. Indian J. Exp. Biol. 20: 534 - 36.

Ebisch IM, Thomas CM, Peters WH, Braat DD, Steegers-Theunissen RP (2007). The importance of folate, zinc and antioxidants in the pathogenesis and prevention of subfertility. Hum. Reprod. Update. 13: 163 - 174.

Eslamian G, Amirjannati N, Rashidkhani B, Sadeghi MR, Hekmatdoost A (2012). Intake of food groups and idiopathic asthenozoospermia: a case-control study. Hum Reprod. 27 (11): 3328 - 36.

Estienne MJ, Harper AF, Crawford RJ (2008). Dietary supplementation with a source of omega-3 fatty acids increases sperm number and the duration of ejaculation in boars. Theriogenology. 70 (1): 70 - 76.

Farnsworth NR, Bingel AS, Cordell GA, Crane FA, Fong HS (1975). Potential value of plants as sources of new anti-fertility agents II. J. Pharm. Sci. 64 (4 & 5): 535 - 98; 717 - 54.

Farnsworth NR, Waller DP (1982). Current status of plant products reported to inhibit sperm. Res. Front. Fertil. Regul. 2 (1): 1 - 16.

Fingerová H, Oborná I, Petrová P, Budíková M, Jezdínský J (2003). [Does grapefruit juice increase the bioavailability of orally administered sex steroids?]. Ceska. Gynekol. 68 (2): 117 - 21. [Article in Czech].

Feurt SD, Fox LE (1955). Report on Wax from Several Species of *Tillandsia* and from *Ananas comosus* (L.) Merr. Science. 121 (3132): 42.

Garg SK (1975). Anti-fertility effect of some chromatographic fractions of *Daucus carota.* Indian J. Pharmacol. 7 (1, 2): 40 - 42.

Garg SK, Garg GP (1970). Anti-fertility screening of plants part –VII-effect of 5 indigenous plants on early pregnancy in albino rats. Indian J. Med. Res. 59 (2): 302 - 306.

Garg S, Doncel G, Chabra S, Upadhyay SN, Talwar GP (1994). Synergistic spermicidal activity of neem seed extract, reetha saponins and quinine hydrochloride. Contraception. 50 (2): 185 - 90.

Garg S, Talwar GP, Upadhyay SN (1998). Immunocontraceptive activity guided fractionation and characterization of active constituents of neem (*Azadirachta indica*) seed extracts. Ethnopharmacol. 60 (3): 235 - 46.

Gaskins AJ, Colaci DS, Mendiola J, Swan SH, Chavarro JE (2012a). Dietary patterns and semen quality in young men. Hum. Reprod. 27 (10): 2899 - 907.

Gaskins AJ, Mumford SL, Chavarro JE, Zhang C, Pollack AZ, Wactawski-Wende J, Perkins NJ,Schisterman EF (2012b). The impact of dietary folate intake on reproductive function in premenopausal women: a prospective cohort study. PLoS One. 7 (9): e46276.

Gbotolorun SC, Osinubi AA, Noronha CC, Okanlawon AO (2008). Anti-fertility potential of Neem flower extract on adult female Sprague-Dawley rats. Afr. Health Sci. 8 (3): 168 - 73.

Gopalakrishnan M, Rajasekharasetty MR (1978). Effect of papaya (*Carica papaya* Linn.) on pregnancy and estrous cycle in albino rats of Wistar strain. Indian J. Physiol. Pharmacol. 22 (1): 66-70.

Gujaral ML, Varma DR, Sareen KN (1960). Oral contraceptives –part I preliminary observations on the antifertility effect of some indigenous drugs. Indian J. Med..Res. 48 (1): 46 – 51.

Gulaya NM, Margitich VM, Govseeva NM, Klimashevsky VM, Gorpynchenko II, Boyko MI (2001). Phospholipid composition of human sperm and seminal plasma in relation to sperm fertility. Arch. Androl. 46 (3): 169 - 75.

Gupta G (2005). Microbicidal spermicide or spermicidal microbicide? Eur J Contracept. Reprod. Health Care. 10 (4): 212 - 18.

Gupta RS, Saxena P, Gupta R, Kachhawa JB (2011). Evaluation of reversible contraceptive activities of *Cuminum cyminum* in male albino rats. Contraception. 84 (1): 98 - 107.

Hammami I, Amara S, Benahmed M, El May MV, Mauduit C (2009). Chronic crude garlic-feeding modified adult male rat testicular markers: mechanisms of action. Reprod. Biol. Endocrinol. 7: 65.

Hammami I, El May MV (2012). Impact of garlic feeding (*Allium sativum*) on male fertility. Andrologia. 2012 Sep 3. doi: 10.1111/and.12009. [Epub ahead of print].

Hammami I, Nahdi A, Atig F, Kouidhi W, Amri M, Mokni M, May AE, May ME (2013). Effects of garlic fractions consumption on male reproductive functions. J. Med. Food. 16 (1): 82 - 87.

Hammami I, Nahdi A, Mauduit C, Benahmed M, Amri M, Ben Amar A, Zekri S, El May A, El May MV (2008). The inhibitory effects on adult male reproductive functions of crude garlic (*Allium sativum*) feeding. Asian J. Androl. 10 (4): 593 - 601.

Hussain A,Virmani OP, Popli SP, Mujra LN, Gupta MM, Srivastva GN, Abraham Z, Singh AK (1992). Dictionary of Indian medicinal plants. Director, Central Institute of Medicinal and Aromatic Plants. Lucknow. 161 - 62.

Jacobson M (1995). Anti-fertility effects and population control agents. In: Schmutterer. (Ed). The Neem Tree - *Azadirachta indica* A. Juss and other Meliaceous plants. Published jointly by: VCH Verlagsgescll Schaft, Weinheim, Federal Republic of Germany, and VCH Publishers Inc., New York, 526 - 30.

Jensen TK, Heitmann BL, Jensen MB, Halldorsson TI, Andersson AM, Skakkebæk NE, Joensen UN, Lauritsen MP, Christiansen P, Dalgård C, Lassen TH, Jørgensen N (2013). High dietary intake of saturated fat is associated with reduced semen quality among 701 young Danish men from the general population. Am. J. Clin. Nutr. 97 (2): 411 - 18.

Jorsaraei SG, Yousefnia YR, Zainalzadeh M, Moghadamnia AA, Beiky AA, Damavandi MR (2008). The effects of methanolic extracts of ginger (*Zingiber officinale*) on human sperm parameters; an *in vitro* study. Pak. J. Biol. Sci. 11 (13): 1723 - 27.

Joshi J, Virkar K D and Devi P K (1977). Effect of an Ayurvedic preparation on peripheral parameters of the menstrual cycle. Ind. J. Med. Res. 66: 39 - 42.

Juneja SC, Pfeifer T, Williams RS, Chegini N (1994) *Neem* oil inhibits two- cell embryo development and trophoectoderm attachment and proliferation *in- vitro.* J. Assist. Reprod. Genet. 11: 419 - 27.

Juneja SC, Williams RS, Farooq A, Chegini N (1996). Contraception potential of neem oil: effect on pregnancy success in the mouse. J. Assist. Reprod. Genet. 13 (7): 578 - 85.

Kalla NR, Vasudev M (1980). Studies on the male antifertility agent gossypol acetic acid: *in vitro* studies on the effect of gossypol acetic acid on human spermatozoa. IRCS J. Med. Sci. 8 (6): 375 - 76.

Kamboj VP (1988). A review of Indian medicinal plants with interceptive activity. Ind. J. Med. Res. 87: 336 - 55.

Kamboj VP, Dhawan BN (1982). Research on plants for fertility regulation in India. J. Ethnopharmacol. 6 (2): 191 - 226.

Kassem A, Al-Aghbari A, AL-Habori M, Al-Mamary M (2006). Evaluation of the potential anti-fertility effect of fenugreek seeds in male and female rabbits. Contraception. 73 (3): 301 - 306.

Kasturi M, Ahamed RN, Pathan KM, Manivannan B, Aladakatti RH (2002). Ultrastructural changes induced by leaves of *Azadirachta indica* (Neem) in the testis of albino rats. J. Basic Clin. Physiol. Pharmacol. 13: 311 - 28.

Kaushik C, Upadhyay S (1995). Mode of long-term anti-fertility effect of intrauterine neem treatment (IUNT). Contraception. 51 (3): 203 - 207.

Kermani-Alghoraishi M, Anvari M, Talebi AR, Amini-Rad O, Ghahramani R, Miresmaili SM (2010). The effects of acrylamide on sperm parameters and membrane integrity of epididymal spermatozoa in mice. Eur. J. Obstet. Gynecol. Reprod. Biol. 153 (1): 52 - 55.

Khan PK, Awasthy KS (2003). Cytogenetic toxicity of neem. Food Chem. Toxicol., 41: 1325 - 28.

Khillare B, Shrivastav TG (2003). Spermicidal activity of *Azadirachta indica* (neem) leaf extract. Contraception. 68 (3): 225 - 29.

Khory RN, Katrak NN (1999). Materia Medica of India. Komal Prakashan, New Delhi.

Kirtikar, Basu (1984). In: Indian Medicinal Plants. vol1. (2nd edn). Singh B, Singh M (eds). Shastri Publishers, Dehradun.

Kulkarni TR, Kothekar MA, Mateenuddin M (2005). Study of anti-fertility effect of lemon seeds (*Citrus limonum*) in female albino mice. Indian J. Physiol. Pharmacol. 49 (3): 305 - 312.

Kusemiju O, Noronha C, Okanlawon A (2002). The effect of crude extract of the bark of *Carica papaya* on the seminiferous tubules of male Sprague-Dawley rats. Niger. Postgrad. Med. J. 9 (4): 205 - 209.

Lohiya NK, Goyal RB, Jayaprakash D, Ansari AS, Sharma S (1994). Anti-fertility effects of aqueous extract of *Carica papaya* seeds in male rats. *Planta. Med* **60:** 400 - 404.

Lohiya NK, Kothari LK, Manivannan B, Mishra PK, Pathak N (2000). Human sperm immobilization effect of *Carica papaya* seed extracts: an *in vitro* study. Asian J. Androl. 2 (2): 103 - 109.

Lohiya NK, Manivannan B, Garg S (2006). Toxicological investgations on the methanol sub-fraction of the seeds of *Carica papaya* as a male contraceptive in albino rats. *Reprod. Toxicol.* **22**: 461 - 68.

Lohiya NK, Manivannan B, Goyal S, Ansari AS (2008). Sperm motility inhibitory effect of the benzene chromatographic fraction of the chloroform extract of the seeds of *Carica papaya* in langur monkey, *Presbytis entellus entellus. Asian J. Androl.* 10 (2): 298 - 306.

Lohiya NK, Mannivanan B, Mishra PK, Pathak N, Sriram S, Bhande SS, Panneerdoss S (2002). Chloroform extract of *Carica papaya* seeds induces long-term reversible azoospermia in langur monkey. *Asian J. Androl.* 4: 17–26.

Lohiya NK, Mishra PK, Pathak N, Manivannan B, Bhande SS, Panneerdoss S, Sriram S (2005). Efficacy trial on the purified compounds of the seeds of *Carica papaya* for male contraception in albino rat. Reprod. Toxicol. 20 (1): 135 - 48.

Lohiya NK, Mishra PK, Pathak N, Manivannan B, Jain SC (1999a). Reversible azoospermia by oral administration of the benzene chromatographic fraction of the chloroform extract of the seeds of *Carica papaya* in rabbits. *Adv Contracept* **15:** 141 - 61.

Lohiya NK, Pathak N, Mishra PK, Manivannan B (1999b). Reversible contraception with chloroform extract of *Carica papaya* Linn. seeds in male rabbits. *Reprod Toxicol* **13**: 59 - 66.

Makonnen E, Zerihun L, Assefa G, Rostom AA (1999). Anti-fertility activity of *Ricinus communis* seed in female guinea pigs. East Afr. Med. J. 76 (6): 335 - 37.

Malhi BS, Trivedi VP (1972). Quart. J. Crude Drug Res 12: 1922. In: Farnsworth NR, Bingel AS, Cordell GA, Crane FA, Fong HS (1975). Potential value of plants as sources of new anti-fertility agents - I. J. Pharm. Sci. 64(4):535 – 98.

Mankekar K (1973). Techniques of abortion. In: Abortion - A Social Dilemma. Vikas Publishers. New Delhi. Chapter. 6. pp. 41 - 44.

Manivannan B, Mittal R, Goyal S, Ansari AS, Lohiya NK (2009). Sperm characteristics and ultrastructure of testes of rats after long-term treatment with the methanol subfraction of *Carica papaya* seeds. Asian J. Androl. 11 (5): 583 - 99.

Mannivanan B, Mishra PK, Pathak N, Sriram S, Bhande SS, Panneerdoss SS, Lohiya NK (2004). Ultrastructural changes in the testis and epididymis of rats following treatment with the benzene chromatographic fraction of the chloroform extract of the seeds of *Carica papaya. Phytother. Res.* 18 (4): 285 - 89.

Matsui AS, Rogers J, Woo YK, Cutting WC (1967). Effects of some natural products on fertility in mice. Med. Pharmacol. Exp. Int. J. Exp. Med. 16 (5): 414 - 24.

Matte JJ, Girard CL, Brisson GJ (1984). Folic acid and reproductive performances of sows. J. Anim. Sci. 59: 1020 - 25.

Maurya R, Srivastava S, Kulshreshta DK, Gupta CM (2004). Traditional remedies for fertility regulation. Curr. Med. Chem. 11 (11): 1431 - 50.

Mínguez-Alarcón L, Mendiola J, López-Espín JJ, Sarabia-Cos L, Vivero-Salmerón G, Vioque J, Navarrete-Munoz EM, Torres-Cantero AM (2012). Dietary intake of anti-oxidant nutrients is associated with semen quality in young university students. Hum. Reprod. 27 (9): 2807 - 814.

Misago C, Fonseca W (1999). Determinants of induced abortion in north east Brazil. In: Abortion in the Developing World. Mundigo AI, Indviso C (eds). WHO Publication. Vistaar Publishers. Brazil. pp 224 - 225, 298 - 303, 380.

Mishra RK, Singh SK (2005). Effect of aqueous leaf extract of *Azadirachta indica* on the reproductive organs in male mice. Indian J. Exp. Biol. 43 (11): 1093 - 1103.

Mishra RK, Singh SK (2009). Reversible anti-fertility effect of aqueous rhizome extract of *Curcuma longa* L. in male laboratory mice. Contraception. 79 (6): 479 - 87.

Mohan, J., P.K. Tyagi, K.T. Pramad, S.V.S. Verma and R.P. Mougal (1997). Anti-fertility effect of neem seed kernel meal in chicken. AJAS. 10: 609 - 613.

Mukherjee S, Garg S, Talwar GP (1999). Early post- implantation contraceptive effect of a purified fraction of *Neem (Azadirachta indica)* seeds, given orally in rats: possible mechanism involved. J. Ethnopharmacol. 67: 287 - 96.

Mukherjee S, Talwar GP (1996). Termination of pregnancy in rodents by oral administration of praneem, a purified *Neem* seed extract. Am. J. Reprod. Immunol. 35: 51 - 56.

Naz RK (2011). Can curcumin provide an ideal contraceptive? Mol. Reprod. Dev. 78 (2): 116 - 23.

Nithya RS, Anuja MM, Rajamanickam C, Indira M (2012). Rat sperm immobilisation effects of a protein from *Ricinus communis* (Linn.): an *in vitro* comparative study with nonoxynol-9. Andrologia. 2012 Apr 5. doi: 10.1111/j.1439-0272.2012.01291.x. [Epub ahead of print].

Oderinde O, Noronha C, Oremosu A, Kusemiju T, Okanlawon OA (2002). Abortifacient properties of aqueous extract of *Carica papaya* (Linn.) seeds on female Sprague-Dawley rats. Niger. Postgrad. Med. J. 9 (2): 95 - 98.

Ogbuewu, I.P., I.C. Okoli and M.U. Iloeje (2009). Semen quality characteristics, reaction time, testis weight and seminiferous tubule diameter of buck rabbits fed neem (*Azadirachta indica, A. juss*) leaf meal based diets. Iranian J. Reprod. Med., 7: 23 - 28.

Pathak N, Mishra PK, Manivannan B, Lohiya NK (2000). Sterility due to inhibition of sperm motility by oral administration of benzene chromatographic fraction of the chloroform extract of the seeds of *Carica papaya* in rats. Phytomedicine. 7 (4): 325 - 33.

Paton DM (1968). The contractile response of the isolated rat uterus to noradrenaline and 5-hydroxytryptamine. Eur. J. Pharmacol. 3 (4): 310 - 15.

Penningroth SM (1984). Pharmacological basis of therapeutics: gossypol, an oral male contraceptive? J. Med. Soc. N. J. 81 (8): 663 - 65.

Piyachaturawat P, Glinsukon T, Peugvicha P (1982). Postcoital anti-fertility effect of piperine. Contraception. 26 (6): 625 - 33.

Porat O (1990). Effects of gossypol on the motility of mammalian sperm. Mol Reprod. Dev. 25 (4): 400 - 408.

Prakash AO, Gupta RB, Mathur R (1978). Effect of oral administration of 42 indigenous plant extracts on early and late pregnancy in albino rats. Probe. July – Sept. 315 - 23.

Prakash AO, Mathur R (1976). Screening of Indian plants for antifertrility activity. Ind. J. Exp. Biol. 14: 623.

Prakash AO, Pathak S, Shukla S, Mathur R (1987). Uterine histoarchitecture during pre and post-implantation periods of rats treated with aqueous extract of *Moringa oleifera* Lam. Acta. Eur. Fertil. 18 (2): 129 - 35.

Prakash AO, Tewari RK, Mathur R (1988). Non-hormonal post-coital contraceptive action of neem oil in rats. J. Ethnopharmacol. 23 (1): 53 - 59.

Qian SZ, Wang ZG (1984). Gossypol: a potential anti-fertility agent for males. Annu. Rev. Pharmacol. Toxicol. 24: 329 - 60.

Qian YX, Shen PJ, Xu RY, Liu GM, Yang HQ, Lu YS, Sun P, Zhang RW, Qi LM, Lu QH (1986). Spermicidal effect *in vitro* by the active principle of garlic. Contraception. 34: 295 - 302.

Raghuvanshi P, Bagga R, Malhotra D, Gopalan S, Talwar GP (2001). Spermicidal & contraceptive properties of Praneem polyherbal pessary. Indian J. Med. Res. 113: 135 - 41.

Randel RD, Chase CC Jr, Wyse SJ (1992). Effects of gossypol and cottonseed products on reproduction of mammals. J. Anim. Sci. 70 (5): 1628 - 38.

Riar SS, Devakuma C, Ilavazhagam G, Kain AK, Bardham J (1991). Anti-fertility activities of volatile fraction of Neem oil. Contraception. 44: 319 - 26.

Roop JK, Dhaliwal PK, Guraya SS (2005). Extracts of *Azadirachta indica* and *Melia azedarach* seeds inhibit folliculogenesis in albino rats. Braz. J. Med. Biol. Res., 38: 943 - 47.

Roqueta-Rivera M, Stroud CK, Haschek WM, Akare SJ, Segre M, Brush RS, Agbaga MP, Anderson RE,Hess RA, Nakamura MT (2010). Docosahexaenoic acid supplementation fully restores fertility and spermatogenesis in male delta-6 desaturase-null mice. J. Lipid. Res. 51 (2): 360 - 67.

Roychoudhury S, Massanyi P, Slamecka J, Chlebec I, Trandzik J, Bulla J, Okab AB, Taha TA, Salem MH, Ayoub MA (2009). *In vitro* gossypol induced spermatozoa motility alterations in rabbits. J. Environ. Sci. Health B. 44 (7): 730 - 41.

Sadre NL, Vibhavari Y, Deshpande KN, Mendulkar, Nandak DH (1983). In: Male anti-fertility activity of *Azadirachta indica* in different species. Schmutterer H, Acher KRS, editors. pp. 473 - 82.

Safarinejad MR, Hosseini SY, Dadkhah F, Asgari MA (2010). Relationship of omega-3 and omega-6 fatty acids with semen characteristics, and anti-oxidant status of seminal plasma: a comparison between fertile and infertile men. Clin. Nutr. 29 (1): 100 - 105.

Saha JC, Savini EC, Kashinathan S (1961). Ecbolic properties of Indian Medicinal plants. Ind. J.Med. Res. 49 (1): 130 - 51.

Sahasrabuddhe, De (1943). Curr. Sci. 12:.23. in Wealth of India (1972). A Dictionary of Indian Raw Materials and Industrial Products. CSIR Publication. New Delhi.

SaiRam MS, Ilavazhagan G, Sharma SK, Dhanraj SA, Suresh B, Parida MM, Jana AO (2002). Anitimicrobial activity of a new vaginal contraceptive NIM-76 from neem oil (*Azadirachta indica*). J. Ethnopharmacol., 71: 377 - 82.

Salawu AA, Osinubi AA, Dosumu OO, Kusemiju TO, Noronha CC, Okanlawon AO (2010). Effect of the juice of lime (*Citrus aurantifolia*) on estrous cycle and ovulation of Sprague-Dawley rats. Endocr. Pract. 16 (4): 561 - 65.

Salhab AS, Shomaf MS, Gharaibeh MN, Amer NA (1999). Effects of castor bean extract and ricin A-chain on ovulation and implantation in rabbits. Contraception. 59 (6): 395 - 99.

Sanyal SN (1956). Acta. Endocrinol. Suppl. 28: 72. In Farnsworth NR, Bingel AS, Cordell GA, Crane FA, Fong HS (1975). Potential value of plants as sources of new anti-fertility agents - I. J. Pharm. Sci. 64 (4): 535 - 98.

Sanyal SN (1960). Sci. Cult. 25: 661. In Farnsworth NR, Bingel AS, Cordell GA, Crane FA, Fong HS (1975). Potential value of plants as sources of new anti-fertility agents - I. J. Pharm. Sci. 64 (4): 535 - 98.

Sarkar M, Gangopadhyay P, Basak B, Chakrabarty K, Banerji J, Adhikary P, Chatterjee A (2000). The reversible anti-fertility effect of *Piper betle* Linn. on Swiss albino male mice. Contraception. 62 (5): 271 - 74.

Sethi N, Nath D, Shukla SC, Dyal R (1988). Abortificient activity of a medicinal plant *Moringa oleifera* in rats. Anc. Sci. Life. 7 (3-4): 172 - 74.

Setty BS, Kamboj VP, Garg HS, Khanna NM (1976). Spermicidal potential of saponins isolated from Indian medicinal plants. Contraception. 14 (5): 571 - 78.

Shakti N, Updhyay S, Charu Kaushic, Talwar GP (1990). Anti-fertility effects of *Neem (Azadirachta Indica)* oil by single intrauterine administration. Proc. The Royal Soc. Lond. Series B Sci. 242: 175 - 79.

Sharma SK, SaiRam M, Ilavazhagan G, Devendra K, Shivaji SS, Selvamurthy W (1996). Mechanism of action of NIM-76: a novel vaginal contraceptive from neem oil. Contraception. 54 (6): 373 - 78.

Shukla S, Mathur R, Prakash AO (1988a). Anti-fertility profile of the aqueous extract of *Moringa oleifera* roots. J. Ethnopharmacol. 22 (1): 51 - 62.

Shukla S, Mathur R, Prakash AO (1988b). Biochemical and physiological alterations in female reproductive organs of cyclic rats treated with aqueous extract of *Moringa oleifera*. Lam. Acta. Eur. Fertil. 19 (4): 225 - 32.

Shukla S, Mathur R, Prakash AO (1989). Histoarchitecture of the genital tract of ovariectomized rats treated with an aqueous extract of *Moringa oleifera* roots. J. Ethnopharmacol. 25 (3): 249 - 61.

Sidhu OP, Kumar V, Behl HM (2003). Variability in *Neem (Azadirachta indica)* with respect to azadirachta content. J. Agric. Food Chem. 51: 910 - 15.

Singh A, Singh SK (2009). Evaluation of anti-fertility potential of Brahmi in male mouse. Contraception. 79 (1): 71 - 79.

Singh H, Chawla AS, Kapoor VK (1985). Anti-fertility and Related Activities in medicinal and chemical research in India. Kumar N (ed). National Information Centre for Drugs and Pharmaceuticals – Central Drug Research Institute, Lucknow. Pp. 120 – 136.

Singh MM, Wadhwa V, Gupta DN, Pal R, Khanna NM, Kamboj VP (1984). Postcoital contraceptive efficacy and hormonal profile of *Lepidium capitatum.* Planta. Med. 50 (2): 154 - 57.

Sinha, K.C., S.S. Riar, A.K. Tiwary, A.K. Dhawan, J. Bardhan and P. Thomas (1984). Neem oil as a vaginal contraceptive. Indian J. Med. Res. 79: 131 - 36.

Sotelo A, Montalvo I, de la Luz Crail M, González-Garza MT (1982). Infertility in male rats induced by diets containing whole cotton seed flour. J. Nutr. 112 (11): 2052 - 57.

Stoffel W, Holz B, Jenke B, Binczek E, Günter RH, Kiss C, Karakesisoglou I, Thevis M, Weber AA, Arnhold S, Addicks K (2008). Delta6-desaturase (FADS2) deficiency unveils the role of omega3- and omega6-polyunsaturated fatty acids. . EMBO J. 27 (17): 2281 - 92.

Talwar GP, Shah S, Mukherjee S, Chabra R (1997). Induced termination of pregnancy by purified extracts of *Azadirachta indica (Neem):* mechanism involved. Am. J. Reprod. Immunol. 37: 375 - 78.

Tavilani H, Doosti M, Abdi K, Vaisiraygani A, Joshaghani HR (2006). Decreased polyunsaturated and increased saturated fatty acid concentration in spermatozoa from asthenozoospermic males as compared with normo-zoospermic males. Andrologia. 38 (5): 173 - 78.

Tavilani H, Doosti M, Nourmohammadi I, Mahjub H, Vaisiraygani A, Salimi S, Hosseinipanah SM (2007). Lipid composition of spermatozoa in normozoospermic and astheno-zoospermic males. Prostaglandins Leukot. Essent. Fatty Acids. 77 (1): 45 - 50.

Tewari J (1974). Preliminary Clinical trial of flowers of *Hibiscus rosa-sinensis* as an oral contraceptives; Indian Med. Yoga. Homeopath. 9: 96.

Tso WW, Lee CS (1982). [Cottonseed—a source of vaginal contraceptive (author's transl)]. Contracept. Fertil. Sex (Paris). 10 (7-8): 465 - 68. [Article in French].

Uche-Nwachi EO, Ezeokoli DC, Adogwa AO, Offiah VN (2001). Effect of water extract of *Carica papaya* seed on the germinal epithelium of the seminiferous tubules of Sprague Dawley rats. Kaibogaku. Zasshi. 76 (6): 517 - 21.

Uche-Nwachi EO, Mitchell CV, McEwen C (2011). Steroidogenic enzyme histochemistry in the testis of Sprague Dawley rats following the administration the water extracts from *Carica papaya* seed. Afr. J Tradit. Complement. Altern. Med. 8 (1): 69 - 78.

Udoh P, Essien I, Udoh F (2005). Effects of *Carica papaya* (paw paw) seeds extract on the morphology of pituitary-gonadal axis of male Wistar rats. Phytother. Res. 19 (12): 1065 - 68.

Umapathy E (1993). Antifertility effects of cowpeas on male rats. Cent Afr J Med. 39 (3): 52 - 56.

Upadhyay S, Dhawan S, Sharma MG, Talwar GP (1994). Long-term contraceptive effects of intrauterine neem treatment (IUNT) in bonnet monkeys: an alternate to intrauterine contraceptive devices (IUCD). Contraception. 49 (2): 161 - 69.

Updhyay S, Kaushi C, Talwar GP (1990). Anti-fertility effects of Neem oil by single intrauterine administration: A novel method of contraception. Proc. The Royal Soc. Lond. 242: 175 - 79.

Updhyay SN, Dhavan S, Talwar GP (1992). Immuno-modulatory effects of Neem. Inter. J. Immunopharmacol.14: 1188 - 94.

Vohora SB, Parasar GC (1969). Phytochemical and pharmacological studies on *Ficus bengalensis*, Linn. (Preliminary report). Indian J. Physiol. Pharmacol. 13 (3): 143 - 45.

Waites GM, Wang C, Griffin PD (1998). Gossypol: Reasons for its failure to be accepted as a safe, reversible male anti-fertility drug. Int. J. Androl. 21 (1): 8 - 12.

Warrier PK, Nambiar VP, Ramankutty C (1994). Indian Medicinal Plants - A Compendium of 500 Species -1,2,3. Orient Longman. New Delhi.

Watt JM, Breyer–Brandwijk MG (1962). in the Medicinal and Poisonous plants of Southern and Eastern Africa (2ndEd). London - E and S. Livingston Ltd. in Farnsworth NR, Bingel AS, Cordell GA, Crane FA, Fong HS (1975). Potential value of plants as sources of new anti-fertility agents - I. J. Pharm. Sci. 64 (4): 535 - 98.

Wealth of India (1972). A Dictionary of Indian Raw Materials and Industrial Products. CSIR Publication. New Delhi.

Westphal LM, Polan ML, Trant AS, Mooney SB (2004). A nutritional supplement for improving fertility in women: a pilot study. J. Reprod. Med. 49: 289 - 93.

Willmott M, Bartosik DB, Romanoff EB (1968). The effect of folic acid on superovulation in the immature rat. J. Endocrinol. 41: 439 - 45.

Zalata AA, Christophe AB, Depuydt CE, Schoonjans F, Comhaire FH (1998). The fatty acid composition of phospholipids of spermatozoa from infertile patients. Mol. Hum. Reprod. 4 (2): 111 - 18.

Zatuchni GI, Osborn CK (1981). Gossypol: a possible male antifertility agent. Report of a workshop. Res. Front. Fertil. Regul. (4): 1 - 15.

Zhang X, Han F, Gao P, Yu D, Liu S (2007). Bioassay-guided fractionation of anti-fertility components of castorbean (*Ricinus communis* L.) seed extracts. Nat. Prod. Res. 21 (11): 982 - 89.

Zondek B, Bergmann E (1938). Phenol methyl ethers as oestrogenic agents. Biochem. J. 32 (4): 641 - 45.

Chapter 7
Anti-Hyperlipidemic Foods

Cardio Vascular Disease (CVD) is the largest single contributor to global mortality presently and will continue to dominate mortality trends in the future as predicted by World Health Organization (WHO) way back in 2009. WHO also estimated that about 20 million CVD deaths to occur in 2015, accounting for 30 per cent of all deaths worldwide (WHO, 2005). Further predictions by researchers project that non-communicable diseases will account for more than three-quarters of deaths worldwide By 2030, and CVD alone will be responsible for more deaths in low income countries than infectious diseases (including HIV/AIDS, tuberculosis, and malaria), maternal and perinatal conditions, and nutritional disorders combined (Beaglehole and Bonita, 2008).

Several lifestyle factors contribute to the development of CVD including diet rich in saturated fat and poor in dietary fiber and antioxidants. Abnormal lipid levels contribute significantly to the risk of coronary heart disease. Significant research efforts focusing on the prevention and treatment have identified elevated plasma cholesterol along with triacylglycerol, LDL and lower HDL cholesterol concentrations as risk factors for CVD. The association of hyper-glycemia with an alteration of lipid parameters presents yet another crucial risk factor for cardiovascular complications in diabetes.

Oxidative stress especially in the vasculature and kidneys contributes to hypertension, which is a major risk factor for cardiovascular disease, thus becomes an important element in the etiology of ischemic stroke. Cardio-protection was associated with increased myocardial antioxidant defences. Toufektsian *et al.* (2008) proved that the anthocyanin-rich diet improves resistance to regional ischemia and reperfusion insult suggesting a beneficial effect of nutritional antioxidants.

Atherosclerosis is closely related to oxidative events such as oxidized LDL accumulation in the macrophages. This necessitates regular consumption of nutritional and non nutritional ant-ioxidants through diet as a preventive measure. Several foods exhibit antihyperlidemic effect that might be either due to their dietary fiber, PUFA or anti-oxidants. The extensive research conducted in this area has been discussed below.

Oats

It is well established that consumption of oats or oat bran lowers serum cholesterol concentrations in animal models of hypercholesterolemia (Jonnalagadda *et al.*, 1993; Kahlon *et al.*, 1993). Complex carbohydrates in oats not only lower the risk of heart disease, but also reduce the risk of stroke and certain cancers and helps lower high blood pressure. Oats also contain tryptophan, a nonessential amino acid that improves mood and thus has also been proven to act as an anti-depressant. Cooked oats relieve fat from the body while unrefined oatmeal can reduce stress. Through its high fiber and vitamin B content oats could be suitable for a gluten-free diet. It not only increases palatability but also offers beneficial effects on cardiovascular health (Pulido *et al.*, 2009).

Dietary fiber has been suggested to interfere with endogenous cholesterol synthesis in the liver. Poulter *et al.* (1994) also found slight reduction in LDL cholesterol on oat based cereal in a crossover study. Increased gut viscosity may prevent dietary cholesterol from reaching the intestinal epithelium. The role of viscosity in determining the cholesterol-lowering effect of soluble fiber has been shown in hamsters (Gallaher *et al.*, 1993) and recently in humans (Reppas *et al.*, 2009) with the use of high-dose (15 g/d) hydroxy-propylmethyl-cellulose.

Oda *et al.* (1994) observed oat gum to suppress the elevation of serum and liver triglyceride concentrations along with lowering of serum and liver cholesterol concentratrions. Marlett *et al.* (1994) demonstrated that oat bran lowers serum cholesterol levels in part by altering bile acid metabolism. In addition, the substantial increase in the proportion of the total bile acid pool that was deoxycholic acid is consistent with the hypothesis that oat bran also decreases cholesterol synthesis. On the other hand, Uusitupa *et al.* (1997) reported that the reduction in the serum cholesterol level by oat bran treatment cannot be ascribed to an inhibition of the endogenous cholesterol synthesis as the cholesterol precursors in serum reflecting endogenous cholesterol synthesis remained almost unchanged.

The role of oats consumption in the prevention and treatment of both hypertension and hypercholesterolemia was ascertained by He *et al.* (1995). Beer *et al.* (1995) reported that the cholesterol-lowering capacity of oat gum in healthy young men to be weak. They also suggested that the effect of at bran preparations on serum cholesterol levels cannot be estimated by the beta-glucan content but by measurement of the solubility and viscosity of the beta-glucan. Beta glucan when fed at 1 per cent and 10 per cent by weight showed a significant decrease in total and LDL cholesterol levels in mildly hyper-cholesterolemic subjects (Behall *et al.*, 1997).

The influence of oat bran on the concentration of triglycerides in the blood serum depended on the kind of fats in a diet The diets containing oat bran with lard did not decrease the concentration of these lipids, but the same diets with sunflower oil decreased this concentration significantly by 22 per cent. (Onning *et al.*, 1998; Grajeta, 1999).

Consumption of oats in adequate amounts on a consistent basis may decrease the risk of cardiovascular disease by several potential mechanisms: lowering blood lipid levels, improving arterial compliance, reducing low-density lipoprotein oxidation, decreasing plaque formation, scavenging free radicals, and inhibiting platelet aggregation (Hasler *et al.*, 2000). Oat bran supplemented to Western diet lowered plasma cholesterol, reduced levels of some inflammatory markers, and inhibited atherosclerotic lesion development in LDL-receptor-deficient mice.

Numerous studies (Amudesan *et al.*, 2003; Berg *et al.*, 2003; Braaten *et al.*, 1994; Brown *et al.*, 1999; Davidson *et al.*, 1991; Karmally *et al.*, 2005; Ripsin *et al.*, 1992; Theuwissen and Mensink, 2007) have shown that oat-containing products reduce LDL cholesterol. Within a practical range of intake, oat bran when added to a fat-modified diet significantly reduced the total cholesterol, low-density lipoprotein cholesterol, and apo-lipoprotein B. These beneficial effects could be seen independent of co-variables such as physical activity or caloric and fat restriction in the diet (Berg *et al.*, 2003). Beta-glucan, constituent of soluble fiber of Oats has been proven effective in lowering blood cholesterol thus reducing the risk of cardiovascular disease (CVD) by 10 per cent. In addition to beta-glucan in the soluble fiber, oats also contain avenanthramides (a type of antioxidant). Preliminary studies showed that avenanthramides help prevent free radicals from damageing LDL cholesterol. Beyond its known effect through lowering blood cholesterol in the prevention of coronary heart disease, avenanthramide-c, which is a unique polyphenol found in oats, arrests SMC proliferation at G1 phase by upregulating the p53-p21cip1 pathway and inhibiting pRB phosphorylation (Nie *et al.*, 2006).

The European Food Safety Authority recently issued an opinion that a cause and effect relation has been established between the consumption of oat β-glucan and a reduction in blood cholesterol (EFSA, 2009). The US Food and Drug Administration allow a claim that food products containing oats and that can deliver 3 g β-glucan/d can reduce risk of heart disease. Whereas Queenan and coworkers (2007) demonstrated that 6 grams concentrated oat beta-glucan per day for six weeks produced significant reduction from baseline in total cholesterol (0.3 ± 0.1 mmol/L) and LDL cholesterol (-0.3 ± 0.1 mmol/L);and the reduction in LDL cholesterol was significantly greater than that of the control group ($p = 0.03$). However, Biörklund *et al.* (2008) did not find a significant reduction in TC and LDL-C with a daily dose of 4 g of oat beta-glucans incorporated into a healthy ready meal compared with an equal ready meal without beta-glucans.

Winbald *et al.* (1995) reported that oat bran supplemented diet was effective in lowering serum cholesterol in hyper-cholesterolaemic males who had failed to comply with a conventional lipid lowering diet. An energy-restricted regimen (a new oat-based soup as the main meal once or twice daily) lead to lower plasma insulin, triglyceride, and low-density lipoprotein cholesterol levels but did not significantly affect the plasma enterostatin concentration in over-weight subjects (Rytter *et al.*, 1996). The hypocholesterolemic effect of oats seems to vary with the serum cholesterol status. Hyper-cholesterolemic individuals supplemented with oat bran showed a 28 per cent reduction in plasma triglycerides after 8 weeks (Romero *et al.*, 1998), and the effect was observed to be on par/superior to Psyllium.

Supplementation with oat bran has also been proved to increase plasma HDL-C levels by 11.2 per cent in women (n = 18) (p = 0.01), but decrease the total cholesterol/HDL-C ratio by 7.0 per cent (p = 0.002) (Robitaille *et al.*, 2005). The authors concluded that integration of these foods as part of a healthy diet may, therefore, improve the cardiovascular risk profile of women. Since 1 per cent reduction in LDL cholesterol reduces Coronary artery disease (CAD) risk by 1–2 per cent, the 5–6 per cent LDL cholesterol lowering elicited by 3–4 g oat β-glucan *i.e.* 3 g of high-MW oat β-glucan/d or 4 g medium MW β-glucan/d or 3 g medium-MW oat β-glucan could reduce the risk of CAD by 5–12 per cent.

According to Maki *et al.* (2007) consumption of high-fiber oat cereal influenced postprandial triglyceride and free fatty acid levels, which may have implications regarding cardiovascular disease risk. Six grams of beta-glucan from oats added to the American Heart Association Step II diet and moderate physical activity improved lipid profile and caused a decrease in weight and, thus, reduced the risk of cardiovascular events in overweight male individuals with mild to moderate hypercholesterolemia (Reyna-Villasmil *et al.*, 2007). Oat consumption was found to be associated with 5 per cent and 7 per cent reductions in total and LDL cholesterol levels, respectively, consistent with earlier conclusions made by the US FDA and United Kingdom Joint Health Claims Initiative (Othman *et al.*, 2011). Interestingly, Charlton *et al.* (2012) recently observed 1-5 g/d of oat beta glucan was as effective as 3 g/d delivered in different food formats. Wolever *et al.* (2011) concluded from their study that oat β-glucan reduces LDL-C in both Caucasians and non-Caucasians.

Different physiological effects of beta-glucan such as attenuation of postprandial plasma glucose and insulin responses, high transport of bile acids towards lower parts of the intestinal tract and high excretion of bile acids thereby lowering of serum cholesterol levels are all related to its viscosity (Butt *et al.*, 2008).

The viscosity of β-glucan solutions is determined by its molecular weight (MW) and solubility (Wood *et al.*, 2000), both of which can be altered by normal methods of processing and storage (Regand *et al.*, 2009). An extruded breakfast cereal containing 3 g oat β-glucan/d with a high-MW (2,210,000 g/mol) or medium-MW (530,000 g/mol) lowered LDL cholesterol similarly by 5 per cent, but efficacy was reduced by 50 per cent when MW was reduced to 210,000 g/mol. Hence, Wolever *et al.* (2010) suggests that the physicochemical properties of oat β-glucan should be considered when assessing the cholesterol-lowering ability. Bae *et al.* (2010) found Oat beta-glucan hydrolysate, having average molecular weight of 730,000g/mol to be more effective at increasing the excretion of fecal cholesterol and triglyceride than the native beta-glucan, showing its effectiveness in improving the lipid profile.

Considering the lipid and glucose improvements as well, increased consumption of whole oats may significantly reduce cardiovascular disease risk. According to Saltzman *et al.* (2001) a hypo-caloric diet containing oats consumed over 6 wk resulted in greater improvements in systolic blood pressure and lipid profile than did a hypo-caloric diet without oats. Keenan *et al.* (1991, 2002) found that subjects on oat consumption experienced a significant reduction in both total cholesterol (9 per cent) and low-density lipoprotein cholesterol (14 per cent) and also a 7.5 mm Hg reduction in Systolic BP and a 5.5 mm Hg reduction in Diastolic BP. Further, Pins *et al.* (2002) suggested that a diet containing soluble fiber-rich whole oats can significantly reduce the need for antihypertensive medication and improve BP control. In a double-blind, randomized crossover study in adults total cholesterol decreased by 14 per cent on oat bran consumption as compared 4 per cent in the control group ($P<0.001$). The LDL cholesterol decreased by 16 per cent in the oat bran period compared with 3 per cent in the control period ($P<0.01$), as did total triacylglycerol (21 vs 10 per cent, $P<0.05$) and very-low-density lipoprotein triacylglycerol 33 vs 9 per cent, ($P<0.01$). Fecal volume and dry matter were greater on consumption of oat bran diet compared with the control ($P<0.001$), and energy expenditure increased by 37 per cent (1014 vs 638kJ/day) (Kristensen and Bügel, 2011).

Eussen *et al.* (2011) documented the inhibitory effect of oat bran on the intestinal absorption and the lipid lowering effect of atorvastatin on simultaneous ingestion and suggested future investigations on oat bran focusing on food–drug interaction.

According to Andersson *et al.* (2010) two substrains of mice respond differently to oat bran on plasma cholesterol and this is of practical value and can also help to elucidate mechanisms of the cholesterol-lowering effect of oats. Again Park *et al.* (2009) demonstrated 2,2,6,6-Tetramethyl-1-piperidine oxoammonium ion (TEMPO)-mediated oxidation applied to oat beta-glucans exhibits potential use as an active cholesterol-lowering ingredient.

It is also reported (Onning *et al.*, 1999) that oat milk deprived of insoluble fiber has cholesterol-reducing properties as the consumption of oat milk resulted in significantly lower serum total cholesterol (6 per cent, $p = 0.005$) and LDL cholesterol (6 per cent, $p = 0.036$) levels. The decrease in LDL cholesterol was more pronounced if the starting value was higher ($r = -0.55$, $p < 0.001$). The concentration of high-density lipoprotein cholesterol and serum triglycerides did not change significantly after intake of oat milk.

Flax Seeds (*Linum usitatissimum*)

Lucas *et al.* (2004) showed that flaxseed is beneficial in reducing plasma cholesterol and plaque formation induced by ovarian hormone deficiency in female Golden Syrian hamsters. Human studies have shown that flaxseed can modestly reduce serum total and low-density lipoprotein cholesterol concentrations, reduce postprandial glucose absorption, decrease some markers of inflammation, and raise serum levels of the omega-3 fatty acids- ALA and eicosapentaenoic acid (Bloedon and Szapary, 2004), α-linolenic acid and soluble fiber components (Cunnane *et al.*, 1995; Bierenbaum *et al.*, 1993; Jenkins *et al.*, 1999; Brown *et al.*, 1999; Chen and

Anderson, 1986). ALA appears to decrease CVD risk by inhibiting vascular inflammation and endothelial activation beyond its lipid-lowering effects (Zhao *et al.*, 2004).

In general, flaxseed-enriched diets have been reported to induce anywhere from 0 per cent to 18 per cent decrease in LDL and 0 per cent to 11 per cent decreases in TC (Bloedon *et al.*, 2008), most studies reported no changes in HDL levels in response to dietary flax-seed (Cunnane *et al.*, 1993; Lemay *et al.*, 2002; Arjmandi *et al.*, 1998; Lucas *et al.*, 2002).

Secoisolariciresinol diglucoside (SDG) is a plant lignan isolated from flaxseed. Lignans are platelet-activating factor-receptor antagonists that would inhibit the production of oxygen radicals by polymorphonuclear leukocytes. SDG is an antioxidant. Prasad (1999) observed that SDG reduced hyper-cholesterolemic atherosclerosis and that this effect was associated with a decrease in serum cholesterol, LDL-C, and lipid peroxidation product and an increase in HDL-C and antioxidant reserve. SDG treatment prevented the progression of atherosclerosis on a regular diet following a high cholesterol diet. Prevention of progression is associated with a reduction of aortic oxidative stress and not with reductions in serum lipids. A longer duration of treatment reduced the progression of atherosclerosis to a greater extent, and tended to regress the atherosclerosis (Prasad, 2008).

The hypo-cholesterolemic effects of α-linolenic acid have been reported in both animals and humans (Chan *et al.*, 1991). Cornish *et al.* (2009) found no differences between groups fed flax seed lignan and the placebo for change in bone measures, body composition, lipoproteins, or cytokines. Males taking the flaxseed lignan complex reduced metabolic syndrome score relative to men taking placebo, but a similar trend was not seen in females. Prasad (2005; 2009) also showed that lignan complex isolated from flaxseed reduced the extent of hyper-cholesterolemic atherosclerosis along with marked decreases in oxidative stress, serum total cholesterol, LDL-C and risk ratio, and elevation of serum HDL-C.

Flaxseed (Type I flaxseed) with 51-55 per cent alpha-linolenic acid in its oil and richest source of plant lignans, has been shown to reduce hyper-cholesterolemic atherosclerosis by 46 per cent without lowering serum lipids. But, CDC-flaxseed (Type II flaxseed) having similar oil and lignan content but has very little (2-3 per cent of the total oil) alpha-linolenic acid showed anti-atherogenic activity by decrease in serum TC and LDL-C indicating that anti-atherogenic activity of Type II flax seed is not due to alpha-linolenic acid (Prasad *et al.*, 1998).

It has been suggested that the consumption of up to 50 g flaxseed in its raw form is also safe (Cunnane *et al.*, 1993). Flaxseed given in the form of bread and muffins reduced total cholesterol in postmenopausal women (Arjmandi *et al.*, 1998). Flaxseed consumption was reported to be beneficial as a hypo-lipidemic agent in post menopausal women too. Moreover, the lignan SDG is converted by bacteria in the colon of humans and other animals to enterodiol and enterolactone, referred to as mammalian lignans. These exhibit weak estrogenic activity as they can bind to estrogen receptors on cell membranes (Nesbitt *et al.*, 1999).

Lucas *et al.* (2002) have shown that supplementation of flaxseed to the diets of postmenopausal women can lower concentrations of serum total cholesterol and non-HDL cholesterol. In a crossover study in which hyper-lipidemic men and postmenopausal women were fed 50 g of partially defatted flaxseed daily for 3 weeks, Jenkins *et al.* (1999) observed overall reductions of 5.5 and 9.7 per cent in serum total- and LDL-cholesterol concentrations, respectively and concluded that flaxseed gum is likely the major active ingredient responsible for the lipid-lowering action of flaxseed. They also confirmed that supplementing the diet with partially defatted flaxseed results in reductions in serum LDL-cholesterol concentrations similar to those observed with full-fat flaxseed by Cunnane *et al. (1993*; 1995) and Bierenbaum *et al.* (1993). Dietary flaxseed significantly improves lipid profile in hyper-lipidemic patients and may favorably modify cardiovascular risk factors (Manda°escu *et al.*, 2005).

Patade *et al.* (2008) found that mild to moderate hyper-cholesterolemic native American postmenopausal women who consumed flaxseed (30 g/day) for three months exhibited a reduction of TC by 7 per cent and LDL cholesterol by 10 per cent without changes in HDL cholesterol or TG concentrations. Zhang *et al.* (2008) also found significant reductions in TC (22 per cent) and LDL cholesterol levels (24 per cent) in hyper-cholesterolemic subjects after an eight-week dietary supplementation with 600 mg/day of secoisolariciresinol diglucoside (SDG), a lignan derived from flaxseed. These results suggest that specific subgroups of patients could obtain more beneficial hypo-lipidemic effects from flaxseed or its components.

Dietary flaxseed may also protect against ischemic heart disease by improving vascular relaxation responses and by inhibiting the incidence of ventricular fibrillation (Bassett *et al.*, 2009). Kinniry *et al.* (2006) found dietary FS to decrease lung inflammation and lipid peroxidation, suggesting a protective role against pro-oxidant-induced tissue damage *in vivo*. Two independent studies of healthy subjects have shown that inflammatory markers, such as tumour necrosis factor alpha (TNF-α), IL-1-beta, thromboxane B_5 and prostaglandin E_5, were significantly reduced after administration of an ALA-rich diet (13.7 g/day of ALA from flaxseed) (Caughey *et al.*, 1996), as were VCAM-1 and E-selectin after delivery of 2 g/day of ALA (Thies *et al.*, 2001). ALA intake (8 g/day) from a flaxseed source decreases serum concentrations of serum amyloid A, IL-6 (Rallidis *et al.*, 2003), soluble VCAM-1, soluble intercellular adhesion molecule-1, soluble E-selectin (Zhao *et al.*, 2004) as well as the production of TNF-α, IL-1-beta and prostaglandin E_2 by peripheral blood mononuclear cells (Caughey *et al.*, 1996) over a period of four to 12 weeks with doses of ALA greater than 9 g/day. The cardio-protective effects of ALA are mediated in part by a reduction in the production of inflammatory cytokines.

The study by Barakat and Mahmoud (2011) suggests that both flax/pumpkin and purslane/pumpkin seed mixtures had anti-atherogenic hypo-lipidemic and immuno-modulator effects which were probably mediated by unsaturated fatty acids (including alpha linolenic acid) present in seed mixture.

Interestingly, Flaxseed intake during lactation did not produce histological alterations in prostatic alveolus or in sexual hormones, but programmed to a reduction in lipid profile in adult life with decreased cardiovascular risk (Cardozo *et al.*, 2010).

Similarly, the cardiotoxic effect of isoprenalin was less in flax lignan concentrate pretreated animals, which was confirmed in histopathological alterations. Haemodynamic, biochemical alteration and histopathological results suggest a cardioprotective protective effect of FLC in isoprenalin induced cardiotoxicity (Zanwar *et al.*, 2011).

Barley (*Hordeum vulgare*)

Hordeum vulgare var. Himalaya 292 is a new barley cultivar with altered starch synthesis with more amylose, resistant starch and total and soluble NSP including beta-glucan. Bird *et al.* (2004) proved that barley improves health through plasma cholesterol reduction and increased large-bowel short chain fatty acid production. Total cholesterol was significantly lower when the diet contained 3 or 6 g beta-glucan/d from barley than when it contained no beta-glucan; the greatest change occurred in the men and post-menopausal women (Behall *et al.*, 2004; Ikegami *et al.*, 1996; Newman *et al.*, 1989a; b).

McIntosh *et al.* (1991) showed that a 4-wk diet enriched with barley foods containing 8 g β-glucan per day reduced total and LDL cholesterol in moderately cholesterolemic men by 6.0 and 6.8 per cent, respectively, compared with wheat foods containing 1.5 per cent β-glucan and whole-grain barley flour products containing 9.6 per cent β-glucan per day for 4 wk, showed 12 and 14 per cent reduction in total and LDL cholesterol in cholesterolemic men.

The consumption of dietary fiber, especially water-soluble fiber (5-10g per day), has been shown to be inversely associated with coronary heart disease (Anderson, 1995; Pereira *et al.*, 2004). Biörklund *et al.* (2005) compared barley beta glucan with oat beta glucan found a daily consumption of 5 g of barley beta-glucans in a beverage did not improve the lipid and glucose metabolism, but the oat beta-glucans did.

The use of barley significantly lowered total cholesterol (weighted mean difference -13.38 mg/dL; 95 per cent CI, -18.46 to -8.31 mg/dL), low-density lipoprotein cholesterol -10.02 mg/dL; 95 per cent CI, -14.03 to -6.00 mg/dL) and triglycerides, -11.83 mg/dl; 95 per cent CI, -20.12 to -3.55 mg/dL) but did not appear to significantly alter high-density lipoprotein (HDL) cholesterol (P=.07). According to these results, Talati *et al.* (2009) confirms that barley-derived beta-glucan appears to beneficially affect total cholesterol, LDL-cholesterol, and triglycerides, but not HDL-cholesterol. The cholesterol-lowering activities of oats and barley are commonly attributed to the beta-glucan fractions. As beta-glucan is present in both grains and appears to be chemically similar, Delaney *et al.* (2003) demonstrated that the cholesterol-lowering potency of beta-glucan is approximately identical whether its origin was oats or barley. Barley and β-glucan isolated from barley lowered total and low-density lipoprotein cholesterol by 0.30 mmol/l (95 per cent confidence interval) and 0.27 mmol/l (95 per cent), respectively, compared with control (AbuMweis, 2010).

Aller *et al.* (2004) showed that an increase in soluble fiber intake of 4 g as part of a normal diet reduced LDL cholesterol levels by 12.8 per cent in healthy humans. But Tiwari and Cummins (2011) reported that consumption of 3 g/d of oat or barley β-glucan is sufficient to decrease blood cholesterol, and the FDA concluded that daily consumption of 3 g of soluble β-glucan from whole-grain barley or certain dry milled barley products would produce the same cholesterol-lowering effect as oat products (lowering plasma total cholesterol by 5–8 per cent). The required dosage for a single food is 0.75 g in a single serving (FDA, 2006).

The ability of barley β-glucan soluble fiber to lower serum cholesterol is thought to occur through a combination of factors and mechanisms. Fermentation of β-glucan in the colon, results in the production of short-chain fatty acids, which impede cholesterol biosynthesis (Wilson *et al.*, 2004).

There are various mechanisms by which cholesterol is reduced by dietary fiber. Increased production of short-chain fatty delayed intestinal absorption of glucose and lipids and inhibition of absorption and reabsorption of cholesterol and bile acids accompanied by increased excretion of bile acids (Beer *et al.*, 1995; Bridges *et al.*, 1992; Lia *et al.*, 1995; 1997; Bourdon *et al.*, 1999; Anderson and Bridges, 1993; Pins *et al.*, 2007; Wilson *et al.*, 2004). The reduced absorption may be caused by the high viscosity of β-glucan solutions, which increases the viscosity of the intestinal contents (Wursch and Pi-Sunyer, 1997; Lairon, 2001; Jenkins *et al.*, 2002a; Wood, 2002). According to Wilson *et al.* (2004) barley beta-glucan possesses cholesterol-lowering and anti-atherogenic activities that occur at both lower and higher molecular weight. Oda *et al.* (1994) also reported barley gums to suppress the elevation of serum and liver triglyceride concentrations in diet induced hyper-glyceridemic rats.

Barley diet (25 per cent) lowered serum total cholesterol by 16.4 per cent, but not dose dependent as higher per cent barley diet did not show further lowering of cholesterol (Ranhotra *et al.*, 1998). Madhujith and Shahidi (2007) proved that phenolic extracts from whole barley kernel possess high antioxidant, antiradical, and antiproliferative potentials. Specifically, antioxidants slow down the rate of oxidative damage by scavenging the free radicals that form when body cells use oxygen.

Both the barley protein- and casein-enriched breads, showed no differences in their effects on serum LDL cholesterol or C-reactive protein, measures of oxidative stress, or blood pressure. Nevertheless, because no adverse effects were observed on cardiovascular risk factors, Jenkins *et al.* (2010) suggested barley protein as an additional option for raising the protein content of the diet. Lahouar *et al.* (2011) indicated that the diet enriched with dietary fiber of barley variety "Rihane" could be effective in decreasing the atherogenic risk factors in rats.

The U.S. FDA allowed a claim for β-glucan soluble fiber from whole-grain barley and certain barley milling fractions for reducing plasma cholesterol levels and reducing the risk of heart disease (FDA, 2006). But Ames and Rhymer, (2008) feel that more research is needed to fully understand the mechanism of cholesterol reduction and the role of beta-glucan molecular weight, viscosity, and solubility.

Garlic (*Allium sativum*)

Garlic is reported to be a wonderful medicinal plant not only for its preventive characteristics in cardiovascular diseases, regulating blood pressure, lowering blood sugar and cholesterol levels, Evidence from numerous studies points to the fact that garlic can bring about the normalization of plasma lipids, enhancement of fibrinolytic activity, inhibition of platelet aggregation and reduction of blood pressure and glucose. Animal studies, and some early investigational studies in humans, have suggested possible cardiovascular benefits of garlic. The cardiovascular effects of garlic have been documented in several older publications (Schlesinger, 1926, Taubmann, 1934). However only in late 70's Sainani *et al.* (1976) found that people who regularly eat larger amounts of garlic and onions have lower lipid and cholesterol levels than people who refrain from eating these. Later, Agarwal (1996) demonstrated that garlic ingestion could bring down the blood cholesterol and triglyceride levels significantly. Prasad *et al.* (1997) found garlic to decrease aortic malondialdehyde and chemiluminescence although there was no change in serum cholesterol. This proves that garlic prevents the development of hyper-cholesterolemic atherosclerosis.

A Czech study by Sovova and Sova (2004) found that garlic supplementation reduced accumulation of cholesterol on the vascular walls of animals. Another study had similar results, with garlic supplementation significantly reducing aortic plaque deposits of cholesterol-fed rabbits (Durak *et al.*, 2002). Another study by Durak *et al.* (2004) showed that supplementation with garlic extract inhibited vascular calcification in human patients with high blood cholesterol. The known vasodilative effect of garlic is possibly caused by catabolism of garlic-derived polysulfide to hydrogen sulfide in red blood cells, a reaction that is dependent on reduced thiols in or on the RBC membrane. Hydrogen sulfide is an endogenous cardio protective vascular cell-signaling molecule.

The complete depression of cholesterol synthesis by diallyl disulfide, diallyl trisulfide, and dipropyl disulfide was found to be associated with cyto-toxicity by Liu and Yeh (2000) as indicated by marked increase in cellular LDH release. Judging from maximal inhibition and IC50 (concentration required for 50 per cent of maximal inhibition), S-allyl cysteine, S-ethyl cysteine, and S-propyl cysteine are equally potent in inhibiting cholesterol synthesis. The cholesterol lowering effect was higher in rats fed raw garlic fractions and extracts. LDL decreased significantly with respect to the hyper-cholesterolemic groups fed with raw or frozen. However, HDL was found to increase in those treated with frozen fractions and extracts (Slowing *et al.*, 2001).

Chang *et al.* (2011) reported that treatment Garlic oil significantly inhibits the up-regulation in MAPK (*e.g.*, p38, JNK and ERK1/2) and IL-6/MEK5/ERK5 signaling pathways in the diabetic rat hearts, reducing the levels of cardiac pathologic hypertrophy markers such as ANP and BNP, and improving the cardiac contractile function. His study demonstrated that garlic oil is a potential cardioprotective agent from diabetic cardio-myopathy.

Rahman (2007), Chan *et al.* (2007), Borrelli *et al.* (2007), Steiner and Lin (1998) have found garlic to reduce platelet aggregation and hyper-lipidemia (Kojuri *et al.*, 2007, Mader 1990). However, a randomized clinical trial funded by the National Institutes of Health (NIH) in the United States and published in the Archives of Internal Medicine in 2007 found that the consumption of garlic in any form did not reduce blood cholesterol levels in patients with moderately high baseline cholesterol levels.

On reviewing ten studies Alder *et al.* (2003) found 6 of them to be effective. The average drop in total cholesterol was 24.8 mg/dL (9.9 per cent), LDL 15.3 mg/dL (11.4 per cent), and triglycerides 38 mg/dL (9.9 per cent). The overall average MQI score was 39.6 per cent (18 per cent -70 per cent). Major shortcomings of many of the RCTs included short duration, lack of power analysis and intention to treat analysis, as well as lack of control of diet as a confounding variable.

Recently, it has been observed that aged garlic extract, but not the fresh garlic extract, exhibited radical scavenging activity. Just how much garlic should be consumed to achieve any health benefits is unknown. It takes at least 10 cloves to inhibit blood clotting to the same degree as a daily aspirin. Also, practitioners disagree as to whether cooked or dried garlic confers the same benefits imparted by eating it raw (Thomson and Ali, 2003).

The mean difference in reduction of total cholesterol between garlic-treated subjects and those receiving placebo (or avoiding garlic in their diet) was -0.77 mmol/l (95 per cent CI: -0.65, - 0.89 mmol/l). These changes represent a 12 per cent reduction with garlic therapy beyond the final levels achieved with placebo alone. Dried garlic powder preparations also significantly lowered serum triglyceride by 0.31 mmol/l compared to placebo (Silagy and Neil, 1994).

Primary hepatocyte cultures as used in the present study have been proven useful as tools for screening the anti-cholesterogenic properties of garlic principles (Yeh and Yeh, 1994). Gebhardt (1991) demonstrated that water-soluble garlic extracts diminish hepatic cholesterol biosynthesis, thus contributing to the reduction of blood cholesterol the main target site being HMGCoA-reductase. Gebhardt and Beck (1996) demonstrated that different garlic-derived organosulfur compounds interfere differently with cholesterol biosynthesis and, thus, may provoke multiple inhibition of this metabolic pathway in response to garlic consumption. Diallyl disulfide, diallyl trisulfide and dipropyl disulfide depressed cholesterol synthesis by 10 to 25 per cent at low concentrations (< or =0.5 mmol/l), and abolished the synthesis at high concentrations (> or =1.0 mmol/L (Liu and Yeh, 2000).

The cholesterol-lowering effects of garlic extract stem in part from inhibition of hepatic cholesterol synthesis by water-soluble sulfur compounds, especially S-allylcysteine (Yeh and Liu, 2001), whereas the triacylglycerol-lowering effect appears to be due to inhibition of fatty acid synthesis (Yeh and Yeh, 1994). According to Liu and Yeh (2000; 2001) S-allyl cysteine, S-ethyl cysteine, and S-propyl cysteine inhibit lipid biosynthesis in cultured rat hepatocytes, and they further suggest that these S-alkyl cysteines of garlic impair triglyceride synthesis in part due to decreased de novo fatty acid synthesis. Matsuura (2001) found that the saponin fractions from garlic lowered plasma total and LDL cholesterol concentrations without changing HDL cholesterol levels in a hyper-cholesterolemic animal model. Several steroid saponins occur in both garlic and aged garic extract. These results suggest that special consideration should be given to steroid saponins, as well as organosulfur compounds, in biological and pharmacologic studies of garlic and its preparations.

The mechanisms involved in the cardio-protective effects of polyphenols are numerous and include anti-oxidant, vasodilator, anti-inflammatory, anti-fibrotic, anti-apoptotic and metabolic. Most importantly, recent experimental data demonstrate that polyphenols can exert its cardio-protective effect via the activation of several powerful prosurvival cellular pathways that involve metabolic intermediates, micro RNAs, sirtuins and mediators of the recently described reperfusion injury salvage kinases (RISK) and survivor activating factor enhancement (SAFE) pathways (Lecour and Lamont, 2011).

Monascus Garlic Fermented Extract attenuates hyperlipidemia, suggesting that MGFE is a potent agent for preventing arteriosclerotic diseases (Sumioka *et al.*, 2006). The intake of garlic fermented with *Monascus pilosus* decreased triglyceride and cholesterol in serum with no appreciable adverse effects in normal to mildly hyper-lipidemic individuals, suggesting that it may be effective to improve and prevent the metabolic syndrome (Higashikawa *et al.*, 2011).

Cholesterol-induced steatosis leads to a weakened antioxidant defence system and causes peroxidation in the hepatic tissue. Arhan *et al.* (2009) established that treatment with aqueous garlic extract resulted in a significant increase in antioxidant potential and partly eliminated peroxidation damage in the hepatic tissue. Additionally, the extract reduced the cholesterol levels of blood and hepatic tissues significantly. The histological evaluations confirmed the same.

Ginger (*Zingiber officinale*)

Ginger is now exciting considerable interest for its potential to treat many aspects of cardiovascular disease. Rats fed with ethanolic extract of ginger (200 mg/kg, p.o along with cholesterol showed a significantly lower degree of atherosclerosis as compared to gemfibrozil, a standard orally effective hypolipidaemic drug indicating that ginger is definitely an antihyperlipidaemic agent (Bhandari *et al.*, 1998).

Koo *et al.* (2001) and Nurtjahja-Tjendraputra *et al.* (2003) showed that gingerol compounds and their derivatives are more potent anti-platelet agents than aspirin. [8]-Paradol, a natural constituent of ginger, was found to be the most potent COX-1 inhibitor and anti platelet aggregation agent. The mechanism underlying arachidonic acid-induced platelet aggregation inhibition may be related to attenuation of COX-1/Tx synthase enzymatic activity. Dosages of 5 g or more demonstrated significant anti-platelet activity. More human trials are needed using an appropriate dosage of a standardised extract. If found positive, ginger has the potential to offer not only a cheaper natural alternative to conventional agents but one with significantly lower side effects (Nicoll and Henein, 2009).

Herbalists prescribe ginger after dinner to hypertensive patients. Interestingly, a few studies have been carried out to explore the BP-lowering potential of ginger extract. Previously, Weidner and Sigwart (2000) have observed that the standardized ethanol extract of dried ginger was not active on the systolic BP or heart rate in conscious rats when given orally. On the contrary, the ginger pungent principles, gingerol and shogaol, have been studied for their cardiovascular effects in laboratory animals (Suekawa *et al.*, 1984; 1986) and the precise mode of action remains to be elucidated. Ghayur and Gilani (2005a) observed that the blood pressure lowering effect is mediated through blockade of voltage-dependent calcium channels. Fresh ginger crude extract, when injected intravenously in rats under anesthesia, evoked a dose-dependent fall in arterial BP (Ghayur and Gilani, 2005b) which is in line with its traditional use in hypertension (Duke, 2002).

Ginger might delay blood clotting. Taking ginger along with medications that slower clotting might increase the chances of bruising and bleeding (Backon, 1986). However, there is conflicting evidence related to the effect of ginger constituents on human platelets suggesting that recommended doses (less than 5 g) of ginger do not affect platelet aggregation (Bordia, 1997; Verma *et al.*, 1993; Weidner and Sigwart 2000). Similarly, no significant effect was found by Jiang *et al.* (2005), on platelet aggregation and coagulation in healthy human subjects who received a daily dose of 3.6 g of ginger for 5 days. The authors also suggested that the co-administration of ginger at recommended doses is unlikely to cause problems in healthy persons because, ginger administered in herbal medicine products at recommended doses were found to affect the pharmacokinetics or pharmacodynamics of either S-warfarin or R-warfarin in humans, nor did they affect coagulation status.

In the United States, ginger is used to prevent motion and morning sickness. It is recognized as safe by the Food and Drug Administration and is sold as an unregulated dietary supplement.

Fish Oils

Docosahexaenoic acid (DHA) is an n-3 unsaturated fatty acid derived from fish oils. Kimura (2000) demonstrated that DHA produces an ameliorative effect on cholinergic nerve dysfunction in Stroke-prone spontaneously hypertensive rats (SHRSP). The improved cholinergic nerve function induced by DHA might have an inhibitory effect on stroke-related behavior in SHRSP. Thus he suggests that long term administration of DHA may suppress the development of hypertension and stroke-related behavioral changes in SHRSP. On the other hand, Almendingen *et al.* (1995) indicate that consumption of partially hydrogenated fish oil may unfavorably affect lipid risk indicators for coronary heart disease at least to the same extent as butterfat. To what extent the observed effects are due to the content of monoene trans, diene trans, or to the long chain saturated fatty acids in PHFO remains to be elucidated (Almendingen *et al.*, 1995). Halvorsen *et al.* (1996) did not find any significant differences on either conjugated dienes, lipid peroxides, uptake by macrophages or relative electrophoretic mobility of LDL. Vitamin E level in serum from subjects on the PHFO-diet was significantly higher compared to the two other diets. Furthermore, no significant differences were found in the composition of the LDL particle between the three diet groups.

Diets rich in (n-3) fatty acids have been shown to be cardio-protective; these diets decreased inflammation, platelet aggregation, cardiac arrhythmias, triacylglycerols, number of total LDL, and small dense LDL particles and increased the (n-3) index, endothelial relaxation, and atherosclerotic plaque stability (Harris and Von Schacky, 2004; Breslow, 2006). Most of the earlier studies regarding the effects of long chain (n-3) PUFA on blood lipids were conducted with fish oils that contain a mixture of eicosa pentaenoic acid (EPA) and DHA. Recently a number of studies have been conducted with EPA and DHA individually (Buckley *et al.*, 2004; Conquer *et al.*, 1996; Sanders *et al.*, 2006; Theobald *et al.*, 2004; Geppert *et al.*, 2006; Stark and Holub, 2004; Leigh-Firbank *et al.*, 2002; Cazzola *et al.*, 2007). Results from these studies with individual fatty acids show that EPA and DHA have similar effects on some of the lipid variables, but they are assimilated to different concentrations in tissues and have different effects on lipoprotein particle size, heart rate, and blood pressure (Stark and Holub, 2004; Leigh-Firbank *et al.*, 2002).

Many studies have reported that fish oil lowered total cholesterol (TC), low-density lipoprotein (LDL)-cholesterol, high-density lipoprotein (HDL)-cholesterol, and triacylglycerol (TG) concentrations (Morgado *et al.*, 2005; Qi *et al.*, 2008). Fish oil in combination with fish protein hydrolysate lowered plasma cholesterol increased hepatic cholesterol as compared to either of them alone (Wergedahl *et al.*, 2009). Similarly, simultaneous ingestion of fish oil and sulfur amino acid (L-methionine and L-cystine) supplementation indicated that they have hypo-lipidemic effects in cancer-related hyper-lipidemia. Dietary fish oil suppressed the hepatoma-induced increase in cholesterogenesis in the host liver, and dietary methionine and cystine enhanced bile acid excretion into feces, which were the causes of the hypo-cholesterolemic effect (Kawasaki *et al.*, 2010).

Soya (*Glycine max*)

Anderson *et al.* (1995) reported that ingestion of 47 g soy protein/d reduced serum total cholesterol by 9.3 per cent, LDL cholesterol by 12.9 per cent, and triacylglycerol by 10.5 per cent and increased HDL cholesterol by 2.4 per cent. Weggemans and Trautwein (2003) and Zhan and Ho (2005) found substantially weaker effects on lipid profile with soy protein that contained isoflavones. Anderson *et al.* (1995) and Zhan and Ho (2005) concluded that the effects were related to the initial serum lipid concentrations. Zhuo *et al.* (2004) found that the consumption of soy protein with a high isoflavone content reduced serum LDL-cholesterol concentrations more than consumption of the same soy protein amount with low isoflavone content.

Consumption of isoflavones as a constituent of isolated soy protein resulted in small but significant improvements in the lipid profile in normocholesterolemic and mildly hypercholesterolemic postmenopausal women. Although the effects were small, it is possible that isoflavones may contribute to a lower risk of coronary heart disease if consumed over many years in conjunction with other lipid-lowering strategies (Wangen *et al.*, 2001). The semipurified extract of soy, rich in isoflavones, added to casein-lactalbumin protein did not have the same effects as intact soy protein on plasma lipids and lipoproteins. Other components of soy protein, either alone or in combination with isoflavones, may be involved in the effects (Greaves *et al.*, 1999).

Soy isoflavones significantly reduced serum total and LDL cholesterol but did not change HDL cholesterol and triacylglycerol. Soy protein with enriched or depleted isoflavones also significantly improved lipid profiles. Soy protein with enriched isoflavones did significantly increase HDL cholesterol by 0.04 mmol/L (1.6 mg/dL or 3 per cent. Also, the reductions in LDL cholesterol were larger in hypercholesterolemic than in normocholesterolemic subjects (Zhuo *et al.*, 2004; Taku *et al.*, 2007). Naturally occurring isoflavones with soy protein reduced the plasma concentrations of total and LDL cholesterol without affecting concentrations of triglycerides or high-density lipoprotein cholesterol in mildly hypercholesterolemic volunteers consuming a National Cholesterol Education Program Step I diet. Ethanol-extracted isolated soy protein did not significantly reduce plasma concentrations of total or LDL cholesterol (Crouse *et al.*, 1999).

The mechanism of the cholesterol-lowering effect of isoflavones is not well understood, but it may be a result of the chemical and biological similarity to mammalian estrogens, which were shown to have cholesterol-lowering effects in humans (Rossouw, 1999). Soy protein–rich foods may indirectly reduce cardiovascular disease risk if they replaced animal and dairy products that contain saturated fat and cholesterol (Lichtenstein *et al.*, 2006). Soy-based supplements may therefore play a valuable role in reducing cardiovascular protection.

Green Tea

Regular intake of epigallocatechin-3-gallate (EGCG) had no effect on insulin resistance but did result in a modest reduction in diastolic blood pressure. This antihypertensive effect may contribute to some of the cardiovascular benefits associated with habitual green tea consumption (Brown *et al.*, 2009). EGCG treatment for 7 or 15 days, significantly lowered mean levels of 3,4-methylenedioxyamphetamine, higher mean levels of enzymatic and non-enzymatic anti-oxidants occurred, compared with those in saline-treated rats (Ramesh *et al.*, 2008) and protected against the hepatic abnormalities occurring in Wistar rats fed an atherogenic diet (Ramesh *et al.*, 2009).

Pu-erh tea is a variety of fermented dark tea produced in Yunnan province, China. Fermentation is a tea production style in which the tea leaves undergo microbial fermentation and oxidation after they are dried and rolled. Pu-erh tea extract significantly lowered serum low density lipoprotein-cholesterol and triglyceride levels as compared to the control group. ($p < 0.05$). Conversely, levels of high density lipoprotein-cholesterol (HDL-C) were elevated in the groups given daily doses of tea extract (Hou *et al.*, 2009). This tea significantly reduced the total body weight and the weight of various adipose pads. Pu-erh tea administration also significantly lowered plasma total cholesterol, triglyceride concentrations and low-density lipoprotein-cholesterol levels in rats with high fat diet (HFD)-induced obesity, but did not affect high-density lipoprotein-cholesterol levels.

Kuo *et al.* (2005) evaluated the four major commercial teas, oolong, black, pu-erh, and green teas, for the growth suppressive and hypo-lipidemic effect. They found the fully fermented pu-erh and black tea leaves and partially fermented oolong tea leaves to be more effective on their growth suppressive and hypo-lipidemic effects as compared to the non-fermented green tea leaves. Pu-erh tea significantly increased lipoprotein lipase, hepatic lipase and hormone-sensitive lipase activities in epididymal fat tissue in rats with HFD-induced obesity significantly enhanced mRNA levels of hormone-sensitive lipase in rats with HFD-induced obesity (Cao *et al.*, 2011).

Tea extracts prepared from green, oolong, black and pu-erh tea were tested for their ability to modulate fatty acid synthase expression in rats fed on a high-fructose diet. Interestingly, consuming tea leaves for 12 weeks almost normalized the serum triacylglycerols concentrations. Again, rats fed with fructose/green tea and fructose/pu-erh tea showed the greatest reduction in serum triglycerides, cholesterol, insulin and leptin levels. In contrast, serum cholesterol and insulin concentrations of the fructose/oolong tea-fed rats did not normalize. The relative epididymal adipose tissue weight was lower in all rats supplemented with tea leaves than those fed with fructose alone. Furthermore, supplementation of green, black, and pu-erh tea leaves significantly decreased hepatic fatty acid synthase (FAS) mRNA and protein levels, and increased AMPK phosphorylation, compared with those of rats fed with fructose only. Thus, Huang and Lin (2012) concluded that the intake of green, black, and pu-erh tea leaves ameliorated the fructose-induced hyper-lipidemia and hyper-leptinemia state in part through the suppression of FAS protein levels and increased AMPK phosphorylation.

Fenugreek/Methi Seeds (*Trigonella foenum graecum*)

Studies on methi have shown significant reduction in total cholesterol, LDL cholesterol and Triglycerides concentrations without any change in HDL-cholesterol concentrations. The steroidal saponins (diosgenin, yamogenin, tigogenin and neotigogenin) are thought to inhibit cholesterol absorption and synthesis and hence its potential role in arteriosclerosis. Sharma (1986) reported a decrease in total cholesterol levels in five diabetic patients treated with fenugreek seed powder (25g orally per day) for 21 days. The saponins also help to increase the cholesterol and bile acid excretion. (Sharma *et al.*, 1990; 1991). Stark and Madar (1993) too demonstrated that the hypo-cholesterolemic components *i.e.* saponins interact with bile salts in the digestive tract. Thus fenugreek seeds help in maintaining overall cardiovascular health. Bordia *et al.* (1997) studied the effects of fenugreek seed powder (2.5g administered twice daily for three months) in a sub group of 40 subjects. The subjects with coronary artery disease and type 2 diabetes, showed significant decreases in the TC and TG levels, with no change in HDL-C level.

Bhardwaj *et al.* (1994) administered a powder containing methi seeds, Tundika and Meshasringi to 30 NIDDM Patients twice daily for 4 weeks and found a reduction in total as well as LDL cholesterol along with postprandial blood glucose. Sowmya and Rajyalakshmi (1999) observed significant reductions in TC and LDL-C levels in 20 adults with hypercholesterolemia who received 12.5-18.0 g powdered, germinated fenugreek seeds for one month, although no changes in HDL-C, very-low-density lipoprotein (VLDL) or TG levels were observed.

At a dose of 200 mg/kg body weight alcoholic extract of fenugreek seeds reduced plasma cholesterol by 26.19 per cent and triglycerides by 36.6 per cent in triton treated hyperlipidemic rats. Chronic feeding of the same lowered the plasma and hepatic lipid levels by (47 per cent), due to activation of Lecithin-Acyl-Cholesterol-Transferase Chaturvedi *et al.* (2013) thus demonstrating the anti-dyslipidemic and anti-oxidant properties of the extract. Rats fed ethanol extract of defatted methi seeds (30 or 50 gms/Kg body weight were found to have a reduction of 18-26 per cent in plasma cholesterol and a tendency for lower concentrations of liver cholesterol.

Turmeric (*Curcuma longa*)

Curcumin lowers total cholesterol levels. Perhaps even more important, it prevents peroxidation of LDL cholesterol. Since curcumin is an anti-oxidant it is capable of destroying the free radicals that lead to lipid peroxidation. It raises HDL cholesterol levels, even as it reduces LDL levels. Srivastava *et al.* (1985) have shown turmeric to be able to reduce platelets from clumping together, which in turn improves circulation and may help protect against atherosclerosis. In a small study of human volunteers, Mesa *et al.* (2003) reported a highly significant 29 per cent increase in HDL among subjects who consumed 500 mg of curcumin per day for seven days. Subjects also experienced a decrease in total serum cholesterol of more than 11 per cent, and a decrease in serum lipid peroxides of 33 per cent (Soni and Kuttan, 1992). Though further human studies are needed, these findings are promising. In laboratory tests on animals and *in vitro*, scientists have shown that curcumin prevents lipid peroxidation and the oxidation of cellular and subcellular membranes that are associated with atherosclerosis (Sreejayan and Rao, 1994; Quiles *et al.*, 1998; 2002; Ramirez-Tortosa 1999; Mesa *et al.*, 2003).

Researchers in Egypt noted that curcumin protected rats from oxidative stress injury following experimentally induced stroke (Ghoneim, 2002). But rats fed a diet causing high blood sugar, when received high doses of curcumin actually developed cataracts somewhat faster, (Suryanarayana *et al.*, 2003) possibly due to increased oxidative stress. Mesa *et al.* (2003) also noted that curcumin may prevent the effects caused by a high fat diet on cholesterol during development of atherosclerosis.

Very recently it has been found that curcumin pretreatment attenuates the I/R injury as evidenced by (a) loss of cardiac mechanical work, (b) oxidant stress (increase in lipid peroxidation and decrease in reduced glutathione content) and (c) decrease in the activity of the antioxidant enzymes superoxide dismutase and glutathione reductase in both cardiac tissue and isolated mitochondria, and (d) decrease in mitochondrial respiratory capacity (González-Salazar *et al.*, 2011).

Ajwain (*Trachyspermum ammi*)

Ajwain has been shown to possess hypolipidemic (Kumari and Prameela, 1992) and hypoxtensive (Gilani *et al.*, 2005) effects. An ether extract of omum was found to inhibit platelet aggregation induced by arachidonic acid (AA), epinephrine and collagen. But it was most effective against AA-induced aggregation. Effect of omum on platelet thromboxane production could be explained as (i) Reduced TxB2 formation in intact platelet preparations from added arachidonate, and (ii) Reduced formation of TxB2 from AA-labelled platelets after stimulation with Ca^{2+}-ionophore A23187 by a direct action on cyclooxygenase. Thus an increased formation of lipoxygenase-derived products from exogenous AA in omum-treated platelets was apparently due to redirection of AA from cyclooxygenase to the lipoxygenase pathway (Srivastava, 1988).

Methanol and petroleum ether extracts of ajwain equivalent to its powder (2 g/kg body weight) and simvastatin (0.6 mg/kg body weight) were equally effective in treating hyper-lipidaemia in albino rabbits. In fact, petroleum ether extract appeared to be more potent than methanol extract on the basis of increasing the level of HDL-cholesterol and lowering the LDL-cholesterol more effectively. It also reduced atherogenic index (total cholesterol/HDL-cholesterol) more effectively than methanol extract (Javed *et al.*, 2002; 2006) due to the significant increase in HDL-Cholesterol (42 per cent).

Almonds (*Prunus amygdalus*)

Almonds are a whole food rich in numerous beneficial nutritive and bioactive compounds like fatty acids, dietary fibers, micronutrients and phytochemicals. Almond consumption has been associated with improvements in serum lipid profiles. A growing number of human nutritional studies have revealed that almonds have a cholesterol-lowering effect (Jenkins *et al.*, 2002; Sabate *et al.*, 2003). Diets supplemented with almonds or almond products (*i.e.*, oil and butter) have been shown to produce a moderate, yet significant decrease in plasma total cholesterol (3–11 per cent) and plasma LDL cholesterol (3–18 per cent) (Abbey *et al.*, 1994; Berry *et al.*, 1992; Spiller *et al.*, 1990; 1992; 1998; Kendall *et al.*, 2002; Fulgoni III *et al.*, 2002; Hyson *et al.*, 2002; Kritchevsky *et al.*, 1982; Sabate and Fraser, 1993; Farquhar, 1996; USDA, 1984) which demonstrates a potential benefit from consuming almonds on improving cardiovascular health.

Proteins in almonds have an arginine-rich amino acid profile that is thought to be cardio-protective (USDA, 1984). In addition, they are good sources of dietary fiber and phyto-chemicals, such as plant sterols, which have been shown to contribute to reduced risk of coronary heart disease (NRC, 1989). Almonds are rich in tocopherols, especially α-tocopherol, which has demonstrated potent anti-atherogenic effects. Recently, Hyson *et al.* (2002) postulated that the beneficial effects of almonds might be mediated by the lipid fraction.

However, the fat content and energy density of almonds raise concerns that chronic consumption will promote weight gain. But Hollis and Mattes (2007) confirmed that ten weeks of daily almond consumption did not cause a change in body weight predominantly due to compensation for the energy contained in the almonds through reduced food intake from other sources. Moreover, inefficiency in the absorption of energy from almonds was documented ($P < 0.05$). No changes in resting metabolic rate, thermic effect of food or total energy expenditure were noted. A daily 1440 kJ serving of almonds, sufficient to provide beneficial effects on cardiovascular risk factors, may be included in the diet with limited risk of weight gain. Zaveri and Drummond (2009) also demonstrated that snacking on almonds, in comparison to cereal bars, promoted a higher eating frequency, but not a higher energy intake. Snacking on either almonds or cereal bars did not result in weight gain, suggesting that energy compensation took place. Recently, Foster *et al.* (2012) observed that the hypo-caloric, almond-enriched diet as well as the hypo-caloric nut free diet groups experienced clinically significant and comparable weight loss at 18 months. Despite smaller weight loss in the almond group at 6 months, there were greater improvements in lipid profiles. Ortiz *et al.* (2012) on reviewing the available data concluded that increase in almond intake contributed to the reduction in plasma total cholesterol and plasma LDL-C to a greater extent than a reduction in dietary saturated fatty acid (SFA), but a simultaneous decrease in dietary SFA should further improve lipid profiles. Spiller *et al.* (2003) observed that unblanched almonds-whether raw, dry roasted, or in roasted butter form-can play an effective role in cholesterol-lowering, plant-based diets.

Consumption of plant sterols, soyabean proteins, viscous fibre and nuts are known to modulate the risk of CVD favorably through their cholesterol-lowering properties, both independently and more recently in combination. Jenkins *et al.* (2003a, b), Lamarche *et al.* (2004) and Gigleux *et al.* (2007) assessed the effect of incorporating concurrently plant sterols (1 g/4.2 MJ), soyabean protein (23 g/4.2 MJ), viscous fibre (9 g/4.2 MJ) and almonds (15 g/4.2 MJ) into a diet very low in saturated fat in twelve patients with mildly elevated plasma LDL-C levels. The diet-induced reduction in plasma LDL-C of 30.0 per cent ($P<0.0001$) was attributed to concurrent reductions in the serum cholesterol concentrations of large ($P<0.001$), medium ($P<0.001$) and small ($P<0.01$) LDL particles, with near maximal reductions seen by week 2. The reductions in plasma LDL-cholesterol levels with the combination diet and with statins were comparable. Thus it is quite clear that combining a number of foods and food components in a single dietary portfolio may lower LDL-C similarly to statins and benefit cardiovascular disease risk both by reducing serum lipids and also blood pressure (Jenkins *et al.*, 2002b, 2008).

Walnuts (*Juglans regia*)

Nut consumption, particularly walnut intake, has been inversely related to incident coronary heart disease (CHD) in observational studies and to improved lipid profiles with a decrease in total and LDL cholesterol as well as triglycerides (Abbey *et al.*, 1994; Zambon *et al.*, 2000; Sabate *et al.*, 1993; Chisholm *et al.*, 1998) and an increase in HDL cholesterol and apo-lipoprotein A1 (Lavedrine *et al.*, 1999) in short-term feeding trials. The walnut extracts exhibited a Trolox equivalent activity greater than that of alpha-tocopherol. LC-ELSD/MS analysis of the walnut extracts identified ellagic acid monomers, polymeric ellagitannins and other phenolics, principally non-flavonoid compounds. Walnut poly-phenolics are effective inhibitors of *in vitro* plasma and LDL oxidation. Therefore, Anderson *et al.* (2001) recommended that the poly-phenolic content of walnuts should be considered when evaluating their anti-atherogenic potential. Papoutsi *et al.* (2008) reported that the walnut extract has a high anti-atherogenic potential and a remarkable osteoblastic activity, an effect mediated, at least in part, by its major component ellagic acid. Such findings implicate the beneficial effect of a walnut-enriched diet on cardio-protection and bone loss. The restructured meat products with added walnuts supplied can be considered functional foods for subjects at high risk for CVD, as their regular consumption provokes a reduction in total cholesterol of 4.5 per cent with respect to baseline values (mixed diet) and 3 per cent with respect to the restructured meat without walnuts (Olmedilla-Alonso *et al.*, 2008; Sánchez-Muniz *et al.*, 2012). Rajaram *et al.* (2009) through a randomized cross-over study confirmed that including walnuts and fatty fish in a healthy diet lowered serum cholesterol and triglyceride concentrations, respectively, and thus decreased CHD risk considerably. Canales *et al.* (2009) also demonstrated that meat enriched with walnut paste and low-fat meat consumptions reduced plasma thromboxane A2 (TXB2) levels most (P = 0.050) in obese individuals, while the prostacyclin I2 and the thrombogenic (TXB2/6-keto-PGF1alpha) ratio decreased most (P = 0.066) in volunteers whose serum cholesterol levels were > or = 220 mg/dl.

Grapes (*Vitis vinifera*)

Epidemiological studies suggest that consumption of wine, grape products, and other foods containing polyphenols is associated with decreased risk for cardiovascular disease. Experimental studies indicate that grape polyphenols could reduce atherosclerosis by a number of mechanisms, including inhibition of oxidation of LDL and other favorable effects on cellular redox state, improvement of endothelial function, lowering blood pressure, inhibition of platelet aggregation, reducing inflammation, and activating novel proteins that prevent cell senescence (Dohadwala and Vita, 2009). The flavonoid components of grape products, including red wine and purple grape juice inhibit collagen-mediated platelet aggregation (Renaud *et al.*, 1992; Osman *et al.*, 1998; Keevil *et al.*, 1998; Folts, 1997).

Short-term ingestion of purple grape juice improved flow-mediated vasodilation and reduced LDL susceptibility to oxidation in CAD patients. Stein *et al.* (1999) concluded that improved endothelium-dependent vasodilation and prevention of LDL oxidation are potential mechanisms by which flavonoids in purple grape products may prevent cardiovascular events, independent of alcohol content. According to Fitzpatrick *et al.* (1993) and Flesch *et al.* (1997) *in vitro,* flavonoid components of red wine and purple grape juice induced endothelium-dependent vasodilation of arterial rings, a phenomenon mediated by the nitric oxide-guanosine 32,52 cyclic monophosphate (NO-cGMP) pathway. The cardio-protective mechanism of grape seed proanthocyanidin extract has been attributed to its ability to block anti-death signaling mediated through the pro-aapoptotic transcription factors and genes such as JNK-1 and c-JUN. Grape seed proanthocyanidin extract (GSPE) supplementation to hyper-cholesterolemic subjects significantly inhibited inducible endothelial CD36 expression, a novel cardio-regulatory gene (Bagchi *et al.*, 2003).

Both red wine and purple grape juice improved flow-mediated dilation, but red wine also enhanced endothelium-independent vasodilation in hyper-cholesterolemic patients despite the increased plasma cholesterol. Thus, Coimbra *et al.* (2005) concluded that purple grape juice may protect against coronary artery disease without the additional negative effects of alcohol despite the gender. Castilla *et al.* (2006) confirmed that dietary supplementation with concentrated red grape juice improved the lipoprotein profile, reduced plasma concentrations of inflammatory biomarkers and oxidized LDL, and thus favored a reduction in cardiovascular disease risk.

Pakhale *et al.* (2007) studied the antioxidant potency of Indian grape cultivars varying in their skin color, seed and polyphenol content (Bangalore blue, Pandhari sahebi, Sharad seedless and Thompson seedless) and their components (whole grapes, pulp with skin and seeds). The results indicate that polyphenols extracted from Indian grapes/components (with/without seeds) exhibited free radical scavenging activity. Leifert and Abeywardena (2008) on reviewing the studies available on Grapes, concludes that consumption of grape and grape extracts and/or grape products such as red wine may be beneficial in preventing the development of chronic degenerative diseases such as cardiovascular disease. Ngamukote *et al.* (2011) demonstrated that three major polyphenolic compounds gallic acid, catechin, and epicatechin present in a particular grape seed have cholesterol-lowering activity by inhibiting pancreatic cholesterol esterase, binding of bile acids, and reducing solubility of cholesterol in micelles which may result in delayed cholesterol absorption.

Regular consumption of unripe grape juice was also found to have a dramatic effect on improving HDL-C level of serum but no lipid-lowering effect on TG, total cholesterol, or LDL-C (ZibaeeNezhad *et al.*, 2012).

Interestingly, the grape skin extract 500 mg/kg body weight and resveratrol 20 mg/kg body weight showed a significant improvement in lipid profile. A significant reduction of atherogenic index was also observed with grape skin extract. In addition, the changed levels of hepatic tissue lipid peroxidation, superoxide dismutase, catalase and glutathione peroxidase induced by high-fat diet reverted back to normal levels by grape skin extract (Rajesh *et al.*, 2013).

Blue Berry (*Vaccinium ashei*)

Blueberry extracts have high anti-oxidant potential and increase phase II enzyme activities *in vitro*. In healthy rats, short-term supplementation with freeze-dried whole blueberries, blueberry polyphenols, or blueberry flavonoids did not significantly increase phase II enzyme activities. However, supplementation with 1 per cent blueberry flavonoids did decrease oxidative DNA damage in the liver (Dulebohn *et al.*, 2008).

Lowbush blueberries (*Vaccinium angustifolium*) also have a high antioxidant capacity. Rats on blueberry-supplemented diets lost only 17 +/- 2 per cent of neurons in the ischemic hippocampus. Neuroprotection was observed in the CA1 and CA2 regions, but not CA3 region, of the hippocampus. The blueberry diet had no detectable effects on the plasma or urine oxygen radical absorbance capacity (ORAC) or plasma lipids. From these observations Sweeney *et al.* (2002) concluded that consumption of low bush blueberries by rats confers protection to the brain against damage from ischemia, suggesting that inclusion of blueberries in the diet may improve ischemic stroke outcomes. Again, Wang *et al.* (2005) Animals treated with blueberry, spinach, or spirulina had significantly lower caspase-3 activity in the ischemic hemisphere. In conclusion, our data suggest that chronic treatment with blueberry, spinach, or spirulina reduces ischemia/reperfusion-induced apoptosis and cerebral infarction.

Though blueberry diets had no effect on angiotensin-converting enzyme (ACE) activity in lung, testis, kidney, or aorta, according to Wiseman *et al.* (2011) dietary blueberries may be effective in manageing early stages of hypertension, partially due to an inhibition of soluble ACE activity.

A 3 per cent blue berry diet may be capable of protecting the kidneys from oxidative damage in spontaneously hypertensive stroke-prone rats, thereby reducing the magnitude of hypertension as Shaughnessy *et al.* (2009) found blueberry intake had no effect on urinary excretion of F_2-isoprostanes and thus a systemic antioxidant effect of the berry may not be responsible for the anti hypertensive effects. Blueberry-fed rats had reduced markers of renal oxidative stress, such as proteinuria and kidney nitrites.

Jamun (*Eugenia jambolana*)

Jadeja *et al.* (2012) demonstrated the anti-atherogenic potential of Jamun which has been suggested to be due to its high flavonoid content. Flavanoids in *jamum* were also instrumental in lowering oxidative intra-cellular stress, thus preventing depletion of cellular anti-oxidants and improving cell viability (Devkar *et al.*, 2012).

Chocolate

Epidemiologic investigations support the hypothesis that regular consumption of flavonoid-containing foods can reduce the risk of cardiovascular diseases (CVD). While flavonoids are ubiquitous in plants, cocoa can be particularly rich in a sub-class of flavonoids known as flavanols. A number of human dietary intervention trials with flavanol-containing cocoa products have demonstrated improvements in endothelial and platelet function, as well as blood pressure. A single ingestion of flavanol-containing cocoa was dose-dependently associated with significant acute increases in circulating flavanols. Diets rich in flavanols reverse vascular dysfunction in diabetes, highlighting therapeutic potentials in cardiovascular disease (Balzer *et al.*, 2008).

Wang-Polagruto *et al.* (2006) was the first to identify beneficial vascular effects of flavanol-rich cocoa consumption in hyper-cholesterolemic postmenopausal women. In addition, our results suggest that reductions in plasma soluble vascular cell adhesion molecule-1 after chronic consumption of a flavanol-rich cocoa may be mechanistically linked to improved vascular reactivity. The daily consumption of flavanol-containing dark chocolate was associated with a significant mean reduction of 5.8 mmHg in systolic blood pressure. These human dietary intervention trials provide scientific evidence of the vascular effects of cocoa flavanols and suggest that the regular consumption of cocoa products containing flavanols may reduce risk of CVD (Erdman *et al.*, 2008).

The circulating pool of bioactive NO and endothelium-dependent vasodilation is acutely increased in smokers following the oral ingestion of a flavanol-rich cocoa drink (Heiss *et al.*, 2005). The increase in circulating NO pool may contribute to beneficial vascular health effects of flavanol-rich food.

Cheese

Despite its high content of saturated fatty acids, cheese decreases plasma total and LDL-cholesterol concentrations when compared with an equivalent intake of fat from butter. This effect may be due to the high calcium content of cheese, which results in a higher excretion of fecal fat (Hjerpsted *et al.*, 2011). Similarly, 40 g dairy fat (butter) eaten daily for 4 weeks, raised total and LDL cholesterol significantly but not cheese, as compared to a diet containing significantly less saturated fat. Therefore,

Nestel *et al.* (2005) feel that the dietary advice regarding cheese consumption may require modification.

Asafoetida (*Ferula assafoetida*)

Asafoetida gum extract (0.3-2.2 mg/100g body weight) significantly reduced the mean arterial blood pressure in anaesthetized rats. Fatehi *et al.* (2004) concluded that the relaxant compounds in asafoetida gum extract might interfere with a variety of muscarinic, adrenergic and histaminic receptor activities or with the mobilization of calcium ions required for smooth muscle contraction non-specifically.

Cumin Seeds (*Cuminum cyminum*)

The levels of tissue (liver and kidney) cholesterol and triglycerides decreased when cumin was given along with alcohol and thermally oxidized oil. The level of phospholipids also increased. The activity of phospholipase A and C decreased significantly in the liver of groups fed cumin seeds indicating that cumin can decrease the lipid levels in alcohol and thermally oxidized oil induced hepatotoxicity (Aruna *et al.*, 2005).

Administration to Wistar rats of the cumin essential oil could bring a 17.38 per cent decrease in WBCs count, and 25.77 per cent, 14.24 per cent, and 108.81 per cent increase in hemoglobin concentration, hematocrit, and platelet count, respectively. LDL/HDL ratio was also reduced to half, which adds to the nutritional effects of cumin (Allahghadri *et al.*, 2010).

The liver phospholipids fatty acid concentrations of 16:0, 16:1, 18:0, 18:1 and 20:4 were near normal in cumin-treated rats when *C. cyminum* was administered at a dosage of 250 mg/kg body weight for 45 days (Kode *et al.*, 2005).

Amla (*Emblica officinalis/Phyllanthus emblica*)

Amla is highly nutritious and could be an important dietary source of vitamin C, amino acids, and minerals. The plant also contains phenolic compounds, tannins, phyllembelic acid, phyllembelin, rutin, curcum-inoids, and emblicol. Various parts of the plant show anti-diabetic, hypo-lipidemic, anti-bacterial, anti-oxidant, anti-ulcerogenic, hepato-protective, gastro-protective, and chemo-preventive properties (Krishnaveni and Mirunalini, 2010).

Drumstick (*Moringa oleifera*)

Moringa oleifera is a highly valued plant, distributed in many countries of the tropics and subtropics. It has an impressive range of medicinal uses with high nutritional value. Different parts of this plant contain a profile of important minerals, and are a good source of protein, vitamins, beta-carotene, amino acids and various phenolics. The *Moringa* plant provides a rich and rare combination of zeatin, quercetin, beta-sitosterol, caffeoylquinic acid and kaempferol. Compounds, bearing thiocarbamate, isolated from the leaves of *M. oleifera*, fully acetylated glycoside, very rare in nature showed hypotensive activity

Ethanol extract of drumstick leaves attenuated the development of pulmonary hypertension via direct vasodilatation and a potential increase in antioxidant activity (Chen *et al.,* 2012). Chronic *M. oleifera* treatment resulted in significant favorable modulation of the biochemical enzymes (superoxide dismutase, catalase, glutathione peroxidase, lactate dehydrogenase, and creatine kinase-MB) but failed to demonstrate any significant effect on reduced glutathione compared to the ISP control group. *Moringa* treatment significantly prevented the rise in lipid peroxidation in myocardial tissue. Furthermore, *M. oleifera* also prevented the deleterious histo-pathological and ultra-structural perturbations caused by isoproterenol. Thus *M. oleifera* extract possesses significant cardio-protective effect, which may be attributed to its antioxidant, anti-peroxidative, and myocardial preservative properties (Nandave *et al.,* 2009).

Various parts of this plant such as the leaves, roots, seed, bark, fruit, flowers and immature pods act as cardiac and circulatory stimulants, possess anti-tumor, anti-pyretic, anti-epileptic, anti-inflammatory, anti-ulcer, anti-spasmodic, diuretic, anti-hypertensive, cholesterol lowering, anti-oxidant, anti-diabetic, hepato-protective, anti-bacterial and anti-fungal activities, and are being employed for the treatment of different ailments in the indigenous system of medicine, particularly in South Asia (Anwar *et al.,* 2007).

Cabbage (*Brassica oleracea*)

Red cabbage extract fed to atherogenic diet induced hyper-cholesterolaemic rats significantly prevented elevation in serum and tissue lipids, circulating levels of cardiac and hepatic damage markers, and resulted in excretion of lipids through faeces. Also, the cabbage extract significantly attenuated alterations in the cardiac and hepatic antioxidants, and histopathological changes in cardiac and hepatic tissue (Sankhari *et al.,* 2012). The cabbage leaf extract has been found to posses cardioprotective activity against hydrogen peroxide (H_2O_2) induced cytotoxicity in H9C2 cells. The high content of anthocynins in cabbage seems to be instrumental in lowering the intra-cellular oxidative stress, preventing depletion of cellular anti-oxidants and improving cell viability (Devkar *et al.,* 2012).

Saffron (*Crocus sativus*)

The two active constituents, crocin and safranal from saffron have been found to be hypo-tensive in dose-dependent manner and safranal seems to be more effective than crocin (Imenshahidi *et al.,* 2010).

Tamarind (*Tamarindus indica*)

Treatment of hypercholesterolemic hamsters with the tamarind fruit pulp extract (5 per cent) led to a decrease in the levels of serum total cholesterol (50 per cent), non-HDL cholesterol (73 per cent) and triglyceride (60 per cent), and to an increase of high-density lipoprotein (HDL) cholesterol levels (61 per cent). *In vitro*, the extract presented radical scavenging ability, as assessed by the 2,2-diphenyl-1-picrylhydrazyl (DPPH) and superoxide radicals assays, and led to decreased lipid peroxidation in serum, as assessed by the thiobarbituric acid reactive substances (TBARS) assay. *In vivo*, the extract improved the efficiency of the antioxidant defense system, as assessed by the superoxide dismutase, catalase and glutathione peroxidase activities. Together these results indicate the potential of tamarind extracts in diminishing the risk of atherosclerosis development in humans (Martinello *et al.*, 2006).

Conclusions

Studies on Garlic, Oats, Flax seeds, Fish, Walnuts etc. as Hypo-lipidemic foods are abundant. Interestingly, consumption of these foods has also been on the rise as public awareness of the alarming risk of CVD increased. Surprisingly cheese has been reported to lower the LDL and total cholesterol in spite of its high saturated fat content. It has been postulated that high calcium content or its mobilization could be responsible. Amla being very rich in anti-oxidants could serve as a hypo-lipidemic food as suggested by Krishnaveni and Mrinalini (2010). But no studies are available on this aspect. Foods like Amla, Tamarind, Cheese etc. need further probing. Stress being one of the culprits, the role of anti-stress foods like, coffee, tea, chocolate also need to be explored in connection with CVD.

References

Abbey M, Noakes M, Belling GB, Nestel PJ (1994). Partial replacement of saturated fatty acids with almonds or walnuts lowers total plasma cholesterol and low-density-lipoprotein cholesterol. Am. J. Clin. Nutr. 59: 995 - 99.

AbuMweis SS, Jew S, Ames NP (2010). β-glucan from barley and its lipid-lowering capacity: a meta-analysis of randomized, controlled trials. Eur. J. Clin. Nutr. 64 (12): 1472 - 80.

Agarwal KC (1996). Therapeutic actions of garlic constituents. Med. Res. Rev. 16: 111 - 24.

Alder R, Lookinland S, Berry JA, Williams M (2003). A systematic review of the effectiveness of garlic as an anti-hyper-lipidemic agent. J. Am. Acad. Nurse. Pract. 15 (3): 120 - 29.

Allahghadri T, Rasooli I, Owlia P, Nadooshan MJ, Ghazanfari T, Taghizadeh M, Astaneh SD (2010). Anitimicrobial property, anti-oxidant capacity, and cyto-toxicity of essential oil from cumin produced in Iran. J. Food Sci. 75 (2): H54 - 61.

Aller R, de Luis DA, Izaola O, La Calle F, del Olmo L, Fernandez L, Arranz T, Hernandez JM (2004). Effect of soluble fiber intake in lipid and glucose levels in healthy subjects: a randomized clinical trial. Diabetes Res. Clin. Pract. 65 (1): 7 - 11.

Almendingen K, Jordal O, Kierulf P, Sandstad B, Pedersen JI (1995). Effects of partially hydrogenated fish oil, partially hydrogenated soybean oil, and butter on serum lipoproteins and Lp[a] in men. J. Lipid. Res. 36 (6): 1370 - 84.

Ames NP, Rhymer CR (2008). Issues surrounding health claims for barley. J. Nutr. 138 (6): 1237S - 4.

Amundesan ÅL, Haugum B, Andersson H (2003). Changes in serum cholesterol and sterol metabolites after intake of products enriched with oat bran concentrate within a controlled diet. Scand. J. Clin. Nutr. 47: 68 - 74.

Anderson JW. (1995). Cholesterol-lowering effects of soluble fiber in humans. In: Kritchevsky D, Bonfield C, editors. Dietary fiber in health and disease. St. Paul: Eagan Press. p. 126–136.

Anderson JW, Bridges SR. (1993). Hypo-cholesterolemic effects of oat bran in humans. In: Wood PJ, editor. Oat bran. St. Paul: American Association of Cereal Chemists. p. 139–157.

Anderson JW, Johnstone BM, Cook-Newell ME (1995). Meta-analysis of the effects of soy protein intake on serum lipids. N. Engl. J. Med. 333: 276 - 82.

Anderson KJ, Teuber SS, Gobeille A, Cremin P, Waterhouse AL, Steinberg FM (2001). Walnut polyphenolics inhibit *in vitro* human plasma and LDL oxidation. J. Nutr. 131 (11): 2837 - 42.

Andersson KE, Svedberg KA, Lindholm MW, Oste R, Hellstrand P (2010). Oats (*Avena sativa*) reduce atherogenesis in LDL-receptor-deficient mice. Atherosclerosis. 212 (1): 93 - 99.

Anwar F, Latif S, Ashraf M, Gilani AH (2007). *Moringa oleifera*: a food plant with multiple medicinal uses. Phytother. Res. 21 (1): 17 - 25.

Arhan M, Oztürk HS, Turhan N, Aytac B, Güven MC, Olcay E, Durak I (2009). Hepatic oxidant/anti-oxidant status in cholesterol-fed rabbits: Effects of garlic extract. Hepatol. Res. 39 (1): 70 - 77.

Arjmandi BH, Khan DA, Juma S, Drum ML, Venkatesh S, Sohn E, Wei L, Derman R (1998). Whole flaxseed consumption lowers serum LDL-cholesterol and lipoprotein (a) concentrations in post-menopausal women. Nutr. Res. 18: 1203 - 14.

Aruna K, Rukkumani R, Varma PS, Menon VP (2005). Therapeutic role of *Cuminum cyminum* on ethanol and thermally oxidized sunflower oil induced toxicity. Phytother. Res. 19 (5): 416 - 21.

Backon J (1986) Ginger: Inhibition of thromboxane synthetase and stimulation of prostacyclin: Relevance for medicine and psychiatry Medical Hypotheses. 20 (3): 271 - 78.

Bae IY, Kim SM, Lee S, Lee HG (2010). Effect of enzymatic hydrolysis on cholesterol-lowering activity of oat beta-glucan. N. Biotechnol. 27 (1): 85 - 88.

Bagchi D, Sen CK, Ray SD, Das DK, Bagchi M, Preuss HG, Vinson JA (2003). Molecular mechanisms of cardioprotection by a novel grape seed proanthocyanidin extract. Mutat. Res. 523 - 524: 87 - 97.

Balzer J, Rassaf T, Heiss C, Kleinbongard P, Lauer T, Merx M, Heussen N, Gross HB, Keen CL, Schroeter H, Kelm M. (2008) Sustained benefits in vascular function through flavanol-containing cocoa in medicated diabetic patients a double-masked, randomized, controlled trial. J. Am. Coll. Cardiol. 51 (22): 2141 - 49.

Barakat LA, Mahmoud RH (2011). The anti-atherogenic, renal protective and immuno-modulatory effects of purslane, pumpkin and flax seeds on hyper-cholesterolemic rats. N. Am. J. Med. Sci. 3 (9): 411 - 17.

Bassett CM, Rodriguez-Leyva D, Pierce GN (2009). Experimental and clinical research findings on the cardiovascular benefits of consuming flaxseed. Appl. Physiol. Nutr. Metab. 34 (5): 965 - 74.

Beaglehole R, Bonita R (2008). Global public health: A scorecard. Lancet. 372 (9654): 1988 - 1996.

Beer MU, Arrigoni E, Amado R (1995). Effects of oat gum on blood cholesterol levels in healthy young men. Eur. J. Clin. Nutr. 49: 517 - 22.

Behall KM, Scholfield DJ, Hallfrisch J (1997). Effect of beta-glucan level in oat fiber extracts on blood lipids in men and women. J. Am.Coll. Nutr. 16 (1): 46 - 51.

Behall KM, Scholfield DJ, Hallfrisch J (2004). Diets containing barley significantly reduce lipids in mildly hyper-cholesterolemic men and women. Am. J. Clin. Nutr. N80 (5): 1185-93.

Berg A, König D, Deibert P, Grathwohl D, Berg A, Baumstark MW, Franz IW (2003). Effect of an oat bran enriched diet on the atherogenic lipid profile in patients with an increased coronary heart disease risk. A controlled randomized lifestyle intervention study. Ann. Nutr. Metab. 47 (6): 306 - 11.

Berry EM, Eisenberg S, Haratz D, Friedlander Y, Norman Y, Kaufmann N, Stein Y (1992). Effects of diets rich in monounsaturated fatty acids on plasma lipoproteins-the Jerusalem Nutrition Study. II. Monounsaturated fatty acids vs. carbohydrates. Am. J. Clin. Nutr. 56: 394 - 403.

Bhandari U, Sharma JN, Zafar R (1998). The protective action of ethanolic ginger (*Zingiber officinale*) extract in cholesterol fed rabbits. J. Ethnopharm. 61 (2): 167 - 71.

Bhardwaj PK, Dasgupta DJ, Prashar BS, Kaushal SS (1994). Control of hyperglycaemia and hyper-lipidaemia by plant product. J. Assoc. Physicians India. 42 (1): 33 - 35.

Bierenbaum ML, Reichstein R, Watkins TR (1993). Reducing atherogenic risk in hyper-lipemic humans with flaxseed supplementation: a preliminary report. J. Am. Coll. Nutr. 12: 501 - 504.

Biörklund M, Holm J, Onning G (2008). Serum lipids and postprandial glucose and insulin levels in hyperlipidemic subjects after consumption of an oat beta-glucan-containing ready meal. Ann. Nutr. Metab. 52 (2): 83-90.

Biörklund M, van Rees A, Mensink RP, Onning G (2005). Changes in serum lipids and postprandial glucose and insulin concentrations after consumption of beverages with beta-glucans from oats or barley: a randomised dose-controlled trial. Eur. J. Clin. Nutr. 59 (11): 1272 - 81.

Bird AR, Jackson M, King RA, Davies DA, Usher S, Topping DL (2004). A novel high-amylose barley cultivar (*Hordeum vulgare* var. Himalaya 292) lowers plasma cholesterol and alters indices of large-bowel fermentation in pigs. Br. J. Nutr. 92 (4): 607 - 15.

Bloedon LT, Balikai S, Chittams J, Cunnane S, Berlin J, Rader D, Szapary PO (2008). Flaxseed and cardiovascular risk factors: results from a double blind, randomized, controlled clinical trial. J. Am. Coll. Nutr. 27: 65 - 74.

Bloedon LT, Szapary PO (2004). Flaxseed and cardiovascular risk. Nutr. Rev. 62 (1): 18 - 27.

Bordia A, Verma SK, Srivastava KC (1997). Effect of ginger (*Zingiber officinale* Rosc.) and fenugreek (*Trigonella foenumgraecum L.)* on blood lipids, blood sugar, and platelet aggregation ion patients with coronary heart disease. Prostaglandins. Leukot. Essent. Fatty Acids. 56 (5): 379 - 84.

Borrelli F, Capasso R, Izzo AA (2007). Garlic (*Allium sativum* L.): adverse effects and drug interactions in humans. Mol. Nutr. Food Res. 51 (11): 386 - 97.

Bourdon I, Yokoyama W, Davis P, Hudson C, Backus R, Richter D, Knuckles B, Schneeman BO. (1999). Postprandial lipid, glucose, insulin, and cholecystokinin responses in men fed barley pasta enriched with beta-glucan. Am. J. Clin. Nutr. 69: 55 - 63.

Braaten JT, Wood PJ, Scott FW, *et al.* (1994). Oat β-glucan reduces blood cholesterol concentration in hypercholesterolemic subjects. Eur. J. Clin. Nutr. 48: 465 - 74.

Breslow JL (2006). n-3 fatty acids and cardiovascular disease. Am. J. Clin. Nutr. 83 (6 Suppl): 1477S - 1482S.

Bridges SR, Anderson JW, Deakins DA, Dillon DW, Wood CL. (1992). Oat bran increases serum acetate of hyper-cholesterolemic men. Am. J. Clin. Nutr. 56: 455 - 459.

Brown AL, Lane J, Coverly J, Stocks J, Jackson S, Stephen A, Bluck L, Coward A, Hendricks H. (2009). Effects of dietary supplementation with the green tea polyphenol epigallocatechin-3-gallate on insulin resistance and associated metabolic risk factors: randomized controlled trial. Br. J. Nutr. 101 (6): 886 - 94.

Brown L, Rosner B, Willett WW, Sacks FM (1999). Cholesterol-lowering effects of dietary fiber: a meta-analysis. Am. J. Clin. Nutr. 69 (1): 30 - 42.

Buckley R, Shewring B, Turner R, Yaqoob P, Minihane AM (2004). Circulating triacylglycerol and apoE levels in response to EPA and docosahexaenoic acid supplementation in adult human subjects. Br. J. Nutr. 92 (3): 477 - 83.

Butt SM, Tahir-Nadeem M, Khan MK, Shabir R, Butt MS (2008). Oat: unique among the cereals. Eur. J. Nutr. 47 (2): 68 - 79.

Canales A, Bastida S, Librelottto J, Nus M, Sánchez-Muniz FJ, Benedi J (2009). Platelet aggregation, eicosanoid production and thrombogenic ratio in individuals at high cardiovascular risk consuming meat enriched in walnut paste. A crossover, placebo-controlled study. Br. J. Nutr. 102 (1): 134 - 41.

Cao ZH, Gu DH, Lin QY, Xu ZQ, Huang QC, Rao H, Liu EW, Jia JJ, Ge CR (2011). Effect of pu-erh tea on body fat and lipid profiles in rats with diet-induced obesity. Phytother. Res. 25 (2): 234 - 38.

Cardozo LF, Alves Chagas M, Leal Soares L, Andrade Troina A, Teles Bonaventura G. (2010). Exposure to flaxseed during lactation does not alter prostate area or epithelium height but changes lipid profile in rats. Nutr. Hosp. 25 (2): 250 - 55.

Castilla P, Echarri R, Dávalos A, Cerrato F, Ortega H, Teruel JL, Lucas MF, Gómez-Coronado D, Ortuno J, Lasunción MA (2006). Concentrated red grape juice exerts anti-oxidant, hypo-lipidemic, and anti-inflammatory effects in both hemo-dialysis patients and healthy subjects. Am. J. Clin. Nutr. 84 (1): 252 - 62.

Caughey GE, Mantzioris E, Gibson RA, Cleland LG, James MJ (1996). The effect on human tumor necrosis factor alpha and interleukin 1 beta production of diets enriched in n-3 fatty acids from vegetable oil or fish oil. Am. J. Clin. Nutr. 63 (1): 116 - 22.

Cazzola R, Russo-Volpe S, Miles EA, Rees D, Banerjee T, Roynette CE, Wells SJ, Goua M, Wahle KW, Calder PC, Cestaro B (2007). Age- and dose-dependent effects of an eicosapentaenoic acid-rich oil on cardiovascular risk factors in healthy male subjects. Atherosclerosis. 193 (1): 159 - 67.

Chan JK, Bruce VM, McDonald BE (1991). Dietary α-linolenic acid is as effective as oleic acid and linoleic acid in lowering blood cholesterol in normo-lipidemic men. Am. J. Clin. Nutr. 53 (5): 1230 - 40.

Chan KC, Yin MC, Chao WJ (2007). Effect of diallyl trisulfide-rich garlic oil on blood coagulation and plasma activity of anti-coagulation factors in rats. Food Chem. Toxicol. 45 (3): 502 - 507.

Chang SH, Liu CJ, Kuo CH, Chen H, Lin WY, Teng KY, Chang SW, Tsai CH, Tsai FJ, Huang CY, Tzang BS, Kuo WW (2011). Garlic Oil Alleviates MAPKs- and IL-6-mediated Diabetes-related Cardiac Hypertrophy in STZ-induced DM Rats. Evid. Based Complement. Alternat. Med. 2011: 950150.

Charlton KE, Tapsell LC, Batterham MJ, O'Shea J, Thorne R, Beck E, Tosh SM (2012). Effect of 6 weeks' consumption of β-glucan-rich oat products on cholesterol levels in mildly hyper-cholesterolaemic overweight adults. Br. J. Nutr. 107 (7): 1037 - 47.

Chaturvedi U, Shrivastava A, Bhadauria S, Saxena JK, Bhatia G (2013). A mechanism based pharmacological evaluation of efficacy of *Trigonella-foenom graecum* (fenugreek) seeds in regulation of dyslipidemia and oxidative stress in hyper-lipidemic rats. J. Cardiovasc. Pharmacol. 2013 Feb 20. [Epub ahead of print].

Chen KH, Chen YJ, Yang CH, Liu KW, Chang JL, Pan SF, Lin TB, Chen MJ (2012). Attenuation of the extract from *Moringa oleifera* on monocrotaline-induced pulmonary hypertension in rats. Chin. J. Physiol. 55 (1): 22 – 30.

Chen WJL, Anderson JW (1986). Hypo-cholesterolemic effects of soluble fibers. In: Kritchevsky D, Yahouny GV, eds. Dietary fiber: basic and clinical aspects. Plenum Press. New York. 275 - 89.

Chisholm A, Mann J, Skeaff M, Frampton C, Sutherland W, Duncan A, Tiszavari S (1998). A diet rich in walnuts favorably influences plasma fatty acid profile in moderately hyper-lipidaemic subjects. Eur. J. Clin. Nutr. 52: 12 - 16.

Coimbra SR, Lage SH, Brandizzi L, Yoshida V, da Luz PL (2005). The action of red wine and purple grape juice on vascular reactivity is independent of plasma lipids in hyper-cholesterolemic patients. Braz. J. Med. Biol. Res. 38 (9): 1339 - 47.

Conquer JA, Holub BJ (1996). Supplementation with an algae source of docosahexaenoic acid increases (n-3) fatty acid status and alters selected risk factors for heart disease in vegetarian subjects. J. Nutr. 126 (12): 3032 - 39.

Cornish SM, Chilibeck PD, Paus-Jennsen L, Biem HJ, Khozani T, Senanayake V, Vatanparast H, Little JP, Whiting SJ, Pahwa P (2009). A randomized controlled trial of the effects of flax seed lignan complex on metabolic syndrome composite score and bone mineral in older adults. Appl. Physiol. Nutr. Metab. 34 (2): 89 - 98.

Crouse JR 3rd, Morgan T, Terry JG, Ellis J, Vitolins M, Burke GL (1999). A randomized trial comparing the effect of casein with that of soy protein containing varying amounts of isoflavones on plasma concentrations of lipids and lipoproteins. Arch Intern Med. 159 (17): 2070 - 76.

Cunnane SC, Ganguli S, Menard C, Liede AC, Hamadeh MJ, Chen ZY, Wolever TM, Jenkins DJ (1993). High α linolenic acid flaxseed (*Linum usitatissimum*): some nutritional properties in humans. Br. J. Nutr. 69 (2): 443 - 53.

Cunnane SC, Hamadeh MJ, Leide AC, Thompson LU, Wolever TMS, Jenkins DJA (1995). Nutritional attributes of traditional FS in healthy young adults. Am. J. Clin. Nutr. 61 (1): 62 - 68.

Davidson MH, Dugan LD, Burns JH, Bova J, Story K, Drennan KB (1991). The hypo-cholesterolemic effects of β-glucan in oatmeal and oat bran. JAMA. 265: 1833 - 39.

Delaney B, Nicolosi RJ, Wilson TA, Carlson T, Frazer S, Zheng GH, Hess R, Ostergren K, Haworth J, Knutson N (2003). Beta-glucan fractions from barley and oats are similarly antiatherogenic in hypercholesterolemic Syrian golden hamsters. J. Nutr. 133 (2): 468 - 75.

Devkar RV, Pandya AV, Shah NH (2012). Protective role of *Brassica olerecea* and *Eugenia jambolana* extracts against HO induced cytotoxicity in H9C2 cells. Food Funct. 3 (8): 837 - 43.

Dohadwala MM, Vita JA (2009). Grapes and cardiovascular disease. J. Nutr. 139 (9): 1788S - 93S.

Duke JA (2002). Handbook of Medicinal Herbs. Boca Raton: CRC Press. 327 - 29.

Dulebohn RV, Yi W, Srivastava A, Akoh CC, Krewer G, Fischer JG (2008). Effects of blueberry (*Vaccinium ashei*) on DNA damage, lipid peroxidation, and phase II enzyme activities in rats. J. Agric. Food Chem. 56 (24): 11700 - 706.

Durak A, Ozturk HS, Olcay E, Guven C (2002). Effects of garlic extract supplementation on blood lipid and anti-oxidant parameters and atherosclerotic plaque formation process of cholesterol-fed rabbits. J. Herb. Pharmcother. 2 (2): 19 - 32.

Durak I, Kavutcu M, Aytac B, Avci A, Devrim E, Ozbek H, Oztürk HS. (2004). Effects of garlic extract consumption on blood lipid and oxidant/anti-oxidant parameters in humans with high blood cholesterol. J. Nutr. Biochem. 15 (6): 373 - 77.

EFSA (European Food Safety Authority) (2009). Panel on Dietetic Products. Nutrition and allergies (NDA). Scientific opinion on the substantiation of health claims related to beta-glucans and maintenance of normal blood cholesterol concentrations. EFSA J 7: 1254.

Erdman JW Jr, Carson L, Kwik-Uribe C, Evans EM, Allen RR (2008). Effects of cocoa flavanols on risk factors for cardiovascular disease. Asia. Pac. J. Clin. Nutr.17 Suppl. 1: 284 - 87.

Eussen SR, Rompelberg CJ, Andersson KE, Klungel OH, Hellstrand P, Oste R, van Kranen H, Garssen J (2011). Simultaneous intake of oat bran and atorvastatin reduces their efficacy to lower lipid levels and atherosclerosis in LDLr-/- mice. Pharmacol Res. 64 (1): 36 - 43.

FDA (2006). FDA. CFR 101.81 Health claims: Soluble fiber from certain foods and risk of coronary heart disease (CHD). Washington, DC.

Farquhar JW (1996). Plant sterols: their biological effects in humans. In Spiller G (ed): Handbook of Lipids in Human Nutrition. Boca Raton: CRC Press. pp101 - 105.

Fatehi M, Farifteh F, Fatehi-Hassanabad Z (2004). Antispasmodic and hypotensive effects of *Ferula F. Foetida* gum extract. J. Ethnopharmacol. 91: 321 - 24.

Fitzpatrick DF, Hirschfield SL, Coffey RG (1993). Endothelium-dependent vasorelaxing activity of wine and other grape products. Am. J. Physiol. 265: H774 - 78.

Flesch M, Schwarz A, Boehm M (1997). Divergent effects of red and white wine on endothelium-dependent relaxation of human coronary arteries. Circulation. 96: I - 341.

Folts JD (1997). Three glasses of grape but not orange or grapefruit juice inhibits *ex vivo* platelet aggregation in human volunteers. J. Am. Coll. Cardiol. 29: 226A.

Foster GD, Shantz KL, Vander Veur SS, Oliver TL, Lent MR, Virus A, Szapary PO, Rader DJ, Zemel BS, Gilden-Tsai A (2012). A randomized trial of the effects of an almond-enriched, hypocaloric diet in the treatment of obesity. Am. J. Clin. Nutr. 96 (2): 249 - 54.

Fulgoni III, VL, Abbey M, Davis P, Hyson D, Jenkins D, Lovejoy J, Most M, Sabate J, Spiller GA: Almonds significantly lower elevated blood cholesterol and LDL-cholesterol but not HDL-cholesterol or triglycerides in human subjects: results of a meta-analysis [Abstract]. Proceedings of The Fourth International Congress on Vegetarian Nutrition, April 8 - 14, 2002.

Gallaher DD, Hassel CA, Lee K-J (1993). Relationship between viscosity of hydroxypropyl methylcellulose and plasma cholesterol in hamsters. J. Nutr. 123: 1732 - 38.

Gebhardt R (1991) Inhibition of cholesterol biosynthesis by a water-soluble garlic extract in primary cultures of rat hepatocytes. Arzneimittelforschung. 41 (8): 800 - 804.

Gebhardt R, Beck H (1996). Differential inhibitory effects of garlic-derived organosulfur compounds on cholesterol biosynthesis in primary rat hepatocyte cultures. Lipids. 31 (12): 1269 - 76.

Geppert J, Kraft V, Demmelmair H, Koletzko B (2006). Microalgal docosahexaenoic acid decreases plasma triacylglycerol in normolipidaemic vegetarians: a randomised trial. Br. J. Nutr. 95 (4): 779 - 86.

Ghayur MN, Gilani AH (2005a). Pharmacological basis for the medicinal use of ginger in gastro-intestinal disorders. Dig. Dis. Sci. 50 (10): 1889 - 97.

Ghayur MN, Gilani, AH (2005b). Ginger lowers blood pressure through blockade of voltage-dependent calcium channels. J. Cardiovasc. Pharmacol.45 (1): 74 - 80.

Ghoneim AI, Abdel-Naim AB, Khalifa AE, El-Denshary ES (2002). Protective effects of curcumin against ischaemis-reperfusion insult in rat forebrain. Pharmacol Res. 46 (3): 273 - 79.

Gigleux I, Jenkins DJ, Kendall CW, Marchie A, Faulkner DA, Wong JM, de Souza R, Emam A, Parker TL, Trautwein EA, Lapsley KG, Connelly PW, Lamarche B (2007). Comparison of a dietary portfolio diet of cholesterol-lowering foods and a statin on LDL particle size phenotype in hyper-cholesterolaemic participants. Br. J. Nutr. 98 (6): 1229 – 36.

Gilani AH, Jabeen Q, Ghayur MN, Janbaz KH, Akhtar MS (2005). Studies on the anti-hypertensive, anti-spasmodic, broncho-dilator and hepato-protective activities of the *Carum copticum* seed extract. J. Ethnopharmacol. 98 (1-2): 127 - 35.

González-Salazar A, Molina-Jijón E, Correa F, Zarco-Márquez G, Calderón-Oliver M, Tapia E, Zazueta C, Pedraza-Chaverri J (2011). Curcumin protects from cardiac reperfusion damage by attenuation of oxidant stress and mitochondrial dysfunction. Cardiovasc. Toxicol. 11 (4): 357 – 64.

Grajeta H (1999). Effect of amaranth and oat bran on blood serum and liver lipids in rats depending on the kind of dietary fats. Nahrung. 43 (2): 114 - 17.

Greaves KA, Parks JS, Williams JK, Wagner JD (1999). Intact dietary soy protein, but not adding an isoflavone-rich soy extract to casein, improves plasma lipids in ovariectomized cynomolgus monkeys. J. Nutr. 129 (8): 1585 - 92.

Halvorsen B, Almendingen K, Nenseter MS, Pedersen JI, Christiansen EN (1996). Effects of partially hydrogenated fish oil, partially hydrogenated soybean oil and butter on the susceptibility of low density lipoprotein to oxidative modification in men. Eur. J. Clin. Nutr. 50 (6): 364 - 70.

Harris WS, Von Schacky C (2004). The Omega-3 Index: a new risk factor for death from coronary heart disease? Prev. Med. 39 (1): 212 - 20.

He J, Klag MJ, Whelton PK, Mo JP, Chen JY, Qian MC, Mo PS, He GQ (1995). Oats and buckwheat intakes and cardiovascular disease risk factors in an ethnic minority of China. Am. J. Clin. Nutr. 61 (2): 366 - 72.

Heiss C, Kleinbongard P, Dejam A, Perré S, Schroeter H, Sies H, Kelm M (2005). Acute consumption of flavanol-rich cocoa and the reversal of endothelial dysfunction in smokers. J. Am.Coll. Cardiol. 46 (7): 1276 - 83.

Higashikawa F, Noda M, Awaya T, Ushijima M, Sugiyama M.(2011) Reduction of serum lipids by the intake of the extract of garlic fermented with *Monascus pilosus*: A randomized, double-blind, placebo-controlled clinical trial. Clin. Nutr. 2011 Oct 29. [Epub ahead of print].

Hjerpsted J, Leedo E, Tholstrup T (2011). Cheese intake in large amounts lowers LDL-cholesterol concentrations compared with butter intake of equal fat content. Am. J. Clin. Nutr. 94 (6): 1479 - 84.

Hollis J, Mattes R (2007). Effect of chronic consumption of almonds on body weight in healthy humans. Br. J. Nutr. 98 (3): 651 -56.

Hou Y, Shao W, Xiao R, Xu K, Ma Z, Johnstone BH, Du Y (2009). Pu-erh tea aqueous extracts lower atherosclerotic risk factors in a rat hyperlipidemia model. Exp. Gerontol. 44 (6-7): 434 - 39.

Huang HC, Lin JK (2012). Pu-erh tea, green tea, and black tea suppresses hyper-lipidemia, hyper-leptinemia and fatty acid synthase through activating AMPK in rats fed a high-fructose diet. Food Funct. 3 (2): 170 - 77.

Hyson DA, Schneeman BO, Davis PA (2002). Almonds and almond oil have similar effects on plasma lipids and LDL oxidation in healthy men and women. J. Nutr. 132: 703 - 707.

Ikegami S, Tomita M, Honda S, *et al.* (1996). Effect of boiled barley-rice feeding in hypercholesterolemic and normo-lipemic subjects. Plant Foods Hum. Nutr. 49: 317 - 28.

Imenshahidi M, Hosseinzadeh H, Javadpour Y (2010). Hypotensive effect of aqueous saffron extract (*Crocus sativus* L.) and its constituents, safranal and crocin, in normotensive and hypertensive rats. Phytother. Res. 24 (7): 990 - 94.

Jadeja RN, Thouaojam MC, Sankhari JM, Jain M, Devkar RV, Ramachandran AV (2012). Standardized flavonoid-rich *Eugenia jambolana* seed extract retards *in vitro* and *in vivo* LDL oxidation and expression of VCAM-1 and P-selectin in atherogenic rats. Cardiovasc Toxicol. 12 (1): 73 - 82.

Javed IM, Akhtar T, Khaliq MZ, Khan G, Muhammad M (2002). Anti-hyper-lipidaemic effect of *Trachyspermum ammi* (Ajwain) in rabbits. Proc. 33rd All Pakistan Science Conference, Univ. of Agri. Faisalabad. pp. 80 - 81.

Javed I, Iqbal Z, Rahman ZU, Khan FH, Muhammad F, Aslam B and Ali L (2006). Comparative anti-hyperlipidemic efficacy of *Trachspermum ammi* extracts in albino rabbits. Pakistan. Vet. J. 26 (1): 23 - 29.

Jenkins AL, Jenkins DJA, Zdravkovic U, Wursch P, Vuksan V. (2002a). Depression of the glycemic index by high levels of β-glucan fiber in two functional foods tested in type 2 diabetes. Eur. J. Clin. Nutr. 56: 622 - 28.

Jenkins DJ, Kendall CWC, Marchie A, Parker TL, Connelly PW, Qian W, Haight JS, Faulkner D, Vidgen E, Lapsley KG, Spiller GA (2002b). Dose response of almonds on coronary heart disease risk factors: blood lipids, oxidized low-density lipoproteins, lipoprotein(a), homocystein, and pulmonary nitric oxide : a randomized, controlled, crossover trial. Circulation. 106: 1327 - 32.

Jenkins DJ, Kendall CW, Faulkner DA, Kemp T, Marchie A, Nguyen TH, Wong JM, de Souza R, Emam A,Vidgen E, Trautwein EA, Lapsley KG, Josse RG, Leiter LA, Singer W (2008). Long-term effects of a plant-based dietary portfolio of cholesterol-lowering foods on blood pressure. Eur. J. Clin. Nutr. 62 (6): 781 - 88.

Jenkins DJ, Kendall CW, Marchie A, Faulkner D, Vidgen E, Lapsley KG, Trautwein EA, Parker TL, Josse RG, Leiter LA, Connelly PW (2003a). The effect of combining plant sterols, soy protein, viscous fibers, and almonds in treating hyper-cholesterolemia. Metabolism. 52 (11): 1478 - 83.

Jenkins DJ, Kendall CW, Marchie A, Faulkner DA, Wong JM, de Souza R, Emam A, Parker TL, Vidgen E, Lapsley KG, Trautwein EA, Josse RG, Leiter LA, Connelly PW (2003b). Effects of a dietary portfolio of cholesterol-lowering foods vs lovastatin on serum lipids and C-reactive protein. JAMA. 290 (4): 502 - 10.

Jenkins DJ, Kendall CW, Vidgen E, Agarwal S, Rao AV, Rosenberg RS, Diamandis EP, Novokmet R, Mehling CC, Perera T, Griffin LC, Cunnane SC (1999). Health aspects of partially defatted flaxseed, including effects on serum lipids, oxidative measures, and *ex vivo* androgen and progestin activity: a controlled crossover trial. Am. J. Clin. Nutr. 69 (3): 395 - 402.

Jenkins DJ, Srichaikul K, Wong JM, Kendall CW, Bashyam B, Vidgen E, Lamarche B, Rao AV, Jones PJ, Josse RG, Jackson CJ, Ng V, Leong T, Leiter LA (2010). Supplemental barley protein and casein similarly affect serum lipids in hyper-cholesterolemic women and men. J. Nutr. 140 (9): 1633 - 37.

Jiang X, Williams KM, Liauw WS, Ammit AJ, Roufogalis BD, Duke CC, Day RO and McLachlan AJ (2005). Effect of ginkgo and ginger on the pharmacokinetics and pharmacodynamics of warfarin in healthy subjects. British Journal of Clinical Pharmacology. 59 (4): 4425 - 32.

Jonnalagadda, SS, Thye, FW and Robertson, JL (1993). Plasma total and lipoprotein cholesterol, liver cholesterol and fecal cholesterol excretion in hamsters fed fiber diets. J. Nutr. 123: 1377 - 82.

Kahlon, TS, Chow, FI, Knuckles, BE and Chiu, MM (1993). Cholesterol-lowering effects in hamsters of β-glucan-enriched barley fraction, dehulled whole barley, rice bran, and oat bran and their combinations. Cereal Chem.70:435-440.

Karmally W, Montez MG, Palmas W, Martinez W, Branstetter A, Ramakrishnan R, Holleran SF, Haffner SM, Ginsberg HN (2005). Cholesterol-lowering benefits of oat-containing cereal in Hispanic Americans. J. Am. Diet. Assoc. 105: 967 - 70.

Kawasaki M, Miura Y, Funabiki R, Yagasaki K (2010). Effects of simultaneous dietary fish oil ingestion and sulfur amino acid supplementation on the lipid metabolism in hepatoma-bearing rats with hyperlipidemia. Nutr. Sci. Vitaminol. (Tokyo). 56 (4): 247 - 54.

Keenan JM, Pins JJ, Frazel C, Moran A, Turnquist L (2002). Oat ingestion reduces systolic and diastolic blood pressure in patients with mild or borderline hypertension: a pilot trial. J. Fam. Pract. 51 (4): 369.

Keenan JM, Wenz JB, Myers S, Ripsin C, Huang ZQ (1991). Randomized, controlled, crossover trial of oat bran in hyper-cholesterolemic subjects. J. Fam. Pract. 33 (6): 600 - 608.

Keevil JG, Osman H, Maalej N, Folts JD (1998). Grape juice inhibits human *ex vivo* platelet aggregation while orange and grapefruit juices do not. J. Am. Coll. Cardiol. 31: 192A.

Kendall CWC, Jenkins DJA, Marchie A, Parker T, Connelly PW, Spiller GA (2002). Dose response to almonds in hyperlipidemia: a randomized controlled cross-over trial. Am. J. Clin. Nutr. 75: 384S.

Kimura S (2000). [Anti-hypertensive effect of docosahexaenoic acid in stroke-prone spontaneously hypertensive rats]. Yakugaku Zasshi. 120 (7): 607 - 19. [Article in Japanese].

Kinniry P, Amrani Y, Vachani A, Solomides CC, Arguiri E, Workman A, Carter J, Christofidou-Solomidou M (2006). Dietary flaxseed supplementation ameliorates inflammation and oxidative tissue damage in experimental models of acute lung injury in mice. J. Nutr. 136 (6): 1545 - 51.

Kode A, Rajagopalan R, Penumathsa SV, Menon VP (2005). Effect of ethanol and thermally oxidized sunflower oil ingestion on phospholipid fatty acid composition of rat liver: protective role of *Cuminum cyminum* L. Ann. Nutr. Metab. 49 (5): 300 - 303.

Kojuri J, Vosoughi AR, Akrami M (2007). Effects of *Anethum graveolens* and garlic on lipid profile in hyperlipidemic patients. Lipids. Health. Dis. 6: 5.

Koo KL, Ammit AJ, Tran VH, Duke CC, Roufogalis BD (2001). Gingerols and related analogues inhibit arachidonic acid-induced human platelet serotonin release and aggregation. Thromb. Res. 103: 387 - 97.

Krishnaveni M, Mirunalini S (2010). Therapeutic potential of *Phyllanthus emblica* (amla): the ayurvedic wonder. J. Basic Clin. Physiol. Pharmacol. 21 (1): 93-105.

Kristensen M, Bügel S (2011). A diet rich in oat bran improves blood lipids and hemostatic factors, and reduces apparent energy digestibility in young healthy volunteers. Eur. J. Clin. Nutr. 65 (9): 1053 - 58.

Kritchevsky D, Tepper SA, Czarnecki SK, Klurfeld DM (1982). Atherogenicity of animal and vegetable protein - influence of the lysine to arginine ratio. Atherosclerosis 41: 429 – 31.

Kumari KS, Prameela M (1992). Effect of incorporating *Carum copticum* seeds in a high fat diet for albino rats. Med. Sci. Res. 20: 219 - 20.

Kuo KL, Weng MS, Chiang CT, Tsai YJ, Lin-Shiau SY, Lin JK (2005). Comparative studies on the hypolipidemic and growth suppressive effects of oolong, black, pu-erh, and green tea leaves in rats. J. Agric. Food Chem. 53 (2): 480 - 89.

Lahouar L, Ghrairi F, El Felah M, Salem HB, Miled AH, Hammami M, Achour L (2011). Effect of dietary fiber of "Rihane" barley grains and azoxymethane on serum and liver lipid variables in Wistar rats. J. Physiol. Biochem. 67 (1): 27 - 34.

Lairon D (2001). Dietary fiber and dietary lipids. In: McCleary BV, Prosky L, editors. Advanced dietary fiber technology. Blackwell Science. London. pp. 177 - 85.

Lamarche B, Desroches S, Jenkins DJ, Kendall CW, Marchie A, Faulkner D, Vidgen E, Lapsley KG, Trautwein EA, Parker TL, Josse RG, Leiter LA, Connelly PW (2004). Combined effects of a dietary portfolio of plant sterols, vegetable protein, viscous fibre and almonds on LDL particle size. Br. J. Nutr. 92 (4): 657 - 63.

Lavedrine F, Zmirou D, Ravel A, Balducci F, Alary J (1999). Blood cholesterol and walnut consumption: a cross-sectional survey in France. Prev. Med. 28: 333 - 39.

Lecour S, Lamont KT (2011). Natural Polyphenols and Cardio-protection. Mini Rev Med Chem. 2011 Oct 28. [Epub ahead of print].

Leifert WR, Abeywardena MY (2008). Cardioprotective actions of grape polyphenols. Nutr. Res. 28 (11): 729 - 37.

Lemay A, Dodin S, Kadri N, Jacques H, Forest JC (2002). Flaxseed dietary supplement versus hormone replacement therapy in hyper-cholesterolemic menopausal women. Obstet. Gynecol. 100 (3): 495 - 504.

Lia A, Andersson H, Mekki N, Juhel C, Senft M, Lairon D. (1997). Postprandial lipemia in relation to sterol and fat excretion in ileostomy subjects given oat-bran and wheat test meals. Am. J. Clin. Nutr. 66: 357 - 65.

Lia A, Hallmans G, Sandberg AS, Sundberg B, Aman P, Andersson H. (1995). Oat beta-glucan increases bile acid excretion and a fiber-rich barley fraction increases cholesterol excretion in ileostomy subjects. Am. J. Clin. Nutr. 62: 1245 - 51.

Liu L, Yeh YY (2000). Inhibition of cholesterol biosynthesis by organosulfur compounds derived from garlic. Lipids. 35 (2): 197 - 203.

Liu L, Yeh YY (2001). Water-soluble organosulfur compounds of garlic inhibit fatty acid and triglyceride syntheses in cultured rat hepatocytes. Lipids. 36 (4): 395 - 400.

Lichtenstein AH, Appel LJ, Brands M, *et al.* (2006). Diet and lifestyle recommendations. Revision 2006: a scientific statement from the American Heart Association Nutrition Committee. Circulation 114: 82 - 96.

Lucas EA, Wild RD, Hammond LJ, Khalil DA, Juma S, Daggy BP, Stoecker BJ, Arjmandi BH (2002). Flaxseed improves lipid profile without altering biomarkers of bone metabolism in postmenopausal women. J. Clin. Endocrinol. Metab. 87 (4): 1527 - 32.

Lucas EA, Lightfoot SA, Hammond LJ, *et al.* (2004). Flaxseed reduces plasma cholesterol and atherosclerotic lesion formation in ovariectomized Golden Syrian hamsters. Atherosclerosis. 173: 223 - 29.

Mader FH (1990). Treatment of hyperlipidaemia with garlic-powder tablets. Evidence from the German Association of General Practitioners' multicentric placebo-controlled double-blind study. Arzneimittelforschung 40 (10): 1111 - 16.

Madhujith T, Shahidi F. (2007). Anti-oxidative and anti-proliferative properties of selected barley (*Hordeum vulgarae* L.) cultivars and their potential for inhibition of low-density lipoprotein (LDL) cholesterol oxidation. J Agric Food Chem. 55 (13): 5018 - 24.

Maki KC, Davidson MH, Witchger MS, Dicklin MR, Subbaiah PV (2007). Effects of high-fiber oat and wheat cereals on postprandial glucose and lipid responses in healthy men. Int. J. Vitam. Nutr. Res. 77 (5): 347 - 56.

Manda°escu S, Mocanu V, Dascalipa AM, Haliga R, Nestian I, Stitt PA, Luca V (2005). Flaxseed supplementation in hyperlipidemic patients. Rev. Med. Chir. Soc. Med. Nat. Iasi. 109 (3): 502 - 506.

Marlett JA, Hosig KB, Vollendorf NW, Shinnick FL, Haack VS, Story JA (1994). Mechanism of serum cholesterol reduction by oat bran. Hepatology. 20 (6): 1450 - 57.

Martinello F, Soares SM, Franco JJ, Santos AC, Sugohara A, Garcia SB, Curti C, Uyemura SA (2006). Hypo-lipemic and anti-oxidant activities from *Tamarindus indica* L. pulp fruit extract in hyper-cholesterolemic hamsters. Food Chem. Toxicol. 44 (6): 810 - 18.

Matsuura (2001). Saponins in Garlic as Modifiers of the Risk of Cardiovascular Disease. *J. Nutri.* 2001; 131: 1000S - 1005S.

McIntosh GH, Whyte J, McArthur R, Nestel PJ (1991). Barley and wheat foods: influence on plasma cholesterol concentrations in hyper-cholesterolemic men. Am. J. Clin. Nutr. 53: 1205 - 209.

Mesa MD, Aguilera CM, Ramirez-Tortosa CL (2003). Oral administration of a turmeric extract inhibits erythrocyte and liver micro- some membrane oxidation in rabbits fed with an atherogenic diet. Nutrition. 19 (9): 800 - 804.

Morgado N, Rigotti A, Valenzuela A (2005). Comparative effect of fish oil feeding and other dietary fatty acids on plasma lipoproteins, biliary lipids, and hepatic expression of proteins involved in reverse cholesterol transport in the rat. Ann. Nutr. Metab. 49 (6): 397 - 406.

Nandave M, Ojha SK, Joshi S, Kumari S, Arya DS (2009). *Moringa oleifera* leaf extract prevents isoproterenol-induced myocardial damage in rats: evidence for an anti-oxidant, anti-peroxidative, and cardioprotective intervention. J. Med. Food. 12 (1): 47 - 55.

Nesbitt PD, Lam Y, Thompson LU (1999). Human metabolism of mammalian lignan precursors in raw and processed flaxseed. Am. J. Clin. Nutr. 69: 549 - 55.

Nestel PJ, Chronopulos A, Cehun M (2005). Dairy fat in cheese raises LDL cholesterol less than that in butter in mildly hyper-cholesterolaemic subjects. Eur. J. Clin. Nutr. 59 (9): 1059 - 63.

Newman RK, Lewis SE, Newman CW, Bioik RJ, Ramage RT (1989a) Hypo-cholesterolemic effect of barley foods on healthy men. Nutr. Rep. Int. 39: 749 - 60.

Newman RK, Newman CW, Graham H (1989b). The hypo-cholesterolemic function of barley ß-glucans. Cereal Foods World. 34: 883.

Ngamukote S, Mäkynen K, Thilawech T, Adisakwattana S (2011). Cholesterol-lowering activity of the major polyphenols in grape seed. Molecules. 16 (6): 5054 - 61.

Nicoll R, Henein MY (2009). Ginger (*Zingiber officinale Roscoe*): a hot remedy for cardiovascular disease? Int. J. Cardiol. 131 (3): 408 - 409.

Nie L, Wise M, Peterson D, Meydani M (2006). Mechanism by which avenanthramide-c, a polyphenol of oats, blocks cell cycle progression in vascular smooth muscle cells. Free Radic Biol Med. 41 (5): 702-8.

NRC (1989). National Research Council. Recommended Dietary Allowances. 10th ed. Washington, DC: National Academy Press.

Nurtjahja-Tjendraputra E, Ammit AJ, Roufogalis BD, Tran VH, Duke CC. (2003). Effective anti-platelet and COX-1 enzyme inhibitors from pungent constituents of ginger. *Thromb. Res.* 111 (4-5): 259 - 65.

Oda T, Aoe S, Imanishi S, Kanazawa Y, Sanada H, Ayano Y (1994). Effects of dietary oat, barley, and guar gums on serum and liver lipid concentrations in diet-induced hyper-triglyceridemic rats. J. Nutr. Sci. Vitaminol. (Tokyo). 40 (2): 213 - 17.

Olmedilla-Alonso B, Granado-Lorencio F, Herrero-Barbudo C, Blanco-Navarro I, Blázquez-García S, Pérez-Sacristán B (2008). Consumption of restructured meat products with added walnuts has a cholesterol-lowering effect in subjects at high cardiovascular risk: a randomised, crossover, placebo-controlled study. J. Am. Coll. Nutr. 27 (2): 342 - 48.

Onning G, Akesson B, Oste R, Lundquist I (1998). Effects of consumption of oat milk, soya milk, or cow's milk on plasma lipids and anti-oxidative capacity in healthy subjects. Ann. Nutr. Metab. 42 (4): 211 - 20.

Onning G, Wallmark A, Persson M, Akesson B, Elmståhl S, Oste R.(1999). Consumption of oat milk for 5 weeks lowers serum cholesterol and LDL cholesterol in free-living men with moderate hyper-cholesterclemia. Ann. Nutr. Metab. 43 (5): 301 - 309.

Ortiz RM, Garcia S, Kim AD (2012). Is Almond Consumption More Effective Than Reduced Dietary Saturated Fat at Decreasing Plasma Total Cholesterol and LDL-c Levels? A Theoretical Approach. J. Nutr. Metab. 2012: 265712.

Osman HE, Maalej N, Shanmuganayagam D, Folts JD (1998). Grape juice, but not orange or grapefruit juice inhibit platelet activity in dogs and monkeys (*Macaca fasciularis*). J. Nutr. 128: 2307 - 312.

Othman RA, Moghadasian MH, Jones PJ (2011). Cholesterol-lowering effects of oat β-glucan. Nutr. Rev. 69 (6): 299 - 309.

Pakhale SS, Karibasappa GS, Ramchandani AG, Bhushan B, Sharma A (2007). Scavenging effect of Indian grape polyphenols on 2,2'-diphenyl-1-picrylhydrazyl

(DPPH) radical by electron spin resonance spectrometry. Indian J. Exp. Biol. 45 (11): 968 - 73.

Papoutsi Z, Kassi E, Chinou I, Halabalaki M, Skaltsounis LA, Moutsatsou P (2008). Walnut extract (*Juglans regia* L.) and its component ellagic acid exhibit anti-inflammatory activity in human aorta endothelial cells and osteoblastic activity in the cell line KS483. Br. J. Nutr. 99 (4): 715 - 22.

Park SY, Bae IY, Lee S, Lee HG (2009). Physico-chemical and hypocholesterolemic characterization of oxidized oat beta-glucan. J. Agric. Food Chem. 57 (2): 439 - 43.

Patade A, Devareddy L, Lucas EA, Korlagunta K, Daggy BP, Arjmandi BH (2008). Flaxseed reduces total and LDL cholesterol concentrations in Native American postmenopausal women. J. Women's Health (Larchmt). 17 (3): 355 - 66.

Pereira MA, O'Reilly E, Augustsson K, Fraser GE, Goldbourt U, Heitmann BL, Hallmans G, Knekt P, Liu S, *et al.* (2004). Dietary fiber and risk of coronary heart disease – a pooled analysis of cohort studies. Arch. Intern. Med. 164: 370 - 76.

Pins JJ, Geleva D, Keenan JM, Frazel C, O'Connor PJ, Cherney LM (2002). Do whole-grain oat cereals reduce the need for antihypertensive medications and improve blood pressure control? J. Fam. Pract. 51 (4): 353 - 59.

Pins JJ, Kaur H, Dodds E, Keenan JM (2007). The effects of cereal fibers and barley foods rich in beta-glucan on cardiovascular disease and diabetes risk. In: Marquart L, Jacobs DR Jr, McIntosh GH, Poutanen K, Reicks M, editors. Whole grains and health. Blackwell. London. pp. 75 - 85.

Poulter N, Chang CL, Cuff A, Poulter C, Sever P, Thom S (1994). Lipid profiles after the daily consumption of an oat-based cereal: a controlled crossover trial. Am. J. Clin. Nutr. 59 (1): 66 - 69.

Prasad K (1999). Reduction of serum cholesterol and hyper-cholesterolemic atherosclerosis in rabbits by secoisolariciresinol diglucoside isolated from flaxseed. Circulation. 99 (10): 1355 - 62.

Prasad K (2005). Hypo-cholesterolemic and anti-atherosclerotic effect of flax lignan complex isolated from flaxseed. Atherosclerosis. 179 (2): 269 - 75.

Prasad K (2008). Regression of hyper-cholesterolemic atherosclerosis in rabbits by secoisolariciresinol diglucoside isolated from flaxseed. Atherosclerosis. 197 (1): 34 - 42.

Prasad K (2009). Flaxseed and cardiovascular health. J. Cardiovasc. Pharmacol. 54 (5): 369 - 77.

Prasad K, Mantha SV, Kalra J, Lee P (1997). Prevention of Hyper-cholesterolemic Atherosclerosis by Garlic, an Antixoidant. J. Cardiovasc. Pharmacol. Ther. 2 4): 309 - 320.

Prasad K, Mantha SV, Muir AD, Westcott ND (1998). Reduction of hyper-cholesterolemic atherosclerosis by CDC-flaxseed with very low alpha-linolenic acid. Atherosclerosis. 136 (2): 367 - 75.

Pulido OM, Gillespie Z, Zarkadas M, Dubois S, Vavasour E, Rashid M, Switzer C, Godefroy SB (2009). Introduction of oats in the diet of individuals with celiac disease: a systematic review. Adv. Food Nutr. Res. 57: 235 - 85.

Qi K, Fan C, Jiang J, Zhu H, Jiao H, Meng Q, Deckelbaum RJ (2008). Omega-3 fatty acid containing diets decrease plasma triglyceride concentrations in mice by reducing endogenous triglyceride synthesis and enhancing the blood clearance of triglyceride-rich particles. Clin. Nutr. 27 (3): 424 - 30.

Queenan KM, Stewart ML, Smith KN, Thomas W, Fulcher RG, Slavin JL (2007). Concentrated oat beta-glucan, a fermentable fiber, lowers serum cholesterol in hyper-cholesterolemic adults in a randomized controlled trial. Nutr. J. 6: 6.

Quiles JL, Aguilera C, Mesa MD, Ramirez- Tortosa MC, Baro L, Gil A (1998). An ethanolic- aqueous extract of *Curcuma longa* decreases the susceptibility of liver microsomes and mitochondria to lipid peroxidation in atherosclerotic rabbits. Biofactors. 8 (1- 2): 51 - 57.

Quiles JL, Mesa MD, Ramirez-Tortosa CL (2002). *Curcuma longa* extract supplementation reduces oxidative stress and attenuates aortic fatty acid streak development in rabbits. Arterioscler. Thromb. Vasc. Biol. 22 (7): 1225 - 31.

Rahman K (2007). Effects of garlic on platelet biochemistry and physiology. Mol. Nutr. Food Res. 51 (11): 1335 - 44.

Rajaram S, Haddad EH, Mejia A, Sabaté J (2009). Walnuts and fatty fish influence different serum lipid fractions in normal to mildly hyper-lipidemic individuals: a randomized controlled study. Am. J. Clin. Nutr. 89 (5): 1657S - 1663S.

Rajesh V, Perumal, P, Aruna P (2013). Hypo-lipidemic and anti-oxidant activity of grape skin extract and resveratrol on rats fed with high-fat diet. Oriental Pharmacy and Experimental Medicine. 13 (1): 11 - 20.

Rallidis LS, Paschos G, Liakos GK, Velissaridou AH, Anastasiadis G, Zampelas A (2003). Dietary alpha-linolenic acid decreases C-reactive protein, serum amyloid A and interleukin-6 in dyslipidaemic patients. Atherosclerosis. 167 (2): 237 - 42.

Ramesh E, Elanchezhian R, Sakthivel M, Jayakumar T, Senthil Kumar RS, Geraldine P, Thomas PA (2008). Epigallocatechin gallate improves serum lipid profile and erythrocyte and cardiac tissue antioxidant parameters in Wistar rats fed an atherogenic diet. Fundam. Clin. Pharmacol. 22 (3): 275 - 84.

Ramesh E, Jayakumar T, Elanchezhian R, Sakthivel M, Geraldine P, Thomas PA (2009). Green tea catechins, alleviate hepatic lipidemic-oxidative injury in Wistar rats fed an atherogenic diet. Chem. Biol. Interact. 180 (1): 10 -19.

Ramirez-Tortosa MC, Mesa MD, Aguilera MC (1999). Oral administration of a turmeric extract inhibits LDL oxidation and has hypo-cholesterolemic effects in rabbits with experimental atherosclerosis. Atherosclerosis. 147 (2): 371 - 78.

Ranhotra GS, Gelroth JA, Leinen SD, Bhatty RS (1998). Dose response to soluble fiber in barley in lowering blood lipids in hamster. Plant Foods Hum. Nutr. 52 (4): 329 - 36.

Regand A, Tosh SM, Wolever TMS, Wood PJ (2009). Physico-chemical properties of beta-glucan in differently processed oat foods influence glycemic response. J. Agric. Food Chem. 57: 8831 - 38.

Reppas C, Swidan SZ, Tobey SW, Turowski M, Drressman JB (2009). Hydroxymethylcellulose significantly lowers blood cholesterol in mildly hypercholesterolemic human subjects. Eur. J. Clin. Nutr.63: 71 - 77.

Renaud SC, Beswick AD, Fehily AM, Sharp DS, Elwood PC (1992). Alcohol and platelet aggregation: the Caerphilly prospective heart disease study. Am. J. Clin. Nutr. 55: 1012 - 17.

Reyna-Villasmil N, Bermúdez-Pirela V, Mengual-Moreno E, Arias N, Cano-Ponce C, Leal-Gonzalez E, Souki A, Inglett GE, Israili ZH, Hernández-Hernández R, Valasco M, Arraiz N (2007). Oat-derived beta-glucan significantly improves HDLC and diminishes LDLC and non-HDL cholesterol in overweight individuals with mild hypercholesterolemia. Am. J. Ther. 14(2): 203 - 12.

Ripsin CM, Keenan JM, Jacobs DR, *et al.* (1992). Oat products and lipid lowering – a meta analysis. JAMA. 267: 3317 - 25.

Robitaille J, Fontaine-Bisson B, Couture P, Tchernof A, Vohl MC. (2005). Effect of an oat bran-rich supplement on the metabolic profile of overweight premenopausal women. Ann. Nutr. Metab. 49 (3): 141 - 48.

Romero AL, Romero JE, Galaviz S, Fernandez ML (1998). Cookies enriched with psyllium or oat bran lower plasma LDL cholesterol in normal and hypercholesterolemic men from Northern Mexico. J. Am. Coll. Nutr. 17 (6): 601 - 608.

Rossouw JE (1999). Hormone replacement therapy and cardiovascular disease. Curr. Opin. Lipidol. 10: 429 - 34.

Rytter E, Erlanson-Albertsson C, Lindahl L, Lundquist I, Viberg U, Akesson B, Oste R (1996). Changes in plasma insulin, enterostatin, and lipoprotein levels during an energy-restricted dietary regimen including a new oat-based liquid food. Ann. Nutr Metab. 40 (4): 212 - 20.

Sabate J, Fraser G: (1993). The probable role of nuts in preventing coronary heart disease. Pri. Card. 19: 65 - 72.

Sabate, J., Fraser, G. E., Burke, K., Knutsen, S. F., Bennett, H. and Lindsted, K. D. (1993). Effects of walnuts on serum lipid levels and blood pressure in normal men. N. Engl. J. Med. 328: 603 - 607.

Sabaté J, Haddad E, Tanzman JS, Jambazian P, Rajaram S (2003). Serum lipid response to the graduated enrichment of a Step I diet with almonds: a randomized feeding trial. *American Journal of Clinical Nutrition.* 77 (6): 1379 - 84.

Sainani GS, Desai DB, More KN (1976). Onion, garlic and atherosclerosis. Lancet. 2: 575 - 76.

Saltzman E, Das SK, Lichtenstein AH, Dallal GE, Corrales A, Schaefer EJ, Greenberg AS, Roberts SB (2001). An oat-containing hypocaloric diet reduces systolic blood pressure and improves lipid profile beyond effects of weight loss in men and women. J. Nutr. 131 (5): 1465 - 70.

Sánchez-Muniz FJ, Canales A, Nus M, Bastida S, Guillén M, Corella D, Olmedilla-Alonso B, Granado-Lorencio F, Benedí J (2012). The antioxidant status response to low-fat and walnut paste-enriched meat differs in volunteers at high cardiovascular Risk carrying different PON-1 polymorphisms. J. Am. Coll. Nutr. 31 (3): 194 - 205.

Sanders TAB, Lewis1 F, Slaughter S, Griffin BA, Griffin M, Davies I, Millward DJ, Cooper JA, Miller GJ (2006). Effect of varying the ratio of n″6 to n″3 fatty acids by increasing the dietary intake of α-linolenic acid, eicosapentaenoic and docosahexaenoic acid, or both on fibrinogen and clotting factors VII and XII in persons aged 45–70 y: the OPTILIP Study1·2·3. Am. J. Clin. Nutr. 84 (3) 513 - 22.

Sankhari JM, Thounaojam MC, Jadeja RN, Devkar RV, Ramachandran AV (2012). Anthocyanin-rich red cabbage (*Brassica oleracea* L.) extract attenuates cardiac and hepatic oxidative stress in rats fed an atherogenic diet. J. Sci. Food. Agric. 92 (8): 1688 - 93.

Schlesinger K. (1926). Knoblauch (*Allium sativum*) als Heilmittel bei Arteriosklerose. Wien. Med. Wochenschr. 76:1076-1077.

Sharma R (1986). An evaluation of hypo-cholesterolemic factor of fenugreek seeds (*T. foenum graecum*) in rats. Nutr. Rep. Int. 33: 669 - 77.

Sharma RD, Raghuram TC, Rao NS (1990). Effect of fenugreek seeds on blood glucose and serum lipids in type I diabetes. Eur. J. Clin. Nutr. 44 (4): 301 - 306.

Sharma RD, Raghuram T, Rao V (1991). Hypo-lipidaemic effect of methi seeds. A clinical study. Phytotherapy Research. 5 (3): 145 - 47.

Shaughnessy KS, Boswall IA, Scanlan AP, Gottschall-Pass KT, Sweeney MI (2009). Diets containing blueberry extract lower blood pressure in spontaneously hypertensive stroke-prone rats. Nutr. Res. 29 (2): 130 - 38.

Silagy C, Neil A (1994). Garlic as a lipid lowering agent–a meta-analysis. JR. Coll. Physicians Lond. 28 (1): 39 - 45.

Slowing K, Ganado P, Sanz M, Ruiz E, Tejerina T (2001). Study of Garlic Extracts and Fractions on Cholesterol Plasma Levels and Vascular Reactivity in Cholesterol-Fed Rats. J. Nutr. 131 (3): 9945 - 95.

Soni KB, Kuttan R. (1992). Effect of oral curcumin administration on serum peroxides and cholesterol levels in human volunteers. Indian J. Physiol. Pharmacol. 36 (4): 273 - 75.

Sovova M, Sova P. (2004). Pharmaceutical importance of *Allium sativum* L. 5. Hypolipemic effects *in vitro* and *in vivo*. Ceska. Slov. Farm. 53 (3): 117 - 23.

Sowmya P, Rajyalakshmi P (1999). Hypocholesterolemic effect of germinated fenugreek seeds in human subjects. Plant Foods Hum. Nutr. 53: 359 - 65.

Spiller GA, Miller A, Olivera K, Reynolds J, Miller B, Morse SJ, Dewell A, Farquhar JW (2003). Effects of plant-based diets high in raw or roasted almonds, or roasted almond butter on serum lipoproteins in humans. J. Am. Col. Nutr. 22 (3): 195 - 200.

Spiller GA, Gates JE, Jenkins DA, Bosello O, Nichols S, Cragen LN (1990). Effect of two foods high in mono-unsaturated fat on plasma cholesterol and lipoproteins in adult humans. Am. J. Clin. Nutr. 51: 524.

Spiller GA, Jenkins DA, Cragen LN, Gates JE, Bosello O, Berra K, Rudd C, Stevenson M, Superko R (1992). Effect of a diet high in mono-unsaturated fat from almonds on plasma cholesterol and lipoproteins. J. Am. Coll. Nutr. 11 : 126 - 30.

Spiller GA, Jenkins DA, Bosello O, Gates JE, Cragen LN, Bruce B (1998). Nuts and plasma lipids: an almond-based diet lowers LDL-C while preserving HDL-C. J. Am. Coll. Nutr. 17: 285 - 90.

Sreejayan, N. Rao MN (1994). Curcuminoids as potent inhibitors of lipid peroxidation. J. Indian Physiol. Pharmacol. 46 (12): 1013 - 16.

Srivastava KC (1988). Extract of a spice–omum (*Trachyspermum ammi*)-shows antiaggregatory effects and alters arachidonic acid metabolism in human platelets. Prostaglandins Leukot. Essent. Fatty Acids. 33 (1): 1 - 6.

Srivastava R, Dikshit M, Srimal RC, Dhawan BN (1985). Anti-thrombotic effect of curcumin. Thromb. Res. 40 (3): 413 - 17.

Stark A, Madar Z (1993). The effect of an ethanol extract derived from fenugreek (*Trigonella foenum-graecum*) on bile acid absorption and cholesterol levels in rats. Br. J. Nutr. 69 (1): 277 - 87.

Stark KD, Holub BJ (2004). Differential eicosapentaenoic acid elevations and altered cardiovascular disease risk factor responses after supplementation with docosahexaenoic acid in postmenopausal women receiving and not receiving hormone replacement therapy. Am. J. Clin. Nutr. 79 (5): 765 - 73.

Stein JH, Keevil JG, Wiebe DA, Aeschlimann S, Folts JD (1999). Purple grape juice improves endothelial function and reduces the susceptibility of LDL cholesterol to oxidation in patients with coronary artery disease. Circulation. 100 (10): 1050 - 55.

Steiner M, Lin RS (1998). Changes in platelet function and susceptibility of lipoproteins to oxidation associated with administration of aged garlic extract. J. Cardiovasc. Pharmacol. 31 (6): 904 - 908.

Suekawa M, Aburada M, Hosoya E (1986). Pharmacological studies on ginger. II.Pressor action of [6]-shogaol in anaesthetized rats, or hindquarters, tail and mesenteric beds of rats. J. Pharmacobiodyn. 9: 842 - 52.

Suekawa M, Ishige A, Yuasa K, Sudo K, Aburada M, Hosoya E (1984). Pharmacological studies on ginger.I. Pharmacological actions of pungent constituents, [6]-gingerol and [6]-shogaol. J. Pharmacobiodyn. 7: 836 - 48.

Sumioka I, Hayama M, Shimokawa Y, Shiraishi S, Tokunaga A. (2006). Lipid-lowering effect of monascus garlic fermented extract (MGFE) in hyperlipidemic subjects. Hiroshima J. Med. Sci. 55 (2): 59 - 64.

Suryanarayana P, Krishnaswamy K, Reddy GB (2003). Effects of curcumin on galactose-induced cataractogenesis in rats. Mol. Vis. 9: 223 - 30.

Sweeney MI, Kalt W, MacKinnon SL, Ashby J, Gottschall-Pass KT (2002). Feeding rats diets enriched in low bush blueberries for six weeks decreases ischemia-induced brain damage. Nutr. Neurosci. 5 (6): 427 - 31.

Taku K, Umegaki K, Sato Y, Taki Y, Endoh K, Watanabe S (2007). Soy isoflavones lower serum total and LDL cholesterol in humans: a meta-analysis of 11 randomized controlled trials. Am. Clin. Nutr.85 (4): 1148 -56.

Talati R, Baker WL, Pabilonia MS, White CM, Coleman CI (2009). The effects of barley-derived soluble fiber on serum lipids. Ann. Fam. Med. 7 (2): 157 - 63.

Taubmann G (1934). Therapie mit Drogen. Med. Klin. 32:1067 - 69.

Theobald HE, Chowienczyk PJ, Whittall R, Humphries SE, Sanders TA (2004). LDL cholesterol-raising effect of low-dose docosahexaenoic acid in middle-aged men and women. Am. J. Clin. Nutr. 79 (4): 558 - 63.

Theuwissen E and Mensink RP (2007). Simultaneous intake of β-glucan and plant stanol esters affects lipid metabolism in slightly hypercholesterolemia subjects. J. Nutr. 137: 583 - 88.

Thies F, Miles EA, Nebe-von-Caron G, Powell JR, Hurst TL, Newsholme EA, Calder PC. (2001). Influence of dietary supplementation with long-chain n-3 or n-6 polyunsaturated fatty acids on blood inflammatory cell populations and functions and on plasma soluble adhesion molecules in healthy adults. Lipids. 36 (11): 1183 - 93.

Thomson M, Ali M (2003). Garlic [*Allium sativum*]: a review of its potential use as an anti-cancer agent. Curr. Cancer. Drug Targets. 3 (1): 67 - 81.

Tiwari U, Cummins E (2011). Meta-analysis of the effect of β-glucan intake on blood cholesterol and glucose levels. Nutrition. Apr 5. [Epub ahead of print].

Toufektsian MC, de Lorgeril M, Nagy N, Salen P, Donati MB, Giordano L, Mock HP, Peterek S, Matros A, Petroni K, Pilu R, Rotilio D, Tonelli C, de Leiris J, Boucher F, Martin C (2008). Chronic dietary intake of plant-derived anthocyanins protects the rat heart against ischemia-reperfusion injury. J Nutr. 2008 Apr;138(4):747-52.

USDA (1984). US Department of Agriculture. Composition of Foods: Nuts and Seed Products. (Agricultural Handbook No. 8 - 12). United States Department of Agriculture. Washington, DC.

Uusitupa MI, Miettinen TA, Sarkkinen ES, Ruuskanen E, Kervinen K, Kesäniemi YA (1997). Lathosterol and other non-cholesterol sterols during treatment of hypercholesterolaemia with beta-glucan-rich oat bran. Eur. J. Clin. Nutr. 51 (9): 607 - 611.

Verma SK, Singh J, Khamesra R, Bordia A (1993). Effect of ginger on platelet aggregation in man. Indian J. Med. Res. 98: 240 - 42.

Wang Y, Chang CF, Chou J, Chen HL, Deng X, Harvey BK, Cadet JL, Bickford PC (2005). Dietary supplementation with blueberries, spinach, or spirulina reduces ischemic brain damage. Exp. Neurol. 193 (1): 75 - 84.

Wangen KE, Duncan AM, xu xia and Kurzer MS (2001). Soy isoflavones improve plasma lipids in normo-cholesterolemic and mildly hyper-cholesterolemic postmenopausal women. American Journal of Clinical Nutrition. 73 (2): 225 - 31.

Wang-Polagruto JF, Villablanca AC, Polagruto JA, Lee L, Holt RR, Schrader HR, Ensunsa JL, Steinberg FM, Schmitz HH, Keen CL.(2006). Chronic consumption of flavanol-rich cocoa improves endothelial function and decreases vascular cell adhesion molecule in hyper-cholesterolemic post-menopausal women. J. Cardiovasc. Pharmacol. 47 Suppl. 2: S177 - 86.

Wergedahl H, Gudbrandsen OA, Røst TH, Berge RK (2009). Combination of fish oil and fish protein hydrolysate reduces the plasma cholesterol level with a concurrent increase in hepatic cholesterol level in high-fat-fed Wistar rats. Nutrition. 25 (1): 98 - 104.

Weggemans RM, Trautwein EA (2003). Relation between soy-associated isoflavones and LDL and HDL cholesterol concentrations in humans: a meta-analysis. Eur. J. Clin. Nutr. 57: 940–6.

Weidner MS, Sigwart K (2000). The safety of a ginger extract in the rat. J. Ethnopharmacol. 73: 513 - 20.

WHO (2009). World health statistics 2009. World Health Organization. Geneva.

WHO (2005). Department of Child and Adolescent Health and Development. The current evidence for the burden of group a streptococcal diseases, Discussion papers on child health. World Health Organization. Geneva.

Wilson TA, Nicolosi RJ, Delaney B, Chadwell K, Moolchandani V, Kotyla T, Ponduru S, Zheng GH, Hess R, *et al.* (2004). Reduced and high molecular weight barley β-glucans decrease plasma total and non-HDL-cholesterol in hypercholesterolemic Syrian golden hamsters. J. Nutr. 134: 2617 - 22.

Winblad I, Joensuu T, Korpela H (1995). Effect of oat bran supplemented diet on hypercholesterolaemia. Scand. J. Prim. Health Care. 13 (2): 118 - 21.

Wiseman W, Egan JM, Slemmer JE, Shaughnessy KS, Ballem K, Gottschall-Pass KT, Sweeney MI (2011). Feeding blueberry diets inhibits angiotensin II-converting enzyme (ACE) activity in spontaneously hypertensive stroke-prone rats. Can. J. Physiol. Pharmacol. 89 (1): 67 - 71.

Wolever TM, Gibbs AL, Brand-Miller J, Duncan AM, Hart V, Lamarche B, Tosh SM, Duss R (2011). Bioactive oat β-glucan reduces LDL cholesterol in Caucasians and non-Caucasians. Nutr. J. 10: 130.

Wolever TM, Tosh SM, Gibbs AL, Brand-Miller J, Duncan AM, Hart V, Lamarche B, Thomson BA, Duss R, Wood PJ (2010). Physicochemical properties of oat β-glucan influence its ability to reduce serum LDL cholesterol in humans: a randomized clinical trial. Am. J. Clin. Nutr. 92 (4): 723 - 32.

Wood PJ (2002). Relationships between soluble properties of cereal beta-glucans and physiological effects–a review. Trends. Food Sci. Technol. 13: 313 - 20.

Wood PJ, Beer MU, Butler G (2000). Evaluation of role of concentration and molecular weight of oat β-glucan in determining effect of viscosity on plasma glucose and insulin following an oral glucose load. Br. J. Nutr. 84: 19–23.

Wursch P, Pi-Sunyer FX (1997). The role of viscous soluble fiber in the metabolic control of diabetes. A review with special emphasis on cereal rich in beta-glucan. Diabetes Care. 20: 1774 - 80.

Yeh YY, Liu L (2001). Cholesterol-lowering effect of garlic extracts and organosulfur compounds: human and animal studies. J. Nutr. 131 (3s): 989S - 93S.

Yeh YY, Yeh SM (1994). Garlic reduces plasma lipids by inhibiting hepatic cholesterol and triacylglycerol synthesis. Lipids. 29 (3): 189 - 93.

Zambon D, Sabate J, Munoz S, Campero B, Casals E, Merlos M, Laguna JC, Ros E (2000). Substituting walnuts for mono-unsaturated fat improves the serum lipid profile of hypercholesterolemic men and women. A randomized crossover trial. Ann. Intern. Med. 132: 538 - 46.

Zanwar AA, Hegde MV, Bodhankar SL (2011). Cardio-protective activity of flax lignan concentrate extracted from seeds of *Linum usitatissimum* in isoprenalin induced myocardial necrosis in rats. Interdiscip. Toxicol. 4 (2): 90 - 97.

Zaveri S, Drummond S (2009). The effect of including a conventional snack (cereal bar) and a non-conventional snack (almonds) on hunger, eating frequency, dietary intake and body weight. J. Hum. Nutr. Diet. 22 (5): 461 - 68.

Zhan S, Ho SC (2005). Meta-analysis of the effects of soy protein containing isoflavones on the lipid profile. Am. J. Clin. Nutr. 81: 397–408.

Zhang W, Wang X, Liu Y, Tian H, Flickinger B, Empie MW, Sun SZ (2008). Dietary flaxseed lignan extract lowers plasma cholesterol and glucose concentrations in hyper-cholesterolaemic subjects. Br. J. Nutr. 99 (6): 1301 - 309.

Zhao G, Etherton TD, Martin KR, West SG, Gillies PJ, Kris-Etherton PM (2004). Dietary alpha-linolenic acid reduces inflammatory and lipid cardiovascular risk factors in hypercholesterolemic men and women. J. Nutr. 134 (11): 2991 - 97.

Zhuo XG, Melby MK, Watanabe S (2004). Soy isoflavone intake lowers serum LDL cholesterol: a meta-analysis of 8 randomized controlled trials in humans. J. Nutr. 134: 2395 - 400.

ZibaeeNezhad MJ, Mohammadi E, Beigi MB, Mirzamohammadi F, Salehi O (2012). The effects of unripe grape juice on lipid profile improvement. Cholesterol. 2012: 8902-62.

Chapter 8

Anti-Inflammatory Foods

Inflammation is a pivotal component of a variety of diseases, such as atherosclerosis and tumor progression. The word inflammation comes from the Latin 'inflammo', meaning "I set alight, I ignite". It is a protective attempt by the organism to remove the injurious stimuli and to initiate the healing process and also a reaction of tissues to irritation, injury, or infection sometimes resulting in destruction of the tissues. Inflammation is part of the body's complex biological immune response to harmful stimuli, such as pathogens, damaged cells, or irritants (Ferrero-Miliani *et al.*, 2007). Symptoms of inflammation include pain (dolor), swelling (tumor), red coloration in the affected area (rubor), heat (calor) and sometimes loss of movement or function (functio laesa).

Inflammation can be classified as acute or chronic. Acute inflammation is the initial response of the body to harmful stimuli during which, the movement of plasma and leukocytes (especially granulocytes) from the blood into the injured tissues increases. The process involves local vascular system, immune system, and various cells within the injured tissue. Prolonged inflammation, known as chronic inflammation, leads to a progressive shift in the type of cells present at the site of inflammation and is characterized by simultaneous destruction and healing of the tissue from the inflammatory process. Chronic inflammation can also lead to a host of diseases, such as hay fever, periodontitis, atherosclerosis, rheumatoid arthritis, and even cancer. It is for that reason that the level of inflammatory response is closely regulated by the body.

Inflammatory diseases are widespread globally. Anti-inflammatory effect refers to the property of a substance or treatment that reduces inflammation. The treatment of these illnesses is generally carried out using synthetic and biotechnological anti-inflammatory drugs. Allopathic treatment of inflammation includes use of analgesics (pain reliever), opioids (which affect the central nervous system), steroids, specifically glucocorticoids/corticosteroids, and Non-steroidal anti-inflammatory drugs (NSAIDs). Corticosteroids bind to the glucocorticoid receptors where as the Non-steroidal anti-inflammatory drugs (NSAIDs) counteract the cyclooxygenase (COX) enzyme which catalyses synthesis of inflammatory prostaglandins to alleviate pain.

Various naturally occurring phytochemicals exhibit anti-inflammatory activity and are considered to be potential drug candidates against inflammation-related pathological processes.

Certain foods such as red meat and refined grains were found to be pro-inflammatory. Whereas nature has provided many anti-inflammatory foods which contribute the benefit without inducing any adverse reaction. Besides their ability to reduce inflammation, they also supply essential vitamins and minerals that boost the immunity. The anti-inflammatory foods include Salmon, tuna, mackerel, anchovies, sardines and herring that provide omega-3 fatty acids which are precursors of protective eicosanoids. There is also persuasive epidemiological and experimental evidence that dietary polyphenols found in many dietary plant products, including fruits, vegetables, beverages, herbs, and spices have anti-inflammatory activity.

Recent molecular studies on the function of taurine provide evidence that taurine is a constituent of biologic macromolecules. Specifically, two novel taurine-containing modified uridines have been found in both human and bovine mitochondria. Studies investigating the mechanism of action of Tau-Cl have shown that it inhibits the activation of NF-kappaB, a potent signal transducer for inflammatory cytokines, by oxidation of IkappaB-alpha at Met45 (Schuller-Levis and Park, 2003).

Recently, re-exploration of anti-inflammatory bioactive food components for characterization of their effects on epigenome modifying enzymatic activities (acetylation, methylation, phosphorylation, ribosylation, oxidation, ubiquitination, sumoylation) has been initiated. This may promote healthy ageing by reversing disease prone epi-mutations involved in chronic inflammatory and metabolic disorders (Szarc vel Szic *et al.*, 2010).

Measurement of Inflammation Factor

The **Inflammation Factor (IF) Rating** is now available (Reinagel, 2006) for more than 6,000 foods that help in selection of anti-inflammatory foods in the diet (Table 1). A positive rating indicates that a particular food is anti-inflammatory, while a rating in the negative zone means it's pro-inflammatory. The amount and type of fat; omega-3 to omega-6 ratio; anti-inflammatory compounds such as vitamins, minerals and antioxidants; glycemic load and research evidence for the anti inflammatory effect are taken into consideration in computation of the rating scale.

Positive IF indicates that the food contains known anti-inflammatory nutrients, including monounsaturated fat, selenium, docosahexaenoic acid (DHA) and folate. **Negative IF** indicates that the food contains known inflammatory nutrients, including arachidonic acid and saturated fat.

Table 1: The Inflammation Factor of different Foods

Food	*Quantity*	*IF Rating*
Inflammatory Foods		
Atlantic salmon (farmed), cooked	1/2 fillet (178g)	-386
Yogurt, non-fat	1 cup (245g)	-156
Raisins, seedless	1 small box (43g)	-145
Long-grain brown rice, cooked	1 cup (195g)	-143
Roasted pumpkin and squash seeds	1 ounce (28g)	-79
Toasted sunflower seeds	1 ounce (28g)	-72
Banana	1 medium (118g)	-60
Whole egg, hard-boiled	1 large (50g)	-51
Corn, boiled	1 ear (77g)	-50
Walnuts	1 oz (28g)	-38
Whole-wheat bread	1 slice (28g)	-28
Mango	1 fruit (207g)	-19
Instant oat cooked with water	1 ounce (28g)	-12
Anti-inflammatory Foods		
Olive oil	1 tbsp (14g)	71
Carrot, boiled	1 carrot (46g)	77
Broccoli, boiled	1 stalk (180g)	143
Onion, raw	1 small (70g)	164
Sweet potato, boiled without skin	1 medium (151g)	232
Mollusks oyster, canned	1 cup (162g)	377
Spinach, boiled	1 cup (180g)	466
Atlantic salmon (wild), cooked	1/2 fillet (154g)	895
Ginger, ground	1 tbsp (5g)	1447
Turmeric, ground	1 tbsp (7g)	1523
Fish oil, salmon	1 tbsp (14g)	1875

Reinagel (2006). (Printed with permission). www.nutritionovereasy.com

The Key to read the scale: *Foods with IF Ratings between 1 and 100 are considered to have mild anti-inflammatory effects. Ratings between 101 and 500 indicate increasingly potent anti-inflammatory actions. Foods that have ratings over 500 are strongly anti-inflammatory. On the other end of the scale, foods that have ratings between -1 and -100 are mildly inflammatory. Foods with ratings between -101 and -500 are increasingly inflammatory, and those with ratings of -500 and lower are considered high inflammatory and* if a food scored 0 for IF Rating, it simply means it's neutral, neither inflammatory nor anti-inflammatory.

Anti-inflammatory Nutrients and Phytonutrients

A number of studies have reported that certain nutritional supplements, in combination with a balanced diet and exercise, may allow for improved recovery and anti-inflammatory action (Joseph *et al.*, 2005). Branched chain amino acids, particularly leucine have analgesic properties (Matsumoto *et al.*, 2009) and may inhibit the breakdown of muscle protein and enhance muscle protein synthesis (Buse and Reid, 1975). Taurine, also an amino acid, acts as a powerful anti-inflammatory agent and reduces IL-6 production (Schuller-Levis and Park, 2003). B-vitamins have limited anti-inflammatory properties but as crucial metabolic cofactors, may increase energy availability (especially if diet is poor in it), and may also improve mood and stress (Skarupski *et al.*, 2010; Kennedy *et al.*, 2010).

Quercetin, an anti-inflammatory phytochemical (Comalada *et al.*, 2005), may inhibit mast cell activation (Kandere-Grzybowska *et al.*, 2006) and improve physiological performance, health, and disease resistance along with serving as a psychostimulant (Davis *et al.*, 2009).

Vegetables and fruits in general are great sources of phytonutrients and antioxidants such as flavonoids, carotenoids and vitamins that help fight inflammation. Cruciferous vegetables like cauliflower and broccoli not only provide a whole host of antioxidants, but they also provide sulfur using which the body produces antioxidants. Onions and garlic are rich in vitamin C and have great anti-inflammatory properties.

Essential Fatty Acids (EFA)

Olive oil has a good balance between omega-6 and omega-3 fatty acids, and mainly consists of a monounsaturated omega-9 fatty acid called oleic acid, which inhibits inflammation. It also contains a substance called oleocanthal which fights inflammation like ibuprofen does, by inhibiting the activity of an enzyme called cyclo-oxygenase in the body. Researchers suggest that adding olive oil to the diet lowers the chances of developing colon cancer and inflammation related diseases. Virgin olive oil is Mediterranean's secret of longevity. Its rich supply of polyphenols protects the heart and blood vessels from inflammation. The monounsaturated fats in olive oil are also converted into anti-inflammatory agents by the body that can lower occurrences of asthma and rheumatoid arthritis.

High consumption of omega-6 fatty acids has also been linked to pro-inflammatory response in the body, leading to heart disease and cancer. Whereas consumption of an omega -3 fatty acid, Docosa Hexaenoic Acid (DHA) led to a decreased colon production of PGE(2) and LTB(4,) endothelial VCAM-1 and VEGFR2 in rats with colitis. Similarly, dietary intervention with fish oil rich in EPA and DHA significantly decreased colon production of PGE (2) and LTB(4,) endothelial Vascular Cell Adhesion Molecule (VCAM-1) and Vascular endothelial growth factor receptor 2 (VEGFR2) in rats with colitis (Ibrahim *et al.*, 2011).

It is important to note that EPA and DHA, appear to be more effective than α-linoleic acid in inhibiting inflammation (Yamada *et al.*, 1998), thus partially explaining the superiority of the fish oil diet compared with the olive oil diet. Omega 3 may exert a beneficial effect in the intestinal inflammatory conditions by competing with Omega 6 for the production of lipid inflammatory mediators, by inhibiting the production of various pro-inflammatory mediators, including eicosanoids such as leukotriene B_4 (LTB_4), thromboxane A_2, or prostaglandin E_2, and cytokines (Gil, 2002).

Several clinical studies indicated a potential effectiveness of n-3 fatty acids in the therapy of ulcerative colitis and Crohn's disease as proved in different experimental models of rat intestinal inflammation, induced by acetic acid (Campos *et al.*, 2002), trinitro-benzenesulfonic acid (TNBS) (Nieto *et al.*, 2002; Yuceyar *et al.*, 1999; Andoh *et al.*, 2003) or dextran sodium sulfate (Shimizu *et al.*, 2001). In most of these studies, the reported intestinal anti-inflammatory effect of these fatty acids was associated with a reduction in LTB_4 production (Campos *et al.*, 2002; Nieto *et al.*, 2002; Yuceyar *et al.*, 1999; Shimizu *et al.*, 2001; 2003). Camuesco *et al.* (2005) also confirmed the therapeutic efficacy of dietary supplementation of n-3 fatty acids in intestinal inflammation among humans (Belluzzi *et al.*, 2000; Almallah *et al.*, 2000). The anti-inflammatory effect is enhanced after n-3 PUFA incorporation into the olive oil–based diet, thus modifying the (n-6):(n-3) ratio in the colonic tissue.

Castillero *et al.* (2009) reported that EPA administration decreased the external signs of arthritis and paw volume as well as liver TNF-alpha mRNA but did not modify arthritis-induced decrease in food intake or body weight gain. In addition, EPA treatment also averted muscle wasting and promoted myogenesis.

Among the various food sources of omega-3 fatty acids, Salmon is an excellent source of EPA (eicosapentaenoic acid) and DHA (docosahexaenoic acid). Intake of Atlantic salmon was found to exhibit beneficial effects on mild ulcerative colitis as evident from clinical colitis activity index and anti-inflammatory fatty acid index, and a reduction in C-Reactive Protein and homocysteine levels (Grimstad *et al.*, 2011). Salmon calcitonin released from nano-complexes reduced joint inflammation together with NR4A2 expression, and preserved local bone architecture (Ryan *et al.*, 2013; Abdullahi *et al.*, 1977).

Turmeric (*Curcuma longa*)

Curcumin, the principal curcumoid of the popular Indian spice turmeric, has been demonstrated as an anti-oxidant, anti-inflammatory (Camacho-Barquero *et al.*, 2007; Sugimoto *et al.*, 2002; Claramunt *et al.*, 2009; Hanai *et al.*, 2006) and anti-carcinogenic properties; and has been used to treat cancer, arthritis, digestive and liver abnormalities and respiratory infections (Srimal and Dhawan, 1973; Maheshwari *et al.*, 2006; Sharma, 1976; Stengler and Balch, 2002; Sharma *et al.*, 2004; 2005; Aggarwal and Harikumar, 2009). Although the precise mechanism by which curcumin mediate its beneficial effects in these model systems is not clear, it has been suggested that the modulation of both pro-inflammatory and anti-inflammatory factors may be involved (Sharma *et al.*, 2005; Anand *et al.*, 2008; Aggarwal *et al.*, 2005; Joe *et al.*, 2004).

Ramadan *et al.* (2011) proved the anti-inflammatory/anti-oxidant activity of turmeric over ginger and indomethacin, all of which may have beneficial effects against rheumatoid arthritis -onset/progression as shown in AIA rat model. The anti inflammatory effects of turmeric have been shown to be comparable with drugs such as hydrocortisone and Motrin, but yet without having any of the side effects. Turmeric has been found to be beneficial in various inflammatory diseases. Avasarala *et al.* (2013) strongly supported the role of curcumin in modulating the pathogenesis of viral-induced Acute Respiratory Distress Syndrome in a pre-clinical model through the alteration of inflammation and myofibroblast differentiation.

Koosirirat *et al.* (2010) concluded from his study that curcumin alone may have limited anti-bactericidal effect on *H. pylori,* and on the production of inflammatory cytokines. Taylor and Leonard (2011) on the basis of the database evaluated the use of curcumin in inflammatory bowel disease (including ulcerative colitis and Crohn's disease). The authors concluded that in addition to improvement in ulcerative colitis, curcumin may pose a less-expensive alternative when used in conjunction with conventional medications.

Pruritus is a common symptom of several skin infections. Curcumin supplementation has been proved to successfully alleviate the itching sensation in patients suffering from chronic SM-induced cutaneous complications (Panahi *et al.*, 2012)

Further, the cumulative administration of curcumin and quercetin- flavonoids present in turmeric was reported to be more beneficial in oxidative stress and inflammation than their individual use, thus suggesting their synergistic effect (Heeba *et al.*, 2012).

Obesity and type 2 diabetes are recently recognized as inflammatory conditions. Surprisingly, the oral administration of curcumin was found to reverse the inflammatory responses in obese mouse models while improving glycemic control in Type 2 diabetes models (Weisberg *et al.*, 2008). Moreover, Kunnumakkara *et al.* (2008) have reported curcumin to be pharmacologically quite safe. According to Aggarwal (2010), curcumin directly interacts with adipocytes, pancreatic cells, hepatic stellate cells, macrophages, and muscle cells. In these cells it suppresses the pro-inflammatory transcription factors -kappa B, signal transducer and activators of transcription-3, and Wnt/beta-catenin; and activates peroxisome proliferator-activated receptor-gamma and Nrf2 cell-signaling pathways, thus leading to the down-regulation of adipokines, including tumor necrosis factor (Chan *et al.*, 1995) interleukin-6, resistin, leptin, and monocyte chemotactic protein-1, and the upregulation of adiponectin and other gene products. These curcumin-induced alterations reverse insulin resistance, hyperglyceamia, hyper-lipidemia, and other symptoms linked to obesity. Shehzad *et al.* (2011) recommended that these results enable translation of curcumin to the clinical practice for the treatment and prevention of obesity-related chronic diseases.

Several *in vitro* and *in vivo* studies have demonstrated that curcumin inhibits activation of the TLR-4 and NF-κB pro-inflammatory signaling pathways in diverse cell types including macrophages (Kunnumakkara *et al.*, 2007; Gradisar *et al.*, 2007; Bharti *et al.*, 2004), implicated in the pathogenesis of type 2 diabetes. Woo *et al.* (2007) have shown that curcumin treatment prevents macrophage activation during coculture with adipocytes *in vitro.*

Curcumin inhibited the IL-1beta-induced stimulation of up-stream protein kinase B Akt. These events correlated with down-regulation of NF-kappaB targets including COX-2 and MMP-9. Similar results were obtained in chondrocytes stimulated with TNF-alpha. Curcumin also reversed the IL-1beta-induced down-regulation of collagen type II and beta1-integrin receptor expression. These results indicate that curcumin has nutritional potential as a naturally occurring anti-inflammatory agent for treating OA through suppression of NF-kappaB mediated IL-1beta/TNF-alpha catabolic signalling pathways in chondrocytes (Shakibaei *et al.*, 2007).

Green Tea (*Camellia sinensis*)

Recently, considerable attention has been focused on phytochemicals from dietary and medicinal sources that inhibit, reverse, or retard diseases caused by oxidative and inflammatory processes.

Three cups of tea provides about 300 mg of polyphenols. The polyphenols in green tea such as Epigallocatechin-3-gallate (EGCG) exhibit chelating, anti-inflammatory, anti-bacterial, anti-mutagenic, anti-diabetic, and hypo-cholesterolemic properties (Cabrera *et al.*, 2006). Studies have also shown that EGCG protects cells by inhibiting DNA damage and oxidation of LDL. One of the protective properties of EGCG is its ability to scavenge free radicals. Cysteine conjugates of epigallocatechin 3-gallate (EGCG) retain the growth inhibitory, anti-inflammatory, and pro-oxidant activities of EGCG *in vitro* and may play a role in disease prevention *in vivo* (Lambert *et al.*, 2010). Thereby, Green tea lowers the risk of a wide variety of diseases, including cardiovascular disease and cancer.

Green tea polyphenols also reduce the severity of liver injury in association with lower concentrations of lipid peroxidation and pro-inflammatory nitric oxide-generated mediators (Chen *et al.*, 2004). EGCG can also reduce the inflammatory response associated with local tissue injuries such as the hepato-cellular necrosis in acute liver injury induced by carbon tetrachloride.

The protective effect of EGCG is due to its ability to decrease lipid peroxidation, oxidative stress and production of nitric oxide (NO) radicals by inhibiting the expression of iNOS. EGCG also ameliorates the overproduction of pro-inflammatory cytokines and mediators, reduces the activity of NF-kappaB and AP-1 and the subsequent formation of peroxynitrite with NO and reactive oxygen species (Tipoe *et al.*, 2007). Investigations by Brückner *et al.* (2012) supported the concept of anti-inflammatory properties of EGCG being generally beneficial in the DSS-model of colitis, an effect that may be mediated by its strong anti-oxidative potential.

Bornhoeft *et al.* (2012) reported that green tea supplementation decreased several cardiovascular risk factors, including body composition, dyslipidemia, and inflammatory status in rats fed an atherogenic diet thus supported the fact that green tea as an effective dietary component for sustaining cardiovascular health. In addition, green tea polyphenol supplementation mitigated myocardial fibrosis through suppression of a chronic inflammation innate immune response and lowered red blood cell counts, hematocrit, and hemoglobin, but not the lipid profiles. Supplementation of green tea polyphenols significantly attenuated the lipo-polysaccharide induced fibrosis in coronary vessels (Shen *et al.*, 2011; 2012).

Consumption of green tea polyphenols ameliorated the detrimental effects of high-fructose diet on insulin signaling, lipid metabolism and inflammation in the cardiac muscle of rats (Qin *et al.*, 2010).

A link between inflammation and cancer has long been suspected. In 2004, Greten *et al.*, found that green tea modulated chronic inflammation that would otherwise contribute to prostate carcinogenesis *in vivo*. The EGCG-DPA ester (EGCG-molecule esterified with docosapentaenoic acid) exhibited anti-inflammatory potentials (Zhong *et al.*, 2012). Specific inactivation of the I kappa B kinase (IKK)/NF-kappa B pathway in two different cell types can attenuate formation of inflammation-associated tumors. In addition to suppressing apoptosis in advanced tumors, IKKbeta may link inflammation to cancer. Later, Hsu *et al.* (2010; 2011) found Green tea to decrease prostate inflammatory infiltration, increase Bax/BcL2 ratio and decrease protein expression of tumor necrosis factor-alpha, interleukin (IL)-6 and IL-1β compared to control. The green tea polyphenol EGCG prevented DON-induced cytotoxicity to HT-29 cells in a dose-response manner. EGCG also protect the body against oxidative stress, up regulation of nuclear factor-kB (NF-κB), cyclooxygenase-2 (COX-2) and caspase-3 activated apoptosis (Kalaiselvi *et al.*, 2013). The *in vivo* studies suggested that combination of foods, such as soy and tea, may inhibit hormone-induced pro-inflammatory NFκB signals that contribute to prostate cancer development.

Catechin, epigallocatechin and epigallocatechin-3-gallate decreased the leukocytopenia in mice after irradiation and significantly reduced the elevated serum inflammatory cytokines (TNF-α, IL-1β, and IL-6). The anti-oxidant and anti-inflammatory activities of green tea polyphenol has been attributed to the interaction of the different components through multiple and synergistic mechanisms (Hu *et al.*, 2011). Thus, green tea polyphenols have a potential to offer protection against irradiation-induced toxicity.

Nitic oxide (NO) has been implicated in the pathogenesis of various inflammatory diseases, including sunburn and pigmentation induced by ultraviolet irradiation. EGCG inhibited and down regulated the UVB-induced activation and translocation of NF-kappaB, expression of iNOS mRNA and generation of NO respectively, indicating EGCG may play a protective role from UVB-induced skin damage (Song *et al.*, 2006).

El-Mowafy *et al.* (2011) showed for the first time that EGCG can protect against cisplatin-induced nephro-toxicity at the molecular level, better than resveratrol or quercetin.

Chatterjee *et al.* (2012) concluded from their comparative study that both green and black tea leaves possessed a marked anti-inflammatory effect against the denaturation of protein, *in vitro*, with Green tea being more active than black tea, probably due to the higher flavonoid content.

Onion (*Allium cepa*)

Onion peel extract lowered serum LDL-cholesterol and enhanced HDL-cholesterol through increasing low-density lipoprotein receptor and ATP-binding cassette transporter A1 genes (Lee *et al.*, 2012). Supplementation with quercetin-rich onion peel extract was found to influence adipokine expressions, particularly from mesenteric fat, addressing the modulatory effect of this substance on obesity-induced inflammation (Kim *et al.*, 2012).

Wang *et al.* (2013) reported that administration of an aqueous extract of Welsh onion green leaves (WOE) in the range of 0.25 – 1.0 g/Kg showed a concentration dependent inhibition on paw edema development after carrageenan treatment in mice. The anti-inflammatory effects of WOE were closely attributed to decreased levels of tissue NO and tumor necrosis factor-α (TNF-α) along with reduction in lipid oxidation and increase in antioxidant enzyme activities, including catalase (CAT), superoxide dismutase (SOD), and glutathione peroxidase (GPX) *in vivo*. In addition, there was a decrease in the number of acetic acid-induced writhing responses and formalin-induced pain in the late phase in mice.

Garlic (*Allium sativum*)

Garlic is well known for its anti-oxidant and anti-inflammatory properties. *In vitro* studies have shown that high concentrations of garlic can decrease cytokine production in endothelial cells (Ide and Lau, 2001). Aged garlic extract (ARG) was shown to increase nitric oxide production and decrease the output of inflammatory cytokines from cultured cells in 15 men with coronary artery disease (Williams *et al.*, 2005). Compared to fresh raw garlic, aged red garlic was found to posses higher antioxidant effects. Park *et al.* (2012a) showed that ARG extract has potential effects on prevention and treatment of acute inflammatory lung injury.

Sulfur compounds isolated from garlic exert anti-inflammatory properties. Topical application of thiacremonone, a sulphur compound from garlic suppressed the 12-O-tetradecanoylphorbol-13-acetate-induced ear edema; the carrageenan and mycobacterium butyricum-induced inflammatory and arthritic responses as well as expression of iNOS and COX-2, in addition to NF-kappaB DNA-binding activity. Further *in vitro* study showed inhibition of lipo-polysaccharide-induced nitric oxide (NO) production, and NF-kappa B transcriptional and DNA binding activity in a dose dependent manner by thiacremonone. Thus, Ban *et al.* (2009) recommended that thiacremonone of garlic could be a useful agent for the treatment of inflammatory and arthritic diseases.

Lee *et al.* (2012) identified anti-inflammatory sulfur-containing compounds from garlic, and their chemical structures. They were Z- and E-ajoene and oxidized sulfonyl derivatives of ajoene. The sulfur compounds inhibited the production of nitric oxide and prostaglandin E-2, and the expression of the pro-inflammatory cytokines, tumor necrosis factor-α, interleukin-1β, and interleukin-6 in lipo-polysaccharide (LPS)-activated macrophages.

Dkhil *et al.* (2011) studied the effect of garlic on mice infected with *E. papillata* and proved that garlic treatment significantly attenuated inflammation and injury of the liver. Administration of garlic and onion to fructose-fed rats reduced oxidative stress, increased eNOS activity, and also attenuated vascular cell adhesion molecule-(VCAM-1) expression (Vazquez-Prieto *et al.*, 2011).

Chronic bacterial prostatitis (CBP), which is characterized by recurrent urinary tract infection (UTI), persistence of pathogenic bacteria and evidence of inflammation in the prostatic secretions, is one of the most common causes of relapsing UTI in men. Sohn *et al.* (2009) observed that the garlic significantly decreased the bacterial growth and improved prostatic inflammation and the garlic plus ciprofloxacin group showed better results than the ciprofloxacin group alone suggesting a synergistic effect of garlic with the antibiotic, ciprofloxacin.

Ginger (*Zingiber officinale*)

For the past two or more decades, many researchers have provided scientific support for the long-held belief that ginger contains constituents with anti-inflammatory properties. Ginger suppresses prostaglandin synthesis through inhibition of cyclooxygenase-1 and cyclooxygenase-2. It also suppresses leukotriene biosynthesis by inhibiting 5-lipoxygenase. This pharmacological property distinguishes ginger from non-steroidal anti-inflammatory drugs (Grzanna *et al.*, 2005).

Ginger is reported in Ayurvedic and Tibb systems of medicine to be useful in rheumatic disorders. As early as 1989, Srivastava and Mustafa reported that prolonged use of non-steroidal anti-inflammatory drugs and corticosteroid drugs produce adverse side-effects, and administration of ginger powder was beneficial in relieving pain in the joints of rheumatoid and osteoarthritis arthritis without any side effects. Inhibition of inflammatory eicosanoids (prostaglandin and leukotriene biosynthesis) was suggested as the mechanism involved in the effect.

Penna *et al.* (2003) demonstrated the anti-edematogenic activity of crude extract of ginger through its antagonistic effect on the serotonin receptor and thereby, reduction in the rat paws and skin edema. [6]-gingerol (25 mg/kg-50 mg/kg), the phytochemical isolate of ginger was also found to inhibit paw edema (Young *et al.*, 2005).

Ojewole (2006) confirmed the folkloric ethno-medical uses of ginger in the treatment and/or management of painful, arthritic inflammatory conditions, as well as in the management and/or control of type 2 diabetes mellitus in some rural African communities through pharmacological studies on the ethanol extract of ginger.

Different varieties of ginger were also found to be therapeutically beneficial. Shimoda *et al.* (2010) found a potent suppressive effect of red ginger extract on acute and chronic inflammation through inhibition of macrophage activation. The effect has been attributed to [6]-Shogaol, gingerdiols, and proanthocyanidins.

Cellular studies on synoviocytes from osteoarthritis and rheumatoid arthritis subjects indicated antiinflammatory effect of ginger extract which was comparable with that of an anti inflammatory drug, betamethasone (Ribel-Madsen *et al.*, 2012).

The phytochemical 1-dehydro-[10]-gingerdione (1D10G) has been shown to suppress NF-κB-associated inflammation in autoimmune disorders (Lee *et al.*, 2012), which was also supported by Li *et al.* (2012). The molecular target for anti-inflammatory action of 1D10G was reported to be Myeloid differentiation protein 2, a co-receptor of toll-like receptor 4 for innate immunity (Park *et al.*, 2012b). Inhibition of cyclooxygenase-2 expression was also a suggested anti inflammatory mechanism of ginger extracts (Lantz *et al.*, 2007).

The role of ginger in neuro-degeneration, which is also recognised as an inflammatory condition is worth appreciation. 6-shogaol, one of the most bioactive components of ginger, can significantly attenuate a variety of neuro-inflammatory responses by inducing heat-shock protein (HSP70) that is associated with histone deacetylase (HDAC)1 inhibition in cortical astrocytes (Shim *et al.*, 2011). Ha *et al.* (2012) demonstrated the anti oxidant and anti-inflammatory role of 6-shogaol. The proposed mechanisms included significant inhibition of (1) the release of nitric oxide (NO) and the expression of nitric oxide synthase (iNOS) induced by lipo-polysaccharide (LPS), (2) the production of prostaglandin E(2) and pro-inflammatory cytokines, such as interleukin-1β and tumor necrosis factor-α, and by down-regulating cyclooxygenase-2, mitogen-activated protein kinase and nuclear factor kappa B expression. The effect was found to be better than that of other nitric oxide inhibitors such as 6-gingerol, wogonin, or N-monomethyl-l-arginine. In addition, 6-shogaol was found to suppress the microglial activation *in vitro* as well as *in vivo*. It also showed significant neuro-protective effects *in vivo* in transient global ischemia via the inhibition of microglia.

Again Habib *et al.* (2008) observed a significant correlation between NFkappaB and TNF-alpha in the choline-deficient diet group but not in the choline-deficient diet treated with ginger extract group. Thus, ginger acted as an anti-cancer and anti-inflammatory agent by inactivating NFkappaB through the suppression of the pro-inflammatory TNF-alpha.

Ueda *et al.* (2010) demonstrated the ability of orally administered ginger extract to induce an immune response in RAW 264 cells in mice by increasing the serum corticosterone level after oral administration. It also inhibited arachidonic acid-induced ear edema, but only on repeated administration. The authors concluded that the augmentation of serum corticosterone level on repeated administration of the aqueous constituents of ginger was responsible for its anti-inflammatory activity. According to Han *et al.* (2012) 12-DHGD, a constituent of ginger, is a potent inhibitor of pro-inflammatory mediator production in Raw 264.7 macrophage cells.

Thomson *et al.* (2002) observed a significant reduction in the serum cholesterol at a low dose of ginger (50 mg/kg), only when ginger was administered intra-peritoneally, suggesting that ginger could be used as cholesterol-lowering, antithrombotic and anti-inflammatory agent.

Minghetti *et al.* (2007) reported that a commercial ginger dry extract (GDE) was more effective as an anti inflammatory agent than a gingerol-enriched dry extract (GEDE) in mice, while testing the feasibility of the same in an an anti-inflammatory plaster. The results indicated a possible application in humans.

Drumstick (*Moringa oleifera*)

Drumstick has an impressive range of medicinal uses with high nutritional value. Different parts of this plant contain a profile of important nutrients including protein, minerals, vitamins and various phenolics. The phenolics include a rich and rare combination of zeatin, quercetin, beta-sitosterol, caffeoylquinic acid and kaempferol. Various parts of this plant such as the leaves, roots, seed, bark, fruit, flowers and immature pods act as cardiac and circulatory stimulants, possess anti-tumor, antipyretic, anti-epileptic, anti-inflammatory, anti-ulcer, anti-spasmodic, diuretic, anti-hypertensive, cholesterol lowering, anti-oxidant, anti-diabetic, hepato-protective, anti-bacterial and anti-fungal activities, and are being employed for the treatment of different ailments in the indigenous system of medicine, particularly in South Asia (Anwar *et al.*, 2007).

The anti-inflammatory activity of *M. oleifera* was proved in carrageenan-induced hind paw edema at a dose of 1000 mg/kg (Cáceres *et al.*, 1992). Cheenpracha *et al.* (2010) found that the phenolic glycosides isolated from ethyl acetate extract of *M.oleifera* fruits possessed potent NO-inhibitory activity. Ndiaye *et al.* (2002) reported that an aqueous root extract of *Moringa oleifera* at 750 mg/kg reduces the carrageenin induced oedema to similar extent as the potent anti-inflammatory drug indomethacin. These results provided further evidence that the roots of *M. oleifera* also contain anti-inflammatory principle that may be useful in the treatment of the acute inflammatory conditions.

Hamza (2010) demonstrated that administration of M. seed extract could act against CCl_4-induced liver injury and fibrosis in rats by a mechanism related to its anti-oxidant properties, anti-inflammatory effect, and its ability to attenuate the activation of hepatic stellate cells.

Atawodi *et al.* (2010) identified the methanol extract of the Drumstick leaves to contain chlorogenic acid, rutin, quercetin glucoside, and kaempferol rhamnoglucoside, whereas in the root and stem barks, several procyanidin peaks were detected. Due to its high antioxidant/radical scavenging effects observed by Atawodi *et al.* (2010) with the 2-deoxyguanosine assay model system for different parts of *M. oleifera* seems to provide justification for their widespread therapeutic use in traditional medicine in different continents. A chitin-binding protein Mo-CBP4 in *M. oleifera* seeds exhibited anti-inflammatory and anti-nociceptive properties (Pereira *et al.*, 2011).

Even the methanolic extracts of the root or leaf of *M. oleifera* are found to be effective in the reduction of pain induced by CFA in rats. A comparison of single and combination therapies of root and leaf extracts also showed a synergistic effect on pain reduction (Manaheji *et al.*, 2011).

In addition to the anti-oxidant and anti-inflammatory activity of the ethanolic extract of seeds of *M. oleifera*, Mahajan and his colleagues (2007) reported that histo-pathological observations also reflected a protective as well as preventive effect of immune-mediated inflammatory responses in luene diisocyanate (TDI as antigen)-induced asthma in Wistar rats.

Sashidhara *et al.* (2009) isolated a rare aurantiamide acetate 4 and 1,3-dibenzyl urea 5 from the roots of *M.oleifera* which inhibited the production of TNF-alpha and IL-2. Further the compound showed significant analgesic activities in a dose dependant manner. These findings may help in understanding the mechanism of action of this traditional plant leading to control of activated mast cells on inflammatory conditions like arthritis.

Capsicum (*Capsicum annuum*) and Chillies (*Capsicum baccatum* L. var. *pendulum*)

Capsicum species have been used for the treatment of arthritis, rheumatism, stomach aches, skin rashes, dog/snake bites, and flesh wounds in Indian, Native

American, and Chinese traditional medicine, (Meghvansi *et al.*, 2010; Wyk and Wink, (2010). The hydroalcoholic extracts of both plants at dose level of 100 mg/kg body weight showed demonstrable anti-inflammatory activity in the carrageenan-induced hind paw model in rats. Nevertheless, the overall anti-inflammatory activity exhibited by the extracts is found to be less as compared with that of standard drug Indometacin (Vijayalakshmi *et al.*, 2010).

Capsicum baccatum L. var. pendulum (Wild.) Eshbaugh (Solanaceae) is the most consumed species in Brazil, and its compounds, such as capsaicinoids, have been found to inhibit the inflammatory process. The anti-inflammatory effect induced by red pepper is attributed to inhibition of pro-inflammatory cytokine production at the inflammatory site (Spiller *et al.*, 2008).

These therapeutic applications are related to the capsaicinoid and carotenoid content of peppers (Zimmer *et al.*, 2012; and Park *et al.*, 2010). The carotenoids in dried guajillo peppers have been shown to exhibit significant analgesic and anti-inflammatory benefits and hence could be useful for pain and relief from inflammation (Hernández-Ortega *et al.*, 2012).

Cinnamon (*Cinnamomon zeylanicun*)

Cinnamon bark is one of the most popular herbal ingredients in traditional oriental medicine and possesses diverse pharmacological activities including anti-bacterial, anti-viral, and anti-cancer properties. *Cinnamomum osmophloeum* Kaneh. (Lauraceae) is one of the indigenous tree species in Taiwan. This tree species has been of interest to researchers because the chemical constituents of its essential oil are similar to those of *C. cassia*. Presl bark oil, known as cinnamon oil is commonly used in foods and beverages. Tung *et al.* (2008; 2010) and Chao *et al.*, 2005) demonstrated that the leaf essential oils and their constituents of *C. osmophloeum* as well as the essential oil of *C. osmophloeum* twigs have excellent anti-inflammatory activities and thus have great potential as a source for health products in pharmaceuticals and nutraceuticals.

The polyphenols in cinnamon may be responsible for the anti-inflammatory action (Hong *et al.*, 2012). The biologically active constituents of C. cassia extract were characterized as trans-cinnamaldehyde by spectral analysis. Suppression of inducible nitric oxide synthase expression of cinnamaldehyde was revealed by Western blot analysis. As a naturally occurring therapeutic agent, trans-cinnamaldehyde could be useful for developing new types of NO inhibitors (Lee *et al.*, 2002). According to Kim *et al.* (2007) cinnamaldehyde plays a role in the regulation of age-related alterations in signal transduction pathways.

The anti-inflammatory property of cinnamon metabolite, sodium benzoate (NaB) has been demonstrated in microglia and astrocytes. It was found to inhibit LPS-induced expression of NO synthase (iNOS), pro-inflammatory cytokines (TNF-alpha and IL-1beta) and surface markers (CD11b, CD11c, and CD68) in mouse microglia. NaB exerts its anti-inflammatory effect through the inhibition of NF-kappa B. Depletion of intermediates of the mevalonate pathway is involved in the anti-inflammatory effect of NaB (Brahmachari *et al.*, 2009).

Oral administration of water extract of cinnamon (CWE) to mice significantly decreased the serum levels of TNF-α and IL-6. CWE treatment *in vitro* decreased the mRNA expression of TNF-α. CWE blocked the lipo-polysaccharide-induced degradation of IκBα as well as the activation of JNK, p38 and ERK1/2. Furthermore, the fraction of CWE containing highest level of total polyphenols was found to be responsible for the beneficial effect.

Oral treatment with cinnamon extract resulted in significant reduction in the expression of the mast cell proteases MCP6 and MC-CPA *in vitro* and *in vivo* (Hagenlocher *et al.*, 2013).

Berries

An antioxidant powerhouse, blueberry is high in phytonutrients that confer anti-inflammatory protection against many diseases such as cancer and dementia.

The American cranberry (*Vaccinium macrocarpon*) is one of the three commercially important fruits native to North America. Cranberries are a particularly rich source of phenolic phytochemicals, including phenolic acids (benzoic, hydroxyl-cinnamic, and ellagic acids) and flavonoids (anthocyanins, flavonols, and flavan-3-ols). McKay and Blumberg (2007) on reviewing the literature found a growing body of evidence suggesting that polyphenols, including those found in cranberries, may contribute to reduced risk of cardiovascular disease (CVD) by increasing the resistance of LDL to oxidation, inhibiting platelet aggregation, reducing blood pressure, and via other anti-thrombotic and anti-inflammatory mechanisms.

Red Currant (*Rhus chirindensis*)

Ojewole (2007) scientifically evaluated some of the anecdotal, folkloric, ethnomedical uses of *Rhus chirindensis* and confirmed the analgesic, anti-inflammatory and hypo-glycaemic effects of the plant's stem-bark aqueous extract (RCE) in mice and rats. These results suggest use of the Red currant in the treatment and/or management of painful arthritic, inflammatory conditions, as well as in the management and/or control of type 2 diabetes mellitus.

Fenugreek (*Trigonella foenum graecum*)

Trigonella foenum graecum is used in the treatment of rheumatoid arthritis and inflammation. Fenugreek was found to significantly decrease the IL-1α, IL-1β, IL-2, IL-6 and TNF-α and LPO ($P < 0.05$); and increase the SOD and GSH levels in cartilage tissue. 400-mg/kg dose of *T. foenum graecum* showed more prominent results compared to the 200-mg/kg dose suggesting that its anti-inflammatory and anti-oxidant activities may be dose dependent (Suresh *et al.*, 2012). Fenugreek mucilage exhibited maximum percentage of edema inhibition at a dose of 75 mg/kg on 21st day of adjuvant arthritis, with the effect being higher than that of standard drug indomethacin. Inhibition of inflammation was evident from the histopathological changes of paw tissue with fenugreek mucilage. Thus the results demonstrated the potential beneficiary effect of fenugreek mucilage on adjuvant induced arthritis in rats (Sindhu *et al.*, 2012).

Colocasia (*Colocasia esculenta*)

South African medicinal plants used traditionally for the treatment of pain-related ailments were evaluated for anti-inflammatory activity and other pharmacological properties such as anti-cholinesterase and antioxidant activities. The highest COX-1 percentage inhibition (100 per cent) was shown by Aloe ferox leaf PE and *Colocasia anti-quorum* tuber DCM extracts, while colocasia tuber PE extract exhibited the highest (92.7 per cent) percentage inhibition against COX-2. Crinum moorei bulb DCM extract showed the lowest EC (50) value (2.9 microg/ml) in the AChE assay (Fawole *et al.*, 2010).

Sweet Potato

Sweet potato is often over shadowed by other exotic vegetables and fruits. But it is also a good source of complex carbohydrate, beta-carotene, manganese, vitamin B_6 and C as well as dietary fiber. Working in concert, these nutrients are powerful anti-oxidants that help to heal inflammation in the body. According to Wang *et al.* (2010) the purple sweet potato color which is natural anthocyanin may be useful for mitigating inflammatory brain diseases by the inhibition of pro-inflammatory molecule production, at least in part, through blocking ERK, JNK and NF-kappa B signaling. Ju *et al.* (2011) showed that the extract of purple sweet potatoes has anti-lipogenic, anti-inflammatory, and lipolytic effects on adipocytes along with free radical scavenging activity.

Papaya (*Carica papaya*)

Coined by Christopher Columbus as the 'fruit of the angels', papaya contains papain, a protein-digesting enzyme. Together with other nutrients such as vitamin C and E, papain helps to reduce inflammation. Treatment with the phyto-preparation from papaya accelerated wound healing and reduced the severity of local inflammation in rats with burn wounds. The effect of this phyto-preparation can be related to an increase in the effectiveness of intracellular death of bacteria by tissue phagocytes due to the inhibition of bacterial catalase. Anti-oxidant activity of the preparation decreases the risk of oxidative damage to tissues (Mikhal'chik *et al.*, 2004). Extracts of bromelain derived from papaya have also proven to be as effective as some non-steroidal anti-inflammatory drugs and are used in a number of natural anti-inflammatory supplements for arthritis.

Yeast fermented papaya preparation (FPP) has a long track record of safe human consumption. Collard and Roy (2010) observed that FPP supplementation influences the response of wound-site macrophages and the subsequent angiogenic response in diabetic-wound. FPP as a food supplement favorably modulates the parameters related to immunological, hematological, inflammatory, vascular and oxidative stress damage in chronic and degenerative disease conditions (such as thalassemia, cirrhosis, diabetes and ageing) and performance sports (Aruoma *et al.*, 2010). Thus it is a novel, economically feasible nutraceutical supplement for the management of diabetes and for those at risk for cardiovascular disease, neurological disease and other conditions worsened by overt inflammation and oxidative stress (Somanah *et al.*, 2012).

Rice Bran

Islam *et al.* (2009) observed that phytosteryl ferulates in rice bran are responsible for the anti-oxidant and anti-inflammatory activity via ROS scavenging and inhibition of ROS production. *In vivo* and *in vitro* studies have clarified that rice bran phytosteryl ferulates mediate anti-inflammatory effects by down-regulating the inflammatory transcription factor, nuclear factor κB (NF-κB), which in turn reduces expression of inflammatory enzymes such as COX-2 and iNOS, and pro-inflammatory cytokines such as IL-1β, IL-6 and TNF-α. Moreover, rice bran phytosteryl ferulates up-regulate blood adiponectin levels via indirect activation of peroxisomal proliferator-activated receptor γ (PPARγ) through NF-κB inhibition (Islam *et al.*, 2011).

Cocoa

Cocoa and its flavonoids have potential anti-inflammatory properties *in vitro* and in acute inflammation models *in vivo*. Although arthritic cocoa-fed rats showed a similar hind-paw swelling time course as the arthritic animals fed a standard diet. Similarly, the cocoa-enriched diets were not able to significantly decrease joint inflammation in adjuvant arthritic rats but modified Th-cell proportions and prevented specific anti-body synthesis. The cocoa intake was able to decrease specific IgG2a, IgG2b and IgG2c titres. Moreover, cocoa intake in collagen-induced arthritic rats reduced ROS production, TNFα and NO release from peritoneal macrophages, and decreased the Th:cytotoxic T cell ratio in inguinal lymph nodes. Thus a cocoa-enriched diet could be a good adjuvant therapy in disorders with oxidative stress or auto-immune pathogenesis (Ramos-Romero *et al.*, 2012 a and b). Clinically, joint swelling in arthritic rats was not reduced by cocoa flavonoids. But, the 5 per cent cocoa diet and quercetin administration reduced ROS production while normalizing the activities of superoxide dismutase and catalase (Ramos-Romero *et al.*, 2012c).

Wild/Dog Mustard *(Cleome viscose)*

Cleome viscosa Linn. (Capparidaceae), commonly known as 'wild or dog mustard', is an annual, sticky herb found as a common weed all over the plains of India and throughout the tropics of the world. The whole plant and its parts (leaves, seeds, and roots) are widely used in traditional and folkloric systems of medicine where, the plant is reported to possess beneficial effects as an anthelmintic, antiseptic, carminative, antiscorbutic, sudorific, febrifuge, cardiac stimulant, anitimicrobial, analgesic, anti-inflammatory, immuno-modulatory, antipyretic, psychopharmacological, antidiarrheal, and hepato-protective activities. A wide variety of phyto-principles have been isolated from the plant (Mali, 2010).

Oral administration of the ethanolic extract (200 and 400 mg/kg, p.o) and its fractions (200 mg/kg each) of the aerial parts of *Cleome rutidosperma* produced significant analgesic activity in acetic acid-induced writhing and tail immersion tests, anti-inflammatory effect against carrageenin induced inflammation and adjuvant induced poly-arthritis and anti-pyretic activity against yeast-induced pyrexia. Fractionation of the ethanolic extract potentiated the activities (Bose *et al.*, 2007).

Resveratrol

Osteoarthritis is an inflammatory disease of load-bearing synovial joints. The drugs that are currently used not only cause numerous side effects but also give only temporary relief from pain, the main symptom of the disease. Resveratrol is a phytoalexin stilbene produced naturally by plants including red grapes, peanuts and various berries. Recent research in various cell models has demonstrated that resveratrol is a safe and potent anti-inflammatory agent. Shakibaei *et al.* (2007) found that resveratrol significantly reduced the IL-1beta-induced inhibition of expression of cartilage-specific collagen type II and signal transduction receptor beta1-integrin in a time-dependent manner. Shakibaei *et al.* (2008) also provided experimental evidence that resveratrol inhibits the expression of VEGF, MMP-3, MMP-9 and COX-2 in human articular chondrocytes stimulated by the pro-inflammatory cytokine IL-1beta. Resveratrol thus suppresses apoptosis and inflammatory signaling through its actions on the NF-kappaB pathway in human chondrocytes.

Treatment with curcumin and resveratrol suppressed NF-kappaB-regulated gene products involved in inflammation (cyclooxygenase-2, matrix metalloproteinase (MMP)-3, MMP-9, vascular endothelial growth factor), inhibited apoptosis (Bcl-2, Bcl-xL, and TNF-alpha receptor-associated factor 1) and prevented activation of caspase-3. IL-1beta-induced NF-kappaB activation was suppressed directly by cocktails of curcumin and resveratrol through inhibition of Ikappakappa and proteasome activation, inhibition of IkappaB alpha phosphorylation and degradation, and inhibition of nuclear translocation of NF-kappaB (Csaki *et al.*, 2009).

Conclusions

The traditional therapies for inflammation associated with various clinical conditions such as arthritis, obesity, Type 2 diabetes, with ginger, garlic, drumstick etc. have all been scientifically confirmed. Green tea seems to be another potent therapeutic agent for several disorders. Since altered inflammatory response of the body has been implicated in several degenerative diseases, the specific role of anti-inflammatory foods in these diseases has been discussed in the relevant chapters.

The attempt of Reinagel (2006) to devise an Inflammatory Factor Rating (IF) Scale is worth appreciation as it facilitates selection and inclusion of anti-inflammatory foods in the diet. It would be worthwhile expanding the list of foods in this scale by each country for wider use.

References

Abdullahi SE, Martelli EA, Bramm E, Franco L, Velo GP (1977). Effect of calcitonin on different inflammatory models. Agents. Actions. 7 (5 - 6): 533 - 38.

Aggarwal BB (2010). Targeting inflammation-induced obesity and metabolic diseases by curcumin and other nutraceuticals. Annu. Rev. Nutr. 30: 173 - 99.

Aggarwal BB, Harikumar KB (2009). Potential therapeutic effects of curcumin, the anti-inflammatory agent, against neurodegenerative, cardiovascular, pulmonary, metabolic, autoimmune and neoplastic diseases. Int. J. Biochem. Cell. Biol. 41: 40 - 59.

Aggarwal BB, Kumar A, Aggarwal MS, *et al.* (2005). Curcumin derived from turmeric (*Curcuma longa*): a spice for all seasons;. Preuss PDDBHG, editor. CRC Press. New York. pp 350 - 78.

Almallah, Y. Z., Ewen, S. W., El-Tahir, A., Mowat, N.A.G., Brunt, P. W., Sinclair, T. S., Heys, T. S. and Eremin, O (2000). Distal proctocolitis and n-3 polyunsaturated fatty acids (n-3 PUFAs): the mucosal effect in situ. J. Clin. Immunol. 20: 68 - 76.

Anand P, Thomas SG, Kunnumakkara AB, Sundaram C, Harikumar KB, *et al.* (2008). Biological activities of curcumin and its analogues (Congeners) made by man and Mother Nature. Biochem. Pharmacol. 76: 1590 - 611.

Andoh A, Tsujikawa T, Ishizuka I, Araki Y, Sasaki M, Koyama S, Fujiyama Y (2003). n-3 Fatty acid-rich diet prevents early response of interleukin-6 elevation in trinitrobenzene sulfonic acid-induced enteritis. Int. J. Mol. Med. 12: 721 - 25.

Anwar F, Latif S, Ashraf M, Gilani AH (2007). *Moringa oleifera*: a food plant with multiple medicinal uses. Phytother. Res. 21 (1): 17 - 25.

Aruoma OI, Hayashi Y, Marotta F, Mantello P, Rachmilewitz E, Montagnier L (2010). Applications and bioefficacy of the functional food supplement fermented papaya preparation. Toxicology. 278 (1): 6 - 16.

Atawodi SE, Atawodi JC, Idakwo GA, Pfundstein B, Haubner R, Wurtele G, Bartsch H, Owen RW (2010). Evaluation of the polyphenol content and anti-oxidant properties of methanol extracts of the leaves, stem, and root barks of *M.oleifera* Lam. J. Med. Food. 13 (3): 710 - 16.

Avasarala S, Zhang F, Liu G, Wang R, London SD, London L (2013). Curcumin Modulates the Inflammatory Response and Inhibits Subsequent Fibrosis in a Mouse Model of Viral-induced Acute Respiratory Distress Syndrome. PLoS. One. 8 (2): e57285.

Ban JO, Oh JH, Kim TM, Kim DJ, Jeong HS, Han SB, Hong JT (2009). Anti-inflammatory and arthritic effects of thiacremonone, a novel sulfur compound isolated from garlic via inhibition of NF-kappaB. Arthritis. Res. Ther. 11 (5): R145.

Belluzzi A, Boschi S, Brignola C, Munarini A, Cariani G, Miglio F (2000). Polyunsaturated fatty acids and inflammatory bowel disease. Am. J. Clin. Nutr. 71: 339S - 342S.

Bharti AC, Takada Y, Aggarwal BB (2004). Curcumin (diferuloylmethane) inhibits receptor activator of NF-kappa B ligand-induced NF-kappa B activation in osteoclast precursors and suppresses osteoclastogenesis. J Immunol. 172 (10): 5940 - 47.

Bornhoeft J, Castaneda D, Nemoseck T, Wang P, Henning SM, Hong MY (2012). The protective effects of green tea polyphenols: lipid profile, inflammation, and anti-oxidant capacity in rats fed an atherogenic diet and dextran sodium sulfate. J. Med. Food. 15 (8): 726 - 32.

Bose A, Mondal S, Gupta JK, Ghosh T, Dash GK, Si S (2007). Analgesic, anti-inflammatory and antipyretic activities of the ethanolic extract and its fractions of Cleome rutidosperma. Fitoterapia. 78 (7-8): 515 - 20.

Brahmachari S, Jana A, Pahan K (2009). Sodium benzoate, a metabolite of cinnamon and a food additive, reduces microglial and astroglial inflammatory responses. J. Immunol. 183 (9): 5917 - 27.

Brückner M, Westphal S, Domschke W, Kucharzik T, Lügering A (2012). Green tea polyphenol epigallocatechin-3-gallate shows therapeutic antioxidative effects in a murine model of colitis. J. Crohns. Colitis. 6 (2): 226 - 35.

Buse MG, Reid SS (1975). Leucine. A possible regulator of protein turnover in muscle. *J. Clin. Invest.* 56 (5): 1250 - 61.

Cabrera C, Artacho R, Gimenez R (2006). Beneficial effects of green tea–a review. *J. Am. Coll. Nutr.* 25 (2): 79 - 99.

Cáceres A, Saravia A, Rizzo S, Zabala L, De Leon E, Nave F (1992). Pharmacologic properties of *Moringa oleifera*. 2: Screening for antispasmodic*, anti-inflammatory* and diuretic activity. J. Ethnopharmacol. 36 (3): 233 - 37.

Camacho-Barquero L, Villegas I, Sánchez-Calvo JM, Talero E, Sanches-Fidalgo S, Motilva V, Alarcón de la Lastra C (2007). Curcumin, a *Curcuma longa* constituent, acts on MAPK p38 pathway modulating COX-2 and iNOS expression in chronic experimental colitis. Int. Immunopharmacol. 3: 333 - 42.

Campos FG, Waitzberg DL, Habr-Gama A, Logullo AF, Noronha IL, Jancar S, Torrinhas RS, Furst P (2002). Impact of parenteral n-3 fatty acids on experimental acute colitis. Br. J. Nutr. 87 (suppl. 1): S83 - S88.

Camuesco D, Gálvez J, Nieto A, Comalada M, Rodríguez-Cabezas ME, Concha A, Xaus J, Zarzuelo A (2005). Dietary olive oil supplemented with fish oil, rich in EPA and DHA (n-3) polyunsaturated fatty acids, attenuates colonic inflammation in rats with DSS-induced colitis. J. Nutr. 135 (4): 687 - 94.

Castillero E, Martín AI, López-Menduina M, Villanúa MA, López-Calderón A (2009). Eicosapentaenoic acid attenuates arthritis-induced muscle wasting acting on atrogin-1 and on myogenic regulatory factors. Am. J. Physiol. Regul. Integr. Comp. Physiol. 297 (5): R1322 - 31.

Chan MM, Ho CT, Huang HI (1995). Effects of three dietary phytochemicals from tea, rosemary and turmeric on inflammation-induced nitrite production. Cancer. Lett. 96 (1): 23 - 29.

Chao LK, Hua KF, Hsu HY, Cheng SS, Liu JY, Chang ST (2005). Study on the anti-inflammatory activity of essential oil from leaves of *Cinnamomum osmophloeum*. J Agric Food Chem. 2005 Sep 7;53 (18): 7274 - 78.

Chatterjee P, Chandra S, Dey P, Bhattacharya S (2012). Evaluation of anti-inflammatory effects of green tea and black tea: A comparative *in vitro* study. J. Adv. Pharm. Technol. Res. 3 (2): 136 - 38.

Cheenpracha S, Park EJ, Yoshida WY, Barit C, Wall M, Pezzuto JM, Chang LC.(2010) Potential anti-inflammatory phenolic glycosides from the medicinal plant *M.oleiferafruits*. Bioorg. Med. Chem. 18 (17): 6598 - 602.

Chen JH, Tipoe GL, Liong EC, So HS, Leung KM, Tom WM, Fung PC, Nanji AA (2004). Green tea polyphenols prevent toxin-induced hepato-toxicity in mice by down-regulating inducible nitric oxide-derived pro-oxidants. Am. J. Clin. Nutr. 80 (3): 742 - 51.

Claramunt RM, Bouissane L, Cabildo MP, Cornago MP, Elguero J, Radziwon A, Medina C (2009). Synthesis and biological evaluation of curcuminoid pyrazoles as new therapeutic agents in inflammatory bowel disease: effect on matrix metallo-proteinases. Bioorg. Med. Chem. 171: 290 - 96.

Collard E, Roy S (2010). Improved function of diabetic wound-site macrophages and accelerated wound closure in response to oral supplementation of a fermented papaya preparation. Antioxid. Redox. Signal. 13 (5): 599 - 606.

Comalada M Camuesco D, Sierra S, Ballester I, Xaus J, Gálvez J, Zarzuelo A (2005). *In vivo* quercitrin anti-inflammatory effect involves release of quercetin, which inhibits inflammation through down-regulation of the NF-kappaB pathway. Eur. J. Immunol. 35 (2): 584 - 92.

Csaki C, Mobasheri A, Shakibaei M (2009). Synergistic chondroprotective effects of curcumin and resveratrol in human articular chondrocytes: inhibition of IL-1beta-induced NF-kappaB-mediated inflammation and apoptosis. Arthritis Res Ther. 11 (6): R165.

Davis JM, Murphy EA, Carmichael MD (2009). Effects of the dietary flavonoid quercetin upon performance and health. *Curr. Sports Med. Rep.* 8 (4): 206 - 13.

Dkhil MA, Abdel-Baki AS, Wunderlich F, Sies H, Al-Quraishy S (2011). Anti-coccidial and anti-inflammatory activity of garlic in murine *Eimeria papillata* infections. Vet. Parasitol. 175 (1-2): 66 - 72.

El-Mowafy AM, Salem HA, Al-Gayyar MM, El-Mesery ME, El-Azab MF (2011). Evaluation of renal protective effects of the green-tea (EGCG) and red grape resveratrol: role of oxidative stress and inflammatory cytokines. Nat. Prod. Res. 25 (8): 850 - 56.

Fawole OA, Amoo SO, Ndhlala AR, Light ME, Finnie JF, Van Staden J.(2010). Anti-inflammatory, anti-cholinesterase, anti-oxidant and phytochemical properties of medicinal plants used for pain-related ailments in South Africa. J. Ethnopharmacol. 127 (2): 235 - 41.

Ferrero-Miliani L, Nielsen OH, Andersen PS, Girardin SE (2007). Chronic inflammation: importance of NOD2 and NALP3 in interleukin-1beta generation. Clin. Exp. Immunol. 147 (2): 061127015327006.

Gil, A (2002). Polyunsaturated fatty acids and inflammatory diseases. Biomed. Pharmacother. 56: 388 - 93.

Gradisar H, Keber MM, Pristovsek P, Jerala R (2007). MD-2 as the target of curcumin in the inhibition of response to LPS. J. Leukoc. Biol. 82 (4): 968 - 74.

Greten FR, Eckmann L, Greten TF, Park JM, Li ZW, Egan LJ, Kagnoff MF, Karin M (2004). IKKbeta links inflammation and tumorigenesis in a mouse model of colitis-associated cancer. Cell. 118 (3): 285 - 96.

Grimstad T, Berge RK, Bohov P, Skorve J, Gøransson L, Omdal R, Aasprong OG, Haugen M, Meltzer HM, Hausken T (2011). Salmon diet in patients with active ulcerative colitis reduced the simple clinical colitis activity index and increased the anti-inflammatory fatty acid index–a pilot study. Scand. J. Clin. Lab. Invest. 71 (1): 68 - 73.

Grzanna R, Lindmark L, Frondoza CG (2005). Ginger - an herbal medicinal product with broad anti-inflammatory actions. J. Med. Food. 8 (2): 125 - 32.

Ha SK, Moon E, Ju MS, Kim DH, Ryu JH, Oh MS, Kim SY (2012). 6-Shogaol, a ginger product, modulates neuro-inflammation: a new approach to neuroprotection. Neuropharmacology. 63 (2): 211 - 23.

Habib SH, Makpol S, Abdul Hamid NA, Das S, Ngah WZ, Yusof YA (2008). Ginger extract (*Zingiber officinale*) has anti-cancer and anti-inflammatory effects on ethionine-induced hepatoma rats. Clinics (Sao Paulo). 63 (6): 807 - 813.

Hagenlocher Y, Bergheim I, Zacheja S, Schäffer M, Bischoff SC, Lorentz A (2013). Cinnamon extract inhibits degranulation and de novo synthesis of inflammatory mediators in mast cells. Allergy. 2013 Feb 15. doi: 10.1111/all.12122. [Epub ahead of print].

Hamza AA (2010). Ameliorative effects of *M. oleifera* Lam seed extract on liver fibrosis in rats. Food Chem. Toxicol. 48 (1): 345 - 55.

Han YA, Song CW, Koh WS, Yon GH, Kim YS, Ryu SY, Kwon HJ, Lee KH (2012). Anti-inflammatory Effects of the *Zingiber officinale* roscoe Constituent 12-Dehydrogingerdione in Lipopolysaccharide-stimulated Raw 264.7 Cells. Phytother Res. 2012 Oct 2. [Epub ahead of print].

Hanai H, Iida T, Takeuchi K, Watanabe F, Maruyama Y, Andoh A, Tsujikawa T, Fujiyama Y, Mitsuyama K, Sata M, Yamada M, Iwaoka Y, Kanke K, Hiraishi H, Hirayama K, Arai H, Yoshii S, Uchijima M, Nagata T, Koide Y (2006). Curcumin maintenance therapy for ulcerative colitis: randomized, multicenter, double-blind, placebo-controlled trial. Clin. Gastroenterol. Hepatol. 12: 1502 - 506.

Heeba GH, Mahmoud ME, El Hanafy AA (2012). Anti-inflammatory potential of curcumin and quercetin in rats: Role of oxidative stress, heme oxygenase-1 and TNF-α. Toxicol. Ind. Health. Pharm. Biol. 49 (2): 146 - 51.

Hernández-Ortega M, Ortiz-Moreno A, Hernández-Navarro MD, Chamorro-Cevallos G, Dorantes-Alvarez L, Necoechea-Mondragón H (2012). Anti-oxidant, anti-nociceptive, and anti-inflammatory effects of carotenoids extracted from dried pepper (*Capsicum annuum* L.). J. Biomed. Biotechnol. 2012: 524019.

Hong JW, Yang GE, Kim YB, Eom SH, Lew JH, Kang H (2012). Anti-inflammatory activity of cinnamon water extract *in vivo* and *in vitro* LPS-induced models. BMC Complement Altern. Med. 12: 237.

Hsu A, Bray TM, Ho E (2010). Anti-inflammatory activity of soy and tea in prostate cancer prevention. Exp. Biol. Med. (Maywood). 235 (6): 659 - 67.

Hsu A, Bruno RS, Löhr CV, Taylor AW, Dashwood RH, Bray TM, Ho E (2011). Dietary soy and tea mitigate chronic inflammation and prostate cancer via NFκB pathway in the Noble rat model. J. Nutr. Biochem. 22 (5): 502 - 510.

Hu Y, Guo DH, Liu P, Cao JJ, Wang YP, Yin J, Zhu Y, Rahman K (2011), Bioactive components from the tea polyphenols influence on endogenous anti-oxidant defense system and modulate inflammatory cytokines after total-body irradiation in mice. Phytomedicine.18 (11): 970 - 75.

Ibrahim A, Mbodji K, Hassan A, Aziz M, Boukhettala N, Coëffier M, Savoye G, Déchelotte P, Marion-Letellier R.(2011) Anti-inflammatory and anti-angiogenic effect of long chain n-3 polyunsaturated fatty acids in intestinal microvascular endothelium. Clin. Nutr. 30 (5): 678 - 87.

Ide N, Lau BH (2001). Garlic compounds minimize intracellular oxidative stress and inhibit nuclear factor-kappaB activation. J.Nutr.131 (suppl). 1020S - 6S.

Islam MS, Yoshida H, Matsuki N, Ono K, Nagasaka R, Ushio H, Guo Y, Hiramatsu T, Hosoya T, Murata T, Hori M, Ozaki H (2009). Anti-oxidant, free radical-scavenging, and NF-kappaB-inhibitory activities of phytosteryl ferulates: structure-activity studies. J. Pharmacol. Sci. 111 (4): 328 - 37.

Islam MS, Nagasaka R, Ohara K, Hosoya T, Ozaki H, Ushio H, Hori M (2011). Biological abilities of rice bran-derived antioxidant phytochemicals for medical therapy. Curr. Top. Med. Chem. 11 (14): 1847 - 53.

Joe B, Vijaykumar M, Lokesh BR (2004). Biological properties of curcumin-cellular and molecular mechanisms of action. Crit. Rev. Food Sci. Nutr. 44: 97 - 111.

Joseph JA, Shukitt-Hale B, Casadesus G, Fisher D (2005). Oxidative stress and inflammation in brain ageing: nutritional considerations. *Neurochem. Res.* 30 (6-7): 927 - 35.

Ju JH, Yoon HS, Park HJ, Kim MY, Shin HK, Park KY, Yang JO, Sohn MS, Do MS (2011). Anti-obesity and anti-oxidative effects of purple sweet potato extract in 3T3-L1 adipocytes *in vitro*. Med Food. 14 (10): 1097 - 106.

Kalaiselvi P, Rajashree K, Bharathi Priya L, Padma VV (2013). Cytoprotective effect of epigallocatechin-3-gallate against deoxynivalenol-induced toxicity through anti-oxidative and anti-inflammatory mechanisms in HT-29 cells. Food Chem. Toxicol. pii: S0278-6915 (13) 00090 - 92.

Kandere-Grzybowska K Kempuraj D, Cao J, Cetrulo CL, Theoharides TC (2006). Regulation of IL-1-induced selective IL-6 release from human mast cells and inhibition by quercetin. *Br. J. Pharmacol.* 148 (2): 208 - 215.

Kennedy DO, Veasey R, Watson A, Dodd F, Jones E, Maggini S, Haskell CF (2010). Effects of high-dose B vitamin complex with vitamin C and minerals on subjective mood and performance in healthy males. *Psychopharmacology (Berl)* 211 (1): 55 - 68.

Kim DH, Kim CH, Kim MS, Kim JY, Jung KJ, Chung JH, An WG, Lee JW, Yu BP, Chung HY (2007). Suppression of age-related inflammatory NF-kappaB activation by cinnamaldehyde. Biogerontology. 8 (5): 545 - 54.

Kim OY, Lee SM, Do H, Moon J, Lee KH, Cha YJ, Shin MJ (2012). Influence of quercetin-rich onion peel extracts on adipokine expression in the visceral adipose tissue of rats. Phytother. Res. 26 (3): 432 - 37.

Koosirirat C, Linpisarn S, Changsom D, Chawansuntati K, Wipasa J (2010). Investigation of the anti-inflammatory effect of *Curcuma longa* in H. pylori-infected patients. Int. Immunopharmacol. 10 (7): 815 - 18.

Kunnumakkara AB, Diagaradjane P, Guha S, Deorukhkar A, Shentu S, Aggarwal BB, Krishnan S (2008). Curcumin sensitizes human colorectal cancer xenografts in nude mice to gamma-radiation by targeting nuclear factor-kappaB-regulated gene products. Clin. Cancer Res. 14 (7): 2128 - 36.

Kunnumakkara AB, Guha S, Krishnan S, Diagaradjane P, Gelovani J, Aggarwal BB (2007). Curcumin potentiates antitumor activity of gemcitabine in an orthotopic model of pancreatic cancer through suppression of proliferation, angiogenesis, and inhibition of nuclear factor-κB-regulated gene products. Cancer Res. 67: 3853 - 61.

Lambert JD, Sang S, Hong J, Yang CS (2010). Anti-cancer and anti-inflammatory effects of cysteine metabolites of the green tea polyphenol, (-)-epigallocatechin-3-gallate. J. Agric. Food Chem. 58 (18): 10016 - 19.

Lantz RC, Chen GJ, Sarihan M, Sólyom AM, Jolad SD, Timmermann BN (2007). The effect of extracts from ginger rhizome on inflammatory mediator production. Phytomedicine. 14 (2-3): 123 - 28.

Lee HS, Kim BS, Kim MK (2002). Suppression effect of *Cinnamomum cassia* bark-derived component on nitric oxide synthase. J. Agric. Food Chem. 50 (26): 7700 - 703.

Lee da Y, Li H, Lim HJ, Lee HJ, Jeon R, Ryu JH (2012). Anti-inflammatory activity of sulfur-containing compounds from garlic. J. Med. Food. 15(11): 992 - 99.

Li XH, McGrath KC, Nammi S, Heather AK, Roufogalis BD (2012). Attenuation of liver pro-inflammatory responses by *Zingiber officinale* via inhibition of NF-kappa B activation in high-fat diet-fed rats. Basic Clin. Pharmacol. Toxicol. 110 (3): 238 - 44.

Mahajan SG, Mali RG, Mehta AA (2007). Protective effect of ethanolic extract of seeds of *Moringa oleifera* Lam. against inflammation associated with development of arthritis in rats. J. Immunotoxicol. 4 (1): 39 - 47.

Maheshwari RK, Singh AK, Gaddipati J, Srimal RC (2006). Multiple biological activities of curcumin: a short review. Life Sci. 78: 2081 - 87.

Mali RG (2010). *Cleome viscosa* (wild mustard): a review on ethnobotany, phytochemistry, and pharmacology. Pharm. Biol. 48 (1): 105 - 12.

Manaheji H, Jafari S, Zaringhalam J, Rezazadeh S, Taghizadfarid R (2011). Analgesic effects of methanolic extracts of the leaf or root of *Moringa oleifera* on complete Freund's adjuvant-induced arthritis in rats. Zhong. Xi. Yi. Jie. He. Xue. Bao. 9 (2): 216 - 22.

Matsumoto K, Koba T, Hamada K, Sakurai M, Higuchi T, Miyata H (2009). Branched-chain amino acid supplementation attenuates muscle soreness, muscle damage and inflammation during an intensive training program. J. Sports Med. Phys. Fitness. 49 (4): 424 - 31.

McKay DL, Blumberg JB (2007). Cranberries (*Vaccinium macrocarpon*) and cardiovascular disease risk factors. Nutr. Rev. 65 (11): 490 - 502.

Meghvansi MK, Siddiqui S, Khan MH, *et al.* (2010). Naga chilli: a potential source of capsaicinoids with broad-spectrum ethno-pharmacological applications. *Journal of Ethnopharmacology.* 132 (1): 1 - 14.

Mikhal'chik EV, Ivanova AV, Anurov MV, Titkova SM, Pen'kov LY, Kharaeva ZF, Korkina LG (2004). Wound-healing effect of papaya-based preparation in experimental thermal trauma. Bull. Exp. Biol. Med. 137 (6): 560 - 62.

Minghetti P, Sosa S, Cilurzo F, Casiraghi A, Alberti E, Tubaro A, Loggia RD, Montanari L (2007). Evaluation of the topical anti-inflammatory activity of ginger dry extracts from solutions and plasters. Planta. Med. 73 (15): 1525 - 30.

Ndiaye M, Dieye AM, Mariko F, Tall A, Sall Diallo A, Faye B (2002). [Contribution to the study of the anti-inflammatory activity of *Moringa oleifera* (moringaceae)]. Dakar. Med. 47 (2): 210 - 12. [Article in French].

Nieto N, Torres, MI, Rios A, Gil A (2002). Dietary polyunsaturated fatty acids improve histological and biochemical alterations in rats with experimental ulcerative colitis. J. Nutr. 132: 11 - 19.

Ojewole JA (2006). Analgesic, anti-inflammatory and hypoglycaemic effects of ethanol extract of *Zingiber officinale* (Roscoe) rhizomes (Zingiberaceae) in mice and rats. Phytother. Res. 20 (9): 764 - 72.

Ojewole JA (2007). Analgesic, anti-inflammatory and hypo-glycaemic effects of *Rhus chirindensis* (Baker F.) [Anacardiaceae] stem-bark aqueous extract in mice and rats. J. Ethnopharmacol. 113 (2): 338 - 45.

Panahi Y, Sahebkar A, Parvin S, Saadat A (2012). A randomized controlled trial on the anti-inflammatory effects of curcumin in patients with chronic sulphur mustard-induced cutaneous complications. Ann. Clin. Biochem. 49 (Pt 6): 580 - 88.

Park JS, Chyun JH, Kim YK, Line LL, Chew BP (2010). Astaxanthin decreased oxidative stress and inflammation and enhanced immune response in humans. *Nutrition and Metabolism.* 7 (1, article 18).

Park HJ, Jeon BT, Kim HC, Roh GS, Shin JH, Sung NJ, Han J, Kang D (2012a). Aged red garlic extract reduces lipo-polysaccharide-induced nitric oxide production in RAW 264.7 macrophages and acute pulmonary inflammation through haeme oxygenase-1 induction. Acta. Physiol. (Oxf). 205 (1): 61 - 70.

Park SH, Kyeong MS, Hwang Y, Ryu SY, Han SB, Kim Y (2012b). Inhibition of LPS binding to MD-2 co-receptor for suppressing TLR4-mediated expression of inflammatory cytokine by 1-dehydro-10-gingerdione from dietary ginger. Biochem. Biophys. Res. Commun. 419 (4): 735 - 40.

Penna SC, Medeiros MV, Aimbire FS, Faria-Neto HC, Sertié JA, Lopes-Martins RA (2003). Anti-inflammatory effect of the hydralcoholic extract of *Zingiber officinale* rhizomes on rat paw and skin edema. Phytomedicine. 10 (5): 381 - 85.

Pereira ML, de Oliveira HD, de Oliveira JT, Gifoni JM, Rocha Rde O, de Sousa Dde O, Vasconcelos IM (2011). Purification of a chitin-binding protein from *Moringa oleifera* seeds with potential to relieve pain and inflammation. Protein Pept. Lett. 18 (11): 1078 - 85.

Qin B, Polansky MM, Harry D, Anderson RA (2010). Green tea polyphenols improve cardiac muscle mRNA and protein levels of signal pathways related to insulin and lipid metabolism and inflammation in insulin-resistant rats. Mol. Nutr. Food Res. 54 Suppl. 1: S14 - 23.

Ramadan G, Al-Kahtani MA, El-Sayed WM (2011). Anti-inflammatory and anti-oxidant properties of *Curcuma longa* (turmeric) versus *Zingiber officinale* (ginger) rhizomes in rat adjuvant-induced arthritis. Inflammation. 34 (4): 291 - 301.

Ramos-Romero S, Pérez-Cano FJ, Castellote C, Castell M, Franch À (2012a). Effect of cocoa-enriched diets on lymphocytes involved in adjuvant arthritis in rats. Br. J. Nutr. 107 (3): 378 - 87.

Ramos-Romero S, Pérez-Cano FJ, Pérez-Berezo T, Castellote C, Franch A, Castell M (2012b). Effect of a cocoa flavonoid-enriched diet on experimental autoimmune arthritis. Br. J. Nutr. 107 (4): 523 - 32.

Ramos-Romero S, Pérez-Cano FJ, Ramiro-Puig E, Franch A, Castell M (2012c). Cocoa intake attenuates oxidative stress associated with rat adjuvant arthritis. Pharmacol. Res. 66 (3): 207 - 212.

Reinagel, M (2006). Editor: Julius Torelli. *The Inflammation Free Diet Plan*. The McGraw-Hill Companies, Inc.

Ribel-Madsen S, Bartels EM, Stockmarr A, Borgwardt A, Cornett C, Danneskiold-Samsøe B, Bliddal H (2012). A synoviocyte model for osteoarthritis and rheumatoid arthritis: response to Ibuprofen, betamethasone, and ginger extract-a cross-sectional *in vitro* study. Arthritis. 2012: 505842.

Ryan SM, McMorrow J, Umerska A, Patel HB, Kornerup KN, Tajber L, Murphy EP, Perretti M, Corrigan OI, Brayden DJ (2013). An intra-articular salmon calcitonin-based nano complex reduced experimental inflammatory arthritis. J. Control. Release. 167 (2): 120 - 129.

Sashidhara KV, Rosaiah JN, Tyagi E, Shukla R, Raghubir R, Rajendran SM (2009). Rare dipeptide and urea derivatives from roots of *M.oleifera* as potential anti-inflammatory and anti-nociceptive agents. Eur. J. Med. Chem. 44 (1): 432 - 36.

Schuller-Levis GB, Park E (2003). Taurine: new implications for an old amino acid. FEMS. Microbiol. Lett. 226 (2): 195 - 202.

Shakibaei M, Csaki C, Nebrich S, Mobasheri A (2008). Resveratrol suppresses interleukin-1beta-induced inflammatory signaling and apoptosis in human articular chondrocytes: potential for use as a novel nutraceutical for the treatment of osteoarthritis. Biochem. Pharmacol. 76 (11): 1426 - 39.

Shakibaei M, John T, Seifarth C, Mobasheri A (2007). Resveratrol inhibits IL-1 beta-induced stimulation of caspase-3 and cleavage of PARP in human articular chondrocytes *in vitro.* Ann. N. Y. Acad. Sci. 1095: 554 - 63.

Sharma OP (1976). Anti-oxidant activity of curcumin and related compounds. Biochem. Pharmacol. 25: 1811 - 12.

Sharma RA, Gescher AJ, Steward WP (2005). Curcumin: the story so far. Eur. J, Cancer. 41: 1955 - 68.

Sharma RA, Euden SA, Platton SL, Cooke DN, Shafayat A, Hewitt HR, Marczylo TH, Morgan B, Hemingway D, Plummer SM, Pirmohamed M, Gescher AJ, Steward WP (2004). Phase I clinical trial of oral curcumin: biomarkers of systemic activity and compliance. Clin. Cancer. Res. 10: 6847 - 54.

Shehzad A, Ha T, Subhan F, Lee YS (2011). New mechanisms and the anti-inflammatory role of curcumin in obesity and obesity-related metabolic diseases. Eur. J. Nutr. 50 (3): 151 - 61.

Shen CL, Samathanam C, Graham S, Dagda RY, Chyu MC, Dunn DM (2012). Green tea polyphenols and 1-α-OH-vitamin D attenuate chronic inflammation-induced myocardial fibrosis in female rats. J, Med. Food. 15 (3): 269 – 77.

Shen CL, Samathanam C, Tatum OL, Graham S, Tubb C, Cao JJ, Dunn DM, Wang JS (2011). Green tea polyphenols avert chronic inflammation-induced myocardial fibrosis of female rats. Inflamm. Res. 60 (7): 665 - 72.

Shim S, Kim S, Choi DS, Kwon YB, Kwon J (2011). Anti-inflammatory effects of [6]-shogaol: potential roles of HDAC inhibition and HSP70 induction. Food Chem. Toxicol. 49 (11): 2734 - 40.

Shimizu T, Fujii T, Suzuki R, Igarashi J, Ohtsuka Y, Nagata S, Yamashiro Y (2003). Effects of highly purified eicosapentaenoic acid on erythrocyte fatty acid composition and leukocyte and colonic mucosa leukotriene B_4 production in children with ulcerative colitis. J. Pediatr. Gastroenterol. Nutr. 37: 581 - 85.

Shimizu T, Igarashi J, Ohtuka Y, Oguchi S, Kaneko K, Yamashiro Y (2001). Effects of n-3 polyunsaturated fatty acids and vitamin E on colonic mucosal leukotriene generation, lipid peroxidation, and microcirculation in rats with experimental colitis. Digestion. 63: 49 - 54.

Shimoda H, Shan SJ, Tanaka J, Seki A, Seo JW, Kasajima N, Tamura S, Ke Y, Murakami N (2010). Anti-inflammatory properties of red ginger (*Zingiber officinale* var. Rubra) extract and suppression of nitric oxide production by its constituents. J. Med. Food. 13 (1): 156 - 62.

Sindhu G, Ratheesh M, Shyni GL, Nambisan B, Helen A (2012). Anti-inflammatory and anti-oxidative effects of mucilage of *Trigonella foenum graecum* (Fenugreek) on adjuvant induced arthritic rats. Int. Immunopharmacol. 12 (1): 205 - 11.

Skarupski KA, Tangney C, Li H, Ouyang B, Evans DA, Morris MC (2010). Longitudinal association of vitamin B-6, folate, and vitamin B-12 with depressive symptoms among older adults over time. Am. J. Clin. Nutr. 92 (2): 330 - 35.

Sohn DW, Han CH, Jung YS, Kim SI, Kim SW, Cho YH (2009). Anti-inflammatory and antimicrobial effects of garlic and synergistic effect between garlic and ciprofloxacin in a chronic bacterial prostatitis rat model. Int. J. Antimicrob. Agents. 34 (3): 215 - 19.

Somanah J, Aruoma OI, Gunness TK, Kowelssur S, Dambala V, Murad F, Googoolye K, Daus D, Indelicato J, Bourdon E, Bahorun T (2012). Effects of a short term supplementation of a fermented papaya preparation on biomarkers of diabetes mellitus in a randomized Mauritian population. Prev. Med. 54 Suppl: S90 - 97.

Song XZ, Bi ZG, Xu AE (2006). Green tea polyphenol epigallocatechin-3-gallate inhibits the expression of nitric oxide synthase and generation of nitric oxide induced by ultraviolet B in HaCaT cells.Chin.Med.J.(Engl).119 (4):282 - 87.

Spiller F, Alves MK, Vieira SM, Carvalho TA, Leite CE, Lunardelli A, Poloni JA, Cunha FQ, de Oliveira JR (2008). Anti-inflammatory effects of red pepper (*Capsicum baccatum*) on carrageenan- and antigen-induced inflammation. J Pharm Pharmacol. 60 (4): 473 - 78.

Srimal RC, Dhawan BN (1973). Pharmacology of diferuloyl methane (curcumin), a non-steroidal anti-inflammatory agent. J. Pharm. Pharmacol. 25: 447 - 52.

Srivastava KC, Mustafa T (1989). Ginger (*Zingiber officinale*) and rheumatic disorders. Med. Hypotheses. 29 (1): 25 - 28.

Srivastava KC, Mustafa T (1992). Ginger (*Zingiber officinale*) in rheumatism and musculoskeletal disorders. Med. Hypotheses. 39 (4): 342 - 48.

Stengler M, Balch JF (2002). Natural Physician's Healing Therapies. Prentice Hall Publishers, USA. pp. 444 - 46.

Sugimoto K, Hanai H, Tozawa K, Aoshi T, Uchijima M, Nagata T, Koide Y. (2002). Curcumin prevents and ameliorates trinitrobenzenesulfonic acid-induced colitis in mice. Gastroenterology. 123: 1912 - 22.

Suresh P, Kavitha ChN, Babu SM, Reddy VP, Latha AK (2012). Effect of ethanol extract of *Trigonella foenum graecum* (Fenugreek) seeds on Freund's adjuvant-induced arthritis in albino rats. Inflammation. 35 (4): 1314 - 21.

Szarc vel Szic K, Ndlovu MN, Haegeman G, Vanden Berghe W (2010). Nature or nurture: let food be your epigenetic medicine in chronic inflammatory disorders. Biochem. Pharmacol. 80 (12): 1816 - 32.

Taylor RA, Leonard MC (2011). Curcumin for inflammatory bowel disease: a review of human studies. Altern. Med. Rev. 16 (2): 152 - 56.

Thomson M, Al-Qattan KK, Al-Sawan SM, Alnaqeeb MA, Khan I, Ali M (2002). The use of ginger (*Zingiber officinale* Rosc.) as a potential anti-inflammatory and antithrombotic agent. Prostaglandins Leukot. Essent. Fatty Acids. 67 (6): 475 - 78.

Tipoe GL, Leung TM, Hung MW, Fung ML (2007). Green tea polyphenols as an anti-oxidant and anti-inflammatory agent for cardiovascular protection. Cardiovasc. Hematol. Disord. Drug Targets. 7 (2): 135 - 44.

Tung YT, Chua MT, Wang SY, Chang ST (2008). Anti-inflammation activities of essential oil and its constituents from indigenous cinnamon (*Cinnamomum osmophloeum*) twigs. Bioresour. Technol. 99 (9): 3908 - 13.

Tung YT, Yen PL, Lin CY, Chang ST (2010). Anti-inflammatory activities of essential oils and their constituents from different provenances of indigenous cinnamon (*Cinnamomum osmophloeum*) leaves. Pharm. Biol. 48 (10): 1130 - 36.

Ueda H, Ippoushi K, Takeuchi A (2010). Repeated oral administration of a squeezed ginger (*Zingiber officinale*) extract augmented the serum corticosterone level and had anti-inflammatory properties. Biosci. Biotechnol. Biochem. 74 (11): 2248 - 52.

Vazquez-Prieto MA, Rodriguez Lanzi C, Lembo C, Galmarini CR, Miatello RM. (2011) Garlic and onion attenuates vascular inflammation and oxidative stress in fructose-fed rats. J. Nutr. Metab. 2011: 475216.

Vijayalakshmi K, Shyamala R, Thirumurugan V, Sethuraman M, Rajan S, Badami S, Mukherjee PK (2010). Physico-Phytochemical investigation and Anti-inflammatory screening of *Capsicum annum* L. and *Hemidesmus indicus* (Linn.) R. Br. Anc. Sci. Life. 29 (4): 35 - 40.

Wang YJ, Zheng YL, Lu J, Chen GQ, Wang XH, Feng J, Ruan J, Sun X, Li CX, Sun QJ. (2010). Purple sweet potato color suppresses lipo-polysaccharide-induced acute inflammatory response in mouse brain. Neurochem. Int. 56 (3): 424 - 30.

Wang BS, Huang GJ, Lu YH, Chang LW (2013). Anti-inflammatory effects of an aqueous extract of Welsh onion green leaves in mice. Food Chem. 138 (2-3): 751 - 56.

Weisberg SP, Leibel R, Tortoriello DV (2008). Dietary curcumin significantly improves obesity-associated inflammation and diabetes in mouse models of diabesity. Endocrinology. 149 (7): 3549 - 58.

Williams MJ, Sutherland WH, McCormick MP, Yeoman DJ, de Jong SA (2005). Aged garlic extract improves endothelial function in men with coronary artery disease. Phytother. Res. 19 (4): 314 - 19.

Woo HM, Kang JH, Kawada T, Yoo H, Sung MK, Yu R (2007). Active spice-derived components can inhibit inflammatory responses of adipose tissue in obesity by suppressing inflammatory actions of macrophages and release of monocyte chemoattractant protein-1 from adipocytes. Life Sci. 80: 926 - 31.

Yamada, N., Shimizu, J., Wada, M., Takita, T. and Innami, S (1998). Changes in platelet aggregation and lipid metabolism in rats given dietary lipids containing different n-3 polyunsaturated fatty acids. J. Nutr. Sci. Vitaminol. 44: 279 - 89.

Young HY, Luo YL, Cheng HY, Hsieh WC, Liao JC, Peng WH (2005). Analgesic and anti-inflammatory activities of [6]-gingerol. J. Ethnopharmacol. 96 (1-2): 207 - 10.

Yuceyar H, Ozutemiz O, Huseyinov A, Saruc M, Alkanat M, Bor S, Coker I, Batur Y (1999). Is administration of n-3 fatty acids by mucosal enema protective against trinitrobenzene-induced colitis in rats?. Prostaglandins Leukot. Essent. Fatty Acids. 61: 339 - 45.

Zhong Y, Chiou YS, Pan MH, Shahidi F (2012). Anti-inflammatory activity of lipophilic epigallocatechin gallate (EGCG) derivatives in LPS-stimulated murine macrophages. Food Chem. 134 (2): 742 - 48.

Zimmer AR, Leonardi B, Miron D, Schapoval E, Oliveira JR, Gosmann G (2012). Antioxidant and anti-inflammatory properties of *Capsicum baccatum*: from traditional use to scientific approach. *Journal of Ethnopharmacology*. 139 (1): 228 - 33.

Chapter 9

Antimicrobial Foods

Infectious diseases, also known as transmissible diseases or communicable diseases comprise of clinically evident illness (*i.e.* characteristic medical signs and/ or symptoms of disease) resulting from an infection *i.e.* presence and growth of pathogenic biological agents in an individual host organism. An infection is not synonymous with an infectious disease, as some infections do not cause illness in a host (Ryan and Ray, 2004). Infectious pathogens include some viruses, bacteria, fungi, protozoa, multicellular parasites, and aberrant proteins known as prions.

Bacteria are single-celled micro-organisms that grow throughout the human body, mainly on the skin and in the digestive tract. Majority of them, interestingly, are either beneficial or are rendered harmless by the immune system. Some of these beneficial bacteria also help fight the harmful pathogens.

Anti-biotics are commonly prescribed to treat harmful bacterial infections. Most antibiotics do not discriminate between healthy bacteria and unhealthy bacteria. As a consequence of frequent consumption of antibiotics, many people no longer possess adequate levels of beneficial bacteria in their digestive tracts, thus increasing the risk of infections.

The increasing incidence of food borne diseases, the side effects of antibiotics along with the continuous escalation of resistant bacteria against a wide range of antibiotics necessitate discovering novel unconventional sources of antibiotics.

Most of the anitimicrobial compounds are found in plant foods especially in spices. The bioactive components of many foods including spices, allium vegetables (garlic and onions), chillies, coconuts, and oils contain potential anti-oxidant, anti-mutagenic, anti-inflammatory, and anitimicrobial/anti-bacterial properties (Pehowich *et al.*, 2000; Bianchini and Vainio, 2001; Surh, 2002; Lampe, 2003; Larsson *et al.*, 2004; Sengupta *et al.*, 2004; Psota *et al.*, 2006; Slimestad *et al.*, 2007; Kaefer and

Milner, 2008; Krishnaswamy, 2008; Powolny and Singh, 2008; Aggarwal and Sung, 2009; Butt *et al.*, 2009; Iciek *et al.*, 2009; Russo, 2009; Ganguly, 2010; Prasad *et al.*, 2010). If isolated, the antimicrobial compounds of foods can be coated with edible films for fruits and vegetables for easy and safe consumption.

The anitimicrobial properties of food extracts are well researched in the field of food preservation and infectious diseases in humans. The potential anitimicrobial benefits of various foods are discussed below.

Part - A SPICES

Spices and plant foods are rich in essential oils and show inhibition against various microorganisms. Anti-bacterial spices include cinnamon, ginger, and garlic. According to Ayurvedic system of medicine, the use of cinnamon in the diet improves immunity against bacteria, viruses and fungi. It also restricts the growth of certain bacteria such as *C. albicans and Helicobacter*. The Environmental Illness Resource reports that ginger inhibits the action of harmful bacteria such as *E.coli, Salmonella, S. aureus and S. viridans*. In addition, garlic contains sulfur compounds that have anti-bacterial properties.

The anitimicrobial properties of essential oils have been known for many centuries. In the recent years (1987-2001), a large number of essential oils and their constituents have been investigated for their anitimicrobial properties. Some essential oils extracted from spices were documented to possess strong anti-bacterial and anti-fungal activities in more than 500 reports (Kalemba and Kunicka, 2003).

In vitro studies have demonstrated anti-bacterial activity of essential oils (EOs) against *L. monocytogenes, S. typhimurium, E. coli* O157:H7, *S. dysenteria, B. cereus* and *S. aureus* at levels between 0.2 and 10 microl ml (-1). According to Burt (2004) the hydrophobicity of EOs enables them to disintegrate in the lipids of cell membrane and mitochondria of microbes and thereby increasing their permeability leading to leakage of cell contents and cell death. Physical conditions that improve the action of EOs are low pH, low temperature and low oxygen levels.

The essential oils of thyme, origanum, clove, and orange were also found to be the most effective inhibitory agents against bacteria and yeasts. Cumin, tea tree, and mint oils inhibited the yeasts actively (Mohsenzadeh, 2007). Thus, some essential oils could be used as potential bio preservatives capable of controlling food borne pathogens and food spoilage yeasts.

Not only the microorganisms differ in their resistance to a given spice or herb but also a given micro-organism differs in its resistance to various spices and herbs. Bacteria are more resistant than fungi. The effect on spores may be different than that on vegetative cells. Gram-negative bacteria are more resistant than gram-positive bacteria. Studies in the past decades confirmed that the growth of both Gram-positive and Gram-negative food borne bacteria, yeast and mold can be inhibited by garlic, onion, cinnamon, cloves, thyme, sage, and other spices, but the fat, protein, water, and salt contents of food influence microbial resistance. It is not certain if the levels of spices added to foods are sufficient to inhibit microbial growth in food as most of these studies are based on cultures (Zaika, 1988).

Spices and herbs can also be contaminated as they serve as substrates for microbial growth and the amounts of spices added to foods are generally too low to prevent spoilage by micro-organisms. Active components of spices/herbs at low concentrations may interact synergistically with other preservatives (salt, acids, and preservatives) to increase preservative effect.

Incorporating essential oils into edible films provides a new way to improve the safety and shelf life of foods, which will provide multiple benefits to consumers. Du *et al.* (2008) demonstrated that edible anitimicrobial tomato films have the potential to prevent adverse effects of contaminated food and promote human health associated with the consumption of tomatoes. Again, apple-based films coated with allspice, cinnamon or clove bud oils were effective against *E. coli, S. enterica* and *L. monocytogenes* (Du *et al.*, 2009 a and b; 2011).

But on the otherhand, nutrients present in spices/herbs may stimulate growth and/or biochemical activities of micro-organisms. Thus, food product safety and shelf life depend in some part on the type, quantity, and nature of spices and herbs added.

Ajwain (*Carum copticum/Trachyspermum ammi*)

The essential oil of ajwain exhibited a broad spectrum of fungitoxic behavior against all tested fungi such as *A. niger, A. flavus, A. oryzae, A. ochraceus, F. monoliforme, F. graminearum, P. citrium, P. viridicatum, P.madriti,* and *C. lunata* through absolute mycelial zone inhibition that was obtained at a 6-microL dose of the oil (Singh *et al.*, 2004, Rasooli *et al.*, 2008). The essential oil has some use in the treatment of intestinal dysbiosis. Its benefit comes from being able to inhibit the growth of undesired pathogens while not adversely affecting the beneficial flora (Hawrelak *et al.*, 2009).

Anti-bacterial efficacy of ajwain shown by Kaur and Arora (2009) provided a scientific basis and thus, validated their traditional uses as home-made remedies. Isolation and purification of different phytochemicals form ajwain may further yield significant anti-bacterial agents.

Lymphatic filariasis is caused by infection with the parasitic filarial nematodes *Wuchereria bancrofti, Brugia malayi* and *B. timori*, transmitted by mosquitoes. The lack of an adulticidal drug poses a challenge to filariasis elimination, hence it is essential to develop an effective anti-filarial drug which could either kill or permanently sterilize the adult worms. Mathew *et al.* (2008) found that the crude extract of ajwain showed significant activity against the adult *S. digitata* by both a worm motility and MTT [3-(4,5-dimethylthiazol-2-yl)-2,5-diphenyltetrazolium bromide] reduction assays. The isolated active principle was chemically characterized by IR, (1) H-NMR and MS analysis and identified as a phenolic monoterpene. It was screened for *in vivo* anti-filarial activity against the human filarial worm *B. malayi* in Mastomys coucha rats. The findings thus provide a new lead for development of a macrofilaricidal drug from ajwain.

The emerging trends of multidrug resistance among several groups of micro-organisms against different classes of antibiotics led different researchers to develop efficient drugs from plant sources to counter multidrug resistant strains. Khan *et al.* (2010c) investigated different solvent extracts of ajwain to determine the efficacy against multidrug resistant microbes. The petroleum ether fraction (least MIC- 625 microg/ml) showed best activity against multidrug resistant strains of *C. glabrata, E. coli* and reference strains of *S. mutans* and *S. bovis* when compared to its other fractions. As mentioned earlier, Khan *et al.* (2010d) reported a novel compound, a naphthalene derivative, isolated first time from ajwain seeds with anti-biofilm activity against *S. mutans.*

Asafoetida (*Ferula assafoetida*)

Asafoetida has a broad range of uses in traditional medicine as an anitimicrobial agent with well documented uses for treating chronic bronchitis and whooping cough, as well as reducing flatulence (Srinivasan, 2005).

Asafoetida was used in 1918 to fight the Spanish influenza pandemic. In 2009, scientists at the Kaohsiung Medical University in Taiwan reported that the roots of Asafoetida produce natural antiviral drug compounds that kill the swine flu virus, H1N1. In an article published in the American Chemical Society's Journal of Natural Products, the researchers said that the compounds "may serve as promising lead components for new drug development" against this type of flu (Lee *et al.*, 2009).

The oleo-gum-resin from asafetida has been known to possess antifungal, anti-diabetic, anti-inflammatory, anti-mutagenic and anti-viral activities. Asafoetida decreased counts and viability of all tested isolates of *Blastocystis* sp. subtype 3 which was confirmed by microscopy. The degree of the inhibitory effect was dependent on the concentration, form, as well as the time of incubation with asafetida extracts. The lowest concentrations of 16 and 40 mg/ml, of asafetida powder and oil respectively caused 100 per cent inhibition of *Blastocystis* growth and 100 per cent inhibition of multiplication (El Deeb *et al.*, 2012).

Asafoetida had a potent anti-parasitic effect on *T. vaginalis* compared to metronidazole, thus, worth further investigation on its applicability in treatment of parasitic infections (Ramadan and Khadrawy, 2003).

A highly significant statistical difference was noticed in the antimicrobial effect of different forms of asafoetida (oil-form and a powder-form in different concentrations) administered to experimentally infected mice with *S. mansoni,* with regard to the mean worm burden and tissue egg count as confirmed histo-pathologically and by ultra-structural profile alteration (Ramadan *et al.*, 2004).

Cinnamon (*Cinnamomon zeylanicun*)

The essential oil of cinnamon has anitimicrobial properties (Lopez *et al.*, 2005). Cinnamon bark is also used extensively as an anitimicrobial material and thus can be used as food preservative. Both cinnamaldehyde and cinnamon oil vapors are potent anti-fungal compounds (Singh *et al.*, 1995). Preliminary human studies confirmed this effect in a clinical trial with AIDS patients suffering from oral candida (thrush) infections that improved with topical application of cinnamon oil (Quale *et al.*, 1996). Antibacterial actions have also been demonstrated for cinnamon (Azumi *et al.*, 1997).

Meades *et al.* (2010) studied the action of cinnamon oil, its major component, trans-cinnamaldehyde, and an analogue, 4-hydroxy-3-methoxy-trans-cinnamaldehyde against bacterial acetyl-CoA carboxylase in an attempt to elucidate and confirm the mechanism of action. It was observed that the carboxyltransferase component of *E. Coli*, acetyl-CoA carboxylase was inhibited, but the activity of the biotin carboxylase component was not affected. The inhibition patterns indicated that these products bound to the biotin binding site of carboxyltransferase with Trans-cinnamaldehyde.

Dugoua *et al.* (2007) on the basis of review of available literature, found good scientific evidence that some species of cinnamon are not effective at eradicating *H. pylori* infection. Common cinnamon showed weak to very weak evidence of efficacy in treating oral candidiasis in HIV patients and chronic salmonellosis. In a 2000 study published in The Indian Journal of Medical Research, it was shown that 16 of the 69 plant species screened were effective against HIV-1 and 4 were against both HIV-1 and HIV-2. *Cinnamomum cassia* (bark) and *Cardiospermum helicacabum* (shoot + fruit) were the most effective extracts against HIV-1 and HIV-2 respectively (Premanathan *et al.*, 2000).

Cloves (*Syzygium aromaticum*)

The anitimicrobial activity of clove is attributable to eugenol, oleic acids and lipids found in its essential oils (Hammer *et al.*, 1999). The biological activity of *Eugenia caryophyllata* has been investigated on several pathogenic and spoilage microorganisms and parasites, *Herpes simplex* and *hepatitis* C viruses and also the anitimicrobial activity against a large number of multi-resistant *Staphylococcus* species isolated from dialysis biomaterials (Chaieb *et al.*, 2007 a). Cloves displayed an important antifungal effect against the tested 53 human pathogenic yeasts using a disc paper diffusion method. It is clear that clove oil shows powerful anti-fungal activity (Chaieb *et al.*, 2007 b). The essential oil of cloves and Eugenol showed inhibitory activity against all the tested *Candida*, and *Aspergillus*. Clove oil and eugenol also caused a considerable reduction in the quantity of ergosterol, a specific fungal cell membrane component. Nzeako *et al.* (2006) showed that the place of cultivation has no effect on clove's anitimicrobial activity as there was no significant difference in antimicrobial activity between cloves obtained from Sri Lanka or Zanzibar or thyme obtained from Iran or Oman.

Clove essential oil and eugenol, the antifungal constituent of clove oil presented prominent anti-fungal action with MIC of 1 per cent and 4 per cent, respectively on fungal strains isolated from onychomycosis (Gayoso *et al.*, 2005). Eugenol was the most effective antifungal agent against the dermatophytes *T. mentagrophytes* and *M. canis*, *T. rubrum*, *E. floccosum*, and *M. gypseum* (Park *et al.*, 2007).

The activities of clove oil against the dermatophytes tested were highest at a concentration of 0.2 mg/ml, with an effectiveness of more than 60 per cent hyphal growth completely inhibited in *T. mentagrophytes*, *T. rubrum*, and *M. gypseum*.

Germ tube formation by *Candida albicans* was almost completely inhibited by clove oil and eugenol concentrations below the MIC values (Pinto *et al.*, 2009). Presence of anti- quorum sensing (QS) activity in clove oil and other essential oils has indicated new anti-infective activity. The identification of anti-QS phytoconstituents is needed to assess the mechanism of action against both *C. violaceum* and *P. aeruginosa*. Because of its anti-QS activity, clove bud essential oil might be important in reducing virulence and pathogenicity of drug-resistant bacteria *in vivo* (Khan *et al.*, 2009).

The anti-bacterial activity of the clove oil and its major compounds, eugenol and β-caryophyllene were compared, the same was higher for clove oil than β-caryophyllene but was similar to eugenol against all tested oral bacteria suggesting that the clove oil and eugenol could be employed as a natural anti-bacterial agent against cariogenic and periodontopathogenic bacteria (Moon *et al.*, 2011).

The anitimicrobial activity of combinations of the two essential oils from clove and rosemary indicated their additive, synergistic or antagonistic effects against individual micro-organisms. The time-kill curves of clove and rosemary essential oils towards *Staphylococcus epidermidis, Escherichia coli* and *Candida albicans* showed clearly the bactericidal and fungicidal processes (Fu *et al.*, 2007). Cinnamon oil and clove oil strongly inhibited the growth of *E. coli* O157:H7 at neutral and acidic pH. A synergistic effect between the essential oils and the lower pH of the growth medium was evident by consistently lower MICs at pH 4.5. The addition of either essential oil (cinnamon and clove oils at 0.01 per cent vol/vol) resulted in lower D-values of *E. coli* O157:H7 than those for cider alone, suggesting a synergistic effect and the potential efficacy of a mild heat treatment for apple cider (Knight and McKellar, 2007).

Mixtures of cinnamon and clove oils were tested for inhibitory activity against important spoilage micro-organisms of intermediate moisture foods. *Aspergillus flavus* and *Eurotium sp*. proved to be the most resistant micro-organisms out of four fungal species (*A. flavus, P. roqueforti, M. plumbeus* and *Eurotium* sp.). Cinnamon and clove oil added between 1000 and 4000 microL at a ratio of 1:1 were tested for minimum inhibitory volume (MIV) against molds and four yeasts species (*D. hansenii, P. membranaefaciens, Z. rouxii* and *C. lipolytica*). The gas phase above 1000 microL of the oil mixture inhibited growth of *C. lipolytica* and *P. membranaefaciens*; 2000 microL inhibited growth of A. flavus, *P. roqueforti, M. plumbeus*, Eurotium sp., *D. hansenii*, and *Z. rouxii*, while inhibition of *A. flavus* required the addition of 4000 microL. Higher ratios of cinnamon oil/clove oil were more effective for inhibiting the growth of *A. flavus* (Matan *et al.*, 2006).

Oregano and clove oils have been shown to possess a broad spectrum of anitimicrobial activity. Chami *et al.* (2005) observed these two essential oils to effect yeast cell lysis by the release of substances absorbing at 260 nm. In addition, scanning electron microscopy analyses revealed that the surface of treated cells by oregano and clove oils was significantly damaged.

Eugenol from clove inactivated *S. typhi* within 60 min exposure. The chemo-attractant property of eugenol combined with the observed high anti-bacterial activity at alkaline pH favors the fact that the compound can work more efficiently when given *in vivo*. Eugenol increased the permeability of the membrane and thus Devi *et al.* (2010) confirmed the disruptive action of eugenol on cytoplasmic membrane.

The anitimicrobial activities of allspice, cinnamon, and clove bud oils in apple puree film-forming solutions formulated into edible films at 0.5 per cent to 3 per cent (w/w) concentrations showed higher influence against *L. monocytogenes* than against the *S. enterica*. The antimicrobial activities against the 3 pathogens, *E. coli* O157:H7, *S. enterica*, and *L. monocytogenes* were in the following order: cinnamon oil > clove bud oil > allspice oil (Du *et al.*, 2009a; b).

Rattanachaikunsopon and Phumkhachorn (2009) indicated that clove oil has a higher protective effect on experimental *L. garvieae* infection in tilapia and better potential to replace antibiotics for controlling the disease when compared to cinnamon, ginger and holy basil oils.

C. albicans was found to be the most susceptible organism to the influence of thyme and clove oil with concentration end-points of 0.1 per cent (1024) and 0.2 per cent (512) respectively. Clove water extract showed inhibitions with all the organisms tested except with *S. pyogenes*, *B. fragilis* and *C. albicans* (Hili *et al.*, 1997; Panizzi *et al.*, 1993; Piccaglia *et al.*, 1993).

An extract from the flower buds of *E. caryophyllus* (Spreng.) and the essential oil, eugenol, were evaluated by Tragoolpua and Jatisatienr (2007) for their anti-*Herpes simplex* virus properties on standard HSV-1(F), standard HSV-2(G) and ten HSV isolates. The plaque reduction assay showed that HSV-1(F), HSV-2(G), two HSV-1 isolates (2, 30) and four HSV-2 isolates (1, 2, 3, 21) were inhibited by *E. caryophyllus*. Only HSV-1 isolates 1 and 30 were inhibited by eugenol. The anti-HSV activity of eugenol against HSV-1(F) and HSV isolates was stronger than with the *E. caryophyllus* crude extract. However, the percentage inhibition was more pronounced on HSV-1(F) than on HSV-2(G). Moreover, HSV-1(1) and HSV-2(1, 32) could not replicate when eugenol was included in the assay.

Essential oils of clove, basil and the oil constituents (eugenol and linalool) inhibited parasite growth, with clove essential being the most effective one. Ultrastructural alterations were observed mainly in the nucleus (Santoro *et al.*, 2007). Essential oil of clove, dispersed (0.4 per cent v/v) in a concentrated sugar solution, had a marked germicidal effect against various bacteria *e.g. C. albicans. S. aureus* (five strains), *K. pneumoniae*, *P. aeruginosa*, *C. perfringens*, *E. coli* and *C. albicans* inoculated in laboratory broth supplemented with 63 per cent (v/w) of sugar, and containing 0.4 per cent (v/w) of essential oil of clove were killed. The concentrated sugar solution provided a good vehicle for obtaining an oil dispersion that is relatively stable for certain practical applications (Briozzo *et al.*, 1989).

Clove oil was found to possess strong antifungal activity against opportunistic fungal pathogens such as *C. albicans*, *C. neoformans*, *A. fumigatus*, etc. The oil was found to be extremely successful in the treatment of experimental murine vaginitis in model animals. On evaluating various formulations, topical administration of the liposomized clove oil was found to be most effective against treatment of vaginal candidiasis (Ahmad *et al.*, 2005).

Role in Food Preservation

Mycelial growth of the four test pathogens namely *P. vagabunda, P. expansum, B. cinerea* and *M. fructigena* was completely inhibited when treated with 150 microl l(-1) of volatile eugenol whether at 4 or 20° C. Ethoxylate- and Tween 80-eugenol formulations applied at room temperature were ineffective in reducing disease incidence. When heated to 50° C, both formulations induced phytotoxicity on apple surface and caused cuticle damages as revealed by scanning electronic microscopic observations. The application of heated lecithin-formulated eugenol could become a successful alternative to the traditional fungicides used in postharvest disease management of apple fruit (Amiri *et al.*, 2008).

Cava *et al.* (2007) indicated the possibility of using three essential oils (EOs) *i.e.* the oil of the cinnamon bark, clove and cinnamon leaf in milk beverages as natural anitimicrobials, especially because milk beverages flavored with cinnamon and clove are consumed worldwide and have been receiving high popularity in recent years. A crude methonolic extract of clove exhibited preferential growth-inhibitory activity against Gram-negative anaerobic periodontal oral pathogens, including *P. gingivalis* and *P. intermedia*. Also the flavones, kaempferol and myricetin, isolated from cloves showed potent growth-inhibitory activity against the periodontal pathogens *P. gingivalis* and *P. intermedia* (Cai and Wu, 1996).

Clove oil was found to be fungistatic and fungicidal against *L. theobromae, C. musae* and *F. proliferatum*, (responsible for crown rot in banana) and anthracnose and crown rot pathogens within a range of 0.03-0.11 per cent (v/v). It was therefore suggested that clove essential oil could be used as an alternative post-harvest treatments which is chemically safe and acceptable to consumers. Where as Benomyl (Benlate), which is currently used to manage fungal pathogens in banana, can cause adverse health effects (Ranasinghe *et al.*, 2002).

But no anitimicrobial effect of 1 per cent (w/w) clove powder on *L. monocytogenes* was observed in cheese after 1 or 2 weeks either at lower or higher temperature (Leuschner and Ielsh, 2003). Hence, the antimicrobial effect of cloves could be organism specific.

Coriander Leaves/Seeds (*Coriandrum sativum*)

Chemicals derived from coriander leaves were found to have antibacterial activity against *S. choleraesuis*. Coriander essential oil also showed a delay in *E. coli* growth, suggesting possible agricultural anti-bacterial applications (Kubo *et al.*, 2004).

Cumin Seeds (*Cuminum cyminum*)

It is encourageing that there is currently a quest for safe and effective anitimicrobial agents.

The anti-bacterial activity of *C. cyminum* essential oil is perhaps attributable to the high levels of cuminaldehyde (16.1 per cent), followed by *a*-pinene (11.4 per cent). (Iacobellis *et al.*, 2005; Helander *et al.*, 1998). Fabio *et al.* (2007) reported the zone diameter of inhibition (ZDI) of 24 and 18 mm, respectively for *C. zeylanicum* and *S aromaticum* against *S. aureus*. Agaoglu *et al.* (2007) also reported *C. zeylanicum* as the most effective spice against *S. aureus*.

Cumin seeds showed excellent *in vitro* anti-bacterial activity against methicillin-resistant *S. aureus* (MRSA). The *C. cyminum* exhibited bactericidal activity at a concentration of 300 μg/ml, hence, could be a potential anti- MRSA agent. It will also be of great benefit in combating antibiotic resistance of *S. aureus* (Mandal *et al.*, 2011).

Recently, many anitimicrobial/resistant organisms such as *K. pneumoniae* (Maroncle *et al.*, 2002) are emerging. *K. pneumoniae* is an important Gram-negative pathogen, usually associated with nosocomially acquired infections in addition to its involvement in urinary tract infections, pneumonia, bacteremia, septicemia, and infections of surgical wounds. Biofilm growth enhances its resistance to antibiotic therapies, as well as host defense mechanisms (Boddicker *et al.*, 2006). Derakhshan *et al.* (2008) reported that the essential oil of cumin seeds has a significant anti-bacterial activity against *K. pneumoniae in vitro*. The essential oil decreased biofilm formation and enhanced the activity of the ciprofloxacin disk. The incubation of the R-plasmid DNA with essential oil could not induce plasmid DNA degradation. The results of this study by Derakhshan *et al.* (2010) suggest the potential use of cumin seed essential oil against *K. pneumoniae in vitro* while suggesting its potential contribution to the *in vivo* efficacy. The mechanism by which the cumin seed essential oil acts to enhance the activity of ciprofloxacin against *K. pneumoniae*, as indicated by an increased inhibition zone diameter, is not known; but some cell wall damage or alteration in the outer membrane proteins may be caused by the cumin seed essential oil, which sensitizes cells to ciprofloxacin as well as resists cells to trimethoprim-sulfamethoxazole (Gutmann *et al.*, 1985; Huovinen, 1987). The enhancement of anti-bacterial efficacy of ciprofloxacin by the essential oil is significant.

C. cyminum essential oil may be considered as an interesting source of anti-bacterial, anti-fungal and anti-oxidant components used as potent agents in food preservation and for therapeutic or nutraceutical industries (Hajlaoui *et al.*, 2010). The seed essential oil in combination with nisin can inhibit growth of food-borne pathogens in food. Cumin seed showed the most bactericidal effects on *B. cereus* at 8°C. Ultrastructural studies of vegetative cells confirmed the synergistic destructive effects of the essential oil and nisin on membrane and utilization ofcell wall of the bacteria (Pajohi *et al.*, 2011). The cumin seed oil exhibited anti-bacterial and antifungal activities (Romagnoli *et al.*, 2010) with a high effectiveness against *Vibrio* spp. strains with a diameter of inhibition zones growth ranging from 11 to 23 mm, and MIC and MBC values ranging from (0.078-0.31 mg/ml) to (0.31-1.25mg/ml), respectively.

Keskin and Toroglu (2011) studied the anitimicrobial activity of cumin seed and the inhibition zone was found to be 7-15 mm 30microl (-1). All cumin oils and cuminic aldehyde exhibited a considerable inhibitory effect against all the organisms tested, (Gram-positive and Gram-negative bacteria isolated from different sources of food (pork fillet, minced meat and sausages) except *Pseudomonas* spp. (Wanner *et al.*, 2010). According to Khosravi *et al.* (2011) the essential oil of *C. cyminum*, could be used as natural inhibitor in foods at low concentrations to protect from fungal and toxin contaminations by *A. parasiticus*.

The anti-bacterial activity of 1-(2-Ethyl, 6-Heptyl) Phenol (EHP) was studied against four Gram-negative and four Gram-positive bacterial pathogens. It was more effective against the Gram negative than Gram positive bacteria. The most sensitive bacterial strain was *S. aureus* where an inhibition zone of 0.8, 1.6, 2.8, and 3.5 cm was obtained when applying EHP at concentrations of 1, 2.5, 5.0, and 1.0 µg/ml respectively. *S. aureus* was followed by *B. subtilis, S. pneumoniae* and *B. thuringiensis*. The largest zone of inhibition in Gram-negative bacteria was observed against *E. coli*; where, 1.5 and 1.8 cm inhibition diameters were reported at 5 and 10 µg/ml EHP concentration respectively. *E. coli* was followed by *S. typhi, S. marcescens* and least for *P. aeruginosa* (Mekawey *et al.*, 2009). Similar results were seen in another study where cumin was more effective against the Gram positive bacteria as compared to the Gram negative bacteria. Amongst the Gram negative bacteria, the anitimicrobial activity of cumin was seen in case of *E.coli* and not much against any other strain. (Sheikh *et al.*, 2010)

In another study carried out by Chaudhary and Tariq (2008) also cumin was found to be more effective against the gram negative bacteria as compared to the Gram positive bacteria and the largest inhibitory zone was found against *E. coli* (23.8mm ± 1.2SD). The aqueous decoction of cumin also exhibited significant inhibitory activity against *M. roseus* (20.8mm ± 2.3SD), *P. shigelloides* (18.5mm ± 8.3SD), *Alcaligenes spp.* (17.1mm ± 2.9SD), *Citrobacter spp.* (16.2mm ± 0.5SD), *K. pneumoniae* (15.9mm ± 0.8SD), *A. hydrophila* (15.8mm ± 1.3SD), *K. ozaenae* (15.2mm ± 1.3SD), *P. aeruginosa* (12.3mm ± 3.3SD), *E. aerogenes* (12.0mm ± 0.1SD) and *S. aureus* (8.9mm ± 5.6SD).

Cumin oil was also found to be effective against various fungal organisms such as *A.flavus, C.albicans etc.* responsible for food spoilage. Hajlaoui *et al.* (2010) in the light of their findings suggested that *C. cyminum* essential oil may be considered as a source of anti-bacterial, anti-fungal and anti-oxidant components to be potent agents in food preservation and for therapeutic or nutraceutical industries.

Garlic (*Allium sativum*)

Louis Pasteur in 1858, observed garlic's anti-bacterial activity. It was used as an antiseptic to prevent gangrene during World War I and World War II (Ellen, 2005). It is an effective anitimicrobial agent against bacterial, viral, fungal, protozoal and parasitic infections. While enhancing the immune system, garlic also showed anti-tumoral and anti-oxidant features (Ayaz and Alpsoy, 2007; Harris *et al.*, 2001). It may also play an important role in the ecological control of pathogenic micro-organisms in nature (Adetumbi and Lau, 1983). Garlic is renowned for the compound allicin, which exerts anti-bacterial and anti-fungal effects. It is effective in curing common diseases such as dysentery, diarrhea, tuberculosis etc. Garlic oil was found to have significant inhibition of microbial growth on fresh-cut tomatoes.

Garlic extract showed greater activity against Gram-positive organisms, Gram-negative organisms and fungi as compared to the extract of onion (Elnima *et al.*, 1983). Thirty strains of mycobacteria, consisting of 17 species, were inhibited by various concentrations of garlic extract incorporated in Middlebrook 7H10 agar. The concentration required ranged from 1.34 mg/ml to 3.35 mg/ml of media. Six strains of *M. tuberculosis* required a mean inhibitory concentration of 1.67 mg/ml of media (Delaha and Garagusi, 1985).

The anti-fungal activity of six fractions derived from garlic in an *in vitro* system showed that Ajoene had the strongest activity among all other fractions. The growth of both *A. niger* and *C. albicans* was inhibited by ajoene at less than 20 µg/ml. (Yoshida *et al.*, 1987).

Steroid saponins have been found to have some interesting biological and pharmacologic activities including anti-fungal, anti-bacterial, anti-inflammatory and hypo-cholesteremic influences (Lacaille-Dubois and Wagner, 1996). Plants of the genus *Allium* are known for their production of steroid saponins, as well as organosulfur compounds (Kravets *et al.*, 1990). The genuine saponin proto-eruboside-B was inactive against *C. albicans.* Interestingly, when raw garlic bulbs are crushed, the enzymatic conversion of compound 1 into compound 2 by ß-glucosidase is similar to the conversion of alliin into allicin by alliinase, and both end-products exhibit anti-fungal properties (Matsuura, 2001).

Garlic destroys the micro-organisms *E. coli* and *S. albus*. However, the antibacterial effect of garlic decreases after a 30-minute exposure to heat. In addition to garlic, members of the *Allium* genus such as onions, leeks, shallots and chives show antibiotic effects. Bachrach *et al.* (2011) demonstrated that planktonic growth of the tested Gram-negative periopathogenic species *Aggregatibacter actinomycetemcomitans* and *Fusobacterium nucleatum* was inhibited by a minimum allicin concentration of 300 µg/mL. *P. gingivalis*, an anaerobic, Gram-negative pathogen and the bacterium most associated with chronic periodontitis, demonstrated the lowest sensitivity to allicin (2,400 µg/mL). A gingipain-inactivated mutant demonstrated high sensitivity to allicin (<300 µg/mL), revealing that gingipains confer resistance to allicin.

Fresh extract of garlic showed greater anitimicrobial activity as compared to similar extracts of onion (Amin and Kapadnis, 2005; Elnima *et al.*, 1983). At comparable concentrations, freshly reconstituted dehydrated onion and garlic powders exhibited that growing cultures of *E. coli* were as susceptible to garlic, but apparently more resistant to onion, than were those of *S. typhimurium* (Johnson and Vaught, 1969).

Although garlic has been used for its medicinal properties for thousands of years, investigations into its mode of action are relatively recent. Garlic showed anitimicrobial activity against *Mutans streptococci* and other oral microorganisms, and hence, might be an alternative to chlorhexidine (Groppo *et al.*, 2002).

Periodontal disease is the collective term given to a variety of inflammatory conditions in the tissue that supports and secures the teeth to the jawbone. The inflammatory response is to bacterial products and/or bacteria that enter the tissue from the dental plaque. The dental plaque is a complex microbial community containing over 190 different taxa that exist on the tooth surfaces. In periodontitis the majority of the plaque bacteria are anaerobes including the black pigmented bacteroides species and motile forms such as spirochetes.

Garlic extract is effective against *S. mutans* when tested both *in vitro* and *in vivo* (Chavan *et al.*, 2010). Thus garlic extract mouth rinse might be used as an effective remedy in the prevention of dental caries. According to Bakri and Douglas (2005), Time-kill curves for *S. mutans* and *P. ginigvalis*, showed that killing of the latter started almost immediately, whereas there was a delay before *S. mutans* was killed. The garlic extract also inhibited the trypsin-like and total protease activity of *P. gingivalis* by 92.7 per cent and 94.88 per cent, respectively indicating that garlic extract inhibits the growth of oral pathogens and certain proteases and so may have therapeutic value, particularly for periodontitis. All isolates, MDR and non-MDR of *S. mutans* were sensitive to garlic extract. Considering these beneficial effects of garlic, mouthwashes or toothpastes containing optimum concentration of garlic extract could be used for prevention of dental caries (Fani *et al.*, 2007). *In vitro* study by Groppo *et al.* (2007) revealed the Minimum inhibitory concentration ranged from 0.5 to 32.0 mg ml (-1) for White garlic extract and from 8 to 64.0 mg ml (-1) for Purple garlic. Minimum bactericidal concentration ranged from 1.0 to 128.0 ml (-1) and from 8.0 to 128.0 ml (-1) regarding white and purple garlic respectively. *In vivo* experiment showed that 2.5 per cent garlic mouthwash solution had good antimicrobial activity against mutans streptococci and oral microorganisms. The reduced salivary levels of streptococci were maintained even after 2 weeks after mouthwash discontinued.

There is a need for alternate solutions to decrease the burden of drug resistance and cost in the management of diseases. The use of garlic against emergence of multi-drug resistant (MDR) -TB may be of great importance regarding public health. The minimum inhibitory concentration of garlic extract ranged from 1 to 3 mg/ml; showed inhibitory effects against both non-MDR and MDR M. tuberculosis isolates (Hannan *et al.*, 2011).

Helicobacter pylori is a bacterium implicated in the etiology of stomach cancer and ulcers. The incidence of stomach cancer is lower in populations with a high intake of allium vegetables, probably due to the sensitivity of *H. pylori* to garlic (Sivam *et al.*, 1997). Sivam (2001) has demonstrated *in vitro* that *H.pylori*, including the antibiotic-resistant strains is susceptible to garlic extract at a fairly moderate concentration.

Aqueous extract of garlic and onion showed significant growth inhibition against Gram-positive organisms, Gram-negative organisms and fungi. The activity of the garlic extract on the mouth flora of volunteers was investigated by Elnima *et al.* (1983) and they observed a drastic reduction in the number of oral bacteria by a mouth wash containing 10 per cent garlic in quarter Ringer solution.

In addition to its health benefits in humans, garlic has also been found to be an efficient antimicrobial agent in other species. The protozoan parasite *Eimeria* causes coccidiosis which leads to enormous economic losses particularly in poultry farms. Toulah and Al-Rawi (2007) found that treatment of *E. stiedae* in infected garlic resulted in regaining of normalcy in the liver, where as the untreated group continued to show histopathological alterations in liver tissue, marked cytoplasmic vacuolations in hepatocytes with clear signs of karyolysis, and dilatation of sinusoids with increase in Kupffer cells. Dkhil *et al.* (2011) reported that garlic counteracted the *E. papillata*-

induced loss of glutathione and the activities of catalase and superoxide dismutase and significantly attenuated inflammation and injury of the liver induced by the infection.

Spironucleus is a genus of small, flagellated parasites, many of which can infect a wide range of vertebrates and are a significant problem in aquaculture. Following the ban on the use of metronidazole in edible fish due to toxicity problems, no satisfactory chemotherapies for the treatment of spironucleosis are currently available. Millet *et al.* (2011) demonstrated that of all the allium-derived compounds from garlic, the ajoene-free mixture of dithiins and thiosulfinates was the most effective with a minimum inhibitory concentration (MIC) of 107 μg/ml(-1) and an inhibitory concentration at 50 per cent (IC(50 per cent)) of 58 μg ml(-1). These concentrations are much higher than those reported to be required for the inhibition of most bacteria, protozoa and fungi previously investigated, indicating an unusual level of tolerance for allium-derived products in *S. vortens*.

Onion (*Allium cepa*)

Onion is an exceptionally strong antibiotic and antiseptic food. It was used to treat infections in wounded Russian soldiers during World War II. Latest researches have confirmed the bactericidal properties of onion. A significant growth inhibition was shown in most of the organisms, tested (Gram-positive organisms, Gram-negative organisms and fungi) at random by garlic and onion (Elnima *et al.*, 1983).

Cholera is a major public health problem in developing countries of the world. The spread of microbial drug resistance is a global public health challenge that results in increased illness and death rate. Bacterial resistance, lack of surveillance data and proper microbiological facilities are major problems regarding diagnosis of cholera. Thirty-three clinical isolates of *Vibrio cholerae* tested were sensitive to onion (*Allium cepa*) extracts of two types (purple and yellow). Purple type of extract had MIC range of 19.2-21.6 mg/ml. The extract of yellow type onion had an MIC range of 66-68.4 mg/ml (Hannan *et al.*, 2010).

Ginger

Ginger has been used for centuries to treat many infectious diseases like cholera, diarrhoea and chest congestion. Its use has been found especially effective in whooping cough. A teaspoon of the fresh ginger juice, mixed with a cup of fenugreek decoction and honey to taste, acts as an expectorant and diaplioretic in this disease. Its gingerol-related components have been reported to possess antimicrobial and anti-fungal properties. Park *et al.* (2008) revealed that the ethanol and n-hexane extracts of ginger exhibited anti-bacterial activities against three anaerobic Gram-negative bacteria, *P. gingivalis, P. endodontalis* and *P. intermedia*, causing periodontal diseases. Two highly alkylated gingerols, [10]-gingerol and [12]-gingerol effectively inhibited the growth of these oral pathogens at a minimum inhibitory concentration (MIC) range of 6-30 μg/ml. These ginger compounds also killed the oral pathogens at a minimum bactericidal concentration (MBC) range of 4-20 μg/ml.

Throat swabs were collected from 333 individuals with running nostrils, cough and/or catarrh and *S. aureus, S. pyogenes, S.pneumoniae* and *H. influenzae* were isolated from the specimens using standard microbiological procedures. Ginger extracts exhibited anti-bacterial activity against the pathogens. The Minimum Inhibitory Concentration ranged from 0.0003 to 0.7 μg/ml while Minimum Bactericidal Concentration ranged from 0.1.35 μg/ml to 2.04 μg/ml (Akoachere *et al.*, 2002).

Earlier Goto *et al.* (1990) reported that an extract from *Zingiber officinale*, traditionally eaten along with raw fish and used in traditional Chinese medicine, effectively destroyed Anisakis larvae *in vitro*. Further experiments showed that [6]-Shogaol and [6]-gingerol, known neutral components of ginger, could kill Anisakis larvae at a minimal effective dose of 62.5 and 250 μg/ml, respectively.

Martins *et al.* (2001) reported that the essential oils of ginger showed anitimicrobial activity against all Gram-positive and Gram-negative bacteria tested, as well as against yeasts and filamentous fungi, using the agar diffusion method. Also, Norajit *et al.* (2007) found the essential oil of ginger extracted by hydrodistillation had the highest efficiency against three positive strains of bacteria (*S. aureus, B. cereus* and *L. monocytogenes*), with a minimum concentration to inhibit *B. cereus* and *L. monocytogenes* of 6.25 mg/mL.

Mango-ginger (*Curcuma amada*) is very similar to ginger with a raw mango taste. Difurocumenonol, a compound isolated and purified from mango-ginger extracts demonstrated high antibacterial activity against gram-negative and gram-positive bacteria. This novel compound can be used as food preservative to control the growth of food-borne pathogens and as a source of mango flavor in food products (Policegoudra *et al.*, 2007).

Mustard Seeds

An 18.9 kDa anti-fungal protein designated juncin was isolated from seeds of the Japanese takana (*Brassica juncea* var. integrifolia) by Ye and Ng (2009). The protein exhibited antifungal activity toward the phytopathogens *F. oxysporum, H. maydis,* and *M. arachidicola* with IC-50 values of 13.5, 27, and 10 μM, respectively. It inhibited the proliferation of hepatoma (HepG2) and breast cancer (MCF7) cells with IC(50) values of 5.6 and 6.4 μM, respecitvely, and the activity of HIV-1 reverse transcriptase with an IC(50) of 4.5 μM. Its N-terminal sequence differed from those of anti-fungal proteins of *Brassica campestris* and *Brassica alboglabra*.

Luciano *et al.* (2011) found the autoclaved mustard powder to result in more rapid bactericidal action against *E. coli*, yielding a >5 log CFU/g reduction in 18 days. This effect may have been due to the formation and/or release of anitimicrobial substances from mustard by the autoclave treatment. Hence, autoclaved mustard powder could potentially solve an important challenge faced by the meat industry in manufacturing safe dry fermented sausages.

Compounds generated by the enzymatic hydrolysis of glucosinolates naturally present in mustard powder are potently bactericidal against *E. coli*. Because *E. coli* can survive the dry fermented sausage manufacturing process, 2, 4, and 6 per cent (wt/wt) heated mustard powder or 6 per cent (wt/wt) deheated (cold) mustard powder were added to dry sausage batter inoculated with *E. coli* at about 7 log CFU/g to evaluate the antimicrobial effectiveness of the powders. The 6 per cent deheated mustard powder treatment provided the most rapid reductions of *E. coli* (yielding <0.20 log CFU/g after 24 days) by an unknown mechanism and was the least detrimental ($P < 0.05$) to sausage texture (Graumann and Holley, 2008).

An anitimicrobial edible film was developed from defatted mustard meal (*Sinapis alba*) (DMM), a byproduct from the bio-fuel industry, without incorporating external antimicrobials. The film-coating retarded the growth of *L. monocytogenes* in smoked salmon at 5, 10, and 15°C and the anitimicrobial effect during storage was more noticeable when the coating was applied before inoculation. The tensile strength, percentage elongation, solubility in water cxu, and water vapor permeability of the anitimicrobial film were 2.44 ± 0.19 MPa, 6.40 ± 1.13 per cent, 3.19 ± 0.90 per cent, and 3.18 ± 0.63 gmm/kPa hm(2), respectively. Thus, the antimicrobial DMM films have been shown to have potential as food wraps or coatings to control the growth of *L. monocytogenes* (Lee *et al.*, 2012).

Turmeric

Recently, some remarkable studies have been conducted on the effects of curcumin (Turmeric), the phenolic form of *Curcuma longa* plant, on virulence factors of *P.aeruginosa*. Karaman *et al.* (2013) used two strains of *P.aeruginosa* isolated from deep oropharyngeal swab from two cystic fibrosis patients to assess the effect of curcumin on biofilm formation. No increase in biofilm optical density was observed, thus supporting the promising inhibitory effect of curcumin on *P. aeruginosa* biofilms.

Lee *et al.* (2011) found that turmeric essential oil inhibited the growth and acid production of *S. mutans* at concentrations from 0.5 to 4 mg/mL. The essential oil also exhibited significant inhibition of *S. mutans* adherence to saliva-coated hydroxyapatite beads at concentrations higher than 0.5 mg/mL. The minimum inhibitory concentration (MIC) at which curcumin completely inhibited bacterial growth was 128 μg/mL. The addition of curcumin below the MIC diminished bacterial adherence onto both collagen- and fibronectin-coated glass surfaces and human tooth surfaces. It appears that the anti-adhesive effect of curcumin against *S. mutans* is mediated through collagen and fibronectin. These results support the widespread use of curcumin as a food-based anitimicrobial agent (Song *et al.*, 2011).

Dermal application of turmeric oil on the 7th day following dermatophytosis induction with *T. rubrum*, resulted in an improvement in infective skin lesions with in 2-5 days and the lesions disappeared 6-7 days after the application (Apisariyakul *et al.*, 1995). The anti-fungal activity of the 2 fractions of turmeric oil when tested against *A. flavus*, *A. parasiticus*, *F. moniliforme* and *P. digitatum* showed the fration II with turmerone and curlone to be more active (Negi *et al.*, 1999; Jayaprakasha *et al.*, 2001). Turmeric essential oil and the curcumin standard interfered with mycotoxin production. Both the essential oil and curcumin significantly inhibited the production of aflatoxins; the 0.5 per cent level had greater (>96 per cent) inhibitory effect. The levels of aflatoxin B(1) production were 1.0 and 42.7 μg/mL, respectively, for the samples treated with the essential oil of C. longa and curcumin at a concentration of 0.5 per cent (Ferreira *et al.*, 2013).

A varietal difference was observed in the anitimicrobial activity of turmeric. The essential oils of *C. aeruginosa*, *C. mangga* and *Z. cassumunar* displayed varying degrees of anitimicrobial activity against all tested micro-organisms. *C. mangga* oil had the highest and most broad-spectrum activity by inhibiting all micro-organisms tested, with *C. neoformans* being the most sensitive micro-organism by having the lowest minimum inhibitory concentration and minimum fungicidal concentration values of 0.1 μL/mL. *C. aeruginosa* oil showed mild anitimicrobial activity, whereas *Z. cassumunar* had very low or weak activity against the tested microorganisms. Thus, Kamazeri *et al.* (2012) demonstrated promising antimicrobial properties of *C. mangga* and *C. aeruginosa*, which may be useful for food preservation, pharmaceutical treatment and natural therapies.

Na *et al.* (2011) reported that the cytotoxicity of *V. vulnificus* to HeLa cells was significantly inhibited by curcumin (at 10 or 30 μM). Curcumin inhibited both bacterial adhesion and RTX toxin binding to the host cells, which can be considered the major protective mechanisms against the *V. vulnificus* cytotoxicity. Curcumin may thus be an alternative anitimicrobial agent against fatal bacterial infections.

Kim *et al.* (2009) reported that turmeric extract represses *hepatitis B* virus replication by enhancing the level of p53 protein. Thus, it is confirmed that turmeric extract can be used as a safe and specific drug for patients with liver diseases caused by *hepatitis B* virus.The therapeutic effect of curcumin against *H. pylori* infection, suggests its potential as an alternative therapy, and opens the way for further studies on identification of novel antimicrobial targets of curcumin (De *et al.*, 2009). However, Koosirirat *et al.* (2010) reported that curcumin alone may have limited anti-bactericidal effect on *H. pylori*, and on the production of inflammatory cytokines revealing a need for a stronger anti microbial agent along with turmeric.

Curcumin exhibited broad spectrum inhibitory effect against all organisms. Its anti-bacterial activity was more pronounced against Gram-positive bacteria than Gram-negative bacteria. Furthermore, its anti-fungal activity is much better than anti-bacterial activity. Micro-encapsulation of curcumin extract can improve its stability, solubility and retention of antimicrobial activities, and hence can be a potential colorant and preservative in food industry (Wang *et al.*, 2009a).

Bhawana *et al.* (2011) found that the aqueous dispersion of nanocurcumin was much more effective than curcumin against *S. aureus, B. subtilis, E. coli, P. aeruginosa, P. notatum*, and *A. niger*. These results demonstrated that the water solubility and anitimicrobial activity of curcumin markedly improved by particle size reduction up to the nano range. For the selected microorganisms, the activity of nanocurcumin was more pronounced against Gram-positive bacteria than Gram-negative bacteria. Furthermore, its anti-bacterial activity was much better than anti-fungal activity. Transmission electron micrograph analysis revealed that these particles entered inside the bacterial cell by completely breaking the cell wall, leading to cell death.

Xanthorrhizol isolated from the rhizome of *Curcuma xanthorrhiza* showed (*in vitro*) activity against opportunistic filamentous fungi. The susceptibility of six species of filamentous fungi to xanthorrhizol was comparable to that of the commercial anti-fungal; amphotericin B. Xanthorrhizol also inhibited the conidial germination of all tested species. The results strongly suggested that xanthorrhizol can be developed as a natural anti-fungal agent (Rukayadi and Hwang, 2007).

Tulasi (*Ocimum sanctum*)

The increasing incidence of drug-resistant pathogens and host toxicity of existing anti-fungals attract attention toward the efficacy of natural anti-fungal products in muco-cutaneous infections and combinational therapies. The leaves of *Ocimum sanctum* are found to be antiseptic in nature. Basil essential oils and their principal constituents were found to exhibit anitimicrobial activity against a wide range of Gram-negative and Gram-positive bacteria, yeast, and mold (Suppakul *et al.*, 2003) and also possess anti-viral properties. It inhibits the growth of *E. coli*, *B. anthracis* and *M. tuberculosis*. Its anti-tubercular activity is one-tenth the potency of streptomycin and one-fourth that of isoniazid. *In vitro* studies have shown the volatile oil of basil to possess anti-bacterial, antifungal, and antiviral activity. It is also believed to act as a carminative, relieving intestinal gas, and as a mild diuretic, though these actions have yet to be definitively proven (Farnsworth and Bunyapraphatsara, 1992). The essential oils of the aerial parts of *Ocimum basilicum*, an endemic medicinal plant growing in China was found to be of potential use as an anitimicrobial agent to control *S. Enteritidis* in food (Rattanachaikunsopon and Phumkhachorn, 2010).

Preparations containing tulsi extract significantly shorten the course of illness, clinical symptoms and the biochemical parameters in patients with viral hepatitis and viral encephalitis. The anti-bacterial action of tulsi on the pathogenic organisms - *Streptococcus, Staphylococcus, P. pyrogenes, E.coli* and *Cornyebacterium* has also been proved. It has been mentioned that irrigating the wound with infusion of leaves of *Ocimum sanctum* destroys the infective organisms in the wound and hastens the healing process. Oil obtained from leaves has a bactericidal property and kills certain maggots. The leaves of the basil yield an essential oil, which contains eugenol, carvacrol, methyl eugenol and caryophyllene. It has the property of destroying bacteria and insects. Anitimicrobial activity of the essential oil has been shown against *M. tuberculosis* and *S. aureus in vitro* and other bacteria and fungi. An excellent study of oils from four types of *Ocimum species*, reported inspite of certain variation, all the oils were found to have anitimicrobial activity at fairly low dilutions.

Two concentrations of these extracts (30 mg and 60 mg) were tried against the enteric pathogens and *C. albicans* by Agar diffusion method. Wide zones of inhibition were observed at 60 mg concentration of extract. Aqeous extract showed wider zone of inhibition for *Klebisella, E. coli, Proteus* and *S. aureus* when compared to alcoholic extract which showed wider zone for *Vibrio cholerae* (Geeta *et al.*, 2001).

The essential oil obtained from *Ocimum sanctum* with a high content of methyl chavicol (44.63 per cent) and linalool (21.84 per cent) have significant anti-fungal activity against *Candida,* including azole-resistant strains, advocating further investigation for clinical applications in the treatment of fungal infections (Khan *et al.*, 2010a). In another report Khan *et al.* (2010b) found linalool to be the most active constituent of essential oil of tulasi against two of the most prevalent *Candida* species causing candidiasis, *C. albicans* and *C. tropicalis.* Inhibition of H+ extrusion appeared to be a synergistic function of the lead molecules. Similarly, at the 4 per cent concentration of tulsi extract, the widest zone of inhibition of 22 mm against *S. mutans* was observed among all the 15 different concentrations of tulsi that were investigated by Agarwal *et al.* (2010).

The selection of certain combinations of EOs could help to reduce the required amount of essential oils and consequently reduce any adverse sensory impact in food. Bassole *et al.* (2010) found that the essential oils from leaves of *Lippia multiflora, Mentha x piperita* and *Ocimum basilicum* with high phenolic contents were the most effective anitimicrobials.

Suppakul *et al.* (2003) suggested the possible future use of basil in food preservation as the active slow release anitimicrobial coating component of an active package.

Part - B
FRUITS

Amla (*Phyllanthus emblica syn. Emblica officinalis/Phyllanthus niruri*)

Saeed and Tariq (2007) demonstrated *in vitro* anti-viral and anitimicrobial properties of Amla against *E. coli, K. pneumoniae, K. ozaenae, P. mirabilis, P. aeruginosa, S. typhi, S. paratyphi A, S. paratyphi B and S. marcescens* but did not show any anti-bacterial activity against Gram-negative urinary pathogens. This may be due to higher sensitivity of Gram-positive bacteria to the oils than Gram-negative bacteria. Similarly, Liu *et al.* (2009) found the essential oil of amla to show a broad spectrum of anitimicrobial activity against all the tested micro-organisms. The essential oil obtained by supercritical fluid extraction exhibited a higher anti-fungal activity compared to the one obtained by hydro-distillation.

But Rahman *et al.* (2009) observed the chloroform soluble fraction of the methanolic extract of amla to exhibit significant anitimicrobial activity against some Gram-positive and Gram-negative pathogenic bacteria with strong cytotoxicity (LC50 of 10.257 ± 0.770 mcg/ml (-1)). It is thus shown that the chloroform soluble fraction of the ripe fruits of Amla containing alkaloids is biologically more active.

Aqueous extract of amla exhibited potent antimicrobial activity against *E. cloacae* followed by *E. coli*. The minimum inhibitory concentration of aqueous extract of amla was most active against *K. pneumonia*, whereas that of methanol extract showed maximum activity against *E. coli* (Kumar *et al.*, 2011).

Srikumar *et al.* (2007) reported that both individual and combined aqueous and ethanol extracts of Triphala which also contains amala, have anti-bacterial activity against the bacterial isolates (*P. aeruginosa, K. pneumoniae, S. sonnei, S. flexneri, S. aureus, V. cholerae, S. paratyphi-B, E. coli, E. faecalis, S. typhi*) tested.

Besides being antibacterial, amla also showed antiviral properties. Coxsackie virus B3 (CVB3) is believed to be a major contributor to viral myocarditis since virus-associated apoptosis plays a role in the pathogenesis of experimental myocarditis. Wang *et al.* (2009b) showed that Phyllaemblicin B exerts significant antiviral activities against CVB3 and thus is proved to be a potential therapeutic agent for viral myocarditis.

Berries

Phenolic compounds present in berries selectively inhibit the growth of human gastro-intestinal pathogens. Especially cranberry (*Vaccinium macrocarpon*), cloudberry, raspberry, strawberry and bilberry possess clear anitimicrobial effects against *Salmonella* and *Staphylococcus*. Complex phenolic polymers, such as ellagitannins, are strong anti-bacterial agents present in cloudberry, raspberry and strawberry. Berry phenolics seem to affect the growth of different bacterial species with different mechanisms. The most sensitive bacteria on berry phenolics were found to be *H. pylori* and *B. cereus* while *C. jejuni* and *C. albicans* were inhibited only with phenolic extracts of cloudberry, raspberry, and strawberry, (rich in ellagitannins). Cloudberry extract gave strong microbicidic effects on the basis of plate count with all the strains tested (Nohynek *et al.*, 2006).

Anitimicrobial activity of berries may also be related to their anti-adherence activity. Utilization of enzymes in berry processing increases the amount of phenolics and thereby the antimicrobial activity of berry products (Puupponen-Pimiä *et al.*, 2005 a). Phenolic compounds, especially ellagitannins, were strong inhibitory compounds against *Staphylococcus bacteria. Salmonella bacteria* were only partly inhibited by the berry phenolics, and most of the inhibition seemed to originate from other compounds, such as organic acids. *Listeria* strains were not affected by berry compounds, with the exception of cranberry (Puupponen-Pimiä *et al.*, 2005 b). Anitimicrobial activity of berries and other anthocyanin-containing fruits is likely to be caused by multiple mechanisms and synergies because they contain various compounds including anthocyanins, weak organic acids, phenolic acids, and their mixtures of different chemical forms (Cisowska *et al.*, 2011).

Proanthocyanidins with unique molecular structures have been isolated from cranberry fruit that exhibited potent bacterial anti-adhesion activity which in turn is responsible for bacteriostatic effect of cranberries (Howell, 2002). In elderly patients, cranberry consumption reduces the incidence of bacteriuria, although this is often not treated with antibiotics (Raz *et al.*, 2004).

Heinonen (2007) opines that tannin-containing berries exhibit anitimicrobial properties against pathogenic bacteria, thus offering many new applications for food industry. The phenolics in cranberries as well as cultivated and wild blueberries have gained attention. Cranberries contain 2 compounds with anti-adherence properties that prevent fimbriated *E. coli* from adhering to uroepithelial cells in the urinary tract (Raz *et al.*, 2004). Among cranberry compounds, a group of proanthocyanidins (PACs) with A-type linkages were isolated which exhibit bacterial anti-adhesion activity against uropathogenic *E. coli* strains. These PAC inhibit P-fimbriae synthesis and induce a bacterial deformation and on both antibiotic susceptible and resistant bacteria (Lavigne *et al.*, 2007) as well.

Kylli *et al.* (2010) found both wild and cultivated rowanberry phenolics exhibited a bacteriostatic effect toward *Staphylococcus aureus* and the amount of phenolic compounds decreased in all berries stored frozen for a year, but their antimicrobial activity was not influenced accordingly. Cloudberry, in particular, showed constantly strong antimicrobial activity during the storage.

Blueberries can eradicate micro-organisms for the prevention of symptomatic urinary tract infections in women (Chen *et al.*, 2010). In pre-menopausal women, of trimethoprim-sulfamethoxazole 480 mg once daily, is more effective than cranberry capsules, 500 mg twice daily, to prevent recurrent urinary tract infections, at the expense of emerging antibiotic resistance (Beerepoot *et al.*, 2011).

Guava (*Psidium guajava*)

Guava extract contain compounds that possess anti-bacterial properties suggesting that guava could be useful in controlling food borne pathogens (*L. monocytogenes, S. aureus, E. coli, S. enteritidis, V. parahaemolyticus*, and *B. cereus*), and spoilage organisms *P. aeruginosa, P. putida, A. faecalis*, and *Aeromonas hydrophila* (Hoque *et al.*, 2007).

Jamun (*Syzygium jambolanum*)

Jamun fruit pulp as well as seeds have been found to possess several health benefits and suggested as remedy for various clinical conditions.The water and methanolic extracts of *S. jambolanum* seeds showed activity against Gram positive bacteria (*B. subtilis, S. aureus*), Gram negative bacteria (*S. typhimurium, P. aeruginosa, K. pneumoniae* and *E. coli*) and fungal strains: *C. albicans, C. neoformans, A. flavus, A. fumigatus, A. niger, Rhizopus sp., T. rubrum, T. mentagrophytes* and *M. gypseum* (Chandrasekaran and Venkatesalu, 2004).

Vegetables

Broccoli (*Brassica oleracea*)

Oral consumption of broccoli sprouts was associated with eradication of *H. pylori* infection in three of nine patients (Galan *et al.*, 2004), the effect has been confirmed by many researchers later and the active components responsible for the same have been identified.

In vitro and *in vivo* experiments have shown that sulforaphane (SFN), an isothiocyanate compound found abundantly in broccoli and other cruciferous vegetables, inhibits the growth of the bacterial pathogen *H. pylori*. Among 18 sulforaphane and related compounds synthesized (6 amines, 6 isothiocyanates, and 6 nitriles) in brocolli, 2 amines, 6 isothiocyanates, and 1 nitrile exhibited >5 cm inhibitory zones for *H. pylori* strain. The results strongly indicated that broccoli sprouts can be an excellent food source for medicinal substances (Moon *et al.*, 2010) and confirmed the previous findings. The anti *H. pylori* property of brocolli sprouts was further strenghened through reduction of certain metabolic markers such as urease measured by the urea breath test and *H. pylori* stool antigen (both biomarkers of *H. pylori* colonization); and serum pepsinogens I and II (biomarkers of gastric inflammation). Intervention with broccoli sprouts decreased the levels of these markers. Values reached normal levels 2 months after treatment was discontinued.

Daily intake of sulforaphane-rich broccoli sprouts for 2 months reduces *H. pylori* colonization in mice and improves the sequelae of infection in infected mice and in humans. The treatment also seems to enhance chemoprotection of the gastric mucosa against *H. pylori*-induced oxidative stress (Yanaka *et al.*, 2009).

In addition *H. pylori*, SFN was found to inhibit 23 out of 28 different microbial species with a minimal inhibitory concentration ranging from 1-4 µg/mL (Johansson *et al.*, 2008). However, five pathogens - *P. aeruginosa*, 3 methicillin-resistant *S. aureus* (MRSA) isolates and *C. albicans* were found to be resistant to SFN, having MICs e"16-32 µg/mL.

Red Cabbage (*Brassica oleracea*)

Red cabbage is a rich source of phenolic compounds, anthocyanins being the most abundant class, which might explain its potent antimicrobial action. The methanolic crude extract of red cabbage showed remarkable, antibacterial activity that was evident particularly against highly infectious micro-organisms such as Methicillin-resistant *S.aureus, E. coli, P. aeruginosa, K. pneumoniae, S. aureus*, and *Salmonella enterica* subspecies 1 *serovar Typhimurium* as well as against human fungal pathogens, *Trichophyton rubrum* and *Aspergillus terreus* (Hafidh *et al.*, 2011).

Drumstick (*Moringa oleifera*)

Drumstick leaves as well as seeds are considered very nutritious. In addition, drumstick seeds and root possess anitimicrobial activity due to its principle component pterygospermin. The fresh leaf juice was found to inhibit the growth of human pathogens as *S. aureus* and *P. aeruginosa* (Das *et al.*, 1957; Eilert *et al.*, 1981; Caceres *et al.*, 1991; Nikkon *et al.*, 2003; Oliveira *et al.*, 1999; The Weath of India, 1960).

Other Foods

Yogurt

Probiotics, which include *L. acidophilus* and *bifidobacteria*, have an indirect antiobiotic effect. They help increase the number of good bacteria in the gastro-intestinal tract, which in turn, helps fight against invasive microorganisms. Bifidobacteria are the primary organisms found in mothers' milk and are effective inhibitors against many disease-causing organisms.

Besides being a probiotic, the fermented dairy product yogurt has been well known as an inhibitor of *S. Mutans*. A study at Hiroshima University, School of Dentistry, Japan, and at the University of Hong Kong, showed that the *L. reuteri* strain in fermented yogurt was effective in combating the dental bacteria. However, the effect has been shown only by *L. reuteri* but no other lactobaccilli species. The results of clinical trial also demonstrated that eating yogurt with *L. reuteri* significantly reduced the oral carriage of *Mutans streptococci*, compared with the placebo yogurt (Nikawa *et al.*, 2004).

Neutralized extracellular culture filtrate obtained from isolates of *Lactobacillus acidophilus, Lactobacillus delbruecki* ssp. *bulgaricus, Lactobacillus salivarius* and *Lactococcus lactis* ssp. *lactis* from 'dahi' showed weak to moderate inhibition of *Staphylococcus aureus, Bacillus cereus, Escherichia coli, Bacillus brevis, Bacillus circulans, Bacillus coagulans, Bacillus laterosporus, Bacillus subtilis* and *Pseudomonas aeruginosa* when tested by the diffusion agar well assay method. Thus Varadaraj *et al.* (1993) reported the antimicrobial activity of dahi and the potential of using neutralized extracellular culture filtrate of lactic acid bacteria in the biopreservation of foods.

Mayan Mool (*Decalepis hamiltonii roots*)

Mayanmool as it is known in Maharshtra, exhibited strong anitimicrobial activity against *B. cereus, B. megaterium, C. albicans, E. coli, M. luteus, M.roseus*, and *S. aureus* at a concentration range of 1:0 with inhibitory activities of 27, 23, 16, 19, 22, 19, and 23 mm, respectively, which are comparable to those of the standards (Thangadurai *et al.*, 2002). The extract was found to contain a flavor compound 2-hydroxy-4-methoxybenzaldehyde (2H4MB) responsible for the effect (Phadke *et al.*, 1994).

Isolated HMBA was also found to inhibit the growth of *H. pylori*, a potential ulcerogen in a dose dependent manner with MIC of <"39 µg/ml as opposed to that of amoxicillin (MIC - 26 µg/ml) to which *H. pylori* is susceptible (Srikanta *et al.*, 2011).

Honey

Honey is increasingly valued for its anti-bacterial activity as it has been known since the 19th century. According to Haffejee and Moosa (1985) honey shortens the duration of bacterial diarrhoea, does not prolong the duration of non-bacterial diarrhoea, and may safely be used as a substitute for glucose in an oral rehydration solution containing electrolytes. Klein *et al.* (2000) confirms that honey has proven anitimicrobial activity.

Honey has also been used to treat adult and neo-natal post-operative infections, burns, boils, necrotizing fasciitis, venous ulcers and diabetic foot ulcers (Al-waili *et al.*, 2011). Varietal differences were noticed in the anitimicrobial property as well as the physicochemical characteristics, and thereby suitability for use in certain conditions. The Tualang honey has a bactericidal as well as bacteriostatic effect. It is used in the dressings as it is easier to apply and is less sticky compared to Manuka honey.

Tualang honey exhibited variable activities against different micro-organisms, but they were within the same range as those for manuka honey. Thus Tan *et al.* (2009) suggest that tualang honey could potentially be used as an alternative therapeutic agent against certain microorganisms, particularly *A. baumannii* and *S. maltophilia*. Kuncic *et al.* (2012) found Slovenian honey to be effective against four bacterial species (*E. coli, E. faecalis, P. aeruginosa and S. aureus*) and against eight fungal species (*A. niger, A. pullulans, C. albicans, C. parapsilosis, C. tropicalis, C. cladosporioides, P. chrysogenum and R. mucilaginosa*) and thus supported the concept that Slovenian honeys can be applied for medicinal purposes.

Nasir *et al.* (2010) reported that Tualang honey is not as effective as other products such as silver-based dressing or medical grade honey dressing for Gram- positive bacteria. Mohapatra *et al.* (2011) proved that honey's bacteriostatic and bactericidal effect are similar to antibiotics, against Gram-positive bacteria (*S. aureus, B. subtilis, B. cereus, E. faecalis*, and *M. luteus*) and Gram-negative bacteria (*E. coli, P. aeruginosa*, and *S. typhi*) organisms and provide alternative therapy against certain bacteria.

The good control of infection is attributed to the high osmolarity, but honey can have additional anti-bacterial activity because of its content of hydrogen peroxide and unidentified substances acquired from certain floral sources. The non-peroxide antibacterial activity of manuka honey at a concentration of 1.8 per cent (v/v) completely inhibited the growth of *S. aureus* during incubation for 8 h. The growth of all seven major wound-infecting species of bacteria was completely inhibited by both types of honey (non-peroxide antibacterial activity of manuka honey and a honey in which the antibacterial activity was primarily due to hydrogen peroxide) at concentrations below 11 per cent (v/v) (Willix *et al.*, 1992).

Voidarou *et al.* (2011) studied the anitimicrobial activity of sixty samples of honey of various botanical origins against 16 clinical pathogens and their respective reference strains. All honey samples, despite their origin (coniferous, citrus, thyme or polyfloral), showed anti-bacterial activity against the pathogens and their respective reference strains at variable levels. Coniferous and thyme honeys showed the highest activity with an average minimum dilution of 17.4 and 19.2 per cent (w/v) followed by citrus and polyfloral honeys with 20.8 and 23.8 per cent respectively. Fangio *et al.* (2007) found that honeys from the southeast region of Buenos Aires province are active against *E. coli* at 25 and 50 per cent (w/v) concentrations. A reduction of microbial growth of 96 per cent in Mueller-Hinton broth and of 90 per cent in Mac Conkey broth by honey solutions containing 50 per cent and 25 per cent (w/v) respectively was observed.

Elbagoury and Rasmy (1993) on testing two samples of natural Honey for their anti-bacterial effect on Bacteroides, mainly the pathogenic black pigmented *B. melaninogenicus* isolated from ten cases of dental infections (dental abscesses and chronic osteomyelitis) observed that the inhibitory effect of honey was not due to its high sugar content or to its acidic pH, when using Schaedler's broth adjusted to the same pH as control. Badet and Quero (2011) who worked on oral bacteria found Manuka honey to be able to reduce oral pathogens within dental plaque and also to be able to control dental biofilm deposit.

Malaysian honeys, namely gelam, kelulut and tualang, have high anti-bacterial potency derived from total and non-peroxide activities, which implies that both peroxide and other constituents are mutually important as contributing factors to the anti-bacterial property of honey (Zainol *et al.*, 2013). Kwakman *et al.* (2011) reported the differences between two medical honeys. Revamil source (RS) honey killed *B. subtilis*, *E. coli* and *P. aeruginosa* within 2 hours, whereas manuka honey had such rapid activity only against *B. subtilis*. After 24 hours of incubation, both honeys killed all tested bacteria, including methicillin-resistant *S. aureus*, but manuka honey retained activity up to higher dilutions than RS honey. Methylglyoxal was a major bactericidal factor in manuka honey, but after neutralization of this compound manuka honey retained bactericidal activity due to several unknown factors. RS and manuka honey have highly distinct compositions of bactericidal factors, resulting in large differences in bactericidal activity.

Australia has unique native flora and produces honey with a wide range of different physic-chemical properties. Irish *et al.* (2011) analysed 477 honey samples and found potentially therapeutically useful antibacterial activity level in 57 per cent of the honey samples, with exceptional activity in samples derived from marri (*Corymbia calophylla*), jarrah (*Eucalyptus marginata*) and jellybush (*Leptospermum polygalifolium*). They attributed the anti-bacterial activity to hydrogen peroxide produced by the bee-derived enzyme glucose oxidase. Non-hydrogen peroxide activity was detected in 80 (16.8 per cent) samples, and was most consistently seen in honey produced from *Leptospermum* spp.

The anti-bacterial effect of honey was found to be more pronounced on *E. coli* than on *S. typhimurium in vitro*, by Badawy *et al.* (2004). Water content, pH value, HMF and the presence of H_2O, all played an important role in the potency of honey as an anti-bacterial agent. The anti-bacterial activity of honey decreased on storage and high concentrations of honey proved more effective as anti-bacterial agents. Badawy *et al.* (2004) also reported lower mortality due to infections among mice treated with honey.

Chronically infected wounds are a costly source of suffering. An important factor in the failure of a sore to heal is the presence of multiple species of bacteria, living cooperatively in highly organized biofilms. The biofilm protects the bacteria from antibiotic therapy and the patient's immune response. Honey has been used as a wound treatment for millennia. Alandejani *et al.* (2009) used a previously established biofilm model to assess antibacterial activity of honey against 11 methicillin-susceptible SA (MSSA), 11 methicillin-resistant SA (MRSA), and 11 PA isolates. Honeys were tested against both planktonic and biofilm-grown bacteria and were found to be effective in killing 100 per cent of the isolates in the planktonic form. The bactericidal rates for the Sidr and Manuka honeys against MSSA, MRSA, and *P. aeruginosa* biofilms were 63-82 per cent, 73-63 per cent, and 91 per cent, respectively. These rates were significantly higher ($P<0.001$) than those seen with single antibiotics commonly used against and *Staphylococcus aureus*.

The anti-bacterial activity of honey is highly complex due to the involvement of multiple active constituents and due to the large variation in the concentrations of these compounds among honey varieties. All bacteria tested, including *B. subtilis*, methicillin-resistant S. aureus, extended-spectrum beta-lactamase producing *E. coli*, ciprofloxacin-resistant *P. aeruginosa*, and vancomycin-resistant *E. faecium*, were killed by 10-20 per cent (v/v) honey (Kwakman *et al.*, 2010). Kwakman *et al.* (2011) found the bactericidal activity differed between the Manuka honey and Revamil® source (RS) honey due to their highly distinct compositions of bactericidal factors. Methyl glyoxal and anitimicrobial peptide bee defensin-1 were identified as important anti-bacterial compounds in honey. Besides the chemical constituents, the high sugar concentration, hydrogen peroxide and low pH are well known anti-bacterial factors in honey (Kwakman and Zaat, 2012).

Several scientists tried to elucidate the mechanism of antimicrobial action of honey. Jenkins *et al.* (2011) observed enlarged cells containing septa in methicillin-resistant *S. aureus* exposed to inhibitory concentrations of manuka honey, suggesting that interruption of cell division was responsible for the effect. The authors believed that these changes were not caused either by the sugars or methylglyoxal in honey but indicated the presence of additional anti-bacterial components in manuka honey. Boukraâ and Amara (2008) speculated that the amylase present in honey hydrolyzed the starch chains of the media to dextrin and maltose which increased the osmotic effect of the media and consequently increased the anti-bacterial effects.

Flaxseeds *(Linum usitatissimum)*

Fungi-static activity of flaxseed flour was investigated using the test micro-organisms of strains of *P. chrysogenum*, *A. flavus*, *F. graminearum*, and a *Penicillium* sp. isolated from molded noodles. Though there were differences in the degree of mold inhibition among flaxseeds obtained from different sources and cultivars. Xu *et al.* (2008) suggested that flaxseed could be used as a multifunctional food ingredient as it possesses fungi-static activity.

Sesame Seeds (*Sesamum indicum*)

A novel anitimicrobial protein -SiAMP2 belonging to the 2S albumin family was isolated from sesame seeds and evaluated its effect against several bacteria and fungi. SiAMP2 specifically inhibited *Klebsiella* sp. reinforcing the hypothesis that plant storage proteins might also play as pathogen protection providing an insight into the mechanism of action for this novel 2S albumin anitimicrobial proteins and evolutionary relations between the two (Maria-Neto *et al.*, 2011).

Asafoetida

β-pinene (47.1 per cent), α-pinene (21.36 per cent), and 1, 2-dithiolane (18.6 per cent) were the main components of asafoetida oil which has shown anitimicrobial activity against *S. typhi*, *E. coli*, *S. aureus*, *B. subtilis*, *A. niger*, and *C. albicans*. Ferula oils could be used as safe and effective natural antioxidants to improve the oxidative stability of fatty foods during storage and to preserve foods against food burn pathogens (Kavoosi *et al.*, 2013).

Conclusions

It is very interesting to understand that several foods not only offer nutritional benefits but also protect the consumers from several infections. Besides, all these are natural agents without any side effects and hence worth further exploitation as anitimicrobial agents against newer varieties of pathogens. Research could also throw light on development of resistance among the pathogens against the foods as well as anitimicrobial constituents of foods.

References

Adetumbi MA, Lau BH (1983). *Allium sativum* (garlic) - a natural anti-biotic. Med. Hypotheses. 12 (3): 227 - 37.

Agarwal P, Nagesh L; Murlikrishnan (2010). Evaluation of the anitimicrobial activity of various concentrations of Tulsi (*Ocimum sanctum*) extract against *Streptococcus mutans*: an *in vitro* study. Indian J Dent Res. 21(3):357-9.

Aggarwal BB, Sung B (2009). Pharmacological basis for the role of curcumin in chronic diseases: an age-old spice with modern targets. Trends. Pharmacol. Sci. 30 (2): 85 - 94.

Agaoglu S, Dostbil N, Alemdar S (2007). Anitimicrobial activity of some spices used in the meat industry. *Bull. Vet. Inst. Pulawy.* 51: 53 - 57.

Ahmad N, Alam MK, Shehbaz A, Khan A, Mannan A, Hakim SR, Bisht D, Owais M (2005). Anitimicrobial activity of clove oil and its potential in the treatment of vaginal candidiasis. J. Drug Target. 13 (10): 555 - 61.

Akoachere JF, Ndip RN, Chenwi EB, Ndip LM, Njock TE, Anong DN (2002). Antibacterial effect of *Zingiber officinale* and *Garcinia kola* on respiratory tract pathogens. East, Afr. Med. J. 79 (11): 588 - 92.

Al-Waili N, Salom K, Al-Ghamdi AA (2011). Honey for wound healing, ulcers, and burns; data supporting its use in clinical practice. Scientific World Journal. 11: 766 - 87.

Alandejani T, Marsan J, Ferris W, Slinger R, Chan F (2009). Effectiveness of honey on *Staphylococcus aureus* and *Pseudomonas aeruginosa* biofilms. Otolaryngol. Head. Neck. Surg. 141 (1): 114 - 18.

Amin M, Kapadnis BP (2005). Heat stable anitimicrobial activity of *Allium ascalonicum* against bacteria and fungi. Indian J. Exp. Biol. 43 (8): 751 - 54.

Amiri A, Dugas R, Pichot AL, Bompeix G (2008). *In vitro* and *in vivo* [corrected] activity of eugenol oil (*Eugenia caryophylata*) against four important postharvest apple pathogens. Int. J. Food Microbiol. 126 (1-2): 13 - 19.

Apisariyakul A, Vanittanakom N, Buddhasukh D (1995). Anti-fungal activity of turmeric oil extracted from *Curcuma longa* (Zingiberaceae). J Ethnopharmacol. 49 (3): 163 - 69.

Ayaz E, Alpsoy HC (2007). Garlic (*Allium sativum*) and traditional medicine. Turkiye. Parazitol. Derg. 31 (2): 145 - 49. [Article in Turkish].

Azumi S, Tanimura A, Tanamoto K (1997). A novel inhibitor of bacterial endotoxin derived from cinnamon bark. *Biochem. Biophys. Res. Commun.* 234: 506 - 10.

Bachrach G, Jamil A, Naor R, Tal G, Ludmer Z, Steinberg D (2011). Garlic allicin as a potential agent for controlling oral pathogens. J. Med. Food. 2011 May 6. [Epub ahead of print].

Badawy OF, Shafii SS, Tharwat EE, Kamal AM (2004). Anti-bacterial activity of bee honey and its therapeutic usefulness against *Escherichia coli* O157:H7 and *Salmonella typhimurium* infection. Rev. Sci. Tech. 23 (3): 1011 - 22.

Badet C, Quero F (2011). The *in vitro* effect of manuka honeys on growth and adherence of oral bacteria. Anaerobe. 17 (1): 19 - 22.

Bakri IM, Douglas CW (2005). Inhibitory effect of garlic extract on oral bacteria. Arch. Oral. Biol. 50 (7): 645 - 51.

Bassolé IH, Lamien-Meda A, Bayala B, Tirogo S, Franz C, Novak J, Nebié RC, Dicko MH (2010). Composition and anitimicrobial activities of *Lippia multiflora Moldenke, Mentha x piperita* L. and *Ocimum basilicum* L. essential oils and their major monoterpene alcohols alone and in combination. Molecules. 15 (11): 7825 - 39.

Beerepoot MA, ter Riet G, Nys S, van der Wal WM, de Borgie CA, de Reijke TM, Prins JM, Koeijers J, Verbon A, Stobberingh E, Geerlings SE (2011). Cranberries vs antibiotics to prevent urinary tract infections: a randomized double-blind non-inferiority trial in pre-menopausal women. Arch. Intern. Med. 171 (14): 1270 - 78.

Bhawana, Basniwal RK, Buttar HS, Jain VK, Jain N (2011). Curcumin nanoparticles: preparation, characterization, and anitimicrobial study. J. Agric. Food Chem. 59 (5): 2056 - 61.

Bianchini F, Vainio H (2001). *Allium* vegetables and organosulfur compounds: do they help prevent cancer? Environ. Health. Perspect. 109 (9): 893 - 902.

Boddicker JD, Anderson RA, Jagnow J, Clegg S (2006). Signature-tagged mutagenesis of *Klebsiella pneumoniae* to identify genes that influence biofilm formation on extracellular matrix material. *Infect. Immun.* 74: 4590 - 97.

Boukraâ L, Amara K (2008). Synergistic effect of starch on the anti-bacterial activity of honey. J. Med. Food. 11 (1): 195 - 98.

Briozzo J, Núnez L, Chirife J, Herszage L, D'Aquino M (1989). Anitimicrobial activity of clove oil dispersed in a concentrated sugar solution. J. Appl. Bacteriol. 66 (1): 69 - 75.

Burt S (2004). Essential oils: their anti-bacterial properties and potential applications in foods–a review. Int. J. Food Microbiol. 94 (3): 223 - 53.

Butt MS, Sultan MT, Butt MS, Iqbal J (2009). Garlic: nature's protection against physiological threats. Crit. Rev. Food Sci. Nutr. 49 (6): 538 - 51.

Caceres A, Cabrera O, Morales O, Mollinedo P, Mendia P (1991). Pharmacological properties of *Moringa oleifera*. 1: preliminary screening for antimicrobial activity. *Journal of Ethnopharmacology*. 33 (3): 213 - 16.

Cai L, Wu CD (1996). Compounds from *Syzygium aromaticum* possessing growth inhibitory activity against oral pathogens. J. Nat. Prod. 59 (10): 987 - 90.

Cava R, Nowak E, Taboada A, Marin-Iniesta F (2007). Anitimicrobial activity of clove and cinnamon essential oils against *Listeria monocytogenes* in pasteurized milk. J. Food Prot. 70 (12): 2757 - 63.

Chaieb K, Hajlaoui H, Zmantar T, Kahla-Nakbi AB, Rouabhia M, Mahdouani K, Bakhrouf A (2007a). The chemical composition and biological activity of clove essential oil, *Eugenia caryophyllata* (*Syzigium aromaticum L. Myrtaceae*): a short review. Phytother. Res. 21 (6): 501 - 506.

Chaieb K, Zmantar T, Ksouri R, Hajlaoui H, Mahdouani K, Abdelly C, Bakhrouf A (2007b). Anti-oxidant properties of the essential oil of *Eugenia caryophyllata* and its anti-fungal activity against a large number of clinical *Candida* species. Mycoses. 50 (5): 403 - 406.

Chami F, Chami N, Bennis S, Bouchikhi T, Remmal A (2005). Oregano and clove essential oils induce surface alteration of *Saccharomyces cerevisiae*. Phytother. Res. 19 (5): 405 - 408.

Chandrasekaran M, Venkatesalu V (2004). Anti-bacterial and anti-fungal activity of *Syzygium jambolanum* seeds. J. Ethnopharmacol. 91 (1): 105 - 108.

Chaudhary N and Tariq P (2008) *In vitro* anti-bacterial activities of kalonji, cumin and poppy seed. Pak. J. Bot. 40 (1): 461 - 67.

Chavan SD, Shetty NL, Kanuri M (2010). Comparative evaluation of garlic extract mouthwash and chlorhexidine mouthwash on salivary *Streptococcus mutans* count - an *in vitro* study. Oral Health Prev. Dent. 8 (4): 369 - 74.

Chen CF, Li YD, Xu Z (2010). Chemical principles and bioactivities of blueberry. Yao. Xue. Xue. Bao. 45 (4): 422 - 29. [Article in Chinese].

Cisowska A, Wojnicz D, Hendrich AB (2011). Anthocyanins as anitimicrobial agents of natural plant origin. Nat. Prod. Commun. 6 (1): 149 - 56.

Das BR, Kurup PA, Rao PL (1957). Antibiotic principle from *Moringa pterygosperma*. VII. Antibacterial activity and chemical structure of compounds related to pterygospermin. The Indian Journal of Medical Research. 45(2):191 - 96.

De R, Kundu P, Swarnakar S, Ramamurthy T, Chowdhury A, Nair GB, Mukhopadhyay AK (2009). Anitimicrobial activity of curcumin against *Helicobacter pylori* isolates from India and during infections in mice. Anitimicrob. Agents Chemother. 53 (4): 1592 - 97.

Delaha EC, Garagusi VF (1985). Inhibition of mycobacteria by garlic extract (*Allium sativum*). Anitimicrob. Agents Chemother. 27 (4): 485 - 86.

Derakhshan S, Sattari M, Bigdeli M (2008). Effect of sub-inhibitory concentrations of cumin (*Cuminum cyminum* L.) seed essential oil and alcoholic extract on the morphology, capsule expression and urease activity of *Klebsiella pneumoniae. Int. J. Anitimicrob. Agents*. 32: 432 - 36.

Derakhshan S, Sattari M, Bigdeli M (2010). Effect of cumin (*Cuminum cyminum*) seed essential oil on biofilm formation and plasmid Integrity of *Klebsiella pneumoniae*. Pharmacogn. Mag. 6 (21): 57 - 61.

Devi KP, Nisha SA, Sakthivel R, Pandian SK (2010). Eugenol (an essential oil of clove) acts as an anti-bacterial agent against *Salmonella typhi* by disrupting the cellular membrane. J. Ethnopharmacol. 130 (1): 107 - 15.

Dkhil MA, Abdel-Baki AS, Wunderlich F, Sies H, Al-Quraishy S (2011). Anti-coccidial and anti-inflammatory activity of garlic in murine *Eimeria papillata* infections. Vet. Parasitol. 175 (1-2): 66 - 72.

Du WX, Olsen CW, Avena-Bustillos RJ, McHugh TH, Levin CE, Friedman M (2008). Anti-bacterial activity against *E. coli* O157:H7, physical properties, and storage stability of novel carvacrol-containing edible tomato films. J. Food Sci. 73 (7): M 378 - 83.

Du, WX, Olsen Avena-Bustillos, McHugh, Levin, Mandrell, R. Friedman, M (2009a). Anti-bacterial effects of allspice, garlic, and oregano essential oils in tomato films determined by overlay and vapor-phase methods. J. Food Sci. 74 (7): M 390 - 97 (1).

Du WX, Olsen CW, Avena-Bustillos RJ, McHugh TH, Levin CE, Friedman M (2009b). Effects of allspice, cinnamon, and clove bud essential oils in edible apple films on physical properties and anitimicrobial activities. J. Food Sci. 74 (7): M 372 - 78.

Du WX, Olsen CW, Avena-Bustillos RJ, Friedman M, McHugh TH (2011). Physical and anti-bacterial properties of edible films formulated with apple skin polyphenols. J. Food Sci. 76 (2): M 149 - 55.

Dugoua JJ, Seely D, Perri D, Cooley K, Forelli T, Mills E, Koren G (2007). From type 2 diabetes to anti-oxidant activity: a systematic review of the safety and efficacy of common and cassia cinnamon bark. Can. J. Physiol. Pharmacol. 85 (9): 837 - 47.

Eilert U, Wolters B, Nahrstedt A (1981). The antibiotic principle of seeds of *Moringa oleifera* and *Moringa Stenopetala. Planta Medica.* 42 (1): 55 -61.

El Deeb HK, Al Khadrawy FM, El-Hameid AK (2012). Inhibitory effect of *Ferula asafoetida L. Umbelliferae)* on *Blastocystis sp.* subtype 3 growth *in- vitro.* Parasitol. Res. [Epub ahead of print].

Elbagoury EF, Rasmy S (1993). Anti-bacterial action of natural honey on anaerobic bacteroides. Egypt. Dent. J. 39 (1): 381 - 86.

Ellen Tattelman (American Family Physician) July 1, (2005). Health effects of garlic.

Elnima EI, Ahmed SA, Mekkawi AG, Mossa JS (1983). The anitimicrobial activity of garlic and onion extracts. Pharmazie. 38 (11): 747 - 48.

Fabio A, Cermelli C, Fabio G, Nicoletti P, Quaglio P (2007). Screening of the anti-bacterial effects of a variety of essential oils on micro-organisms responsible for respiratory infections. *Phytother. Res.* 21 (4): 374 - 77.

Fangio MF, Iurlina MO, Fritz R (2007). Anitimicrobial activity of honey the southeast of Buenos Aires province against *Escherichia coli*. Rev. Argent. Microbiol. 39 (2): 120 - 23.

Fani MM, Kohanteb J, Dayaghi M (2007). Inhibitory activity of garlic (*Allium sativum*) extract on multidrug-resistant *Streptococcus mutans*. J. Indian Soc. Pedod. Prev. Dent. 25 (4): 164 - 68.

Farnsworth NR, Bunyapraphatsara N (eds) (1992). *Thai Medicinal Plants*. Bangkok: Medicinal Plant Information Center, 180 - 82.

Ferreira FD, Kemmelmeier C, Arrotéia CC, da Costa CL, Mallmann CA, Janeiro V, Ferreira FM, Mossini SA, Silva EL, Machinski M Jr (2013). Inhibitory effect of the essential oil of *Curcuma longa* L. and curcumin on aflatoxin production by *Aspergillus flavus* Link. Food Chem. 136 (2): 789 - 93.

Fu Y, Zu Y, Chen L, Shi X, Wang Z, Sun S, Efferth T (2007). Anitimicrobial activity of clove and rosemary essential oils alone and in combination. Phytother. Res. 21 (10): 989 - 94.

Galan MV, Kishan AA, Silverman AL (2004). Oral broccoli sprouts for the treatment of *Helicobacter pylori* infection: a preliminary report. Dig. Dis. Sci. 49 (7-8): 1088 - 90.

Ganguly C (2010). Flavoring agents used in Indian cooking and their anti-carcinogenic properties. Asian Pac. J. Cancer Prev. 11 (1): 25 – 28.

Gayoso CW, Lima EO, Oliveira VT, Pereira FO, Souza EL, Lima IO, Navarro DF (2005). Sensitivity of fungi isolated from onychomycosis to *Eugenia cariophyllata* essential oil and eugenol. Fitoterapia. 76 (2): 247 - 49.

Geeta, Vasudevan DM, Kedlaya R, Deepa S, Ballal M (2001). Activity of *Ocimum sanctum* (the traditional Indian medicinal plant) against the enteric pathogens. Indian J. Med. Sci. 55 (8): 434 - 38, 472.

Goto C, Kasuya S, Koga K, Ohtomo H, Kagei N.(1990) Lethal efficacy of extract from *Zingiber officinale* (traditional Chinese medicine) or [6]-shogaol and [6]-gingerol in Anisakis larvae *in vitro*. Parasitol Res. 76 (8): 653 - 56.

Graumann GH, Holley RA (2008). Inhibition of *Escherichia coli* O157:H7 in ripening dry fermented sausage by ground yellow mustard. J. Food Prot. 71 (3): 486 - 93.

Groppo FC, Ramacciato JC, Motta RH, Ferraresi PM, Sartoratto A (2007). Anitimicrobial activity of garlic against oral *streptococci*. Int. J. Dent. Hyg. 5 (2): 109 - 115.

Groppo FC, Ramacciato JC, Simoes RP, Flório FM, Sartoratto A (2002). Anitimicrobial activity of garlic, tea tree oil, and chlorhexidine against oral micro-organisms. Int. Dent. J. 52 (6): 433 - 37.

Gutmann L, Williamson R, Moreau N, Kitzis MD, Collatz E, Acar JF, Goldstein FW (1985). Cross-resistance to nalidixic acid, trimethoprim, and chloramphenicol associated with alterations in outer membrane proteins *of Klebsiella, Enterobacter,* and *Serratia. J. Infect. Dis.* 151: 501 - 507.

Haffejee IE, Moosa A (1985). Honey in the treatment of infantile gastro-enteritis. Br. Med. J. (Clin. Res. Ed). 290 (6485): 1866 - 67.

Hafidh RR, Abdulamir AS, Vern LS, Abu Bakar F, Abas F, Jahanshiri F, Sekawi Z (2011). Inhibition of growth of highly resistant bacterial and fungal pathogens by a natural product. Open Microbiol. J. 5: 96 - 106.

Hajlaoui H, Mighri H, Noumi E, Snoussi M, Trabelsi N, Ksouri R, Bakhrouf A (2010). Chemical composition and biological activities of Tunisian *Cuminum cyminum* L. essential oil: a high effectiveness against *Vibrio* spp. strains. Food Chem. Toxicol. 48 (8-9): 2186 - 92.

Hammer KA, Carson CF, Riley TV (1999). Anitimicrobial activity of essential Oils and Other Plant Extracts. J. Appl. Microbiol. 86: 985 - 90.

Hannan A, Humayun T, Hussain MB, Yasir M, Sikandar S (2010). *In vitro* anti-bacterial activity of onion (*Allium cepa*) against clinical isolates of Vibrio cholerae. J. Ayub. Med. Coll. Abbottabad. 22 (2): 160 - 63.

Hannan A, Ikram Ullah M, Usman M, Hussain S, Absar M, Javed K (2011). Anti-mycobacterial activity of garlic (*Allium sativum*) against multi-drug resistant and non-multi-drug resistant *Mycobacterium tuberculosis*. Pak. J. Pharm. Sci. 24 (1): 81 - 85.

Harris JC, Cottrell SL, Plummer S, Lloyd D (2001). Anitimicrobial properties of *Allium sativum* (garlic). Appl. Microbiol. Biotechnol. 57 (3): 282 - 86.

Hawrelak JA, Cattley T, Myers SP (2009). Essential oils in the treatment of intestinal dysbiosis: A preliminary *in vitro* study. Altern. Med. Rev. 14 (4): 380 - 84.

Heinonen M (2007). Anti-oxidant activity and anitimicrobial effect of berry phenolics - a Finnish perspective. Mol. Nutr. Food Res. 51 (6): 684 - 91.

Helander IM, Alakomi HL, Latva-Kala K, Mattila-Sandholm T, Pol I, Smid EJ, Gorris LGM, Wright A (1998). Characterization of the action of selected essential oil components on Gram-negative bacteria. *J. Agric. Food Chem.* 46: 3590 - 95.

Hili P, Evans CS, Veness RG (1997). Anitimicrobial action of essential oils: The effect of dimethylsulphoxide on the activity of cinnamon oil. Lett. Appl. Microbiol. 24: 269 - 75.

Hoque MD, Bari ML, Inatsu Y, Juneja VK, Kawamoto S (2007). Anti-bacterial activity of guava (*Psidium guajava* L.) and Neem (*Azadirachta indica* A. Juss.) extracts against foodborne pathogens and spoilage bacteria. Foodborne Pathog. Dis. 4 (4): 481 - 88.

Howell AB (2002). Cranberry proanthocyanidins and the maintenance of urinary tract health. Crit. Rev. Food Sci. Nutr. 42 (3 Suppl): 273 - 78.

Huovinen P (1987). Trimethoprim resistance. *Anitimicrob. agents chemother.* 31: 1451 - 56.

Iacobellis NS, Lo Cantore P, Capasso F, Senatore F (2005). Anti-bacterial activity of *Cuminum cyminum* L. and *Carum carvi* L. essential oils. *J. Agric. Food Chem.* 53 (1): 57 - 61.

Iciek M, Kwiecien I, Wlodek L (2009). Biological properties of garlic and garlic-derived organosulfur compounds. Environ. Mol. Mutagen. 50 (3): 247 - 65.

Irish J, Blair S, Carter DA (2011). The antibacterial activity of honey derived from Australian flora. PLoS. ONE. 6 (3): e18229.

Jayaprakasha GK, Negi PS, Anandharamakrishnan C, Sakariah KK (2001). Chemical composition of turmeric oil - a byproduct from turmeric oleoresin industry and its inhibitory activity against different fungi. Z. Naturforsch.C. 56 (1-2): 40 - 44.

Jenkins R, Burton N, Cooper R (2011). Manuka honey inhibits cell division in methicillin-resistant *Staphylococcus aureus.* J. Anitimicrob. Chemother. 66 (11): 2536 - 42.

Johansson NL, Pavia CS, Chiao JW (2008). Growth inhibition of a spectrum of bacterial and fungal pathogens by sulforaphane, an isothiocyanate product found in broccoli and other cruciferous vegetables. Planta. Med. 74 (7): 747 - 50.

Johnson MG, Vaught RH (1969). Death of *Salmonella typhimurium* and *Escherichia coli* in the presence of freshly reconstituted dehydrated garlic and onion. Appl. Microbiol. 17: 903 - 905.

Kaefer CM, Milner JA (2008). The role of herbs and spices in cancer prevention. J. Nutr. Biochem. 19 (6): 347 - 61.

Kalemba D, Kunicka A (2003). Anti-bacterial and anti-fungal properties of essential oils. Curr. Med. Chem. 10 (10): 813 - 29.

Kamazeri TS, Samah OA, Taher M, Susanti D, Qaralleh H (2012). Anitimicrobial activity and essential oils of *Curcuma aeruginosa*, *Curcuma mangga*, and *Zingiber cassumunar* from Malaysia. Asian Pac J Trop Med. 5 (3): 202 - 209.

Karaman M, Firinci F, Arikan Ayyildiz Z, Bahar IH (2013). Effects of imipenem, tobramycin and curcumin on biofilm formation of *Pseudomonas aeruginosa* Strains. Mikrobiyol. Bul. 47 (1): 192 - 94. [Article in Turkish].

Kavoosi G, Tafsiry A, Ebdam AA, Rowshan V (2013). Evaluation of antioxidant and anitimicrobial activities of essential oils from *Carum copticum* seed and *Ferula assafoetida* latex. J. Food Sci. 78 (2): T356 - 61.

Kaur GJ, Arora DS (2009). Anti-bacterial and phytochemical screening of *Anethum graveolens, Foeniculum vulgare* and *Trachyspermum ammi.* BMC. Complement. Altern. Med. 9: 30.

Keskin D, Toroglu S (2011). Studies on anitimicrobial activities of solvent extracts of different spices. J. Environ. Biol. 32 (2): 251 - 56.

Khan A, Ahmad A, Akhtar F, Yousuf S, Xess I, Khan LA, Manzoor N (2010a). *Ocimum sanctum* essential oil and its active principles exert their anti-fungal activity by disrupting ergosterol biosynthesis and membrane integrity. Res. Microbiol. 161 (10): 816 - 23.

Khan A, Ahmad A, Manzoor N, Khan LA. (2010b). Anti-fungal activities of *Ocimum sanctum* essential oil and its lead molecules. Nat. Prod. Commun. 5 (2): 345 - 49.

Khan R, Zakir M, Afaq SH, Latif A, Khan AU (2010c). Activity of solvent extracts of *Prosopis spicigera, Zingiber officinale* and *Trachyspermum ammi* against multidrug resistant bacterial and fungal strains. J. Infect. Dev. Ctries. 4 (5): 292 - 300.

Khan MS, Zahir M, Hasan S, Husain FM, Ahmad I (2009). Inhibition of quorum sensing regulated bacterial functions by plant essential oils with special reference to clove oil. Lett. Appl. Microbiol. 49 (3): 354 - 60.

Khan R, Zakir M, Khanam Z, Shakil S, Khan AU (2010d). Novel compound from *Trachyspermum ammi (Ajowan caraway)* seeds with anti-biofilm and anti-adherence activities against *Streptococcus mutans*: a potential chemotherapeutic agent against dental caries. J. Appl. Microbiol. 109 (6): 2151 - 59.

Khosravi AR, Shokri H, Minooeianhaghighi M (2011). Inhibition of aflatoxin production and growth of *Aspergillus parasiticus* by *Cuminum cyminum, Ziziphora clinopodioides*, and *Nigella sativa* essential oils. Foodborne Pathog. Dis. 8 (12): 1275 - 80.

Kim HJ, Yoo HS, Kim JC, Park CS, Choi MS, Kim M, Choi H, Min JS, Kim YS, Yoon SW, Ahn JK (2009). Anti-viral effect of *Curcuma longa* Linn. extract against *hepatitis B virus* replication. J. Ethnopharmacol. 124 (2): 189 - 96.

Klein C, Sato T, Meguid MM, Miyata G (2000). From food to nutritional support to specific nutraceuticals: a journey across time in the treatment of disease. J. Gastroenterol. 35 Suppl. 12: 1 - 6.

Knight KP, McKellar RC (2007). Influence of cinnamon and clove essential oils on the D- and z-values of *Escherichia coli* O157:H7 in apple cider. J. Food Prot. 70 (9): 2089 - 94.

Koosirirat C, Linpisarn S, Changsom D, Chawansuntati K, Wipasa J (2010). Investigation of the anti-inflammatory effect of *Curcuma longa* in *Helicobacter pylori*-infected patients. Int. Immunopharmacol. 10 (7): 815 - 18.

Kravets SD, Vollerner YuS, Gorovits MB & Abubakirov NK (1990). Steroids of the spirostan and furostan series from plants of the genus *Allium*. Chemistry of Natural Compounds 1990. publ. 1991. 26 (4): 359 - 73.

Krishnaswamy K (2008). Traditional Indian spices and their health significance. Asia. Pac. J. Clin. Nutr. 17 (Suppl 1): 265 - 68.

Kubo I, Fujita KI, Kubo A, Nihei KI, Ogura T (2004). Anti-bacterial activity of coriander volatile compounds against *Salmonella choleraesuis*. Journal of Agricultural and Food Chemistry 52 (11): 3329 - 32.

Kumar A, Tantry BA, Rahiman S, Gupta U (2011). Comparative study of anitimicrobial activity and phytochemical analysis of methanolic and aqueous extracts of the fruit of *Emblica officinalis* against pathogenic bacteria. J. Tradit. Chin. Med. 31 (3): 246 - 50.

Kuncic MK, Jaklic D, Lapanje A, Gunde-Cimerman N (2012). Anti-bacterial and anti-mycotic activities of Slovenian honeys. Br. J. Biomed. Sci. 69 (4): 154 - 58.

Kwakman PH, te Velde AA, de Boer L, Speijer D, Vandenbroucke-Grauls CM, Zaat SA (2010). How honey kills bacteria. FASEB. J. 24 (7): 2576 - 82.

Kwakman PH, Te Velde AA, de Boer L, Vandenbroucke-Grauls CM, Zaat SA (2011). Two major medicinal honeys have different mechanisms of bactericidal activity. PLoS. One. 6 (3): e17709.

Kwakman PH, Zaat SA (2012). Anti-bacterial components of honey. IUBMB Life. 64 (1): 48 - 55.

Kylli P, Nohynek L, Puupponen-Pimiä R, Westerlund-Wikström B, McDougall G, Stewart D, Heinonen M (2010). Rowanberry phenolics: compositional analysis and bioactivities. J. Agric. Food Chem. 58 (22): 11985 - 92.

Lacaille-Dubois MA, and Wagner H (1996). A review of the biological and pharmacological activities of saponins. Phytomedicine. 2: 363 - 86.

Lampe JW (2003). Spicing up a vegetarian diet: chemopreventive effects of phytochemicals. Am. J. Clin. Nutr. 78 (3 Suppl): 579S - 83S.

Larsson SC, Kumlin M, Ingelman-Sundberg M, Wolk A (2004). Dietary long-chain n-3 fatty acids for the prevention of cancer: a review of potential mechanisms. Am. J. Clin. Nutr. 79 (6): 935 - 45.

Lavigne JP, Bourg G, Botto H, Sotto A (2007). Cranberry (*Vaccinium macrocarpon*) and urinary tract infections: study model and review of literature. Pathol. Biol. (Paris). 55 (8-9): 460 - 64. [Article in French].

Lee CL, Chia-Lin Lee, Lien-Chai Chiang, Li-Hung Cheng, Chih-Chuang Liaw, Mohamed H. Abd El-Razek, Fang-Rong Chang, Yang-Chang Wu (2009). Influenza A (H1N1) anti-viral and cytotoxic agents from *Ferula assa-foetida*. Journal of Natural Products. 72 (9): 1568 - 72.

Lee HB, Noh BS, Min SC (2012). *Listeria monocytogenes* inhibition by defatted mustard meal-based edible films. Int. J. Food Microbiol. 153 (1-2): 99 - 105.

Lee KH, Kim BS, Keum KS, Yu HH, Kim YH, Chang BS, Ra JY, Moon HD, Seo BR, Choi NY, You YO (2011). Essential oil of *Curcuma longa* inhibits *Streptococcus mutans* biofilm formation. J. Food Sci. 76 (9): H226 - 30.

Leuschner RG, Ielsch V (2003). Anitimicrobial effects of garlic, clove and red hot chilli on *Listeria monocytogenes* in broth model systems and soft cheese. Int. J. Food Sci. Nutr. 54 (2): 127 - 33.

Liu X, Zhao M, Luo W, Yang B, Jiang Y (2009). Identification of volatile components in *Phyllanthus emblica* L. and their anitimicrobial activity. J. Med. Food. 12 (2): 423 - 28.

López P, Sánchez C, Batlle R, Nerín C (2005). Solid- and vapor-phase anitimicrobial activities of six essential oils: susceptibility of selected foodborne bacterial and fungal strains. J. Agric. Food Chem. 53 (17): 6939 - 46.

Luciano FB, Belland J, Holley RA (2011). Microbial and chemical origins of the bactericidal activity of thermally treated yellow mustard powder toward *Escherichia coli* O157:H7 during dry sausage ripening. Int. J. Food Microbiol. 145 (1): 69 - 76.

Mandal S, Mandal MD Saha K, Pal NK (2011). *In vitro* anti-bacterial activity of three Indian spices against methicillin-resistant *Staphylococcus aureus*. Oman. Med. J. 26 (5): 319 - 23.

Maria-Neto S, Honorato RV, Costa FT, Almeida RG, Amaro DS, Oliveira JT, Vasconcelos IM, Franco OL (2011). Bactericidal activity identified in 2S Albumin from sesame seeds and in silico studies of structure-function relations. Protein J. 30 (5): 340 - 50.

Maroncle N, Balestrino D, Rich C, Forestier C (2002). Identification of *Klebsiella pneumoniae* genes involved in intestinal colonization and adhesion using signature-tagged mutagenesis. *Infect. Immun.* 70: 4729 - 34

Martins AP, Salgueiro L, Gonçalves MJ, da Cunha AP, Vila R, Canigueral S, Mazzoni V, Tomi F, Casanova J (2001). Essential oil composition and anitimicrobial activity of three Zingiberaceae from S.Tomé e Príncipe. Planta. Med. 67 (6): 580 - 84.

Matan N, Rimkeeree H, Mawson AJ, Chompreeda P, Haruthaithanasan V, Parker M (2006). Anitimicrobial activity of cinnamon and clove oils under modified atmosphere conditions. Int. J. Food Microbiol. 107 (2): 180 - 85.

Matsuura H (2001). Saponins in garlic as modifiers of the risk of cardiovascular disease. J. Nutr. 131 (3): 1000S - 1005S.

Meades G Jr, Henken RL, Waldrop GL, Rahman MM, Gilman SD, Kamatou GP, Viljoen AM, Gibbons S (2010). Constituents of cinnamon inhibit bacterial acetyl CoA carboxylase. Planta. Med. 76 (14): 1570 - 75.

Mathew N, Misra-Bhattacharya S, Perumal V, Muthuswamy K (2008). Anti-filarial lead molecules isolated from *Trachyspermum ammi*. Molecules. 13 (9): 2156 - 68.

Mekawey A, Mokhtar M. and Farrag R (2009). Anti-tumor and Anti-bacterial Activities of [1-(2-Ethyl, 6-Heptyl) Phenol] from *Cuminum cyminum* Seeds, Journal of Applied Sciences Research. 5 (11): 1881- 88.

Millet CO, Lloyd D, Williams C, Williams D, Evans G, Saunders RA, Cable J (2011). Effect of garlic and allium-derived products on the growth and metabolism of *Spironucleus vortens*. Exp. Parasitol. 127 (2): 490 - 99.

Mohapatra DP, Thakur V, Brar SK (2011). Anti-bacterial efficacy of raw and processed honey. Biotechnol. Res. Int. 2011: 917505. Epub 2010 Dec 29.

Mohsenzadeh M (2007). Evaluation of anti-bacterial activity of selected Iranian essential oils against *Staphylococcus aureus* and *Escherichia coli* in nutrient broth medium. Pak. J. Biol. Sci. 10 (20): 3693 - 97.

Moon JK, Kim JR, Ahn YJ, Shibamoto T (2010). Analysis and anti-*Helicobacter* activity of sulforaphane and related compounds present in broccoli (*Brassica oleracea* L.) sprouts. J. Agric. Food Chem. 58 (11): 6672 - 77.

Moon SE, Kim HY, Cha JD (2011). Synergistic effect between clove oil and its major compounds and antibiotics against oral bacteria. Arch. Oral Biol. 56 (9): 907 - 16.

Na HS, Cha MH, Oh DR, Cho CW, Rhee JH, Kim YR (2011). Protective mechanism of curcumin against *Vibrio vulnificus* infection. FEMS Immunol. Med. Microbiol. 63 (3): 355 - 62.

Nasir NA, Halim AS, Singh KK, Dorai AA, Haneef MN (2010). Anti-bacterial properties of tualang honey and its effect in burn wound management: a comparative study. BMC. Complement. Altern. Med. 10: 31.

Negi PS, Jayaprakasha GK, Jagan Mohan Rao L, Sakariah KK (1999). Anti-bacterial activity of turmeric oil: a byproduct from curcumin manufacture. J. Agric. Food Chem. 47 (10): 4297 - 300.

Nikawa H, Makihira S, Fukushima H, Nishimura H, Ozaki Y, Ishida K, Darmawan S, Hamada T, Hara K, Matsumoto A, Takemoto T, Aimi R (2004). *Lactobacillus reuteri* in bovine milk fermented decreases the oral carriage of *Mutans streptococci*. International Journal of Food Microbiology 95: 219 - 23.

Nikkon F, Saud ZA, Rehman MH, Haque ME (2003). *In vitro* anitimicrobial activity of the compound isolated from chloroform extract of *Moringa oleifera* Lam. *Pakistan Journal of Biological Sciences*. 22: 1888 - 90.

Nohynek LJ, Alakomi HL, Kähkönen MP, Heinonen M, Helander IM, Oksman-Caldentey KM, Puupponen-Pimiä RH (2006). Berry phenolics: anitimicrobial properties and mechanisms of action against severe human pathogens. Nutr. Cancer. 54 (1): 18 - 32.

Norajit K, Laohakunjit N, Kerdchoechuen O (2007). Anti-bacterial effect of five Zingiberaceae essential oils. Molecules. 12 (8): 2047 - 60.

Nzeako BC, Al-Kharousi ZS, Al-Mahrooqui Z (2006). Anitimicrobial activities of clove and thyme extracts. Sultan. Qaboos. Univ. Med. J. 6 (1): 33 - 39.

Oliveira JTA, Silveira SB, Vasconcelos IM, Cavada BS, Moreira RA (1999). Compositional and nutritional attributes of seeds from the multiple purpose tree *Moringa oleifera* Lamarck. Journal of the Science of Food and Agriculture. 79 (6): 815 - 20.

Pajohi MR, Tajik H, Farshid AA, Hadian M (2011). Synergistic anti-bacterial activity of the essential oil of *Cuminum cyminum* L. seed and nisin in a food model. J. Appl. Microbiol. 2011 Jan 12. doi: 10.1111/j.1365 - 2672. 2011. 04946.x. [Epub ahead of print].

Panizzi L, Flamini G, Cioni PL, Morelli I (1993). Composition and anitimicrobial properties of essential oils of four Mediterranean Lamiaceae. J. Ethnopharmacol. 39: 167 - 70.

Park M, Bae J, Lee DS (2008). Anti-bacterial activity of [10]-gingerol and [12]-gingerol isolated from ginger rhizome against periodontal bacteria. Phytother Res. 22 (11): 1446 - 49.

Park MJ, Gwak KS, Yang I, Choi WS, Jo HJ, Chang JW, Jeung EB, Choi IG (2007). Anti-fungal activities of the essential oils in *Syzygium aromaticum* (L.) Merr. Et Perry and *Leptospermum petersonii* Bailey and their constituents against various dermatophytes. J. Microbiol. 45 (5): 460 - 65.

Pehowich DJ, Gomes AV, Barnes JA (2000). Fatty acid composition and possible health effects of coconut constituents. West. Indian Med. J. 49 (2): 128 - 33.

Phadke NY, Gholap AS, Ramakrishnan K, Subbulakshmi G (1994). Essential oil of *Decalepis hamiltonii* as an anitimicrobial agent. J. Food Sci. Technol. 31 (6): 472 - 75.

Piccaglia R, Marotti M, Giovanelli E, Deans SG, Eaglesham E (1993). Anti-bacterial and anti-oxidant properties of Mediterranean aromatic plants. Indust. Crops Prod. 2: 47 - 50.

Pinto E, Vale-Silva L, Cavaleiro C, Salgueiro L (2009). Anti-fungal activity of the clove essential oil from *Syzygium aromaticum* on Candida, Aspergillus and dermatophyte species. J. Med. Microbiol. 58 (Pt 11): 1454 - 62.

Policegoudra RS, Divakar S, Aradhya SM (2007). Identification of difurocumenonol, a new anitimicrobial compound from mango ginger (*Curcuma amada* Roxb.) rhizome. J. Appl. Microbiol. 102 (6):1594 - 602.

Powolny AA, Singh SV (2008). Multitargeted prevention and therapy of cancer by diallyl trisulfide and related allium vegetable-derived organosulfur compounds. Cancer Lett. 269 (2): 305 - 14.

Prasad S, Phromnoi K, Yadav VR, Chaturvedi MM, Aggarwal BB (2010). Targeting inflammatory pathways by flavonoids for prevention and treatment of cancer. Planta. Med. 76 (11): 1044 - 63.

Premanathan M, Rajendran S, Ramanathan T, Kathiresan K, Nakashima H, Yamamoto N (2000). A survey of some Indian medicinal plants for anti-human immunodeficiency virus (HIV) activity. The Indian journal of medical research. 112: 73 - 77.

Psota TL, Gebauer SK, Kris-Etherton P (2006). Dietary omega-3 fatty acid intake and cardiovascular risk. Am. J. Cardiol. 98 (4A): 3i - 18i.

Puupponen-Pimiä R, Nohynek L, Alakomi HL, Oksman-Caldentey KM (2005 a). The action of berry phenolics against human intestinal pathogens. Biofactors. 23 (4): 243 - 51.

Puupponen-Pimiä R, Nohynek L, Hartmann-Schmidlin S, Kähkönen M, Heinonen M, Maatta-Riihinen K, Oksman-Caldentey KM (2005 b). Berry phenolics selectively inhibit the growth of intestinal pathogens. J. Appl. Microbiol. 98 (4): 991 - 1000.

Quale JM, Landman D, Zaman MM, Burney S, Sathe SS (1996). *In vitro* activity of *Cinnamomum zeylanicum* against azole resistant and sensitive *Candida* species and a pilot study of cinnamon for oral candidiasis. *Am. J. Chin. Med.* 24: 103 - 109.

Rahman S, Akbor MM, Howlader A, Jabbar A (2009). Anitimicrobial and cytotoxic activity of the alkaloids of Amlaki (*Emblica officinalis*). Pak. J. Biol. Sci. 12 (16): 1152 - 55.

Ramadan NI, Abdel-Aaty HE, Abdel-Hameed DM, El Deeb HK, Samir NA, Mansy SS, Al Khadrawy FM (2004). Effect of *Ferula assafoetida* on experimental murine *Schistosoma mansoni* infection. J. Egypt. Soc. Parasitol. 34 (3 Suppl): 1077 - 94.

Ramadan NI, Al Khadrawy FM (2003). The *in vitro* effect of Assafoetida on *Trichomonas vaginalis*. J. Egypt. Soc. Parasitol. 33 (2): 615 - 30.

Ranasinghe L, Jayawardena B, Abeywickrama K (2002). Fungicidal activity of essential oils of *Cinnamomum zeylanicum* (L.) and *Syzygium aromaticum* (L.) Merr et L.M. Perry against crown rot and anthracnose pathogens isolated from banana. Lett. Appl. Microbiol. 35 (3): 208 - 211.

Rasooli I, Fakoor MH, Yadegarinia D, Gachkar L, Allameh A, Rezaei MB (2008). Anti-mycotoxigenic characteristics of *Rosmarinus officinalis* and *Trachyspermum copticum* L. essential oils. Int. J. Food Microbiol. 122 (1-2): 135 - 39.

Rattanachaikunsopon P, Phumkhachorn P (2009). Protective effect of clove oil-supplemented fish diets on experimental *Lactococcus garvieae* infection in tilapia. Biosci. Biotechnol. Biochem. 73 (9): 2085 - 89.

Rattanachaikunsopon P, Phumkhachorn P (2010). Anitimicrobial activity of basil (*Ocimum basilicum*) oil against *Salmonella enteritidis in vitro* and in food. Biosci. Biotechnol. Biochem. 74 (6): 1200 - 204.

Raz R, Chazan, B, Dan M (2004). Cranberry juice and urinary tract infection. Clinical Infectious Diseases. 38 (10): 1413 - 19.

Romagnoli C, Andreotti E, Maietti S, Mahendra R, Mares D (2010). Anti-fungal activity of essential oil from fruits of Indian *Cuminum cyminum*. Pharm. Biol. 48 (7): 834 - 38.

Rukayadi Y, Hwang JK (2007). *In vitro* antimycotic activity of xanthorrhizol isolated from *Curcuma xanthorrhiza* Roxb. against opportunistic filamentous fungi. Phytother. Res. 21 (5): 434 - 38.

Russo GL (2009). Dietary n-6 and n-3 polyunsaturated fatty acids: from biochemistry to clinical implications in cardiovascular prevention. Biochem. Pharmacol. 77 (6): 937 - 46.

Ryan KJ, Ray CG (editors) (2004). Sherris Medical Microbiology. (4th ed.). McGraw Hill. ISBN. 0 - 8385 – 8529 - 9.

Saeed S, Tariq P (2007). Anti-bacterial activities of *Emblica officinalis* and *Coriandrum sativum* against Gram negative urinary pathogens. Pak. J. Pharm. Sci 20 (1): 32 - 35.

Santoro GF, Cardoso MG, Guimaraes LG, Mendonça LZ, Soares MJ (2007). *Trypanosoma cruzi*: activity of essential oils from *Achillea millefolium* L., *Syzygium aromaticum* L. and *Ocimum basilicum* L. on epimastigotes and trypomastigotes. Exp. Parasitol. 116 (3): 283 - 90.

Sengupta A, Ghosh S, Bhattacharjee S (2004). Allium vegetables in cancer prevention: an overview. Asian. Pac. J. Cancer Prev. 5 (3): 237 - 45.

Sheikh M, Islam S, Rahman A, Rahman M, Rahman M, Rahman M, Rahim A, Alam F (2010). Control of some human pathogenic bacteria by seed extracts of cumin (*Cuminum cyminum* L.) Agric. conspec. sci. 75 (1):

Singh G, Maurya S, Catalan C, De Lampasona MP (2004). Chemical constituents, anti-fungal and anti-oxidative effects of ajwain essential oil and its acetone extract. J. Agric. Food Chem. 52 (11): 3292 - 96.

Singh HB, Srivastava M, Singh AB, Srivastava AK (1995). Cinnamon bark oil, a potent fungi-toxicant against fungi causing respiratory tract mycoses. *Allergy*. 50: 995 - 99.

Sivam GP (2001). Protection against *Helicobacter pylori* and other bacterial infections by garlic. J. Nutr. 131 (3s): 1106S - 1108S.

Sivam GP, Lampe JW, Ulness B, Swanzy SR, Potter JD (1997). H*elicobacter pylori in vitro* susceptibility to garlic (*Allium sativum*) extract. Nutr. Cancer. 27 (2): 118 - 21.

Slimestad R, Fossen T, Vagen IM (2007). Onions: a source of unique dietary flavonoids. J. Agric. Food Chem. 55 (25): 10067 - 80.

Song J, Choi B, Jin EJ, Yoon Y, Choi KH (2011). Curcumin suppresses *Streptococcus mutans* adherence to human tooth surfaces and extracellular matrix proteins. Eur J Clin Microbiol Infect Dis. 2011 Oct 19. [Epub ahead of print].

Srikanta BM, Nayaka MA, Dharmesh SM (2011). Inhibition of *Helicobacter pylori* growth and its cytotoxicity by 2-hydroxy 4-methoxy benzaldehyde of *Decalepis hamiltonii* (Wight and Arn); a new functional attribute. Biochimie. 93 (4): 678 - 88.

Srikumar R, Parthasarathy NJ, Shankar EM, Manikandan S, Vijayakumar R, Thangaraj R, Vijayananth K, Sheeladevi R, Rao UA (2007). Evaluation of the growth inhibitory activities of Triphala against common bacterial isolates from HIV infected patients. Phytother. Res. 21 (5): 476 - 80.

Srinivasan K (2005). Role of Spices Beyond Food Flavoring: Nutraceuticals with Multiple Health Effects. Food Reviews International. 21 (2): 167 - 88.

Suppakul P, Miltz J, Sonneveld K, Bigger SW (2003). Anitimicrobial properties of basil and its possible application in food packageing. J. Agric. Food Chem. 51 (11): 3197 - 207.

Surh YJ (2002). Anti-tumor promoting potential of selected spice ingredients with anti-oxidative and anti-inflammatory activities: a short review. Food Chem. Toxicol. 40 (8): 1091 - 97.

Tan HT, Rahman RA, Gan SH, Halim AS, Hassan SA, Sulaiman SA, Kirnpal-Kaur B. (2009). The antibacterial properties of Malaysian tualang honey against wound and enteric microorganisms in comparison to manuka honey. BMC. Complement. Altern. Med. 9: 34.

Thangadurai D, Anitha S, Pullaiah T, Reddy PN, Ramachandraiah OS (2002). Essential oil constituents and *in vitro* anitimicrobial activity of *Decalepis hamiltonii* roots against foodborne pathogens. J. Agric. Food Chem. 50 (11): 3147 - 49.

The Wealth of India (A Dictionary of Indian Raw Materials and Industrial Products) (1960). *Raw Materials.* Council of Scientific and Industrial Research. New Delhi, India.

Toulah FH, Al-Rawi MM (2007). Efficacy of garlic extract on hepatic coccidiosis in infected rabbits (*Oryctolagus cuniculus*): histological and biochemical studies. J. Egypt. Soc. Parasitol. 37 (3): 957 - 68.

Tragoolpua Y, Jatisatienr A (2007). Anti-herpes simplex virus activities of *Eugenia caryophyllus* (Spreng.) Bullock and S. G. Harrison and essential oil, eugenol. Phytother. Res. 21 (12): 1153 - 58.

Varadaraj MC, Devi N, Keshava N, Manjrekar SP (1993). Antimicrobial activity of neutralized extracellular culture filtrates of lactic acid bacteria isolated from a cultured Indian milk product ('dahi'). Int. J. Food Microbiol. 20 (4): 259 - 67.

Voidarou C, Alexopoulos A, Plessas S, Karapanou A, Mantzourani I, Stavropoulou E, Fotou K, Tzora A, Skoufos I, Bezirtzoglou E (2011). Anti-bacterial activity of different honeys against pathogenic bacteria. Anaerobe. Apr 16. [Epub ahead of print].

Wang Y, Lu Z, Wu H, Lv F (2009a). Study on the antibiotic activity of microcapsule curcumin against foodborne pathogens. Int. J. Food Microbiol. 136 (1): 71 - 74.

Wang YF, Wang XY, Ren Z, Qian CW, Li YC, Kaio K, Wang QD, Zhang Y, Zheng LY, Jiang JH, Yang CR, Liu Q, Zhang YJ, Wang YF (2009b). Phyllaemblicin B inhibits Coxsackie virus B3 induced apoptosis and myocarditis. Anti-viral Res. 84 (2): 150 - 58.

Wanner J, Bail S, Jirovetz L, Buchbauer G, Schmidt E, Gochev V, Girova T, Atanasova T, Stoyanova A (2010). Chemical composition and anitimicrobial activity of cumin oil (*Cuminum cyminum*, Apiaceae). Nat. Prod. Commun. 5 (9): 1355 - 58.

Willix DJ, Molan PC, Harfoot CG (1992). A comparison of the sensitivity of wound-infecting species of bacteria to the anti-bacterial activity of manuka honey and other honey. J. Appl. Bacteriol. 73 (5): 388 - 94.

Xu Y, Hall C 3rd, Wolf-Hall C, Manthey F (2008). Fungistatic activity of flaxseed in potato dextrose agar and a fresh noodle system. Int. J. Food Microbiol. 121 (3): 262 - 67.

Yanaka A, Fahey JW, Fukumoto A, Nakayama M, Inoue S, Zhang S, Tauchi M, Suzuki H, Hyodo I, Yamamoto M (2009). Dietary sulforaphane-rich broccoli sprouts reduce colonization and attenuate gastritis in *Helicobacter pylori*-infected mice and humans. Cancer. Prev. Res. (Phila). 2 (4): 353 - 60.

Ye X, Ng TB (2009). Isolation and characterization of juncin, an anti-fungal protein from seeds of Japanese Takana (*Brassica juncea* Var. integrifolia). J. Agric. Food Chem. 57 (10): 4366 - 71.

Yoshida S, Kasuga S, Hayashi N, Ushiroguchi T, Matsuura H, Nakagawa S (1987). Anti-fungal activity of ajoene derived from garlic. Appl. Environ. Microbiol. 53 (3): 615 - 17.

Zaika LL (1988). Spices and herbs: Their anitimicrobial activity and its determination. J. Food Safety. 9: 97 - 118.

Zainol MI, Mohd Yusoff K, Mohd Yusof MY (2013). Anti-bacterial activity of selected Malaysian honey. BMC. Complement. Altern. Med. 13 (1): 129.

Chapter 10
Anti-Obesity Foods

Overweight and obesity, often attributed to a higher calorie intake than expenditure (sedentary life style), are global health problems contributing to an ever increasing non- communicable disease burden. Obesity, an excessive weight for height due to an enlarged fat deposition such as adipose tissue is increasingly prevalent.

Liver plays an important role in various aspects of lipid metabolism and fat accumulation. Since fatty liver is closely associated with obesity-related physiological features, including hyperlipidemia, hyperglyceamia, and hepatic lipid accumulation (Kantartzis *et al.*, 2010), hepatic triglyceride (TG) synthesis is an important factor in the development of obesity. In other words, obesity is associated with cardiovascular disease, diabetes, certain forms of cancer etc.

As a growing number of people suffer from obesity, understanding the mechanisms by which various hormones and neurotransmitters influence the energy balance has been a subject of intensive research. Leptin, discovered in 1994, is synthesized and secreted primarily by adipocytes. It is present in blood serum in direct proportion to the amount of adipose tissue. As fat cells become enlarged in obesity, they secrete more leptin. This hormone communicates with the central nervous system to regulate energy intake and energy stores in the body so that the hypothalamus can efficiently maintain a stable body weight. Girls have higher leptin concentrations than boys at all stages of biological development and this is also seen in the state of obesity (Reiterer *et al.*, 1999).

In obese subjects the circulating level of the anorexigenic hormone leptin is increased, whereas surprisingly, the level of the orexigenic hormone ghrelin is decreased (Klok *et al.*, 2007). Plasma leptin concentrations reflect not only total fat mass but also adipose tissue distribution, especially peripheral fat. But plasma leptin values per kilogram of fat mass do not change significantly with modest weight loss (Rissanen *et al.*, 1999).

Obese children who showed significantly higher leptin and obestatin, and lower total ghrelin concentrations than control subjects at baseline, showed significantly diminished plasma leptin and insulin levels, and increased ghrelin and obestatin concentrations after weight loss (Arrigo *et al.*, 2012).

Leptin resistance is often reported in obesity due to which the serum leptin levels increase without suppressing the food intake, resulting in further weight gain. Accordingly, Savoye *et al.* (2002) reported 18 per cent of the weight gain in girls with high basal leptin levels.

Adiponectin is another hormone synthesized by the adipose tissue which facilitates utilization of fat by the body. Abbenhardt *et al.* (2013) confirmed an inverse association between the degree of weight loss and concentration of adiponectin; and a direct association of the same and leptin. One proposed mechanism linking obesity to chronic diseases is an alteration in adipose-derived adiponectin and leptin levels.

Total cholesterol along with plasma leptin were found to be predictive of weight gain over 12 months in a cohort of pre-pubertal children. These two potential predictors can be readily measured in clinical practice and these findings may represent a method of defining the 'at risk of obesity' state in childhood (Byrnes *et al.*, 1999).

Several strategies have been developed and adopted to induce weight loss which include dietary modification, exercise, drugs and surgery. The pharmaceutical industry has invested many efforts in producing anti-obesity drugs; but only a lipid digestion inhibitor obtained from an action of bacterium is currently approved and authorized in Europe for obesity treatment. This compound inhibits the activity of pancreatic lipase, which is one of the enzymes involved in fat digestion. In a similar way, hundreds of extracts are currently being isolated from plants, fungi, algae, or bacteria, and screened for their potential inhibition of pancreatic lipase activity. Among them, extracts isolated from common foodstuffs such as tea, soybean, ginseng, peanut, apple, or grapevine have been documented. Some of the components responsible are polyphenols and saponins with an inhibitory effect on pancreatic lipase activity, which could be applied in the management of the obesity epidemic (de la Garza *et al.*, 2011). Structurally homologous nutraceuticals, derived from red chili, cinnamon, cloves, black pepper, and ginger, also exhibited effects against obesity and insulin resistance.

Several of these components are also potential antioxidants. Oxidative stress is highly correlated with a wide variety of inflammatory and metabolic diseases, including obesity (Furukawa *et al.*, 2004; Sonta *et al.*, 2004; Reaven *et al.*, 2004). The role of nutritional and non nutritional anti-obesity food constituents and foods has been discussed below.

Nutrients and Obesity

Calorie Intake and Prevention of Obesity

Prevention and adequately timed treatment of obesity can lead to successful body mass regulation. The key strategy to combat obesity is to prevent chronic positive impairments in the energy equation. However, it is often difficult to maintain energy balance, because many available foods are high-energy yielding, the consumption of which is usually accompanied by low levels of physical activity.

Calorie restriction can achieve short-term weight loss, but the loss has not been shown to be sustainable in the long-term. An alternative approach to calorie restriction is to lower the fat content of the diet. However, the long-term effects of fat-restricted diets on weight loss have not been established.

The review study of Summerbell *et al.* (2008) using all available randomized clinical trials suggests that fat-restricted diets are no better than calorie restricted diets in achieving long term weight loss in overweight or obese people. A combination of a hypo-caloric diet with fiber rich foods and exercise has been reported to be beneficial in weight reduction more effectively than a hypo-caloric diet alone (Melanson *et al.*, 2006).

Dietary Fat and Obesity

High fat diet-induced obesity is accompanied by increased oxidative stress in liver, heart, and kidney, which is characterized by reduction in the antioxidant enzyme activities and levels that correlated with the increase in MDA and PCO levels in most tissues. This may probably contribute to the occurrence of obesity related problems (Noeman *et al.*, 2011). Interestingly, Astrup *et al.* (2000a) observed that a reduction in dietary fat without intentional restriction of energy intake causes weight loss, which is more substantial in heavier subjects. In fact, reduction in dietary fat without restriction of total energy intake prevents weight gain in subjects of normal weight and produces weight loss in overweight subjects, which is highly relevant for public health (Astrup *et al.*, 2000b). Low fat diets with a high content of complex carbohydrates and protein do not produce any adverse effect on cardiovascular risk factors when weight loss is allowed to occur, and they have been shown to decrease mortality among high risk subjects (Astrup, 2001).

Agents Influencing Fat Metabolism

Inhibition of intestinal absorption of dietary fat has been suggested as a strategy to prevent obesity (Han *et al.* (1999a). Orlistat, a weight-loss agent with a novel mechanism of action was approved by the Food and Drug Administration for the treatment of obesity. It inhibits gastric and pancreatic lipases in the lumen of the gastrointestinal tract to decrease systemic absorption of dietary fat. In several trials lasting up to 2 years, orlistat was found to be more effective than diet alone for weight reduction and also for maintenance of lost weight. Orlistat treatment also results in modest improvements in total cholesterol, low-density lipoprotein, blood pressure, and fasting glucose and insulin concentrations in the blood (Heck *et al.*, 2000). The potential for severe gastrointestinal discomfort and the modest degree of weight loss may limit the agent's clinical utility. Its long-term safety and effectiveness for weight maintenance, cost-effectiveness of treatment, and overall reduction in obesity-related morbidity and mortality are all questionable. Thus there has been a scientific quest for natural and safe antiobesity agents.

Okuda and Han (2001) observed that certain components of foods were capable of reducing absorption of fat and elucidated their mechanism of action *e.g.* (a) Tea saponin and chitosan through inhibiting pancreatic lipase activity, (b) Chondroitin sulfate through inhibiting both pancreatic lipase activity and fatty acid absorption, and (c) Lactosucrose through inhibiting beta-monoglyceride absorption. All these functional substances reduced plasma triglyceride levels too. Chitosan, a deacetylated chitin, is a widely available dietary supplement purported to decrease body weight and serum lipids through binding of fat in the gastrointestinal tract (Mhurchu *et al.*, 2004). Han *et al.* (2005) further confirmed that the anti-obesity effects of tea saponin as well as the the saponin fractions of *P. japonicus* rhizomes in high-fat diet-treated mice probably by inhibiting pancreatic lipase activity, and thus, supported the traditional use of *P. japonicus* rhizomes as a substitute drug for ginseng roots.

Salacia reticulata, a Hippocrateaceae plant distributed in Sri Lankan and Indian forests, has been used as a supplementary food in Japan to prevent obesity and diabetes. Polyphenolic compounds isolated from the roots of *S. reticulata* may be involved in the anti-obesity effects of the hot water-soluble extract in rats through inhibition of fat metabolizing enzymes such as pancreatic lipase, lipoprotein lipase and glycerophosphate dehydrogenase; and also enhanced lipolysis (Yoshikawa *et al.*, 2002).

A review of existing data on effects of weight loss on these variables suggests that benefits occur early in weight reduction and are at least in part due to negative energy balance and that lipid-lowering effects may partially wane over time despite continued weight loss or maintenance (Mertens and Van Gall, 2000; Trials of Hypertension Prevention Collaborative Research Group, 1992; Wadden *et al.*, 1999). Further investigation is required to determine whether effects on lipids and blood pressure would persist after weight stabilization.

Low Glycemic Index Foods

Lowering the glycaemic load of the diet appears to be an effective method of promoting weight loss and improving lipid profiles (Thomas *et al.*, 2007). Body mass, total fat mass, body mass index, total cholesterol and LDL-cholesterol all decreased significantly more in the low glycemic index/load group. Overweight or obese people on low glycemic index diets lost more weight and had more improvement in lipid profiles than those receiving control diets.

Whole Grains

Whole grain (WG)-rich diets are purported to have a variety of health benefits, including a favorable role in body weight regulation. Epidemiological studies consistently demonstrated that higher intakes of WG, but not refined Grains, are associated with lower BMI and/or reduced risk of obesity (Karl and Saltzman, 2012; Liu *et al.*, 2003). BMI and weight gain were inversely associated with intake of breakfast cereals (major source of whole and refined grains, independently of other risk factors (Bazzano *et al.*, 2005). Slavin (2003; 2004) reported that the few whole-grain feeding studies that are available show improvements in biomarkers with whole-grain consumption, such as weight loss, blood lipid improvement and anti-oxidant protection.

Moreover, whole-grain RTE oat cereal as part of a dietary program for weight loss had favorable effects on fasting lipid levels and waist circumference also (Maki *et al.*, 2010). O'Neil *et al.* (2010) confirmed that adults who consumed the most servings of whole grains had lower body weight measures. They also suggested that fiber in whole grain foods may mediate associations with weight measures in adults. and hence intake of whole grain foods should be encouraged by health professionals (Kaul and Nidiry, 1993).

Fordyce-Baum *et al.* (1989) found that an air-expanded whole-wheat protein product (SNW) consumed by moderately obese women as a meal substitute for 12 weeks resulted in safe and effective weight reduction and serum lipid modification.

Red Cowpea (*Adzuki Bean*)

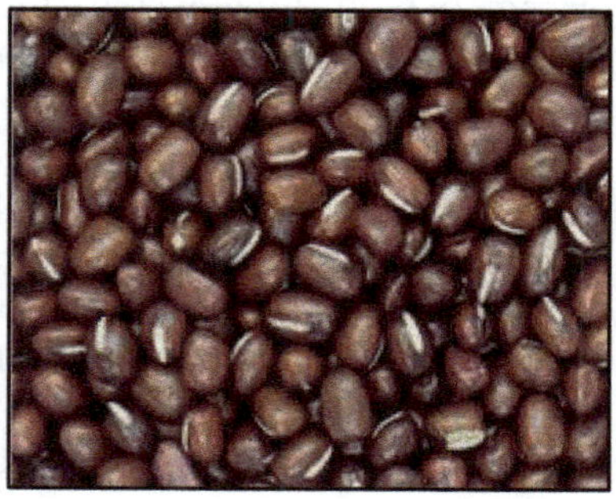

The animal study by Kitano-Okada *et al.* (2012) showed that adzuki bean extracts improved lipid metabolism in both normal and high-fat diet groups. Adzuki bean extract treatment in the high-fat group resulted in significant reductions in total hepatic lipid accumulation and lipid secretion into the feces. Incubation of adipocytes with adzuki bean extract significantly decreased triglyceride accumulation, glycerol phosphate dehydrogenase activity and inflammatory responses without affecting cell viability thus demonstrating that adzuki bean extract has high potential to serve as a natural anti-obesity agent.

Oats (*Avena sativa*)

Recent research suggests that children in the age group of 2-18 years old who have a constant intake of oatmeal lowered their risk of obesity. Research also confirmed that the children who ate oatmeal were 50 per cent less likely to become overweight, when compared to those children that did not. Some studies suggested that protein has a thermogenic effect that boosts metabolism, which may aid weight loss. Beck *et al.* (2009) found a significant dose response, with a positive correlation between the amount of beta-glucan consumed and PYY area under the curve ($r(2) = 0.994$, $P = 0.003$). The optimal dose of beta-glucan appears to lie between 4 and 6 g, with the effects on PYY (an anorexigenic hormone) mediated by viscosity and concentration. Subsequent meal intake decreased by greater than 400 kJ with higher beta-glucan dose (>5 g). Improved satiety by beta-glucan and release of cholecystokinin are likely to be part of the mechanisms.

The average energy intake (-13 per cent, $p<0.05$) and body weight gain were lower with increasing β-glucan over 6 wk with acute suppression of energy intake over 4 h. The highest β-glucan diet significantly increased plasma PYY, with suppression of Arc NPY mRNA (Huang *et al.*, 2011).

Pearl Millet/Fox Tail Millet/Finger Millet (*Panicum miliaceum* L.)

Dietary intake of whole grains reduces the incidence of chronic diseases such as obesity, diabetes, cardiovascular disease, and cancer. Consumption of whole-grain RTE oat cereal as part of a dietary program for weight loss had favorable effects on fasting lipid levels and waist circumference (Maki *et al.*, 2010). Whole grains such as foxtail millet, hog millet, sorghum, Job's tears, and barley have been used as ingredients in traditional Korean food. In a preliminary study hog millet (*Panicum miliaceum* L.) extract showed the highest anti-adipogenic activity by effectively inhibiting lipid synthesis, as measured by lipid-detecting Oil Red O staining, among extracts of nine types of cereal grains in a 3T3-L1 cell system (Park *et al.*, 2011a). Panicum miliaceum L. extract (PME) exhibited the highest antilipogenic activity in 3T3-L1 cells among extracts of nine different cereal grains tested. Also effectively decreased body weight, liver weight, blood triglyceride and total cholesterol levels ($P < 0.05$) compared to obese ob/ob mice on a normal diet. Hepatic lipogenic-related gene (PPARα, L-FABP, FAS, and SCD1) expression decreased, whereas lipolysis-related gene (CPT1) expression increased in animals fed the 1 per cent PME diet ($P < 0.05$). Long chain fatty acid content and the ratio of C18:1/C18:0 fatty acids decreased significantly in adipose tissue of animals fed the 1 per cent PME diet. PME is useful in the chemoprevention or treatment of obesity and obesity-related disorders (Park *et al.*, 2011b). Thus they suggest that PME is useful in the chemoprevention or treatment of obesity and obesity-related disorders.

Flaxseeds (*Linum usitatissimum*)

Dietary fibers have been proposed to play a role in cardiovascular risk as well as body weight management. Flaxseeds are a good source of dietary fibers, and a large proportion of these are water-soluble viscous fibers. Kristensen *et al.* (2012) observed that both flax drink and flax bread decreased plasma total and LDL-cholesterol and increased fat excretion, but suggested that the food matrix and/or processing may be of importance. Viscous flaxseed dietary fibers may be a useful dietary agent for lowering blood cholesterol and potentially play a role in energy balance.

Soya (*Glycine max*)

Soybean (SB) is known to have an anti-obesity effect. A tetrapeptide in soy protein isolate and hydrolysate showed antiobesity effect in genetically obese mice by reducing perirenal fat mass and plasma glucose level. The beneficial effects of this protein food are attributed to its high content of isoflavones mainly genistein and daidzein (Bhatena and Velaquez, (2002). According to them the anti-obesity effect of soy protein and its isoflavones appears to be due to the modulation of pancreatic insulin and antioxidative actions and through long-term substitution of animal proteins by vegetable proteins in low-calorie diet.

Kwon *et al.* (2007) indicated that the anthocyanins in black soybean seed coats have an anti-obesity effect, which can reverse the effects of HFD on body weight, adipose tissue weight, and serum lipid contents. The black soybean anthocyanins suppressed the high fat diet (HFD)-induced weight gain in liver and tended to decrease the weights of epididymal and perirenal fat pads. They improved the lipid profile, by significantly reducing the levels of serum triglyceride and cholesterol, while increasing the high-density lipoprotein-cholesterol concentration. Blake *et al.* (2011) confirmed that the consumption of dietary isoflavones in rats has body weight controlling effects.

A double-blind, randomized clinical trial on the effect of consumption of supplemental whey protein (WP), soy protein (SP), and an isoenergetic amount of carbohydrate (CHO) on body weight and composition in free-living overweight and obese but otherwise healthy participants showed (Baer *et al.*, 2011) the body weight and fat mass of the group consuming the WP to be lower by 1.8 kg ($P < 0.006$) and 2.3 kg ($P < 0.005$), respectively than the group consuming CHO. Lean body mass did not differ among any of the groups. Waist circumference was smaller in the participants consuming WP than in the other groups.

Compared with the high GI/low-protein SB, a high soy protein meal replacement with a low GI was associated with lower glycemia and insulinemia and relatively higher fat oxidation in the postprandial period. Together with a favorable course of appetite-regulating hormones, this could further help to explain the beneficial role of meal replacement regimens high in soy protein for weight reduction and improvement of metabolic risk factors (König *et al.*, 2012).

Recent studies suggest that calcium metabolism and perhaps other components of dairy products may contribute to shifting the energy balance and thus play a role in weight regulation. Faghih *et al.* (2011) observed that weight reductions in high milk, soy milk, calcium supplement and control groups to be 4.43±1.93(kg), 3.46±1.28(kg), 3.89±2.40(kg) and 2.87±1.55(kg), respectively. The greatest changes were seen in the high dairy group in all variables as compared to soya milk or calcium groups. On the other hand Lukaszuk *et al.* (2007) suggested that 720 mL of either soy milk or skim milk daily is needed to optimize the weight loss effects of calcium. In their study, the subjects followed an energy-restricted diet. Soya milk as well as skim milk groups experienced reductions in kilogram weight (4.27±2.05 vs 3.76±2.25; $p=0.668$), body fat per cent (1.30±1.37 vs 1.87±1.45; $p=0.464$), and abdominal circumference (11.28±5.23 vs 8.66±2.51; $p=0.259$) while attenuating losses of fat-free mass (1.12±1.29 vs 0.43±1.12; $p=0.299$) during the 8-week study. There were no significant differences in weight, fat per cent, abdominal circumference, and fat-free mass between groups.

Kwak *et al.* (2012) confirmed that Doenjang (a fermented soya product) was more effective than non fermented soybeans in preventing diet-induced visceral fat accumulation, possibly because of its greater effects on stimulation of carnitine palmitoyltransferase -1 activity and suppression of fatty acid synthase activity. These effects may be due in part to the higher content of aglycone isoflavones in doenjang. Soy-derived isoflavones potentially protect against obesity and depression.

High Protein Diet

The high protein high fiber diet had a satiating effect as evidenced by reduced voluntary intake and has the potential to lead to greater compliance in weight-loss programs (Weber *et al.*, 2007). German *et al.* (2010) reported the percentage weight loss to be greater and mean rate of weight loss to be faster on high protein, high fiber diet. High protein diets are further proved to be offering greater satiety and in some studies are also associated with greater weight loss compared with high carbohydrate diets especially in an ad libitum design (Clifton, 2012).

Green Tea (*Camellia sinensis*, Theaceace)

Green tea is the second most popular beverage in the world and has been extensively studied for its putative disease preventive effects. Green tea is characterized by the presence of a high concentration of polyphenolic compounds known as catechins, with (-)-epigallocatechin-3-gallate (EGCG) being the most abundant and most well-studied. During the last decade, the traditional notion that green tea consumption benefits health has received significant scientific attention.

According to Wang and Tian (2001) epigallocatechin gallate from green tea is a strong inhibitor of fatty acid synthase (FAS) both by reversible fast binding and irreversible slow binding. The inhibitory effects were comparable to that of established FAS inhibitors such as cerulenin and C75, a synthetic FAS inhibitor.

Green tea, green tea catechins, and epigallocatechin gallate (EGCG) have been demonstrated in cell culture and animal models of obesity to reduce adipocyte differentiation and proliferation, lipogenesis, fat mass, body weight, fat absorption, plasma levels of triglycerides, free fatty acids, cholesterol, glucose, insulin and leptin, as well as to increase beta-oxidation and thermogenesis (Kao *et al.*, 2006).

Adipose tissue, liver, intestine, and skeletal muscle are target organs of green tea, mediating its anti-obesity effects (Wolfram *et al.*, 2006). Metabolic syndrome (MetS) is a complex condition that is defined by the presence of elevated waist circumference, dysglycemia, elevated blood pressure, decrease serum high-density lipoprotein-associated cholesterol, and increased serum triglycerides. Studies in both *in vitro* and laboratory animal models have examined the preventive effects of green tea and EGCG against the symptoms of MetS. Overall, the results of these studies have been promising and demonstrated that green tea and EGCG have preventive effects in both genetic and dietary models of obesity, insulin resistance, hypertension, and hypercholesterolemia. According to Bose *et al.* (2008) long-term polyphenol, (-)-epigallocatechin-3-gallate (EGCG) treatment attenuated the development of obesity, symptoms associated with the metabolic syndrome, and fatty liver. Short-term EGCG treatment appeared to reverse preexisting high-fat-induced metabolic pathologies in obese mice. These effects may be mediated by decreased lipid absorption, decreased inflammation, and other mechanisms. Green tea EGCG effectively reduces adipose tissue mass and ameliorates plasma lipid profiles in high-fat diet-induced obese mice. These effects might be at least partially mediated via regulation of the expression of multiple genes involved in adipogenesis, lipolysis, beta-oxidation and thermogenesis in white adipose tissue (Lee *et al.*, 2009).

Chen *et al.* (2009) demonstrated the mechanisms by which tea and EGCG may improve glucose tolerance and support role for these compounds in obesity prevention. These include suppression of adipocyte differentiation and fatty acid uptake into adipose tissue, while increasing fat synthesis and oxidation by the liver, without inducing hepatic fat accumulation by green tea as well as black tea. In contrast,

EGCG increased markers of thermogenesis and differentiation in adipose tissue, while having no effect on liver or muscle tissues at this dose.

Various other mechanisms have also been proposed for the action of green tea components on body fat such as modulation of dietary fat absorption and metabolism, increased glucose utilization, decreased de novo lipogenesis, enhanced vascular responsiveness, and anti oxidative effects (Sae-tan *et al.*, 2011). While reviewing the evidence for the mechanism of action of green tea catechin on weight loss, Rains *et al.* (2011) finds the predominating hypothesis to be its influence on sympathetic nervous system (SNS) activity, increasing energy expenditure and promoting the oxidation of fat. Caffeine, naturally present in green tea, also influences SNS activity, and may act synergistically with catechin to increase energy expenditure and fat oxidation. Other potential mechanisms include modifications in appetite; up-regulation of enzymes involved in hepatic fat oxidation, and decreased nutrient absorption.

EGCG alone has the potential to increase fat oxidation in men and may thereby contribute to the anti-obesity effects of green tea (Moghaddasi and Kashani, 2012).

Another compound in tea, caffeine has also been found to have an effect on body fat. High caffeine intake was associated with weight loss through thermogenesis and fat oxidation, and with suppressed leptin in women. Whereas among the habitual low caffeine consumers, green tea-caffeine mixture improved weight management, partly through thermogenesis and fat oxidation (Westerterp-Plantenga *et al.*, 2005).

Green tea (epigallocatechin gallate + caffeine) and protein each were shown to improve body weight maintenance after weight loss. The green tea-caffeine mixture, as well as the high protein diet, improved weight maintenance independently through thermogenesis, fat oxidation, sparing fat free mass (Hursel *et al.*, 2009a; 2009b). Catechins or an epigallocatechin gallate (EGCG)-caffeine mixture have a small positive effect on weight loss and weight management. The results suggested that habitual caffeine intake and ethnicity may be moderators, as they may influence the effect of catechins. According to Diepvens *et al.* (2007) both green tea catechins and caffeine, may act through inhibition of catechol O-methyl-transferase, and inhibition of phosphodiesterase. Here, the mechanisms may also operate synergistically. In addition, tea catechins have anti-angiogenic properties that may prevent development of overweight and obesity. Furthermore, the sympathetic nervous system is involved in the regulation of lipolysis (Westerterp-Plantenga, 2010).

Thavanesan (2011) on reviewing the available literature on green tea suggests a multimodel approach, involving simultaneous inhibition of the enzymes catechol-O-methyltransferase, acetyl-CoA carboxylase, fatty acid synthase and impeding absorption of fat via the gut. Though the available evidence supports a role of green tea in weight loss, But the author feels the extent of the effects obtained is still subject to debate, and requires more objective quantification in future research.

The antiobesity effects of green tea could be variety specific. Oolong tea is traditionally reported to have anti-obesity and hypolipidaemic effects as it prevented the obesity and fatty liver induced by a high-fat diet. Caffeine in the water extract of oolong tea enhanced noradrenaline-induced lipolysis in fat cells without a concomitant increase in hormone-sensitive lipase activity and also accelerated the hormone-induced lipolysis in a cell-free system consisting of lipid droplets and HSL, but not in the cell-free system with sonicated lipid droplets and HSL. Oolong tea extract also inhibited pancreatic lipase activity and thereby inhibited lipid digestion. Thus, Han *et al.* (1999b) suggested that oolong tea may be an effective crude drug for the treatment of obesity and fatty liver caused by a high-fat diet.

He *et al.* (2009) observed on feeding with 8 g of oolong tea a day for 6 weeks, a decrease of more than 1 kg in body weight in 70 per cent of the severely obese subjects, including 22 per cent who lost more than 3 kg. Similarly, 64 per cent of the obese subjects and 66 per cent of the overweight subjects lost more than 1 kg during the experiment, and the subcutaneous fat content decreased in 12 per cent of the subjects. Oolong tea could decrease body fat content and reduce body weight by improving lipid metabolism. Thus, prolonged consumption of oolong tea may prevent obesity.

Phellinus baumii extract (PBE) in high-fat diet (HFD)-fed 8-week-old male mice significantly reduced body weight gain, hepatic lipid concentrations, and fat accumulation in epididymal adipocytes. The anti-obesity and hypo-lipidemic effects appear to be partly mediated by suppressing plasma and hepatic fat accumulation through the inhibition of enzymes associated with hepatic and intestinal lipid absorption and synthesis (Noh *et al.*, 2011).

Almonds

The fat content and energy density of almonds raise concerns that chronic consumption will promote weight gain. But Hollis and Mattes (2007) confirmed that ten weeks of daily almond consumption did not cause a change in body weight predominantly due to compensation for the energy contained in the almonds through reduced food intake from other sources. Moreover, inefficiency in the absorption of energy from almonds was documented ($P < 0.05$). No changes in resting metabolic rate, thermic effect of food or total energy expenditure were noted. A daily 1440 kJ serving of almonds, sufficient to provide beneficial effects on cardiovascular risk factors, may be included in the diet with limited risk of weight gain. Zaveri and Drummond (2009) also demonstrated that snacking on almonds, in comparison to cereal bars, promoted a higher eating frequency, but not a higher energy intake, but did not result in weight gain, suggesting the possibility of energy compensation.

Wien *et al.* (2003) compared a formula-based LCD enriched with 84 g/day of almonds (almond low calorie diet-39 per cent total fat, 25 per cent MUFA and 32 per cent carbohydrate as per cent of dietary energy) or self-selected complex carbohydrates (CHO-LCD; 18 per cent total fat, 5 per cent MUFA and 53 per cent carbohydrate as per cent of dietary energy) featuring equivalent calories and protein. The almond-enriched low calorie diet (LCD) improved a preponderance of the abnormalities associated with the metabolic syndrome. Although both dietary interventions were effective in decreasing body weight beyond the weight loss observed during long-term pharmacological interventions. The almond-LCD group experienced a sustained and greater weight reduction for the duration of the 24-week intervention. Thus, almond supplementation of a formula-based LCD is a novel alternative to self-selected complex carbohydrates and has a potential role in reducing the public health implications of obesity.

Walnuts (*Juglans regia*)

Studies consistently show the beneficial effects of eating nuts, but as high-energy foods, their regular consumption may lead to weight gain. Epidemiologic studies indicate an inverse association between frequency of nut consumption and body mass index. In well-controlled nut-feeding trials, no changes in body weight were observed. Some studies on free-living subjects in which no constraints on body weight were imposed showed a non-significant tendency to lower weight while subjects are on the nut diets (Sabaté, 2003).

The weight gain from incorporating walnuts into the diet (controle"walnut sequence) was less than the weight loss from withdrawing walnuts from the diet (walnute"control sequence). Sabaté *et al.* (2005) showed that regular walnut intake resulted in weight gain much lower than expected but the gain became non-significant after controlling for differences in energy intake. Despite its high energy content, it appears that in overweight and obese people it did not exert negative effect upon body weight (Canales *et al.*, 2007).

Gurmar (*Gymnema sylvestre*)

Gymnema sylvestre is a woody climbing plant that grows in the tropical forests of central and southern India. Its active constituents include two resins (soluble in alcohol), gymnemic acids, saponins, stigmasterol, quercitol, and the amino acid derivatives betaine, choline and trimethylamine. The active principle of this plant is gymnemic acid. It is a mild diuretic and has the property of abolishing the taste of sugar and neutralising the excess sugar present in the body.

Preuss *et al.* (2004a; b; 2005) showed that the combination of HCA-SX, NBC and *Gymnema sylvestre* can serve as an effective and safe weight-loss formula that can facilitate a reduction in excess body weight and BMI, while promoting healthy blood lipid levels and increasing serum leptin and serotonin levels and fat oxidation more than placebo. Luo *et al.* (2007) also reported that supplementation with gymnemate from *Gymnema sylvestre* promoted weight loss by its ability to reduce hyper-lipidemia, which was no withdrawal rebound: an important discovery. Thus, supplementation with gymnemate could be considered a novel therapeutic tool for weight management, especially in multifactor syndrome.

Garlic (*Allium sativum*)

Kim and Kim (2011) evaluated the effectiveness of garlic on alleviating obesity. Garlic affected the down regulation of expression patterns of epididymal adipose tissue genes such as peroxisome proliferator-activated receptor γ (PPARγ), acetyl CoA carboxylase, adipose specific fatty acid binding protein (aP2), and glycerol-3-phosphate dehydrogenase (GPDH). These results suggest that garlic may have a potential benefit in preventing obesity. They also found the administration of the same to improve the body weight gain and dyslipidemia through the suppression of body fat and alteration in lipid profiles and antioxidant defense system. The anti-obesity effects of garlic were at least partially mediated via activation of AMPK, increased thermogenesis, and decreased expression of multiple genes involved in adipogenesis (Lee *et al.*, 2011). Lee *et al.* (2012) and Joo *et al.* (2013) investigated the effect of hot water extract of garlic (WEG) and high hydrostatic pressure extract of garlic (HEG) on obesity in rats fed a high-fat (HF) diet. Supplementation with HEG significantly reduced body weight gain and adipose tissue mass compared to those in the HF group, whereas WEG did not. Serum levels of triglycerides, total cholesterol, and LDL-cholesterol were also decreased in the HEG supplemented group compared to those in the HF group. Seo *et al.* (2012) reported that AGE supplementation and exercise alone have anti-obesity, cholesterol lowering, and anti-inflammatory effects, but the combined intervention is more effective in reducing weight gain and triglycerides levels than either intervention alone.

Turmeric (*Curcuma longa*)

There is convincing evidence that a large component of obesity-associated pathophysiology may stem from a low-grade pro-inflammatory state. Several spices have been shown to exhibit activity against obesity through antioxidant and anti-inflammatory mechanisms. Among them, turmeric for example, has been described in the literature of Ayurveda ("science of long life"), dating from about 3000 BC, for a wide variety of ailments including obesity. Curcumin, a yellow pigment derived from turmeric has been investigated most extensively as a treatment for obesity and obesity-related metabolic diseases. Curcumin has been shown to possess potent antioxidant, anticarcinogenic, anti-inflammatory, and hypoglycemic properties. Weisberg *et al.* (2008) observed that orally ingested curcumin reversed many of the inflammatory and metabolic derangements associated with obesity and improved glycemic control in mouse models of type 2 diabetes. Ejaz *et al.* (2009) reported that curcumin suppressed lipogenesis in adipose tissue which contributed to lower body fat and body weight gain suggesting that dietary curcumin may have a potential benefit in preventing obesity. Leray *et al.* (2011) also confirmed that highly bioavailable curcumin extract has beneficial effects, targeted in the liver and could improve the obesity-related inflammatory state.

According to Aggarwal (2010), curcumin directly interacts with adipocytes, pancreatic cells, hepatic stellate cells, macrophages, and muscle cells. There, it suppresses the pro-inflammatory transcription factors nuclear factor-kappa B, signal transducer and activators of transcription-3, and Wnt/beta-catenin signaling, and it activates peroxisome proliferator-activated receptor-gamma and Nrf2 cell-signaling pathways, thus leading to the down regulation of adipokines, including tumor necrosis factor (Chan, 1995) interleukin-6, resistin, leptin, and monocyte chemotactic protein-1, and the upregulation of adiponectin and other gene products. These curcumin-induced alterations reverse insulin resistance, hyperglycemia, hyperlipidemia, and other symptoms linked to obesity. Shehzad *et al.* (2011) thus recommended that these results enable translation of curcumin to the clinical practice for the treatment and prevention of obesity-related chronic diseases.

Shao *et al.* (2012) reported that the beneficial effect of curcumin during high fat diet consumption is mediated through attenuating lipogenic gene expression in the liver and the inflammatory response in the adipose tissue, in the absence of stimulation of Wnt signaling in mature adipocytes.

Kaur and Meena (2012) found that combining curcumin with piperine and quercetin in the high fat diet and low-dose streptozotocin-induced diabetic rats corroborate its potential in the treatment of glucose tolerance associated with excess dietary fat intake, obesity, and type 2 diabetes.

Fetuin-A is synthesized in the liver and is secreted into the bloodstream. Clinical studies suggest involvement of fetuin-A in metabolic disorders such as visceral obesity, insulin resistance, diabetes, and fatty liver. Oner-Ýyidoðan *et al.* (2013) confirmed that curcumin treatment to be effective in reducing liver triglycerides and serum fetuin-A levels suggesting that the reduction of fetuin-A may contribute to the beneficial effects of curcumin in the pathogenesis of obesity.

Recent scientific research reveals that curcumin directly interacts with white adipose tissue to suppress chronic inflammation. Bradford (2013) explains the diverse mechanisms by which curcumin reduces obesity and curtails the adverse health effects of obesity. In adipose tissue, curcumin inhibits macrophage infiltration and nuclear factor κB (NF-κB) activation induced by inflammatory agents. Curcumin reduces the expression of the potent pro-inflammatory adipokines -tumor necrosis factor-α (TNFα), monocyte chemo-attractant protein-1 (MCP-1), and plasminogen activator inhibitor type-1 (PAI-1), and it induces the expression of adiponectin, the principal anti-inflammatory agent secreted by adipocytes. Curcumin inhibits adipocyte differentiation and promote anti-oxidant activities.

Cloves (*Syzygium aromaticum*)

In vitro investigation of the effect of ethanol extract of cloves on 3T3-L1 cells revealed that it had efficiently inhibited the conversion of cells into adipocytes in a dose-dependent manner. *In vivo* investigation revealed that supplementation with ethanol extract of cloves had significantly decreased HFD-induced increases in the body weight, liver weight, white adipose tissue (WAT) mass, and serum TG, TC, lipid, glucose, insulin and leptin levels. Consistent with its effects on liver weight and WAT mass, SAE supplementation was found to have suppressed the expression of lipid metabolism-related proteins, including SREBP-1, FAS, CD36 and PPARγ in the liver and WAT, in addition to down regulating mRNA levels of transcription factors including Srebp and Pparg. SAE inhibits fat accumulation in high fat diet-fed mice via the suppression of transcription factors integral to adipogenesis and lipogenesis, suggesting its potential in preventing obesity (Jung *et al.*, 2012).

Curry Leaves (*Murraya koenigii*)

Ethanolic as well as methanolic extracts of curry leaves were found to exhibit anti-lipase activity more than 80 per cent (Birari *et al.*, 2009). An oral dose of 300 mg/kg/day for 2 weeks of *M. koenigii* leaves extract for 2 weeks significantly reduced the body weight gain, plasma total cholesterol and triglyceride levels of obese rats. The anti-obesity and anti-hyperlipidemic activities correlated well with the carbazole alkaloids present in them. Mahanimbine, a carbazole alkaloid, [3, 5-dimethyl-3-(4-methylpent-3-enyl)-11H-pyrano [5, 6-a] carbazole], isolated from the petroleum ether extract of the leaves of *M. koenigii*. (30 mg/kg/day) also significantly lowered the body weight gain as well as plasma total cholesterol and triglyceride levels (Birari *et al.*, 2010).

Bitter Gourd/Bitter Melon *(Momordica charantia)*

Bitter melon has been shown to ameliorate diet-induced obesity and insulin resistance. Extracts of bitter gourd inhibited the proliferation on 3T3-L1 preadipocytes in a dose-dependent manner having the most toxic effect with an LC_{50} value of 1.7 mg/mL. The extract also inhibited the differentiation of preadipocytes in a time-and dose-dependent manner. These anti-obesity-related bioactivities were again attributed to the potential synergistic effects of flavonoids (Gooda *et al.*, 2011). Bitter gourd seed oil is effective in attenuating body fat accumulation through mechanisms associated with protein kinase activation and programmed cell death in the white adipose tissue (Chen *et al.*, 2012). Rats fed 5 per cent lyophilised BM powder showed significantly lower mRNA levels of fatty acid synthase, acetyl-CoA carboxylase-1, lipoprotein lipase and adipocyte fatty acid-binding protein than the high fat group ($P < 0.05$). Hence, Huang *et al.* (2008) concluded that bitter gourd can suppress the visceral fat accumulation and inhibit adipocyte hypertrophy, which may be associated with markedly down regulated expressions of lipogenic genes in the adipose tissue. Yama *et al.* (2010) also demonstrated that bitter gourd caused dose-dependent reductions in body weight and serum cholesterol concentration in male Sprague-Dawley rats. It may, therefore, be useful in controlling body weight gain in individuals of growing age as well as be a potential agent in the management of overweight and obesity.

Bitter gourd appears to have multiple influences on glucose and lipid metabolism that strongly counteract the untoward effects of a high fat diet (Chen *et al.*, 2003). A general decrease in tissue fat accumulation, mediated in part by enhanced sympathetic activity and lipolysis by bitter gourd.

Bitter gourd reduced adiposity in rats fed a high fat diet. BM-supplemented rats had lower energy efficiency (g weight gained/kJ consumed), visceral fat mass, serum glucose, and insulin resistance index, but higher plasma norepinephrine than unsupplemented rats. Hepatic and skeletal muscle triglyceride concentrations were lower in supplemented HF diet-fed rats than in unsupplemented High Fat diet-fed rats (Chan *et al.*, 2005). According to Chen and Li (2005), chronic feeding of bitter gourd leads to a general decrease in tissue fat accumulation and that such an effect is mediated in part by enhanced sympathetic activity and lipolysis. Bitter gourd or its bioactive ingredient(s) could be used as a dietary adjunct in the control of body weight and blood glucose.

Bitter gourd could influence dual PPAR alpha/PPAR gamma expression and the mediated gene expression. It is effective in ameliorating insulin resistance and visceral obesity (Shih *et al.*, 2008). Its juice is a potent inhibitor of lipogenesis and stimulator of lipolysis activity in human adipocytes. The juice may therefore prove to be an effective complementary or alternative therapy to reduce adipogenesis in humans (Nerurkar *et al.*, 2010).

Fruits

Intake of fruits may contribute to weight loss due to the high fibre content. Conceiçao *et al.* (2003) compared the effect of fruit intake with oats consumption on weight loss. The fruit group lost 1.22 kg (95 per cent confidence interval = 0.44-1.85), whereas the oat group had a non-significant weight loss of 0.88 kg (0.37-2.13). A significantly greater decrease of blood glucose was observed among those who had eaten fruits compared with those who had eaten oat cookies, but the glucose: insulin ratio was not statistically different from baseline to follow-up thus suggesting energy densities of fruits, independent of their fiber amount can reduce energy consumption and body weight over time (de Oliveira *et al.*, 2008).

Tamarind (*Tamarindus indica*)

The ethanolic extract of Tamarindus indica fruit pulp showed a significant weight-reducing and hypo-lipidemic activity in cafeteria diet- and sulpiride-induced obese rats (Jindal *et al.*, 2011). Pulp of fruits has hypo-lipidemic and anti-oxidant properties. Azman *et al.* (2012) confirmed the anti-obesity effects of tamarind extract, as indicated by a significant reduction of adipose tissue weights, and the degree of hepatic steatosis in the obesity-induced rats. The extract also possesses hepato-protective activity, as it reversed the elevation of plasma liver enzymes concentration prior to the high-fat diet. A dose-dependent effect was noticed, where at 50 mg/kg tamarind extract showed the most prominent effect, followed by 25 mg/kg and, subsequently, 5 mg/kg body weight in diet-induced obese Sprague-Dawley rats.

Vriksh Amla (*Garcinia cambogia*)

Garcinia cambogia is a yellowish pumpkin-shaped tropical fruit tree native to India. It is claimed to lower body weight and reduce fat mass in humans. The dried fruit rind of *Garcinia cambogia*, also known as Malabar tamarind, is a unique source of (-)-hydroxycitric acid (HCA), which exhibits a distinct sour taste and has been safely used for centuries in Southeastern Asia.

Supplementation in experimental animals showed that HCA can suppress appetite and inhibit body fat biosynthesis. In rat brain cortex, HCA was shown to increase availability of 5-hydroxytryptamine or serotonin. This neuro-transmitter is implicated in the appetite regulation and control (Ohio *et al.*, 2001).

Hydroxycitric acid (HCA) has been found to limit the synthesis of fatty acids in the muscles and liver by inhibiting the enzyme ATP-citrate lyase (a key enzyme which facilitates the synthesis of fatty acids, cholesterol and triglycerides). As a citrate cleavage enzyme that may play an essential role in *de novo* lipogenesis inhibition, with no further synthesis, the existing fatty acids are gradually used up, resulting in reduction of body fat and body weight. Thus *Garcinia cambogia*-derived (-)-hydroxycitric acid (HCA) could be considered a safe and natural supplement for weight management. Preuss *et al.* (2004b) demonstrated the safety, bioavailability and efficacy of Ca2+/K+ bound HCA salt (HCA-SX or Super Citri Max) in weight management. HCA-SX has been shown to increase serotonin availability, reduce appetite, increase fat oxidation, improve blood lipid levels, reduce body weight, and modulate a number of obesity regulatory genes without affecting the mitochondrial and nuclear proteins required for normal biochemical and physiological functions (Downs *et al.*, 2005).

Roy *et al.* (2004; 2007) confirmed the anti-lipolytic and anti-adipogenic effects of HCA-SX although according to Heymsfield *et al.* (1998) *Garcinia cambogia* failed to produce significant weight loss and fat mass loss beyond that observed with placebo.

Grapes and Grape Seeds (*Vitis vinifera*)

High fat diet fed rats treated with ethanol (GSAE) and water (GSWE) extracts of grape seeds revealed significant ($P<0.01$) decrease in weight gain and food intake when compared with high fat diet rats (HFD) without the treatment. The organ weight of the liver and adipose tissue weights of mesenteric, peri-renal and uterine tissues were significantly decreased along with Serum TG, total cholesterol, HDL-cholesterol, glucose levels in the HFD + GSAE and HFD + GSWE groups as compared with the HFD group (Arora *et al.*, 2011).

Guava (*Psidium guajava*)

Pink guava puree significantly decreased the body weight, systolic blood pressure and blood glucose levels of high fat diet-induced-obese rats as compared to the control rats. Triglycerides and Low density lipoprotein-cholesterol reduced while high density lipoprotein values increased in the treated group as compared to control. Thus, Norazmir Jr. and Ayub (2010) reported that pink guava puree had anti-obesity properties and high glutathione peroxidase and superoxidase dismutase enzyme activities.

Grapefruit (*Citrus x paradisi*)

Fresh grapefruit was found to result in significantly more weight loss than the placebo group. Half of a fresh grapefruit eaten before meals was associated with significant weight loss. Supplementation of grapefruit in different forms produced different degrees of weight loss in metabolic syndrome patients. After 12 weeks, the fresh grapefruit group had lost 1.6 kg, the grapefruit juice group had lost 1.5 kg, the grapefruit capsule group had lost 1.1 kg, and the placebo group had lost 0.3 kg. (Fujioka *et al.*, 2006). Although the mechanism of this weight loss is unknown it would appear reasonable to include grapefruit in a weight reduction diet.

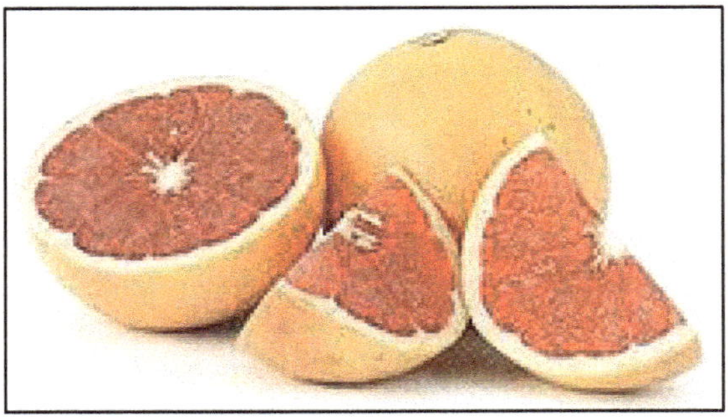

Japanese Pepper (*Zanthoxylum piperitum*)

Zanthoxylum piperitum has been used in Korea as a spice and as a traditional medicine. The fruit and leaves contain terpenoids, flavonoids and other phenolics. Gwon *et al.* (2012) hypothesized that the Japanese pepper contains functional compounds that possess anti-obesity properties. They found that the ethanol extract of the fruit reduced weight gain, white adipose tissue mass, serum triglyceride and cholesterol levels in high fat diet fed mice. A decrease in lipid accumulation and significant attenuation of adipogenic transcription factors, such as PPARγ, C/EBPα, and SREBP-1 in 3T3L1 cells were also observed. Thus they confirmed that *Z. piperitum* exerted an anti-obesity effect by inhibiting adipogenesis through the down regulation of genes involved in the process.

Other Foods

Germinated brown rice (GBR) administration suppressed body weight gain and lipid accumulation in the liver and epididymal adipocytes, and improved serum lipid profiles, probably by controlling adipogenesis through a reduction in transcriptional factors. From these results Ho *et al.* (2012) suggested that GBR is a potential anti-obesity agent.

Recent studies suggest that calcium metabolism and perhaps other components of dairy products may contribute to shifting the energy balance and thus play a role in weight regulation. Faghih *et al.* (2011) found that increasing low fat milk consumption significantly reduces the general and central obesity beyond a low calorie diet.

Both soy and skim milk were observed to induce weight loss in premenopausal women and the effect has been attributed to the calcium content in these products. However, between soy and skim milk groups there were no significant differences in weight, fat per cent, abdominal circumference, and fat-free mass. It was suggested that 720 ml of either soy milk or skim milk must be consumed daily to optimize the weight loss effects of calcium (Lukaszuk *et al.*, 2007).

Conclusions

Several foods and or food constituents have been tested and recommended for controlling obesity. But, further investigations are required to determine whether effects on lipids and blood pressure would persist after weight stabilization. Moreover, the key factors such as fat mass, muscle density, bone density, water mass, their inter-relationships, and impact of anti obesity agents (foods/food components) on energy production, body composition, leptin and overall health and well-being are not yet well understood or addressed in the prevention/cure of obesity.

References

Abbenhardt C, McTiernan A, Alfano CM, Wener MH, Campbell KL, Duggan C, Foster-Schubert KE, Kong A, Toriola AT, Potter JD, Mason C, Xiao L, Blackburn GL, Bain C, Ulrich CM (2013). Effects of individual and combined dietary weight loss and exercise interventions in postmenopausal women on adiponectin and leptin levels. J Intern Med. 2013 Feb 25. doi: 10.1111/joim.12062. [Epub ahead of print].

Aggarwal BB (2010). Targeting inflammation-induced obesity and metabolic diseases by curcumin and other nutraceuticals. Annu. Rev. Nutr. 30: 173 - 99.

Arora P, Ansari S, Nazish (2011). Study of antiobesity effects of ethanolic and water extracts of grapes seeds. J. Complement. Integr. Med. 8 (1). doi: 10.2202/1553-3840.1510.

Arrigo T, Gitto E, Ferraù V, Munafò C, Alibrandi A, Marseglia GL, Salpietro A, Miraglia Del Giudice M, Leonardi S, Ciprandi G, Salpietro C (2012). Effect of weight reduction on leptin, total ghrelin and obestatin concentrations in prepubertal children. J. Biol. Regul. Homeost. Agents. 26 (1 Suppl): S95 - 103.

Astrup A (2001). The role of dietary fat in the prevention and treatment of obesity. Efficacy and safety of low-fat diets. Int. J. Obes. Relat. Metab. Disord. 25 (Suppl 1): S46 - 50.

Astrup A, Grunwald GK, Melanson EL, Saris WH, Hill JO (2000a). The role of low-fat diets in body weight control: a meta-analysis of ad libitum dietary intervention studies. Int. J. Obes. Relat. Metab. Disord. 24 (12): 1545 - 52.

Astrup A, Ryan L, Grunwald GK, Storgaard M, Saris W, Melanson E, Hill JO (2000b). The role of dietary fat in body fatness: evidence from a preliminary meta-analysis of ad libitum low-fat dietary intervention studies. Br. J. Nutr. 83 (Suppl 1): S25 - 32.

Azman KF, Amom Z, Azlan A, Esa NM, Ali RM, Shah ZM, Kadir KK (2012). Anti-obesity effect of *Tamarindus indica* L. pulp aqueous extract in high-fat diet-induced obese rats. J. Nat. Med. 66 (2): 333 - 42.

Baer DJ, Stote KS, Paul DR, Harris GK, Rumpler WV, Clevidence BA (2011). Whey protein but not soy protein supplementation alters body weight and composition in free-living overweight and obese adults. J. Nutr.141 (8): 1489 - 94.

Bazzano LA, Song Y, Bubes V, Good CK, Manson JE, Liu S (2005). Dietary intake of whole and refined grain breakfast cereals and weight gain in men. Obes. Res. 13 (11): 1952 - 60.

Beck EJ, Tosh SM, Batterham MJ, Tapsell LC, Huang XF (2009). Oat beta-glucan increases postprandial cholecystokinin levels, decreases insulin response and extends subjective satiety in overweight subjects. Mol. Nutr. Food Res. 53 (10): 1343 - 51.

Bhatena SJ, Velaquez MT (2002). Beneficial role of dietary phytoestrogens in obesity and diabetes. *The American Journal of Clinical Nutrition.* 76 (6): 1191 - 201.

Birari R, Javia V, Bhutani KK (2010). Anti-obesity and lipid lowering effects of *Murraya koenigii* (L.) Spreng leaves extracts and mahanimbine on high fat diet induced obese rats [J]. Fitoterapia. 81 (8): 1129 - 33.

Birari R, Roy SK, Singh A, Bhutani KK (2009). Pancreatic lipase inhibitory alkaloids of *Murraya koenigii* leaves[J]. Nat. Prod. Commun. 4 (8): 1089 - 92.

Blake C, Fabick KM, Setchell KD, Lund TD, Lephart ED (2011). Neuromodulation by soy diets or equol: anti-depressive and anti-obesity-like influences, age- and hormone-dependent effects. BMC. Neurosci. 12: 28.

Bose M, Lambert JD, Ju J, Reuhl KR, Shapses SA, Yang CS (2008). The major green tea polyphenol, (-)-epigallocatechin-3-gallate, inhibits obesity, metabolic syndrome, and fatty liver disease in high-fat-fed mice. J. Nutr. 138 (9): 1677 - 83.

Bradford PG (2013). Curcumin and obesity. Biofactors. 39 (1): 78 - 87.

Byrnes SE, Baur LA, Bermingham M, Brock K, Steinbeck K (1999). Leptin and total cholesterol are predictors of weight gain in pre-pubertal children. Int. J. Obes. Relat. Metab. Disord. 23 (2): 146 - 50.

Canales A, Benedí J, Nus M, Librelotto J, Sánchez-Montero JM, Sánchez-Muniz FJ (2007). Effect of walnut-enriched restructured meat in the antioxidant status of overweight/obese senior subjects with at least one extra CHD-risk factor. J. Am. Coll. Nutr. 26 (3): 225 - 32.

Chan MM (1995). Inhibition of tumor necrosis factor by curcumin, a phytochemical. Biochem Pharmacol. 49 (11): 1551 - 56.

Chan LL, Chen Q, Go AG, Lam EK, Li ET (2005). Reduced adiposity in bitter melon (*Momordica charantia*)-fed rats is associated with increased lipid oxidative enzyme activities and uncoupling protein expression. J. Nutr. 135 (11): 2517 - 23.

Chen N, Bezzina R, Hinch E, Lewandowski PA, Cameron-Smith D, Mathai ML, Jois M, Sinclair AJ, Begg DP, Wark JD, Weisinger HS, Weisinger RS (2009). Green tea, black tea, and epigallocatechin modify body composition, improve glucose tolerance, and differentially alter metabolic gene expression in rats fed a high-fat diet. Nutr. Res. 29 11): 784 - 93.

Chen PH, Chen GC, Yang MF, Hsieh CH, Chuang SH, Yang HL, Kuo YH, Chyuan JH, Chao PM (2012). Bitter melon seed oil-attenuated body fat accumulation in diet-induced obese mice is associated with cAMP-dependent protein kinase activation and cell death in white adipose tissue. J. Nutr. 142 (7): 1197 - 204.

Chen Q, Chan LL, Li ET (2003). Bitter melon (*Momordica charantia*) reduces adiposity, lowers serum insulin and normalizes glucose tolerance in rats fed a high fat diet. J. Nutr. 133 (4): 1088 - 93.

Chen Q, Li ET (2005). Reduced adiposity in bitter melon (*Momordica charantia*) fed rats is associated with lower tissue triglyceride and higher plasma catecholamines. Br. J. Nutr. 93 (5): 747 - 54.

Clifton P (2012). Effects of a high protein diet on body weight and co-morbidities associated with obesity. Br. J. Nutr. 108 (Suppl. 2): S122 - 29.

Conceiçao de Oliveira M, Sichieri R, Sanchez Moura A (2003). Weight loss associated with a daily intake of three apples or three pears among overweight women. Nutrition. 19 (3): 253 - 56.

de la Garza AL, Milagro FI, Boque N, Campión J, Martínez JA (2011). Natural inhibitors of pancreatic lipase as new players in obesity treatment. Planta. Med. 77 (8): 773 - 85.

de Oliveira MC, Sichieri R, Venturim Mozzer R (2008). A low-energy-dense diet adding fruit reduces weight and energy intake in women. Appetite. 51 (2): 291 - 95.

Diepvens K, Westerterp KR, Westerterp-Plantenga MS (2007). Obesity and thermogenesis related to the consumption of caffeine, ephedrine, capsaicin, and green tea. Am. J. Physiol. Regul. Integr. Comp. Physiol. 292 (1): R77 - 85.

Downs BW, Bagchi M, Subbaraju GV, Shara MA, Preuss HG, Bagchi D (2005). Bioefficacy of a novel calcium-potassium salt of (-)-hydroxycitric acid. Mutat. Res. 579 (1-2): 149 - 62.

Ejaz A, Wu D, Kwan P, Meydani M (2009). Curcumin inhibits adipogenesis in 3T3-L1 adipocytes and angiogenesis and obesity in C57/BL mice. J. Nutr. 139 (5): 919 - 25.

Faghih SH, Abadi AR, Hedayati M, Kimiagar SM (2011). Comparison of the effects of cows' milk, fortified soy milk, and calcium supplement on weight and fat loss in premenopausal overweight and obese women. Nutr. Metab Cardiovasc. Dis. 21 (7): 499 - 503.

Fordyce-Baum MK, Langer LM, Mantero-Atienza E, Crass R, Beach RS (1989). Use of an expanded-whole-wheat product in the reduction of body weight and serum lipids in obese females. Am. J. Clin. Nutr. 50 (1): 30 - 36.

Fujioka K, Greenway F, Sheard J, Ying Y (2006). The effects of grapefruit on weight and insulin resistance: relationship to the metabolic syndrome. J. Med. Food. 9 (1): 49 - 54.

Furukawa S, Fujita T, Shimabukuro M, Iwaki M, Nakajima Y, Nakayama O, Makishima M, Matsuda M, Shimomura I (2004). Increased oxidative stress in obesity and its impact on metabolic syndrome. J. Clin. Investig. 114:.1752 - 61.

German AJ, Holden SL, Bissot T, Morris PJ, Biourge V (2010). A high protein, high fibre diet improves weight loss in obese dogs. Vet. J. 183 (3): 294 - 97.

Gooda SN, Hamid AA, Kitts D, Purnama M, Saari N, Abas F (2011). The effects of *Morinda citrifolia, Momordica charantia* and *Centella asiatica* extracts on lipoprotein lipase and 3T3-L1 preadipocytes. *Journal of Food Biochemistry.* 35 (4): 1186 - 205.

Gwon SY, Ahn JY, Kim TW, Ha TY (2012). *Zanthoxylum piperitum* DC ethanol extract suppresses fat accumulation in adipocytes and high fat diet-induced obese mice by regulating adipogenesis. J. Nutr. Sci. Vitaminol. (Tokyo). 58 (6): 393 - 401.

Han LK, Kimura Y, Okuda H (1999a). Reduction in fat storage during chitin-chitosan treatment in mice fed a high-fat diet. Int. J. Obes. Relat. Metab. Disord. 23 (2): 174 - 79.

Han LK, Takaku T, Li J, Kimura Y, Okuda H (1999b). Anti-obesity action of oolong tea. Int. J. Obes. Relat. Metab. Disord. 23 (1): 98 - 105.

Han LK, Zheng YN, Yoshikawa M, Okuda H, Kimura Y (2005). Anti-obesity effects of chikusetsusaponins isolated from *Panax japonicus* rhizomes. BMC. Complement. Altern. Med. 5: 9.

He RR, Chen L, Lin BH, Matsui Y, Yao XS, Kurihara H (2009). Beneficial effects of oolong tea consumption on diet-induced overweight and obese subjects. Chin. J. Integr. Med. 15 (1): 34 - 41.

Heck AM, Yanovski JA, Calis KA (2000). Orlistat, a new lipase inhibitor for the management of obesity. Pharmacotherapy. 20 (3): 270 - 79.

Heymsfield SB, Allison DB, Vasselli JR, Pietrobelli A, Greenfield D, Nunez C (1998). *Garcinia cambogia* (hydroxycitric acid) as a potential anti-obesity agent: a randomized controlled trial. JAMA. 280 (18): 1596 - 600.

Ho JN, Son ME, Lim WC, Lim ST, Cho HY (2012). Anti-obesity effects of germinated brown rice extract through down-regulation of lipogenic genes in high fat diet-induced obese mice. Biosci. Biotechnol. Biochem. 76 (6): 1068 - 74.

Hollis J, Mattes R (2007). Effect of chronic consumption of almonds on body weight in healthy humans. Br. J. Nutr. 98 (3): 651 -56.

Huang HL, Hong YW, Wong YH, Chen YN, Chyuan JH, Huang CJ, Chao PM (2008). Bitter melon (*Momordica charantia* L.) inhibits adipocyte hypertrophy and down regulates lipogenic gene expression in adipose tissue of diet-induced obese rats. Br. J. Nutr. 99 (2) 230 - 39.

Huang XF, Yu Y, Beck EJ, South T, Li Y, Batterham MJ, Tapsell LC, Chen J (2011). Diet high in oat β-glucan activates the gut-hypothalamic (PYY-NPY) axis and increases satiety in diet-induced obesity in mice. Mol. Nutr. Food Res. 55 (7): 1118 – 21.

Hursel R, Viechtbauer W, Westerterp-Plantenga MS (2009 a). The effects of green tea on weight loss and weight maintenance: a meta-analysis. Int. J. Obes. (Lond). 33 (9): 956 - 61.

Hursel R, Westerterp-Plantenga MS (2009 b). Green tea catechin plus caffeine supplementation to a high-protein diet has no additional effect on body weight maintenance after weight loss. Am. J. Clin. Nutr. 89 (3): 822 - 30.

Jindal V, Dhingra D, Sharma S, Parle M, Harna RK (2011). Hypolipidemic and weight reducing activity of the ethanolic extract of *Tamarindus indica* fruit pulp in cafeteria diet- and sulpiride-induced obese rats. J. Pharmacol. Pharmacother. 2 (2): 80 - 84.

Joo H, Kim CT, Kim IH, Kim Y (2013). Anti-obesity effects of hot water extract and high hydrostatic pressure extract of garlic in rats fed a high-fat diet. Food Chem. Toxicol. 55C: 100 - 105.

Jung CH, Ahn J, Jeon TI, Kim TW, Ha TY (2012). *Syzygium aromaticum* ethanol extract reduces high-fat diet-induced obesity in mice through downregulation of adipogenic and lipogenic gene expression. Exp Ther Med. 4 (3): 409 - 414.

Kantartzis K, Schick F, Häring HU, Stefan N (2010). Environmental and genetic determinants of fatty liver in humans. Dig. Dis. 28 (1): 169 - 78.

Kao YH, Chang HH, Lee MJ, Chen CL (2006). Tea, obesity, and diabetes. Mol. Nutr. Food Res. 50 (2): 188 - 210.

Karl JP, Saltzman E (2012). The role of whole grains in body weight regulation. Adv. Nutr. 3 (5): 697 - 707.

Kaul L, Nidiry J (1993). High-fiber diet in the treatment of obesity and hyper-cholesterolemia. J. Natl. Med. Assoc. 85 (3): 231 - 32.

Kaur G, Meena C (2012). Amelioration of obesity, glucose intolerance, and oxidative stress in high-fat diet and low-dose streptozotocin-induced diabetic rats by combination consisting of curcumin with piperine and quercetin. ISRN. Pharmacol. 2012: 957283.

Kim MJ, Kim HK (2011). Effect of garlic on high fat induced obesity. Acta. Biol. Hung. 62 (3): 244 - 54.

Kitano-Okada T, Ito A, Koide A, Nakamura Y, Han KH, Shimada K, Sasaki K, Ohba K, Sibayama S, Fukushima M (2012). Anti-obesity role of adzuki bean extract containing polyphenols: *in vivo* and *in vitro* effects. J. Sci. Food. Agric. 2012 Apr 11. doi: 10.1002/jsfa. 5680.

Klok MD, Jakobsdottir S, Drent ML (2007). The role of leptin and ghrelin in the regulation of food intake and body weight in humans: a review. Obes. Rev. 2007 Jan. 8 (1): 21 - 34.

König D, Muser K, Berg A, Deibert P (2012). Fuel selection and appetite-regulating hormones after intake of a soy protein-based meal replacement. Nutrition. 28 (1): 35 - 39.

Kristensen M, Jensen MG, Aarestrup J, Petersen KE, Søndergaard L, Mikkelsen MS, Astrup A (2012). Flaxseed dietary fibers lower cholesterol and increase fecal fat excretion, but magnitude of effect depend on food type. Nutr. Metab. (Lond). 9 : 8.

Kwak CS, Park SC, Song KY (2012). Doenjang, a fermented soybean paste, decreased visceral fat accumulation and adipocyte size in rats fed with high fat diet more effectively than non-fermented soybeans. J. Med. Food. 15 (1): 1 - 9.

Kwon SH, Ahn IS, Kim SO, Kong CS, Chung HY, Do MS, Park KY (2007). Anti-obesity and hypolipidemic effects of black soybean anthocyanins. J.Med. Food. 10 (3): 552 - 56.

Lee MS, Kim CT, Kim Y (2009). Green tea (-)-epigallocatechin-3-gallate reduces body weight with regulation of multiple genes expression in adipose tissue of diet-induced obese mice. Ann. Nutr. Metab. 54 (2): 151 - 57.

Lee MS, Kim IH, Kim CT, Kim Y (2011). Reduction of Body Weight by Dietary Garlic Is Associated with an Increase in Uncoupling Protein mRNA Expression and Activation of AMP-Activated Protein Kinase in Diet-Induced Obese Mice. J. Nutr. 141 (11): 1947 - 53.

Lee S, Joo H, Kim CT, Kim IH, Kim Y (2012). High hydrostatic pressure extract of garlic increases the HDL cholesterol level via up-regulation of apolipoprotein A-I gene expression in rats fed a high-fat diet. Lipids Health. Dis. 11: 77.

Leray V, Freuchet B, Le Bloc'h J, Jeusette I, Torre C, Nguyen P. (2011). Effect of citrus polyphenol- and curcumin-supplemented diet on inflammatory state in obese cats. Br. J. Nutr. 106 Suppl. 1: S198 - 201.

Liu S, Willett WC, Manson JE, Hu FB, Rosner B, Colditz G (2003). Relation between changes in intakes of dietary fiber and grain products and changes in weight and development of obesity among middle-aged women. Am. J. Clin. Nutr. 78 (5): 920 - 27.

Lukaszuk JM, Luebbers P, Gordon BA (2007). Preliminary study: soy milk as effective as skim milk in promoting weight loss. J. Am. Diet. Assoc. 107 (10): 1811 - 14.

Luo H, Kashiwagi A, Shibahara T, Yamada K (2007). Decreased bodyweight without rebound and regulated lipoprotein metabolism by gymnemate in genetic multifactor syndrome animal. Mol, Cell Biochem. 299 (1-2): 93 - 98.

Maki KC, Beiseigel JM, Jonnalagadda SS, Gugger CK, Reeves MS, Farmer MV, Kaden VN, Rains TM (2010). Whole-grain ready-to-eat oat cereal, as part of a dietary program for weight loss, reduces low-density lipoprotein cholesterol in adults with overweight and obesity more than a dietary program including low-fiber control foods. J. Am. Diet. Assoc. 110 (2): 205 - 214.

Melanson KJ, Angelopoulos TJ, Nguyen VT, Martini M, Zukley L, Lowndes J, Dube TJ, Fiutem JJ, Yount BW, Rippe JM (2006). Consumption of whole-grain cereals during weight loss: effects on dietary quality, dietary fiber, magnesium, vitamin B-6, and obesity. J. Am. Diet. Assoc. 106 (9): 1380 - 88.

Mertens IL and Van Gall LF (2000). Overweight, obesity, and blood pressure: the effects of modest weight loss. Obes. Res. 8: 270 - 78.

Mhurchu CN, Poppitt SD, McGill AT, Leahy FE, Bennett DA, Lin RB, Ormrod D, Ward L, Strik C, Rodgers A (2004). The effect of the dietary supplement, Chitosan, on body weight: a randomised controlled trial in 250 overweight and obese adults. Int. J. Obes. Relat. Metab. Disord. 28 (9): 1149 - 56.

Moghaddasi MS, Kashani HH (2012). Effect of tea in the treatment of obesity. Scientific Research and Essays. 7 (13): 1381 - 84.

Nerurkar PV, Lee YK, Nerurkar VR (2010). *Momordica charantia* (bitter melon) inhibits primary human adipocyte differentiation by modulating adipogenic genes. BMC. Complement. Altern. Med. 10: 34.

Noeman SA, Hamooda HE, Baalash AA (2011). Biochemical study of oxidative stress markers in the liver, kidney and heart of high fat diet induced obesity in rats. Diabetol. Metab. Syndr. 3 (1): 17.

Noh JR, Lee IK, Ly SY, Yang KJ, Gang GT, Kim YH, Hwang JH, Yun BS, Lee CH (2011). A *Phellinus baumii* extract reduces obesity in high-fat diet-fed mice and absorption of triglyceride in lipid-loaded mice. J. Med. Food. 14 (3): 209 - 218.

Norazmir MN Jr, Ayub MY (2010). Beneficial lipid-lowering effects of pink guava puree in high fat diet induced-obese rats. Malays. J. Nutr. 16 (1): 171 - 85.

Ohio SE, Awe SO, Le Day AM, Opere CA, Bagchi D (2001). Effect of hydroxycitric acid on serotonin release from isolated rat brain cortex. Research Communications in Molecular Pathology and Pharmacology. 109 (3-4): 210 - 16.

Okuda H, Han LK (2001). Medicinal plant and its related metabolic modulators. Nihon. Yakurigaku. Zasshi. 118 (5): 347 - 51. [Article in Japanese].

O'Neil CE, Zanovec M, Cho SS, Nicklas TA (2010). Whole grain and fiber consumption are associated with lower body weight measures in US adults: National Health and Nutrition Examination Survey 1999-2004. Nutr. Res. 30 (12): 815 - 22.

Oner-Ýyidoðan Y, Koçak H, Seyidhanoðlu M, Gürdöl F, Gülçubuk A, Yildirim F, Cevik A, Uysal M (2013). Curcumin prevents liver fat accumulation and serum fetuin-A increase in rats fed a high-fat diet. J Physiol Biochem. 2013 Feb 22. [Epub ahead of print].

Park MY, Jang HH, Kim JB, Yoon HN, Lee JY, Lee YM, Kim JH, Park DS (2011a). Hog millet (*Panicum miliaceum* L.)-supplemented diet ameliorates hyper-lipidemia and hepatic lipid accumulation in C57BL/6J-ob/ob mice. Nutr Res Pract. 5 (6): 511 - 19.

Park MY, Seo DW, Lee JY, Sung MK, Lee YM, Jang HH, Choi HY, Kim JH, Park DS (2011b). Effects of *Panicum miliaceum* L. extract on adipogenic transcription factors and fatty acid accumulation in 3T3-L1 adipocytes. Nutr. Res. Pract. 5: 192 - 97.

Preuss HG, Bagchi D, Bagchi M, Rao CV, Dey DK, Satyanarayana S (2004a). Effects of a natural extract of (-)-hydroxycitric acid (HCA-SX) and a combination of HCA-SX plus niacin-bound chromium and *Gymnema sylvestre* extract on weight loss. Diabetes Obes. Metab. 6 (3): 171 - 80.

Preuss HG, Garis RI, Bramble JD, Bagchi D, Bagchi M, Rao CV, Satyanarayana S (2005). Efficacy of a novel calcium/potassium salt of (-)-hydroxycitric acid in weight control. Int. J. Clin. Pharmacol. Res. 25 (3): 133 - 44.

Preuss HG, Rao CV, Garis R, Bramble JD, Ohia SE, Bagchi M, Bagchi D (2004b). An overview of the safety and efficacy of a novel, natural (-) -hydroxycitric acid extract (HCA-SX) for weight management. J. Med. 35 (1-6): 33 - 48.

Rains TM, Agarwal S, Maki KC (2011). Anti-obesity effects of green tea catechins: a mechanistic review. J. Nutr. Biochem. 22 (1): 1 - 7.

Reaven G, Abbasi F, McLaughlin T (2004). Obesity, insulin resistance, and cardiovascular disease. Recent Prog. Horm. Res. 59: 207 -23.

Reiterer EE, Sudi KM, Mayer A, Limbert-Zinterl C, Stalzer-Brunner C, Füger G, Borkenstein MH (1999). Changes in leptin, insulin and body composition in obese children during a weight reduction program. J. Pediatr. Endocrinol. Metab. 12 (6): 853 - 62.

Rissanen P, Mäkimattila S, Vehmas T, Taavitsainen M, Rissanen A (1999). Effect of weight loss and regional fat distribution on plasma leptin concentration in obese women. Int J Obes Relat Metab Disord. 23 (6): 645 - 49.

Roy S, Rink C, Khanna S, Phillips C, Bagchi D, Bagchi M, Sen CK (2004). Body weight and abdominal fat gene expression profile in response to a novel hydroxycitric acid-based dietary supplement. Gene Expr. 11 (5-6): 251 - 62.

Roy S, Shah H, Rink C, Khanna S, Bagchi D, Bagchi M, Sen CK (2007). Transcriptome of primary adipocytes from obese women in response to a novel hydroxycitric acid-based dietary supplement. DNA Cell. Biol. 26 (9): 627 - 39.

Sabaté J (2003). Nut consumption and body weight. Am. J. Clin. Nutr. 78 (3 Suppl): 647S - 650S. Review.

Sabaté J, Cordero-Macintyre Z, Siapco G, Torabian S, Haddad E (2005). Does regular walnut consumption lead to weight gain? Br. J. Nutr. 94 (5): 859 - 64.

Sae-tan S, Grove KA, Lambert JD (2011). Weight control and prevention of metabolic syndrome by green tea. Pharmacol. Res. 64 (2): 146 - 54.

Savoye M, Dziura J, Castle J, DiPietro L, Tamborlane WV, Caprio S (2002). Importance of plasma leptin in predicting future weight gain in obese children: a two-and-a-half-year longitudinal study. Int. J. Obes. Relat. Metab. Disord. 26 (7): 942 - 46.

Seo DY, Lee S, Figueroa A, Kwak YS, Kim N, Rhee BD, Ko KS, Bang HS, Baek YH, Han J (2012). Aged garlic extract enhances exercise-mediated improvement of metabolic parameters in high fat diet-induced obese rats. Nutr. Res. Pract. 6 (6): 513 - 19.

Shao W, Yu Z, Chiang Y, Yang Y, Chai T, Foltz W, Lu H, Fantus IG, Jin T (2012). Curcumin prevents high fat diet induced insulin resistance and obesity via attenuating lipogenesis in liver and inflammatory pathway in adipocytes. PLoS One. 7 (1): e28784.

Shehzad A, Ha T, Subhan F, Lee YS (2011). New mechanisms and the anti-inflammatory role of curcumin in obesity and obesity-related metabolic diseases. Eur. J. Nutr. 50 (3): 151 - 61.

Shih CC, Lin CH, Lin WL (2008). Effects of *Momordica charantia* on insulin resistance and visceral obesity in mice on high-fat diet. Diabetes Res Clin Pract. 81 (2): 134 - 43.

Slavin J (2003). Why whole grains are protective: biological mechanisms. Proc. Nutr. Soc. 62 (1): 129 - 34.

Slavin J (2004). Whole grains and human health. Nutr. Res. Rev. 17 (1): 99 - 110.

Sonta T, Inoguchi T, Tsubouchi H, Sekiguchi N, Kobayashi K, Matsumoto S, Utsumi H, Nawata H (2004). Evidence for contribution of vascular NAD(P)H oxidase to increased oxidative stress in animal models of diabetes and obesity. Free Radic. Biol. Med. 37 (1): 115 – 23.

Summerbell CD, Cameron C, Glasziou PP (2008). WITHDRAWN: Advice on low-fat diets for obesity. Cochrane. Database Syst. Rev. 16 (3): CD003640.

Thavanesan N (2011). The putative effects of green tea on body fat: an evaluation of the evidence and a review of the potential mechanisms. Br J Nutr. 106 (9): 1297-309.

Thomas DE, Elliott EJ, Baur L (2007). Low glycaemic index or low glycaemic load diets for overweight and obesity. Cochrane Database Syst. Rev. 18 (3): CD005105.

Trials of Hypertension Prevention Collaborative Research Group (1992). The effects of non-pharmacologic interventions on blood pressure of persons with high normal levels: results of the Trials of Hypertension Prevention, phase 1. J. Am. Med. Assoc. 267: 1213 - 20.

Wadden, TA, Anderson, DA and Foster, GD (1999). Two-year changes in lipids and lipoproteins associated with maintenance of a 5 per cent to 10 per cent reduction in initial weight: some findings and some questions. Obes. Res. 7: 170 - 78.

Wang X, Tian W (2001). Green tea epigallocatechin gallate: a natural inhibitor of fatty acid synthase. *Biochemical and Biophysical Research Communication.* 28 (5): 1200 - 206.

Weber M, Bissot T, Servet E, Sergheraert R, Biourge V, German AJ (2007). A high-protein, high-fiber diet designed for weight loss improves satiety in dogs. J. Vet. Intern. Med. 21 (6): 1203 - 208.

Weisberg SP, Leibel R, Tortoriello DV (2008). Dietary curcumin significantly improves obesity-associated inflammation and diabetes in mouse models of diabesity. Endocrinology. 149 (7): 3549 - 58.

Westerterp-Plantenga MS (2010). Green tea catechins, caffeine and body-weight regulation. Physiol. Behav. 100 (1): 42 - 46.

Westerterp-Plantenga MS, Lejeune MP, Kovacs EM (2005). Body weight loss and weight maintenance in relation to habitual caffeine intake and green tea supplementation. Obes. Res. 13 (7): 1195 - 204.

Wien MA, Sabaté JM, Iklé DN, Cole SE, Kandeel FR (2003). Almonds vs complex carbohydrates in a weight reduction program. Int. J. Obes. Relat. Metab. Disord. 27 (11): 1365 - 72.

Wolfram S, Wang Y, Thielecke F (2006). Anti-obesity effects of green tea: from bedside to bench. Mol. Nutr. Food Res. 50 (2): 176 - 87.

Yama OE, Osinubi AA, Noronha CC, Okanlawon AO (2010). Effect of methanolic seed extract of *Momordica charantia* on body weight and serum cholesterol level of male Sprague-Dawley rats. Nig. Q. J. Hosp. Med. 20 (4): 209 - 13.

Yoshikawa M, Shimoda H, Nishida N, Takada M, Matsuda H (2002). *Salacia reticulata* and its polyphenolic constituents with lipase inhibitory and lipolytic activities have mild antiobesity effects in rats. J. Nutr. 132 (7): 1819-24.

Zaveri S, Drummond S (2009). The effect of including a conventional snack (cereal bar) and a non-conventional snack (almonds) on hunger, eating frequency, dietary intake and body weight. J. Hum. Nutr. Diet. 22 (5): 461 - 68.

Chapter 11

Anti-Oxidant Foods

Oxidation is a chemical reaction that transfers electrons or hydrogen from a substance to an oxidizing agent. Oxidation reactions can produce free radicals which in turn start chain reactions in a cell, causing damage or death to the cell. This process is termed as oxidative stress, a major contributor to the development of overt diabetes, its associated complications, cancer, heart attack and stroke. An anti-oxidant is a molecule that inhibits the oxidation of other molecules. Anti-oxidants terminate the chain reactions by removing free radical intermediates, and inhibiting other oxidation reactions. They do this by being oxidized themselves. The body possesses an enzymatic mechanism against oxidative stress, which is made up of free radical scavengers like superoxide dismutase (SOD), catalase (CAT), and the glutathione-dependent enzymes such as glutathione peroxidase (GPx), glutathione S-transferase (GSH), and Glutathione reductase (GR) (Khan and Kour, 2007). GR and enzymatic anti-oxidant mechanisms play an essential role in preventing oxidative damage in cells and tissues (Anderson and Meister, 1983).

Moreover, several nutritional and phytochemical constituents of food also protect the body against oxidative stress. These include vitamins A, C and E, carotenoids and flavonoids, all of which are available from foods. Anti -oxidants are often reducing agents *e.g.* thiols, ascorbic acid or polyphenols (Sies, 1997). Thus, the antioxidant defense system of the body is composed of antioxidant enzymes and food constituents.

Oxidative stress results from a persistent imbalance between antioxidant defenses and the production of highly reactive oxygen species (ROS). Anti-oxidants prevent and protect the body cells from the damage caused by free radicals. Currently, there has been an increased global interest to identify anti-oxidant compounds that are pharmacologically potent and have low or no side effects, for use in preventive medicine. A wide range of nutritional and non nutritional anti-oxidants including vitamins A, C and E, carotenoids and flavonoids are all available from fruits and vegetables.

The importance on anti-oxidant activities of phenolic compounds in fruits and vegetables as natural anti-oxidants has reached a new high in recent years. Vegetables belonging to the Brassicaceae family are rich in polyphenols, flavonoids and glucosinolates, and their hydrolysis products, which may have anti-bacterial, anti-oxidant and anti-cancer properties. Dietary polyphenols may exert their anti-cancer effects through several possible mechanisms, such as removal of carcinogenic agents, modulation of cancer cell signaling and anti-oxidant enzymatic activities, and induction of apoptosis. The pro-oxidant effect of dietary polyphenols may contribute to the activation of anti-oxidant enzymes and protective proteins in cultured cells and animal models because of the adaptation of cells and tissues to mild/moderate oxidative stress (Hu, 2011).

Because of increased safety concerns about synthetic anti-oxidants, exploitation of cheaper and safer sources of anti-oxidants based on natural origin is the focus of research now a days. As plants produce significant amount of anti-oxidants to prevent oxidative stress, they represent a potential source of new compounds with anti-oxidant activity.

A lot of medicinal plants, traditionally used for thousands of years, are present in a group of herbal preparations of the Indian traditional health care system, Ayurveda. Among the medicinal plants used in 'Ayurvedic Rasayana' for their therapeutic action, some have been thoroughly investigated. Plant foods provide more than 25,000 bioactive constituents (World Cancer Research Fund/American Institute for Cancer Research, 2007). Judging the historical, etymological, morphological, phytochemical and pharmacological aspects of *Emblica officinalis* L., *Curcuma longa* L., *Mangifera indica* L., *Momordica charantia* L., *Santalum album* L., *Swertia chirata Buch-Ham, Withania somnifera Dunal*) all of them were found to contain anti-oxidant principles that explain and justify their use in traditional medicine (Scartezzini and Speroni, 2000).

Anti-oxidants and Disease Prevention

Anti-oxidants can eliminate free radicals and other reactive oxygen and nitrogen species which contribute to most chronic diseases, and also induce mechanisms related to anti-oxidant defense, such as radical scavenging ability, complex formation with DNA and direct binding to proteins (Sarma and Sharma, 1999; Lazze *et al.*, 2003; Kong *et al.*, 2003), longevity (Baur *et al.*, 2006; Wood *et al.*, 2004), cell maintenance and DNA repair (Astley *et al.*, 2004), cancer chemopreventive potential (Deep *et al.*, 2005) antibacterial and wound healing properties (Rasool and Sabina, 2007; Srikumar *et al.*, 2007). Antioxidants offer protection against several diseases including CVD, Alzheimer's Disease, asthma, eye disorders, skin disorders, wrinkles, osteoporosis, gall stones, menstrual disorders etc.

The protective effect of antioxidants against certain diseases has been discussed below.

Heart Disease

Deficiencies of vitamins A, C, E, beta carotene and lycopene have been linked to heart disease. A high intake of fruits and vegetables containing beta carotene, lycopene, and other carotenoids may reduce the risk of heart attack. All of these nutrients have anti-oxidant effects and other properties that may benefit the heart (Joshipura *et al.*, 1999 and 2001; Riboli and Norat 2003; Stanner *et al.*, 2004). Mattioli *et al.* (2011) reported high intake of anti-oxidants to be significantly associated with an increasing probability of spontaneous alleviation of arrhythmia ($P < 0.01$).

Vitamin E had an anti-oxidant effect when administered at low doses over short time periods (biweekly intramuscular administration of 100, 300 and 600 mg/kg at a baseline time point, and additionally at 2, 4 and 6 weeks later) increased the activity of anti-oxidant enzymes. However, at higher doses and over longer time periods, it increased the level of lipid peroxidation, and attenuated the activity of anti-oxidant enzymes (Hajiani *et al.*, 2008).

Cancer

Besides preventing heart disease, fresh fruits and vegetables also help fight cancers, including lung, breast, colon, and prostate cancers. Most chemopreventive agents are antioxidant in nature. Examples of important cancer-fighting foods include various cruciferous vegetables (*e.g.*, cabbage, sprouts and broccoli). Although supplements of vitamins A, C, and E appear to have no advantages, studies have reported an association between low blood levels of these anti-oxidant vitamins and a higher risk for cancer. Some studies have suggested that certain vitamin D compounds may inhibit certain cancer cells, specifically prostate cancer, from proliferating. There is some evidence that anti-oxidants including vitamins E and C, beta carotene, isoflavones (found in soy), and quercetin (found in red wine and purple grape juice) may enhance the anti-cancer effects of chemotherapy. Naziroðlu *et al.* (2004) reported that intra-peritoneally injected selenium combined with a high dose of vitamin E produced a significant improvement on anti-oxidant concentrations in rats treated before, simultaneously and after with cisplatin (one of the most active cytotoxic agents in the treatment of cancer). Interestingly, resveratrol, a polyphenol present in grapes and red wine exhibit anti-cancer and chemo-preventive properties due to its pro-oxidant action (de la Lastra and Villegas, 2007).

Lung Disease

Bentley *et al.* (2011) reported that the intake of anti-oxidant nutrients may modulate lung function decline in older adults exposed to cigarette smoke by delaying the rate of forced expiratory volume (FEV1). Kayan *et al.* (2009) investigated the effects of Vitamins C and E administration on X-ray-induced oxidative toxicity in blood of smoker and nonsmoker X-ray technicians and found that both of these vitamins prevented the smoke and X-ray-induced oxidative stress and strengthened anti-oxidant vitamin concentrations in the blood of the technicians. Vitamin E and selenium also have protective effects on the cigarette smoke-induced blood toxicity by supporting the enzymatic anti-oxidant redox systems (Cay *et al.*, 2009).

Epilepsy

Topiramate, a voltage-gated calcium channel inhibitor, has an evident effect in the treatment of childhood epilepsy; however, topiramate may cause nephrotoxicity. But treatment with topiramate combined with vitamin E showed protective effects on pentylenetetrazol-induced nephro-toxicity by inhibition of free radicals and by supporting the anti-oxidant redox system (Armagan *et al.*, 2008). There is convincing evidence for the proposed crucial role of selenium and deficiency of GSH-Px enzyme activity in epilepsy pathogenesis. Just as Vitamin E, selenium also in combination with topiramate showed protective effects on pentylentetrazol (PTZ)-induced brain toxicity (seizures) in rats by inhibiting free radical production, regulating calcium-dependent processes, and supporting the anti-oxidant redox system (Nazirođlu *et al.*, 2008; 2009), and epilepsy (Kutluhan *et al.*, 2009). Demirci *et al.* (2013) have reported that selenium alone could also provide protective effects on oxidative stress in neuronal PC12 cells by modulating cytosolic Ca^{2+} influx and anti-oxidant levels. Selenium induced protective effects on oxidative stress, (Ca^{2+})(c) release and apoptosis in dorsal root ganglion cells since selenium deficiency is a common feature of oxidative stress-induced neurological diseases of sensory neurons (Uđuz and, Nazýrođlu, 2012).

Cataract

The presence of the direct oxidation product of lutein and 3'-epilutein (metabolite of lutein and zeaxanthin) in human retina suggests that lutein and zeaxanthin may act as antioxidants to protect the macula against short-wavelength visible light (Khachik *et al.*, 1997). Oxidized lutein may be highly reactive, since oxidation results in radical ions, which can combine with similar reactive oxidative species that could lead to higher anti-oxidant effect. Lakshminarayana *et al.* (2010) demonstrated that anti-oxidant property of oxidized lutein was higher than lutein that correlated with free radical scavenging activity and cytotoxic effects on HeLa cells. Further, Lakshminarayana *et al.* (2013) reported that oxidation by 2,2'-Azobis (2-methylpropionamidine) dihydrochloride (AAPH) resulted in peroxyl radical ions, which can react with conjugated polyene chain of lutein that could lead to higher anti-oxidant and cytotoxic effects on HeLa cells.

Anti-oxidant Foods

Anti-oxidants are abundant in apples, grapefruit, green grapes, oranges, peach, red plums, strawberries, beetroot, sprouts cauliflower, green cabbage, lettuce, onion, spinach and tomatoes as well as other foods like nuts, grains and some meats, poultry and fish. The health benefits of certain foods are presented below.

Coffee and Tea

Because of the fairly high content of anti-oxidants and the frequent use, coffee and tea are important anti-oxidant sources in many diets. Among beverages, coffee has the greatest total anti-oxidant capacity (TAC), regardless of the method of preparation or analysis, followed by citrus juices, which exhibit the highest value among soft beverages (Pellegrini *et al.*, 2003). Several compounds contribute to coffee's anti-oxidant content, *e.g.*, caffeine, polyphenols, volatile aroma compounds and heterocyclic compounds (Gonthier *et al.*, 2003; Illy, 2002; Nawvrot *et al.*, 2003; Yanagimoto *et al.*, 2002). Many of these are efficiently absorbed, and increase plasma anti-oxidant content after coffee intake (Illy, 2002; Olthof *et al.*, 2001).

Tea is particularly rich in polyphenols, including catechins, theaflavins and thearubigins, which are thought to contribute to the health benefits of tea. Tea polyphenols act as anti-oxidants *in vitro* by scavenging reactive oxygen and nitrogen species and chelating redox-active transition metal ions. Clinical trials employing putative intermediary indicators of disease, particularly biomarkers of oxidative stress status, suggested that tea polyphenols could play a role in the pathogenesis of cancer and heart disease (McKay and Blumberg, 2002). According to Frei and Higdon (2003) they may also function indirectly as anti-oxidants through 1) inhibition of the redox-sensitive transcription factors, nuclear factor-kappaB and activator protein-1; 2) inhibition of "pro-oxidant" enzymes, such as inducible nitric oxide synthase, lipoxygenases, cyclooxygenases and xanthine oxidase; and 3) induction of phase II and anti-oxidant enzymes, such as glutathione S-transferases and superoxide dismutases.

Black tea consumed throughout the world is believed to be not only a popular beverage but also an anti-oxidative agent. In black tea the polymerized catechins theaflavin and thearubigen predominate in addition to quercetin and flavonols (McKay and Blumberg, 2002). Theaflavins have been also proved to inhibit the activity of pro-oxidative enzymes such as xanthine oxidase or nitric oxide synthase (£uczaj and Skrzydlewska, 2005). Black tea extract reversed the changes in the pro-oxidant and anti-oxidant status of the liver, and protected against apoptotic, cytogenetic and hepato-cellular damage. In green tea, the major flavonoids present are the monomer catechins, epigallocatechin gallate, epigallocatechin, epicatechin gallate and epicatechin.

The beneficial effects of green tea have been attributed to the presence of phenolic compounds that are powerful anti-oxidants and free iron scavengers. In green tea, the major flavonoids present are the monomer catechins. Of all the catechins found in green tea, namely (-)-epicatechin-3-gallate, (-)-epigallocatechin, (-)-epicatechin and (-)-epigallocatechin-3-gallate (EGCG), EGCG is the most abundant and powerful antioxidant (Mak, 2012).

Turmeric (*Curcuma longa*)

The biological effects of turmeric have been attributed to its constituent curcumin a phenolic compound and a major component of *Curcuma longa* that has been widely studied for its anti-inflammatory, anti-angiogenic, anti-oxidant, wound healing and anti-cancer effects (Maheshwari *et al.*, 2006). Curcumin showed an effective scavenging of DPPH, ABTS($^+$), DMPD($^+$), superoxide anion radical, hydrogen peroxide, ferric ions (Fe^{3+}) reducing power and ferrous ions (Fe^{2+}) chelating activities (Ak and Gülçin, 2008). Further, curcumin treatment significantly and dose-dependently restored renal function, reduced lipid peroxidation; and enhanced the levels of reduced glutathione and activities of superoxide dismutase and catalase.

Curcumin has a protective effect on cisplatin-induced experimental nephrotoxicity, which is attributed to its direct anti-inflammatory and strong anti-oxidant profile (Kuhad *et al.*, 2007; Noorafshan and Ashkani-Esfahani., 2013). Tharakan *et al.* (2010) observed that curcumin is an inhibitor of vascular hyper-permeability following hemorrhagic shock, with its protective effects mediated through its anti-oxidant properties.

Pomegranate (*Punica granatum*)

Most parts of pomegranate (*Punica granatum*) are known to possess excellent anti-oxidant activity. The methanol extract of pomegranate (*Punica granatum*) peels showed the highest anti-oxidant activity among all other extracts (Singh *et al.*, 2002). Its effect on lipid peroxidation, hydroxyl radical scavenging activity, and human low-density lipoprotein oxidation showed 56, 58, and 93.7 per cent inhibition using the thiobarbituric acid method at 100 ppm. Alcoholic (ethanolic) extract of pomegranate flowers was found to contain a large amount of polyphenols and exhibit enormous reducing ability, both indicative of potent anti-oxidant ability. The extract showed 81.6 per cent anti-oxidant activity in DPPH model system. Therefore, Singh *et al.* (2002) recommended that pomegranate could be exploited for possible application for the preservation of food products as well as their use as health supplements and neutraceuticals. Devatkal *et al.* (2010) confirmed the anti-oxidant effect of extracts of fruit by-products namely pomegranate rind powder and pomegranate seed powder in goat meat patties and their potential to be used as a natural anti- oxidant preservative in meat products.

Pre-treatment with pomegranate flower extract at a dose regimen of 50-150 mg/kg body wt. for a week significantly and dose dependently protected against Fe-NTA induced oxidative stress as well as hepatic injury in mice. The extract showed 60 per cent protection against hepatic lipid peroxidation and preserved glutathione levels and activities of anti-oxidant enzymes *viz.*, catalase, glutathione peroxidase, glutathione reductase and glutathione-S-transferase by 36 per cent, 28.5 per cent, 28.7 per cent, 40.2 per cent and 42.5 per cent respectively. Protection against liver injury resulted by inhibition in the modulation of liver markers *viz.*, aspartate aminotransferase, alanine aminotransferase, alkaline phosphatase bilirubin and albumin in serum. The histo-pathological changes produced by Fe-NTA, such as ballooning degeneration, fatty changes, necrosis were also alleviated by the extract (Kaur *et al.*, 2006).

Similarly Chidambara Murthy *et al.* (2002a) showed that pre-treatment of the rats with a methanolic extract of pomegranate peel at 50 mg/kg (in terms of catechin equivalents) followed by CCl_4 treatment resulted in preservation of catalase, peroxidase, and SOD to values comparable with control values, whereas lipid peroxidation was brought back by 54 per cent as compared to control.

Drumstick (*Moringa oleifera*)

Water, methanol, and ethanol extracts of freeze-dried leaves of *Moringa oleifera* from different agroclimatic regions were found to be a potential source of natural anti-oxidants due to their marked anti-oxidant activity. All leaf extracts of each collection showed similar scavenging activities for the stable 1,1-diphenyl 2-picrylhydrazyl (DPPH) radical. Both methanol and ethanol extracts of Indian origins showed the highest anti-oxidant activities, 65.1 and 66.8 per cent, respectively, in the beta-carotene-linoleic acid system (Siddhuraju and Becker, 2003).

According to Luqman *et al.* (2012) the successive aqueous extract of *Moringa oleifera* exhibited strong scavenging effect on 2, 2-diphenyl-2-picryl hydrazyl (DPPH) free radical, superoxide, nitric oxide radical and inhibition of lipid per oxidation and the effect was comparable with that of the reference anti-oxidants. The anti-oxidant capacity of ethanolic extract of both fruit and leaf was higher in the *in vitro* assay compared to aqueous extract which showed higher potential *in vivo*. They also found the aqueous extract of leaf was able to increase the glutathione and reduce malonaldehyde level in a concentration-dependent manner.

Sreelatha and Padma (2009) observed that both mature and tender leaves extracts of *M. oleifera* have potent anti-oxidant activity against free radicals, prevent oxidative damage to major biomolecules and afford significant protection against oxidative damage. Verma *et al.* (2009) concluded from their study that the different fractions of *Moringa oleifera* leaves possess high phenolic content and potent anti-oxidant properties, which may be mediated through direct trapping of the free radicals and also through metal chelation.

Betel Leaves (*Piper betel*)

Ethanolic extract of *Piper betel* effectively prevented gamma-ray induced lipid peroxidation as assessed by thiobarbituric acid reactive substrates, lipid hydro-peroxide and conjugated diene. Likewise, it prevented radiation-induced DNA strand breaks in a concentration dependent manner. The radioprotective activity of the extract could be attributed to its hydroxyl and superoxide radicals scavenging property along with its lympho-proliferative activity. The radical scavenging capacity of the extract was primarily due to its constituent phenolics, which were isolated and identified as chevibetol and allyl pyrocatechol (Bhattacharya *et al.*, 2005). Betel leaf and its constituents - beta-carotene and alpha-tocopherol decreased the number of papillomas per animal exhibiting maximum protection. Except for beta-carotene, eugenol, hydroxyl-chavicol and alpha-tocopherol increased the levels of reduced glutathione in the liver while glutathione S-transferase activity was enhanced by all except eugenol. Of seven sources, Banarasi betel leaves showed the maximum amounts of beta-carotene and alpha-tocopherol (Bhide *et al.*, 1991).

Walnuts (*Juglans regia*)

Walnuts are ranked second only to rose hips (*Rosa canina*) in their anti-oxidant activity, as determined by the ferric reducing antioxidant power (FRAP) assay (Halvorsen *et al.*, 2002). Most of this anti-oxidant activity can be attributed to the polyphenolic constituents present primarily in the pellicle (Blomhoff *et al.*, 2006). Polyphenols isolated from walnuts, including ellagic acid monomers, polymeric tannins, and other phenolic compounds, are potent inhibitors of plasma and LDL oxidation *in vitro* (Anderson *et al.*, 2001) and have been found to decrease biomarkers of oxidative stress in diabetic mice (Fukuda *et al.*, 2004). Melatonin, another antioxidant constituent present in walnuts, has been positively correlated with increased plasma antioxidant capacity in rats (Reiter *et al.*, 2005). A limited number of human feeding trials, conducted in subjects at high risk for CVD, indicate that walnuts improve endothelial function (Ma *et al.*, 2010), and affect some measures of antioxidant status (Canales *et al.*, 2007).

Walnuts contain even more anti-oxidants than do pomegranates. The high anti-oxidant content of walnuts may be related to the high monounsaturated fatty acids and polyunsaturated fatty acids n–6 (linoleate) and n–3 (linolenate) content unlike fish that also contain high amount of unsaturated fatty acids but low anti-oxidant value (McKay *et al.*, 2010).

Black Pepper (*Piper nigrum*)

Simultaneous supplementation with black pepper or piperine to rats fed a high-fat diet significantly lowered thio-barbituric acid reactive substances and conjugated diene levels and maintained superoxide dismutase, catalase, glutathione peroxidase, glutathione-S-transferase and reduced glutathione levels in the liver, heart, kidney, intestine and aorta as compared to those of unsupplemented control rats (Vijayakumar *et al.*, 2004). Similarly, piperine supplementation to high fat diet and anti-thyroid drug induced hyper-lipidemic rats markedly protected erythrocytes from oxidative stress by improving the anti-oxidant status (Vijayakumar and Nalini, 2006).

Grapes and Grape Seed (*Vitis vinifera*)

The ethyl acetate, methanol, and water extracts of grapes pomace showed 76, 87.1, and 21.7 per cent anti-oxidant activities at 100 ppm, respectively, using the 1,1-diphenyl-2-picrylhydrazyl model system (Chidambara Murthy *et al.*, 2002b). Clinical studies revealed that lipid peroxidation could be restored to values comparable with the control. Histopathological studies of the liver of different groups also support the protective effects exhibited by the methanol extract of grape pomace by restoring the normal hepatic architecture. In humans, Gollücke (2010) demonstrated effects of grape polyphenols as maintenance of endothelial function, increase in anti-oxidant capacity and protection against LDL oxidation.

Pretreatment of the rats with the methanolic extract of grape pomace at 50 mg/kg (in terms of catechin equivalents) followed by CCl(4) treatment causes restoration of catalase, SOD, and peroxidase by 43.6, 73.2, and 54 per cent, respectively, as compared with control, whereas lipid peroxidation was restored to values comparable with the control. Histo-pathological studies of the liver of different groups also support the protective effects exhibited by the methanol extract of grape pomace by restoring the normal hepatic architecture (Chidambara Murthy *et al.*, 2002b).

Pastrana-Bonilla *et al.* (2003) found the anti-oxidant capacity/g of fresh weight for pulps, skins, seeds, and leaves to be 2.4, 12.8, 281.3, and 236.1 microM. Trolox equivalent respectively. Gallic acid, (+)-catechin, and epicatechin were the major phenolics in seeds and skin. Yilmaz and Toledo (2004) reported that dimeric, trimeric, oligomeric, or polymeric procyanidins accounted for most of the superior antioxidant capacity of grape seeds.

The anti-oxidant and hepato-protective roles of the grape seed supplementation on ethanol-induced oxidative stress have been indicated by Dogan and Celik (2012) and suggested that grape seed could be as important as diet-derived anti-oxidant in preventing oxidative damage in the tissues by reducing the lipid oxidation or inhibiting the production of ethanol-induced free radicals in rats.

Dulundu *et al.* (2007) found grape seed extract to protect the liver from oxidative damage following bile duct ligation in rats. This effect possibly involves the inhibition of neutrophil infiltration and lipid peroxidation, thus, restoring the oxidant and anti-oxidant status in the tissue.

On comparing the seeds, skin, and pulp of eight cultivars of Florida-grown muscadine grapes, Sandhu and Gu (2010) found the total phenolic content and anti-oxidant capacity, based on fresh weight, were highest in seeds followed by skin and pulp. On an average, 87.1, 11.3, and 1.6 per cent of phenolic compounds were present in seeds, skin, and pulp, respectively. A total of 88 phenolic compounds of diverse structures were tentatively identified in muscadines, which included 17 in the pulp, 28 in the skin, and 43 in the seeds.

Resveratrol (3,4',5-trihydroxystilbene) is found in grapes, berries and peanuts. It is also present in wines, especially red wines. During the last years, it has been the focus of numerous *in vitro* and *in vivo* studies investigating its biological attributes, which include mainly anti-oxidant and anti-inflammatory activities, anti-platelet aggregation effect, anti-atherogenic property, oestrogen-like growth-promoting effect, growth-inhibiting activity, immuno-modulation and chemo-prevention. Resveratrol can exhibit pro-oxidant properties, leading to oxidative breakage of cellular DNA in the presence of transition metal ions such as copper (de la Lastra and Villegas, 2007).

Date Palm (*Phoenix dactylifera*)

The anti-oxidant and anti-mutagenic activity in date fruit is quite potent and implicates the presence of compounds with potent free-radical-scavenging activity. Concentrations of 1.5 and 4.0 mg/mL of date fruit extract completely inhibited superoxide and hydroxyl radicals, respectively. Aqueous date extract was also found to inhibit significantly the lipid peroxidation and protein oxidation in a dose-dependent manner (Vayalil, 2002). Ethyl acetate extracts from two varieties of date palm flesh and pit Deglet nour and pit Alig showed an important free radical scavenging activity towards 1-1-diphenyl-2-picrylhydrazyl (DPPH) free radical (Chaira *et al.*, 2007).

Amira *et al.* (2012) analyzed four cultivars (Gondi, Gasbi, Khalt Dhahbi, and Rtob Ahmar) of Tunisian date palm (*Phoenix dactylifera* L.) fruits at 3 maturation stages or their antioxidant activities. All the samples showed the highest total phenolic, total flavonoid and condensed tannins. The major phenolic compounds were caffeic, ferulic, protocatechuic, and catechin for the majority of cultivars. Thus, Amira *et al.* (2012) confirmed that common date fruits are rich in natural anti-oxidants as a source of bioactive health promoting phytochemicals. Pujari *et al.* (2011) found 15 days pre-treatment with methanolic extract of dates (100, 300 mg/kg), significantly attenuated the depletion in superoxide dismutase, catalase, glutathione, glutathione reductase and the lipid peroxidation and the severe neuronal damage in the brain induced by the cerebral ischemia. Hence, the authors suggested the possible use of dates against bilateral common carotid artery occlusion induced oxidative stress and neuronal damage. Saafi-Ben Salah *et al.* (2012) also from their study on rats indicated that dates may be useful *in vivo* in preventing oxidative stress induced nephro-toxicity.

Garlic (*Allium sativum*)

Garlic is known to possess preventive properties in cardiovascular diseases, regulating blood pressure, lowering blood sugar and cholesterol levels, anti-platelet activities, and thromboxane formation. It is also effective against bacterial, viral, fungal and parasitic infections, enhancing the immune system and having anti-tumoral and anti-oxidant features. Garlic contains a number of chemicals such as sulfur compounds (allicin, alliin and agoene), volatile oils, enzymes (allinase, peroxidase and miracynase), carbohydrates (sucrose and glucose), minerals (selenium), amino acids (cysteine, glutamine, isoleucine and methionine) which help to protect cells from the ills of free radicals, bioflavonoids such as quercetin and cyanidin, allistatin I and allistatin II, and vitamins C, E and A which help in protecting from oxidative agents and free radicals (Ayaz and Alpsoy, 2007).

Administration of garlic and onion to fructose-fed rats reduced oxidative stress, increased eNOS activity, and also attenuated vascular cell adhesion molecule-(VCAM-1) expression. These results provide new evidence showing the anti-inflammatory and anti-oxidant effect of these vegetables (Vazquez-Prieto *et al.*, 2011). Butt *et al.* (2009) emphasized garlic's ability to ameliorate oxidative stress, core role in cardiovascular cure, chemo-preventive strategies, and prospective effect as immune booster. Aged garlic extract exerts anti-oxidant action by scavenging Reactive Oxygen Species, enhancing the cellular anti-oxidant enzymes superoxide dismutase, catalase and glutathione peroxidase, and increasing glutathione in the cells (Borek 2001). Aged garlic extract also inhibits lipid peroxidation, reducing ischemic/reperfusion damage to the endothelial cells by the oxidized molecules, which, otherwise contributes to atherosclerosis.

Ginger (*Zingiber officinale*)

Animals given orally ginger extract (1.5-5 g/kg) or polaprezinc (30 and 60 mg/kg) once daily for three consecutive days after ulcer induction by 60 per cent acetic acid significantly reduced the gastric ulcer area in a dose-dependent manner, with concomitant attenuation of the elevated activities of xanthine oxidase and myeloperoxidase, as well as malondialdehyde level in the ulcerated mucosa. Ginger extract and polaprezinc both show anti-oxidation that consequently alleviates gastric mucosal damage and promotes ulcer healing, thus together serving as effective mucosal protective agents (Ko and Leung, 2010).

Berries

With their high content of phytochemicals such as flavonoids, tannins, stilbenoids, phenolic acids and lignans (Kahkonen *et al.*, 2001; Maatta-Riihinen *et al.*,

2004a and b), berries and berry products are potentially excellent anti-oxidant sources. Among fruits, the highest anti-oxidant activities were found in berries (*i.e.*, blackberry, redcurrant and raspberry) regardless of the assay used (Pellegrini *et al.*, 2003). Phytochemicals have been demonstrated to be powerful inhibitors of lipid peroxidation when compared to other classic antioxidants. Berry extracts have proven to be effective in preventing the oxidative damage under different pathological conditions (Kong *et al.*, 2003; Zafra-Stone *et al.*, 2007; Rani *et al.*, 2004; Bagchi *et al.*, 2004 and Duthie *et al.*, 2006) and the protective effect of polyphenols against oxidative damage seems to be via glutathione system (Moskaug *et al.*, 2005).

Blue Berries

Among the different species, there is a group classified as blueberries that have a dark color due to anthocyanins and polyphenols as principal pigments with antioxidant activities (Kong *et al.*, 2003).

Previously, it has been demonstrated that blueberry enriched diet reduced the adverse effects of oxidative stress in rat neuron cell lines and brain tissues (Malin *et al.*, 2011). Fuentealba *et al.* (2011) reported that blueberry extract protects neuronal tissue from amyloid-β peptide toxicity mainly through its anti-aggregation property, and its antioxidant properties while mitochondrial membrane potential capacities are secondary mechanisms important in chronic stages. Such extract has shown to cross the blood-brain barrier (Malin *et al.*, 2011; Rendeiro *et al.*, 2012) thus influencing brain homeostasis (Alves *et al.*, 2012). Zepeda *et al.* (2012) demonstrated that blueberry extract significantly reduced the harmful effects of oxidative stress caused by hypobaric hypoxia in rat testis by affecting glutathione reductase and superoxide dismutase activities.

Blackberry (*Rubus* spp.)

Some bioactive compounds present in blackberry have the ability to act as natural anti-oxidants and minimize effects of reactive oxygen species. The blackberry nectar was found to reduce the serum triglyceride levels, total cholesterol and LDL-cholesterol in hyper-cholesterolemic hamsters, without influencing the HDL and blood glucose concentrations (Ferreira *et al.*, 2011). A decrease in the initiation of lipid peroxidation reactions in the blood, brain and small intestine was also observed.

Vegetables

Aqueous methanol extract of Brassica vegetables, including York cabbage, broccoli, Brussels sprouts and white cabbage showed high flavonoid contents in the order of 21.7, 17.5, 15.4 and 8.75 mg QE/g of extract. With regard to total phenolic content, York cabbage extract had the highest total phenolic content, (33.5), followed by 23.6, 20.4 and 18.4 mg GAE/g of dried weight (dw) of the extracts for broccoli, Brussels sprouts and white cabbage, respectively. All the extracts studied showed a rapid and concentration dependent anti-oxidant capacity in diverse anti-oxidant systems (Jaiswal *et al.*, 2011).

Among vegetables, spinach had the highest anti-oxidant capacity in the Trolox equivalence anti-oxidant capacity (TEAC) and ferric ion reducing anti-oxidant power

(FRAP) assays followed by peppers, whereas asparagus had the greatest anti-oxidant capacity in the total radical trapping anti-oxidant parameter (TRAP) assay (Pellegrini *et al.*, 2003). The antioxidant activity of the methanol extracts of carrot (*Daucus carota*) and beetroot (*Beta vulgaris*) pulp waste determined by the DPPH method exhibited 40 per cent and 78 per cent activity respectively (Shyamala and Jamuna, 2010).

Swallow Root (*Decalepis hamiltonii*)

One of the major constituents of the root vegetable *Decalepis hamiltonii* which is responsible for its anti-oxidant activity, is 2-hydroxy-4-methoxy benzaldehyde (2H4MB). Hence Murthy *et al.* (2006) suggested that the extract of *D. hamiltonii* can be utilized for the production of anti-oxidant rich fractions required for various health benefits. Later Srikanta *et al.* (2011) reported that insignificant anti-oxidant attribute of HMBA revealed the anti-*H.pylori* activity via mechanisms other than anti-oxidative routes.

Vanilla Beans (*V. planifolia*)

The word vanilla (a flavoring agent) derived from the diminutive of the Spanish word vaina (vaina itself meaning sheath or pod), simply translates as little pod. The major compounds, viz, vanillic acid, 4-hydroxybenzyl alcohol, 4-hydroxy-3-methoxybenzyl alcohol, 4-hydroxybenzaldehyde and vanillin, in vanilla extract at a concentration of 200 ppm, showed 26 per cent and 43 per cent of anti-oxidant activity by beta-carotene-linoleate and DPPH methods, respectively. Interestingly, 4-hydroxy-3-methoxybenzyl alcohol and 4-hydroxybenzyl alcohol exhibited anti-oxidant activity of 65 per cent and 45 per cent by beta-carotene-linoleate method and 90 per cent and 50 per cent by DPPH methods, respectively. In contrast, pure vanillin exhibited much lower anti-oxidant activity. Thus the authors (Shyamala *et al.*, 2007) revealed the potential use of vanilla extract components as anti-oxidants for food preservation and in health supplements as nutraceuticals.

Wine

Caffeic acid (3,4-dihydroxycinnamic acid) is among the major hydroxyl-cinnamic acids present in wine. At the concentrations of 10 and 30 μg/ml, caffeic acid showed 68.2 and 75.8 per cent inhibition on lipid peroxidation of linoleic acid emulsion, respectively. In addition, caffeic acid is an effective ABTS $^{(+)}$ scavenging, DPPH scavenging, superoxide anion radical scavenging, total reducing power and metal chelating on ferrous ions activities (Gülçin, 2006).

Green Ginger (*Artemisia absinthium*)

Bora and Sharma (2011) found in their *in vivo* studies, oral administration of methanol extract of *Artemisia absinthium* (100 or 200mg/kg) inhibited cerebral I/R-induced oxidative stress by decreasing the thiobarbituric acid reactive substances (TBARS) and restoring levels of superoxide dismutase (SOD) activity and glutathione (GSH).

Jamun (*Eugenia jambolana*)

Eugenia jambolana seed kernel decreased oxidative stress in diabetic rats, which in turn may be due to its hypoglyceamic property (Ravi *et al.*, 2004a). The anti-oxidant effect of *Eugenia jambolana* seed kernel was also compared with glibenclamide, a standard hypoglycemic drug. Diabetic rats treated with seed kernel extract restored almost normal architecture of liver and kidney and were confirmed by histopathological examination (Ravi *et al.*, 2004b).

Honey Mushroom (*Basidiomycete Armillaria mellea*)

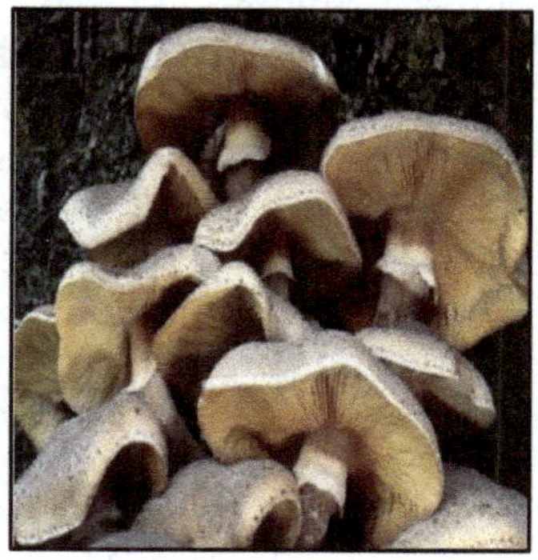

Fermented polysaccharides of edible honey mushrooms in submerged cultures are potential antioxidant source. Lung and Chang (2011) confirmed that the extracts with good anti-oxidant properties from fermenting products by *A. melleaare* are potential good substitutes for synthetic anti-oxidants and can be applied to anti-oxidant-related functional food and pharmaceutical industries.

Watercress (*Nasturtium officinale*)

Watercress is a fast-growing, aquatic or semi-aquatic, perennial plant native to Europe and Asia, and one of the oldest known leaf vegetables consumed by humans. It has been used as a home remedy by the people of south eastern region of Iran as a medicinal plant. This therapeutic application has been attributed to its anti-oxidant capacity as the extract has notable scavenging activity against DPPH radicals as well as potent reducing power in FRAP assay. Treatment of hyper-cholesterolaemic rats with *N. officinale* extract significantly increased the GSH level along with enhanced catalase and superoxide dismutase activities in liver tissues. Furthermore, *N. officinale* extract significantly decreased hepatic malondialdehyde level as well as glutathione peroxidase and glutathione reductase activities in plant-treated rats. Based on the data, Yazdanparast *et al.* (2008) confirmed that *N. officinale* has a high hypo-lipidaemic activity and this may be attributed to its anti-oxidative potential.

Administration of the ethanol extract to rats decreased lipid peroxidation in liver, brain and kidney. Thus Ozen (2009) concluded that *N. officinale* extracts show relevant anti-oxidant activity by means of reducing cellular lipid peroxidation and increasing anti-oxidant activity, reducing power, free radical and superoxide anion radical scavenging activities.

Brahmi (*Bacopa monnieri*)

In rats, bacosides A from *Bacopa monniera* enhanced anti-oxidant defenses, increasing superoxide dismutase, catalase and glutathione peroxidase activity (Anbarasi *et al.*, 2006). The sulfhydryl and polyphenol components of *Bacopa monnieri* extract have also been shown to impact the oxidative stress cascade by scavenging reactive oxygen species, inhibiting lipoxygenase activity and reducing divalent metals. This mechanism of action may explain the effect of *Bacopa monniera* extract in reducing beta amyloid deposits in a mouse model of Alzheimer's disease (Dhanasekaran *et al.*, 2007).

Amrita Bindu (A Salt-Spice-Herbal Mixture)

Amrita Bindu is a salt-spice-herbal mixture containing pepper and ginger along with natural or artificial salt substitute. Shanmugasundaram *et al.* (1994) observed that Amrita Bindu supplementation prevented N-methyl-N'-nitro-N-nitrosoguanidine- induced depletion of the anti-oxidant enzymes and the scavenger anti-oxidants glutathione and vitamins A, C and E. Amrita Bindu provides protection against free radical and reactive oxygen species induced tissue lipid peroxidation and the resultant tissue degeneration. Similarly, Amrita Bindu supplementation for 3 months to asthmatic children resulted in stoppage of all anti-asthmatic medications and the children were free from attacks of asthma (Kumar and Shanmugasundaram, 2004). Co-administration of Amrita Bindu along with 100μg of aflatoxin B_1 (AFB_1) was found to protect lipids and protein against the AFB_1 induced oxidative damage in kidney, liver and brain tissues (Madhusudhanan *et al.*, 2004). The anti-oxidant supplement, Amrita Bindu, has a potential role also in ameliorating the aflatoxin B1-induced DNA damage thus suggesting its applicability in preventing the vital macromolecule DNA (Madhusudhanan *et al.*, 2006). Rats fed diets with Amrita Bindu pretreatment showed significantly lower levels of free radicals, lipid peroxidation and protein carbonyls along with significantly higher levels of anti-oxidants on phenylhydrazine administration as compared to rats without Amrita Bindu pretreatment (Natarajan *et al.*, 2006).

Effect of Cooking on Anti-oxidants

In general, anti-oxidant contents are preserved fairly well during most types of processing, but there are some exceptions. Boari *et al.* (2013) observed that cooking did not always have negative effect on product quality, since in certain cases, it even enhanced the nutritional value of wild edible plants by increasing their total anti-oxidant activity and reducing the nitrate content. The anti-oxidant content increased in products such as carrots, spinach, mushrooms, asparagus, broccoli, cabbage, red cabbage, green and red peppers, potatoes, and tomatoes during microwave cooking, steaming, or boiling. Anti-oxidant values also increased after toasting or baking of bagels, French bread, wheat bread, whole-wheat bread, and pie crust.

Stir-frying increased anti-oxidant capacities in bamboo shoots as compared to boiling and steaming and hence may be considered suitable method of cooking the same (Zhang *et al.*, 2011). On the other hand, Pellegrini *et al.* (2010) demonstrated that fresh brassica vegetables retain phytochemicals and total anti-oxidant capacity better than frozen samples. According to Ng *et al.* (2011) boiling generally improved the overall anti-oxidant activity in all the vegetables while pressure cooking did not cause any significant decline in the anti-oxidant property, thus suggesting that prudence in selecting an appropriate cooking method for different vegetables may improve/preserve their nutritional value.

Measurement of Anti-oxidant Potential

Several assays have been used to assess the total anti-oxidant content of foods, *e.g.* the 6-hydroxy-2,5,7,8-tetramethylchroman-2-carboxylic acid (Trolox) equivalent anti-oxidant capacity (TEAC) assay (Miller and Evans, 1996; Prior *et al.*, 2005; Tian and Schaich, 2013) and the oxygen radical absorbance capacity assay (ORAC) assay (Watanabe *et al.*, 2013) the ferric-reducing ability of plasma (FRAP) (Benzie and Strain, 1996).

Anti-oxidant activity is measured using the linoleic acid system, metal chelating activity, ferric thiocyanate method, and lipid peroxidation, total reducing power by potassium ferricyanide reduction method (Ozen, 2009), scavenging effect on 1,1-diphenyl-2-picrylhydrazyl free radical, and superoxide anion radical scavenging activity as the parameters for assessment of anti-oxidant potential of methanolic extracts (Iqbal *et al.*, 2006). The bioavailability of phytochemical anti-oxidants is influenced by many factors such as, the food matrix, absorption and metabolism (Gonthier *et al.*, 2003: Manach *et al.*, 2004; 2005). The methods measuring total anti-oxidant capacity do not identify single anti-oxidant compound, and thus cannot help in determining the mechanisms involved.

These different anti-oxidant assays for measuring anti-oxidant capacity make it difficult to compare whole lists of foods, products and product categories. But a food that has a high total anti-oxidant capacity (TAC) in one assay will most likely show the same in another assay (Miller *et al.*, 2000; Pellegrini *et al.*, 2003). But, though the exact values differ, the ranking of the products will not differ (Carlsen *et al.*, 2010).

Anti-oxidant Capacity of Different Foods

Foods from all the food groups have been identified with anti-oxidant constituents. Breakfast cereals, grains, legumes, nuts and seeds are poor in anti-oxidant capacity. Among cereal products, whole meal buckwheat and wheat bran had the greatest total anti-oxidant capacity (TAC). Pellegrini *et al*. (2006) expanded the data base for TAC of different foods and reported that among pulses and nuts, broad bean, lentil and walnuts had the highest anti-oxidant capacity, whereas chickpeas, pine nuts and peanuts were less effective. The contribution of bound phytochemicals to the overall TAC was relevant in cereals as well as in nuts and pulses. Among the oils soybean oil has the highest anti-oxidant capacity followed by extra virgin olive oil and groundnut oil having the least capacity (Pellegrini *et al.*, 2003)

Most of the dairy products are low in anti-oxidant content, in the range of 0.0 to 0.8 mmol/100 g. Eggs are almost devoid of anti-oxidants with the highest anti-oxidant values found in egg yolk (0.16 mmol/100 g). Especially high anti-oxidant capacity was found in dried amla (Indian gooseberry, 261.5 mmol/100 g) (Carlsen *et al.*, 2010). Mean anti-oxidant contents increased with increasing content of cocoa in the chocolate product. Chocolate products with cocoa contents of 24-30 per cent, 40-65 per cent and 70-99 per cent had mean anti-oxidant contents of 1.8, 7.2 and 10.9 mmol/100 g, respectively.

Walnuts, with pellicle and nut shell intact contains 33.3 mmol/100 g. Pecans with pellicle, sunflower seeds and chestnuts with pellicle, have mean anti-oxidant content in the range of 4.7 to 8.5 mmol/100 g.

Fresh fruits and vegetables have been considered the most important sources of antioxidants. Examples of anti-oxidant rich berries are fresh, black currants, wild strawberries, blackberries and cranberries. Certain dried fruits and vegetables such as dried apples, lemon skin, plums, apricots, dates, mango, black and green olives, red cabbage, guava, plums, prunes and red beets, paprika, red and green chilli were also found to be rich in antioxidants. However, the antioxidant content in these dried foods was reported to be in the medium range.

Other anti-oxidant rich products are Triphala, Amla and Arjuna from India and Goshuyu-tou, a traditional kampo medicine from Japan, with anti-oxidant values in the range of 132.6 to 706.3 mmol/100 g (Carlsen *et al.*, 2010).

Although spices, herbs and condiments such as fennel seeds are consumed in very small quantities, they may still be important contributors of the total anti-oxidant intake, especially in India where spices and herbs are used in cookery regularly.

Several foods showed improved antioxidant potential when consumed along with individual antioxidant nutrients. *e.g. Phyllanthus emblica* L., *Santalum album* L., *Syzygium cumini* L. and *Trigonella foenum-graecum* L. presented highly significant antiradical efficiency (AE) singly and in combination with either vitamin A, C or E. Further, *Curcuma longa* L., *Momordica charantia* L., *S. cumini*, *T. foenum-graecum*, *Moringa oleifera* Lam. and *S. album* have also shown fairly significant AE in a vitamin combination dose of 0.001mM concentration (Kamal *et al.*, 2011).

Dietary Intake of Anti-oxidants

The relation between dietary anti-oxidants and oxidative stress-induced diseases can be established with the anti-oxidant content coupled with an estimate of anti-oxidant intake (Pellegrini *et al.*, 2003). There are several thousand-fold differences in anti-oxidant content of foods, some with exceptionally high values. A comprehensive food database consisting of the total anti-oxidant content of typical foods as well as other dietary items such as traditional medicinal plants, herbs and spices and dietary supplements (Carlson *et al.*, 2010) is helpful in planning diets. For example, soybean oil has the highest anti-oxidant capacity, followed by extra virgin olive oil, whereas peanut oil is less effective of the oils.

Beverages account for a very high proportion of dietary anti-oxidant intake as compared to intake of anti-oxidant vitamins C and E in the Spanish diet where coffee is the main contributor (61-66 per cent respectively), followed by red wine (16-22 per cent), fruit juices (5-6 per cent), beer (4-5 per cent), tea (3- 5 per cent) and milk (1-4 per cent) (Pulido *et al.*, 2003).

In general, vegetarian diet contains more anti-oxidant vitamins *i.e.* vitamin C, vitamin E, and beta-carotene (Venderley and Campbell, 2006) and copper than that of non vegetarian diet. Intake of zinc in vegetarians is generally comparable to that of non-vegatarians. However, the bioavailability of zinc in vegetarian diets is generally low. Dietary intake of selenium is variable in both groups and depends on the selenium content of the soil. Anti-oxidant status in vegetarians shows higher anti-oxidant vitamin status (vitamin C, vitamin E, beta-carotene) but variable anti-oxidant trace element status as compared to the non-vegetarians (Rauma and Mykkänen, 2000).

In Rural Mexico, Hervert-Hernández and Goni (2011) found soft drinks to be the most commonly consumed beverage (280 ml/d), followed by coffee and fresh fruit beverages among pre-menopausal obese women. Polyphenol intake and dietary anti-oxidant capacity from beverages was 181 mg/person per day and >1000 μmol. Trolox equivalents/person per day respectively. The items that contributed most to this intake were coffee, roselle drink, peach and guava juices and infusions.

Other Applications of Anti-oxidants

Traditionally, the age old practice of improving the stability of ghee (clarified butter) or oils is to use curry leaves or Drumstick leaves as a source of anti-oxidant. The leaves of *M. oleifera* have been reported to be a valuable source of both macro and micro-nutrients, calcium, and potassium and especially β-carotene, vitamin C, and thus act as a good source of natural anti-oxidants; and thus enhance the shelf-life of fat-containing foods (Dillard and German, 2000; Siddhuraju and Becker, 2003). Sánchez de Medina *et al.* (2011) used phenolic extracts from olive tree leaves and olive pomace to enrich refined oils (namely, maize, soy, high-oleic sunflower, sunflower, olive, and rapeseed oils) at two concentration levels (200 and 400 μg/mL, expressed as gallic acid) for their preservation. All the oils experienced either a noticeable or a dramatic improvement of their quality-stability parameters (*e.g.*, peroxide index and Rancimat) as compared with their non-enriched counterparts. According to Mohamad *et al.* (2011) fennel seeds could be used as a safe, effective, and easily accessible source of natural anti-oxidants to improve the oxidative stability of fatty foods during storage.

Fennel seed methanolic extract showed strong free radical-scavenging activity (100 per cent). Thus, fennel seeds may reduce oxidative stress and protect mouse cells from damage caused by reactive oxygen species (Mohamad *et al.*, 2011).

Conclusions

Anti-oxidant nutrients and foods play a fundamental role not only in prevention and cure of CVD but also in anti-ageing along with several other degenerative diseases. Interestingly, the anti-oxidant content in human breast milk is comparable to that in pomegranate juice, strawberries and coffee and on average higher than the anti-oxidant content observed in the commercially available infant formulas analyzed (Carlsen *et al.*, 2010).

The benefits of anti-oxidants have raised commercial and research interest in foods with anti-oxidant components resulting in ascertaining their role in health and disease. Detailed discussion on the clinical applications of anti-oxidant foods is given in respective chapters later in this book.

References

Ak T, Gülçin I (2008). Anti-oxidant and radical scavenging properties of curcumin. Chem. Biol. Interact. 174 (1): 27 - 37.

Alves MG, Oliveira PF, Socorro S, Moreira PI (2012). Impact of diabetes in blood-testis and blood-brain barriers: resemblances and differences. *Current Diabetes Reviews*. 8 (6): 401 - 412.

Amira el A, Behija SE, Beligh M, Lamia L, Manel I, Mohamed H, Lotfi A (2012). Effects of the ripening stage on phenolic profile, phytochemical composition and antioxidant activity of date palm fruit. J. Agric. Food Chem. 60 (44): 10896 - 902.

Anbarasi K, Vani G, Balakrishna K, Devi CS (2006). Effect of bacoside A on brain antioxidant status in cigarette smoke exposed rats. Life Science. 78 (12): 1378 - 84.

Anderson KJ, Teuber SS, Gobeille A, Cremin P, Waterhouse AL, Steinberg FM (2001). Walnut polyphenolics inhibit *in vitro* human plasma and LDL oxidation. J. Nutr. 131 (11): 2837 - 42.

Anderson ME, Meister A (1983). Transport and direct utilization of γ-glutamylcyst(e)ine for glutathione synthesis. Proceedings of the National Academy of Sciences of the United States of America. 80 (3):707 - 711.

Armagan A, Kutluhan S, Yilmaz M, Yilmaz N, Bülbül M, Vural H, Soyupek S, Naziroglu M (2008). Topiramate and vitamin E modulate antioxidant enzyme activities, nitric oxide and lipid peroxidation levels in pentylenetetrazol-induced nephrotoxicity in rats. Basic Clin. Pharmacol. Toxicol. 103 (2): 166 - 70.

Astley SB, Elliott RM, Archer DB, Southon S (2004). Evidence that dietary supplementation with carotenoids and carotenoid-rich foods modulates the DNA damage: repair balance in human lymphocytes. Br. J. Nutr. 91: 63 - 72.

Ayaz E, Alpsoy HC (2007). Garlic (*Allium sativum*) and traditional medicine. Turkiye. Parazitol. Derg. 31 (2):145 - 49 [Article in Turkish].

Bagchi D, Sen CK, Bagchi M, Atalay M (2004). Antiangiogenic, antioxidant, and anticarcinogenic properties of a novel anthocyanin-rich berry extract formula. *Biokhimiya*. 69 (1): 95 - 102.

Baur JA, Pearson KJ, Price NL, Jamieson HA, Lerin C, Kalra A, Prabhu VV, Allard JS, Lopez-Lluch G, Lewis K, Pistell PJ, Poosala S, Becker KG, Boss O, Gwinn D, Wang M, Ramaswamy S, Fishbein KW, Spencer RG, Lakatta EG, Le CD, Shaw RJ, Navas P, Puigserver P, Ingram DK, de CR, Sinclair DA (2006). Resveratrol improves health and survival of mice on a high-calorie diet. Nature. 444: 337 - 42.

Bentley AR, Kritchevsky SB, Harris TB, Holvoet P, Jensen RL, Newman AB, Lee JS, Yende S, Bauer D, Cassano PA (2011). for the Health ABC Study. Dietary Anti-oxidants and FEV1 Decline: the Health, Ageing and Body Composition Study. Eur. Respir. J. 2011 Oct 27. [Epub ahead of print].

Benzie IF, Strain JJ (1996). The ferric reducing ability of plasma (FRAP) as a measure of "antioxidant power": the FRAP assay. Anal. Biochem. 239 (1): 70 - 76.

Bhattacharya S, Subramanian M, Roychowdhury S, Bauri AK, Kamat JP, Chattopadhyay S, Bandyopadhyay SK (2005). Radioprotective property of the ethanolic extract of Piper betel Leaf. J Radiat Res. 46 (2): 165 - 71.

Bhide SV, Zariwala MB, Amonkar AJ, Azuine MA (1991). Chemopreventive efficacy of a betel leaf extract against benzo[a]pyrene-induced forestomach tumors in mice. J. Ethnopharmacol. 34 (2-3): 207 - 13.

Blomhoff R, Carlsen MH, Andersen LF, Jacobs DR Jr. (2006). Health benefits of nuts: potential role of anti-oxidants. Br. J. Nutr. 96 (Suppl 2): S52 - S60.

Boari F, Cefola M, Di Gioia F, Pace B, Serio F, Cantore V (2013). Effect of cooking methods on antioxidant activity and nitrate content of selected wild Mediterranean plants. Int. J. Food Sci. Nutr. 2013 May 24. [Epub ahead of print].

Bora KS, Sharma A (2011). Evaluation of anti-oxidant and free-radical scavenging potential of *Artemisia absinthium*. Pharm. Biol. 49 (12): 1216 - 23.

Borek C (2001). Anti-oxidant health effects of aged garlic extract. Nutr. 131 (3s): 1010S - 5S.

Butt MS, Sultan MT, Butt MS, Iqbal J (2009). Garlic: nature's protection against physiological threats. Crit. Rev. Food Sci. Nutr. 49 (6): 538 - 51.

Canales A, Benedi J, Nus M, Librelotto J, Sánchez-Montero JM, Sánchez-Muniz FJ (2007). Effect of walnut-enriched restructured meat in the antioxidant status of overweight/obese senior subjects with at least one extra CHD-risk factor. J. Am. Coll. Nutr. 26 (3): 225 - 32.

Carlsen MH, Halvorsen BL, Holte MH, Bøhn SK, Dragland S, Sampson L, Willey C, Senoo H, Umezono Y, Sanada C, Barikmo I, Berhe N, Willett WC, Phillips KM, Jacobs Jr DR, and Blomhoff R (2010). The total anti-oxidant content of more than 3100 foods, beverages, spices, herbs and supplements used worldwide. Nutr. J. 9: 3.

Cay M, Naziroðlu M, Köylü H (2009). Selenium and vitamin E modulates cigarette smoke exposure-induced oxidative stress in blood of rats. Biol. Trace Elem. Res. 131 (1): 62 - 70.

Chaira N, Ferchichi A, Mrabet A, Sghairoun M (2007). Chemical composition of the flesh and the pit of date palm fruit and radical scavenging activity of their extracts. Pak J Biol Sci. 10 (13): 2202 – 207.

Chidambara Murthy KN, Jayaprakasha GK, Singh RP (2002a). Studies on anti-oxidant activity of pomegranate (*Punica granatum*) peel extract using *in vivo* models. J. Agric. Food Chem. 50 (17): 4791 - 95.

Chidambara Murthy KN, Singh RP, Jayaprakasha GK (2002b). Anti-oxidant activities of grape (*Vitis vinifera*) pomace extracts. J. Agric. Food Chem. 50 (21): 5909 - 914.

de la Lastra CA, Villegas I (2007). Resveratrol as an anti-oxidant and pro-oxidant agent: mechanisms and clinical implications. Biochem. Soc. Trans. 35 (Pt 5): 1156 - 60.

Deep G, Dhiman M, Rao AR, Kale RK (2005). Chemopreventive potential of Triphala (a composite Indian drug) on Benzo(a)pyrene induced forestomach tumorigenesis in murine tumor model system. J. Exp. Clin. Cancer Res. 24: 555 - 63.

Demirci S, Kutluhan S, Naziroðlu M, Uðuz AC, Yürekli VA, Demirci K (2013). Effects of selenium and topiramate on cytosolic Ca(2+) influx and oxidative stress in neuronal PC12 cells. Neurochem. Res. 38 (1): 90 - 97.

Devatkal SK, Narsaiah K, Borah A (2010). Anti-oxidant effect of extracts of kinnow rind, pomegranate rind and seed powders in cooked goat meat patties. Meat Sci. 85 (1): 155 - 59.

Dhanasekaran, M.; Tharakan, B.; Holcomb, L. A.; Hitt, A. R.; Young, K. A.; Manyam, B. V. (2007). Neuro-protective mechanisms of ayurvedic anti-dementia botanical *Bacopa monniera*. Phytotherapy Research. 21: 965 - 69.

Dillard CJ, German JB (2000). Phytochemicals: nutraceuticals and human health. Journal of the Science of Food and Agriculture. 80 (12): 1744 - 56.

Dogan A, Celik I (2012). Hepato-protective and anti-oxidant activities of grapeseeds against ethanol-induced oxidative stress in rats. Br. J. Nutr. 107 (1): 45 - 51.

Dulundu E, Ozel Y, Topaloglu U, Toklu H, Ercan F, Gedik N, Sener G (2007). Grape seed extract reduces oxidative stress and fibrosis in experimental biliary obstruction. J. Gastroenterol. Hepatol. 22 (6): 885 - 92.

Duthie SJ, Jenkinson AM, Crozier A, Mullen W, Pirie L, Kyle J, Yap LS, Christen P, Duthie GG (2006). The effects of cranberry juice consumption on anti-oxidant status and biomarkers relating to heart disease and cancer in healthy human volunteers. European Journal of Nutrition. 45 (2): 113 - 22.

Ferreira de Araujo PR, da Silva Santos V, Rodrigues Machado A, Gevehr Fernandes C, Silva JA, da Silva Rodrigues R (2011). Benefits of blackberry nectar (*Rubus* spp.) relative to hyper-cholesterolemia and lipid peroxidation. Nutr. Hosp. 26 (5): 984 - 90.

Frei B, Higdon JV (2003). Anti-oxidant activity of tea polyphenols *in vivo*: evidence from animal studies. J. Nutr. 133 (10): 3275S - 84S.

Fuentealba J, Dibarrart AJ, Fuentes-Fuentes MC, Saez-Orellana F, Quinones K, Guzmán L, Perez C, Becerra J, Aguayo LG (2011). Synaptic failure and adenosine triphosphate imbalance induced by amyloid-β aggregates are prevented by blueberry-enriched polyphenols extract. Journal of Neuroscience Research. 89 (9):1499 - 508.

Fukuda T, Ito H, Yoshida T (2004). Effect of the walnut polyphenol fraction on oxidative stress in type 2 diabetes mice. Biofactors. 21 (1-4): 251 - 53.

Gollücke AP (2010). Recent applications of grape polyphenols in foods, beverages and supplements. Recent Pat. Food Nutr. Agric. 2 (2): 105 - 109.

Gonthier MP, Verny MA, Besson C, Remesy C, Scalbert A (2003). Chlorogenic acid bioavailability largely depends on its metabolism by the gut microflora in rats. J. Nutr. 133: 1853 - 59.

Gülçin I (2006). Anti-oxidant activity of caffeic acid (3, 4-dihydroxycinnamic acid). Toxicology. 217 (2-3): 213 - 20.

Hajiani M, Golestani A, Shariftabrizi A, Rastegar R, Payabvash S, Salmasi AH, Dehpour AR, Pasalar P (2008). Dose-dependent modulation of systemic lipid peroxidation and activity of anti-oxidant enzymes by vitamin E in the rat. Redox Rep. 13 (2): 60 - 66.

Halvorsen BL, Holte K, Myhrstad MC, Barikmo I, Hvattum E, Remberg SF, Wold AB, Haffner K, Baugerod H, Andersen LF, Moskaug O, Jacobs DR Jr, Blomhoff R (2002). A systematic screening of total anti-oxidants in dietary plants. J. Nutr. 132: 461 - 71.

Hervert-Hernández D, Goni I (2011). Contribution of beverages to the intake of polyphenols and anti-oxidant capacity in obese women from rural Mexico. Public Health Nutr. 2: 1 - 7.

Hu ML (2011). Dietary polyphenols as anti-oxidants and anticancer agents: more questions than answers. Chang. Gung. Med. J. 34 (5): 449 - 60.

Illy E (2002). The complexity of coffee. Sci. Am. 286: 86 - 91.

Iqbal S, Bhanger MI, Akhtar M, Anwar F, Ahmed KR, Anwer T (2006). Antioxidant properties of methanolic extracts from leaves of *Rhazya stricta*. J. Med. Food. 9 (2): 270 - 75.

Jaiswal AK, Rajauria G, Abu-Ghannam N, Gupta S (2011). Phenolic composition, anti-oxidant capacity and antibacterial activity of selected Irish Brassica vegetables. Nat. Prod. Commun. 6 (9): 1299 - 304.

Joshipura KJ, Ascherio A, Manson JE, Stampfer MJ, Rimm EB, Speizer FE, Hennekens CH, Spiegelman D, Willett WC (1999). Fruit and vegetable intake in relation to risk of ischemic stroke. JAMA. 282: 1233 - 39.

Joshipura KJ, Hu FB, Manson JE, Stampfer MJ, Rimm EB, Speizer FE, Colditz G, Ascherio A, Rosner B, Spiegelman D, Willett WC (2001). The effect of fruit and vegetable intake on risk for coronary heart disease. Ann. Intern. Med. 134: 1106 - 114.

Kahkonen MP, Hopia AI, Heinonen M (2001). Berry phenolics and their anti-oxidant activity. J. Agric. Food Chem. 49: 4076 - 82.

Kamal R, Yadav S, Mathur M, Katariya P (2011). Antiradical efficiency of 20 selected medicinal plants. Nat. Prod. Res. 2011 Oct 20. [Epub ahead of print].

Kaur G, Jabbar Z, Athar M, Alam MS (2006). *Punica granatum* (pomegranate) flower extract possesses potent anti-oxidant activity and abrogates Fe-NTA induced hepatotoxicity in mice. Food Chem. Toxicol. 44 (7): 984 - 93.

Kayan M, Naziroðlu M, Celik O, Yalman K, Köylü H (2009). Vitamin C and E combination modulates oxidative stress induced by X-ray in blood of smoker and nonsmoker radiology technicians. Cell. Biochem. Funct. 27 (7): 424 - 29.

Khachik F, Bernstein PS, Garland DL (1997). Identification of lutein and zeaxanthin oxidation products in human and monkey retinas. Invest. Ophthalmol. Vis. Sci. 38 (9): 1802 - 11.

Khan SM, Kour G (2007). Subacute oral toxicity of chlorpyriphos and protective effect of green tea extract. Pesticide Biochemistry and Physiology. 89 (2): 118 - 23.

Ko JK, Leung CC (2010). Ginger extract and polaprezinc exert gastroprotective actions by anti-oxidant and growth factor modulating effects in rats. J. Gastroenterol. Hepatol. 25 (12): 1861 - 68.

Kong JM, Chia LS, Goh NK, Chia TF, Brouillard R (2003). Analysis and biological activities of anthocyanins. Phytochemistry. 64: 923 - 33.

Kuhad A, Pilkhwal S, Sharma S, Tirkey N, Chopra K (2007). Effect of curcumin on inflammation and oxidative stress in cisplatin-induced experimental nephrotoxicity. J. Agric. Food Chem. 55 (25): 10150 - 55.

Kumar SS, Shanmugasundaram KR (2004). Amrita Bindu–an anti-oxidant inducer therapy in asthma children. J. Ethnopharmacol. 90 (1): 105 - 114.

Kutluhan S, Naziroðlu M, Celik O, Yilmaz M (2009). Effects of selenium and topiramate on lipid peroxidation and antioxidant vitamin levels in blood of pentylentetrazol-induced epileptic rats. Biol. Trace Elem. Res. 129 (1-3): 181 - 89.

Lakshminarayana R, Aruna G, Sathisha UV, Dharmesh SM, Baskaran V (2013). Structural elucidation of possible lutein oxidation products mediated through peroxyl radical inducer 2,2'-Azobis (2-methylpropionamidine) dihydrochloride: Antioxidant and cytotoxic influence of oxidized lutein in HeLa cells. Chem. Biol. Interact. 203 (2): 448 - 55.

Lakshminarayana R, Sathish UV, Dharmesh SM, Baskaran V (2010). Antioxidant and cytotoxic effect of oxidized lutein in human cervical carcinoma cells (HeLa). Food Chem. Toxicol. 48 (7): 1811 - 16.

Lazze MC, Pizzala R, Savio M, Stivala LA, Prosperi E, Bianchi L (2003). Anthocyanins protect against DNA damage induced by tert-butyl-hydroperoxide in rat smooth muscle and hepatoma cells. Mutat. Res. 535: 103 - 15.

£uczaj W, Skrzydlewska E (2005). Antioxidative properties of black tea. Prev. Med. 40 (6): 910 - 18.

Luqman S, Srivastava S, Kumar R, Maurya AK, Chanda D (2012). Experimental assessment of *Moringa oleifera* leaf and fruit for its antistress, antioxidant, and scavenging potential using *in vitro* and *in vivo* assays. Evid. Based Complement. Alternat. Med. 2012: 519084.

Lung MY, Chang YC (2011). Anti-oxidant properties of the edible basidiomycete *Armillaria mellea* in submerged cultures. Int. J. Mol. Sci. 12 (10): 6367 - 84.

Ma Y, Njike VY, Millet J, Dutta S, Doughty K, Treu JA, Katz DL (2010). Effects of walnut consumption on endothelial function in type 2 diabetics: A randomized, controlled, cross-over trial. Diabetes Care. 33 (2): 227 - 32.

Madhusudhanan N, Kavithalakshmi SN, Radha Shanmugasundaram K, Shanmugasundaram ER (2004). Oxidative damage to lipids and proteins induced by aflatoxin B(1) in fish (*Labeo rohita*)-protective role of Amrita Bindu. Environ. Toxicol. Pharmacol. 17 (2): 73 - 77.

Madhusudhanan N, Kavithalakshmi SN, Shanmugasundaram ER, Shanmugasundaram KR (2006). Aflatoxin B1-induced DNA damage in Labeo rohita: protective effect of an anti-oxidant supplement, Amrita Bindu. Basic Clin. Pharmacol. Toxicol. 98 (5): 473 - 79.

Maatta-Riihinen KR, Kamal-Eldin A, Mattila PH, Gonzalez-Paramas AM, Torronen AR (2004a). Distribution and contents of phenolic compounds in eighteen Scandinavian berry species. J. Agric. Food Chem. 52: 4477 - 86.

Maatta-Riihinen KR, Kamal-Eldin A, Torronen AR (2004b). Identification and quantification of phenolic compounds in berries of *Fragaria* and *Rubus* species (family Rosaceae). J. Agric. Food Chem. 52: 6178 - 87.

Maheshwari RK, Singh AK, Gaddipati J, Srimal RC (2006). Multiple biological activities of curcumin: a short review. Life Sci. Mar 78 (18): 2081 - 87.

Mak JC (2012). Potential role of green tea catechins in various disease therapies: progress and promise. Clin. Exp. Pharmacol. Physiol. 39 (3): 265 - 73

Malin DH, Lee DR, Goyarzu P, *et al.* (2011). Short-term blueberry-enriched diet prevents and reverses object recognition memory loss in ageing rats. Nutrition. 27 (3): 338 - 42.

Manach C, Scalbert A, Morand C, Remesy C, Jimenez L (2004). Polyphenols: food sources and bioavailability. Am. J. Clin. Nutr. 79: 727 - 47.

Manach C, Williamson G, Morand C, Scalbert A, Remesy C (2005). Bioavailability and bioefficacy of polyphenols in humans. I. Review of 97 bioavailability studies. Am. J. Clin. Nutr. 81: 230S - 242S.

Mattioli AV, Miloro C, Pennella S, Pedrazzi P, Farinetti A (2011). Adherence to Mediterranean diet and intake of anti-oxidants influence spontaneous conversion of atrial fibrillation. Nutr. Metab. Cardiovasc. Dis. 2011 Jul 26. [Epub ahead of print].

McKay DL, Blumberg JB (2002). The role of tea in human health: an update. J. Am. Coll. Nutr. 21 (1): 1 - 13.

McKay DL, Chen CY, Yeum KJ, Matthan NR, Lichtenstein AH, Blumberg JB (2010). Chronic and acute effects of walnuts on anti-oxidant capacity and nutritional status in humans: a randomized, cross-over pilot study. Nutr. J. 9: 21.

Miller HE, Rigelhof F, Marquart L, Prakash A, Kanter M (2000). Anti-oxidant content of whole grain breakfast cereals, fruits and vegetables. J. Am. Coll. Nutr. 19: 312S - 319S.

Miller NJ, Evans RCA (1996). Spectrophotometric determination of anti-oxidant activity. Redox. Report. 2: 161 - 71.

Mohamad RH, El-Bastawesy AM, Abdel-Monem MG, Noor AM, Al-Mehdar HA, Sharawy SM, El-Merzabani MM (2011). Anti-oxidant and anticarcinogenic effects of methanolic extract and volatile oil of fennel seeds (*Foeniculum vulgare*). J. Med. Food. 14 (9): 986 - 1001.

Moskaug JO, Carlsen H, Myhrstad MC, Blomhoff R (2005). Polyphenols and glutathione synthesis regulation.*The American Journal of Clinical Nutrition.* 81 (1): 277S - 83S.

Murthy KN, Rajasekaran T, Giridhar P, Ravishankar GA (2006). Anti-oxidant property of *Decalepis hamiltonii* Wight and Arn. Indian J. Exp. Biol. 44 (10): 832 - 37.

Natarajan KS, Narasimhan M, Shanmugasundaram KR, Shanmugasundaram ER (2006). Anti-oxidant activity of a salt-spice-herbal mixture against free radical induction. J. Ethnopharmacol. 105 (1-2): 76 - 83.

Nawrot P, Jordan S, Eastwood J, Rotstein J, Hugenholtz A, Feeley M (2003). Effects of caffeine on human health. Food Addit. Contam. 20: 1 - 30.

Nazýroglu M (2009). Role of selenium on calcium signaling and oxidative stress-induced molecular pathways in epilepsy. Neurochem. Res. 34 (12): 2181 - 91.

Naziroglu M, Karaoðlu A, Aksoy AO (2004). Selenium and high dose vitamin E administration protects cisplatin-induced oxidative damage to renal, liver and lens tissues in rats. Toxicology. 195 (2-3): 221 - 30.

Naziroðlu M, Kutluhan S, Yilmaz M (2008). Selenium and topiramate modulates brain microsomal oxidative stress values, Ca2+-ATPase activity, and EEG records in pentylentetrazol-induced seizures in rats. J. Membr. Biol. 225 (1-3): 39 – 49.

Naziroðlu M, Kutluhan S, Uðuz AC, Celik O, Bal R, Butterworth PJ (2009). Topiramate and vitamin e modulate the electro-encephalographic records, brain microsomal and blood anti-oxidant redox system in pentylentetrazol-induced seizure of rats. J. Membr. Biol. 229 (3): 131 - 40.

Ng ZX, Chai JW, Kuppusamy UR (2011). Customized cooking method improves total antioxidant activity in selected vegetables. Int. J. Food Sci. Nutr. 62 (2): 158 - 63.

Noorafshan A, Ashkani-Esfahani S (2013). A review of therapeutic effects of curcumin. Curr. Pharm. Des. 19 (11): 2032 - 46.

Olthof MR, Hollman PC, Katan MB (2001). Chlorogenic acid and caffeic acid are absorbed in humans. J. Nutr. 131: 66 - 71.

Ozen T (2009). Investigation of anti-oxidant properties of *Nasturtium officinale* (watercress) leaf extracts. Acta. Pol. Pharm. 66 (2): 187 - 93.

Pastrana-Bonilla E, Akoh CC, Sellappan S, Krewer G (2003). Phenolic content and anti-oxidant capacity of muscadine grapes. J. Agric. Food Chem. 51 (18): 5497 - 503.

Pellegrini N, Chiavaro E, Gardana C, Mazzeo T, Contino D, Gallo M, Riso P, Fogliano V, Porrini M (2010). Effect of different cooking methods on color, phytochemical concentration, and antioxidant capacity of raw and frozen brassica vegetables. J. Agric. Food Chem. 58 (7): 4310 - 21.

Pellegrini N, Serafini M, Colombi B, Del Rio D, Salvatore S, Bianchi M, Brighenti F (2003). Total anti-oxidant capacity of plant foods, beverages and oils consumed in Italy assessed by three different *in vitro* assays. J. Nutr. 133 (9): 2812 - 19.

Pellegrini N, Serafini M, Salvatore S, Del Rio D, Bianchi M, Brighenti F (2006). Total anti-oxidant capacity of spices, dried fruits, nuts, pulses, cereals and sweets consumed in Italy assessed by three different *in vitro* assays. Mol. Nutr. Food Res. 50: 1030 - 38.

Prior RL, Wu X, Schaich K (2005). Standardized methods for the determination of antioxidant capacity and phenolics in foods and dietary supplements. J. Agric. Food Chem. 53 (10): 4290 - 302.

Pujari RR, Vyawahare NS, Kagathara VG (2011). Evaluation of anti-oxidant and neuroprotective effect of date palm (*Phoenix dactylifera* L.) against bilateral common carotid artery occlusion in rats. Indian J. Exp. Biol. 49 (8): 627 - 33.

Pulido R, Hernández-García M, Saura-Calixto F (2003). Contribution of beverages to the intake of lipophilic and hydrophilic anti-oxidants in the Spanish diet. Eur. J. Clin. Nutr. 57 (10): 1275 - 82.

Rani P, Unni KM, Karthikeyan J (2004). Evaluation of antioxidant properties of berries. Indian Journal of Clinical Biochemistry. 19 (2):103 - 110.

Rasool M, Sabina EP (2007). Anti-inflammatory effect of the Indian Ayurvedic herbal formulation Triphala on adjuvant-induced arthritis in mice. Phytother. Res. 21: 889 - 94.

Rauma AL, Mykkänen H (2000). Anti-oxidant status in vegetarians versus omnivores. Nutrition. 16 (2): 111 - 19.

Ravi K, Ramachandran B, Subramanian S (2004a). Effect of *Eugenia jambolana* seed kernel on antioxidant defense system in streptozotocin-induced diabetes in rats. Life Sci. 75 (22): 2717 - 31.

Ravi K, Ramachandran B, Subramanian S (2004b).Protective effect of *Eugenia jambolana* seed kernel on tissue antioxidants in streptozotocin-induced diabetic rats. Biol. Pharm. Bull. 27 (8): 1212 -17.

Reiter RJ, Manchester LC, Tan DX (2005). Melatonin in walnuts: Influence on levels of melatonin and total antioxidant capacity of blood. Nutrition. 21 (9): 920 - 24.

Rendeiro C, Vauzour D, Kean RJ, *et al.* (2012). Blueberry supplementation induces spatial memory improvements and region-specific regulation of hippocampal BDNF mRNA expression in young rats. Psychopharmacology. 223 (3): 319 - 30

Riboli E, Norat T (2003). Epidemiologic evidence of the protective effect of fruit and vegetables on cancer risk. Am. J. Clin. Nutr. 78: 559S - 569S.

Saafi-Ben Salah EB, El Arem A, Louedi M, Saoudi M, Elfeki A, Zakhama A, Najjar MF, Hammami M, Achour (2012). Antioxidant-rich date palm fruit extract inhibits oxidative stress and nephrotoxicity induced by dimethoate in rat. J. Physiol. Biochem. 68 (1): 47 – 58.

Sánchez de Medina V, Priego-Capote F, Jiménez-Ot C, Luque de Castro MD (2011). Quality and stability of edible oils enriched with hydrophilic anti-oxidants from the olive tree: The role of enrichment extracts and lipid composition. J. Agric. Food Chem. 59 (21): 11432 - 41.

Sandhu AK, Gu L (2010). Antioxidant capacity, phenolic content, and profiling of phenolic compounds in the seeds, skin, and pulp of *Vitis rotundifolia* (Muscadine Grapes) As determined by HPLC-DAD-ESI-MS(n). J. Agric. Food Chem. 58 (8): 4681 - 92.

Sarma AD, Sharma R (1999). Anthocyanin-DNA copigmentation complex: mutual protection against oxidative damage. Phytochemistry. 52:.1313 - 18.

Scartezzini P, Speroni E (2000). Review on some plants of Indian traditional medicine with anti-oxidant activity. J. Ethnopharmacol. 71 (1-2): 23 - 43.

Shanmugasundaram KR, Ramanujam S, Shanmugasundaram ER (1994). Amrita Bindu–a salt-spice-herbal health food supplement for the prevention of nitrosamine induced depletion of anti-oxidants. J. Ethnopharmacol. 42 (2): 83 - 93.

Shyamala BN, Jamuna P (2010). Nutritional content and anti-oxidant properties of pulp waste from *Daucus carota* and *Beta vulgaris*. Mal. J. Nutr. 16 (3): 397 - 408.

Shyamala BN, Naidu MM, Sulochanamma G, Srinivas P (2007). Studies on the anti-oxidant activities of natural vanilla extract and its constituent compounds through *in vitro* models. J. Agric. Food Chem. 55 (19): 7738 - 43.

Siddhuraju P, Becker K (2003). Anti-oxidant properties of various solvent extracts of total phenolic constituents from three different agroclimatic origins of drumstick tree (*Moringa oleifera* Lam.) leaves. J. Agric. Food Chem. 51 (8): 2144 - 55.

Sies H (1997). Oxidative stress: Oxidants and anti-oxidants. Experimental physiology. 82 (2): 291 - 95.

Singh RP, Chidambara Murthy KN, Jayaprakasha GK (2002). Studies on the anti-oxidant activity of pomegranate (*Punica granatum*) peel and seed extracts using *in vitro* models. J. Agric. Food Chem. 50 (1): 81 - 86.

Sreelatha S, Padma PR (2009). Anti-oxidant activity and total phenolic content of *Moringa oleifera* leaves in two stages of maturity. Plant Foods Hum. Nutr. 64 (4): 303 - 311.

Srikanta BM, Nayaka MA, Dharmesh SM (2011). Inhibition of *Helicobacter pylori* growth and its cytotoxicity by 2-hydroxy 4-methoxy benzaldehyde of *Decalepis hamiltonii* (Wight and Arn); a new functional attribute. Biochimie. 93 (4): 678 - 88.

Srikumar R, Parthasarathy NJ, Shankar EM, Manikandan S, Vijayakumar R, Thangaraj R, Vijayananth K, Sheeladevi R, Rao UA (2007). Evaluation of the growth inhibitory activities of Triphala against common bacterial isolates from HIV infected patients. Phytother. Res. 21: 476 - 80.

Stanner SA, Hughes J, Kelly CN, Buttriss J (2004). A review of the epidemiological evidence for the 'anti-oxidant hypothesis'. Public Health Nutr. 7: 407 - 422.

Tharakan B, Hunter FA, Smythe WR, Childs EW (2010). Curcumin inhibits reactive oxygen species formation and vascular hyperpermeability following haemorrhagic shock. Clin. Exp. Pharmacol. Physiol. 37 (9): 939 - 44.

Tian X, Schaich KM (2013). Effects of molecular structure on kinetics and dynamics of Trolox Equivalent Antioxidant Capacity (TEAC) Assay with ABTS(+•). J. Agric. Food Chem. 2013 May 9. [Epub ahead of print].

Uðuz AC, Nazýroðlu M (2012). Effects of selenium on calcium signaling and apoptosis in rat dorsal root ganglion neurons induced by oxidative stress. Neurochem. Res. 37 (8): 1631 - 38.

Vayalil PK (2002). Anti-oxidant and anti-mutagenic properties of aqueous extract of date fruit (Phoenix dactylifera L. Arecaceae). J. Agric. Food Chem. 50 (3): 610 - 17.

Vazquez-Prieto MA, Rodriguez Lanzi C, Lembo C, Galmarini CR, Miatello RM (2011). Garlic and onion attenuates vascular inflammation and oxidative stress in fructose-fed rats. J. Nutr. Metab. 475216. Epub 2011 Aug 25.

Venderley AM, Campbell WW (2006). Vegetarian diets: nutritional considerations for athletes. Sports Med. 36 (4): 293 - 305.

Verma AR, Vijayakumar M, Mathela CS, Rao CV (2009). *In vitro* and *in vivo* anti-oxidant properties of different fractions of *Moringa oleifera* leaves. Food Chem. Toxicol. 47 (9): 2196 - 201.

Vijayakumar RS, Nalini N (2006). Efficacy of piperine, an alkaloidal constituent from *Piper nigrum* on erythrocyte antioxidant status in high fat diet and antithyroid drug induced hyperlipidemic rats. Cell. Biochem. Funct. 24 (6): 491 - 98.

Vijayakumar RS, Surya D, Nalini N (2004). Anti-oxidant efficacy of black pepper (*Piper nigrum* L.) and piperine in rats with high fat diet induced oxidative stress. Redox. Rep. 9 (2): 105 - 110.

Watanabe J, Oki T, Takebayashi J, Yamasaki K, Takano-Ishikawa Y, Hino A, Yasui A (2013). Improvement of the Lipophilic-Oxygen Radical Absorbance Capacity (L-ORAC) Method and Single-Laboratory Validation. Biosci. Biotechnol. Biochem. 77 (4): 857 - 59.

Wood JG, Rogina B, Lavu S, Howitz K, Helfand SL, Tatar M, Sinclair D (2004). Sirtuin activators mimic caloric restriction and delay ageing in metazoans. Nature. 430: 686 - 89.

World Cancer Research Fund / American Institute for Cancer Research (2007). Food, Nutrition, Physical Activity and the Prevention of Cancer: a Global Perspective. American Institute of Cancer Research, Washington. DC.

Yanagimoto K, Lee KG, Ochi H, Shibamoto T (2002). Anti-oxidative activity of heterocyclic compounds found in coffee volatiles produced by Maillard reaction. J.Agric. Food Chem. 50:.5480 - 84.

Yazdanparast R, Bahramikia S, Ardestani A (2008). *Nasturtium officinale* reduces oxidative stress and enhances anti-oxidant capacity in hyper-cholesterolaemic rats. Chem. Biol. Interact. 172 (3):176 - 84.

Yilmaz Y, Toledo RT (2004). Major flavonoids in grape seeds and skins: anti-oxidant capacity of catechin, epicatechin, and gallic acid. J. Agric. Food Chem. 52 (2): 255 - 60.

Zafra-Stone S, Yasmin T, Bagchi M, Chatterjee A, Vinson JA, Bagchi D (2007). Berry anthocyanins as novel anti-oxidants in human health and disease prevention. *Molecular Nutrition and Food Research.* 51 (6): 675 - 83.

Zepeda A, Aguayo LG, Fuentealba J, Figueroa C, Acevedo A, Salgado P, Calaf GM, Farías J (2012). Blueberry extracts protect testis from hypobaric hypoxia induced oxidative stress in rats. Oxid. Med. Cell. Longev. 2012: 975870.

Zhang JJ, Ji R, Hu YQ, Chen JC, Ye XQ (2011). Effect of three cooking methods on nutrient components and anti-oxidant capacities of bamboo shoot (*Phyllostachys praecox* C.D. Chu et C.S. Chao). J. Zhejiang. Univ. Sci. B. 12 (9): 752 - 59.

Chapter - 12

Anti-Ulcerogenic Foods

Gastro-intestinal disorders constitute one of the most common diseases world-wide. Peptic ulcer, encompassing gastric and duodenal ulcers is the most prevalent gastro-intestinal disorder. Oxidative stress and *Helicobactor pylori* colonization are considered to be important factors in the pathogenesis of gastric ulcers. The patho-physiology of peptic ulcer involves an imbalance between some endogenous aggressive factors like acid, pepsin refluxed bile, reactive oxygen species, cyto-protective factors like nitric oxide and growth factors, surface active phospholipids, prostaglandins, enzymatic and non-enzymatic anti-oxidants (Bhattacharjee *et al.*, 2002).

Balint (1998) discussed how the elevation of the gastric mucosal Cyclic adenosine monophosphate:Cyclic guanosine monophosphate (cAMP:cGMP) ratio is a useful molecular marker that could provide insights into the effects of anti-ulcerogenic drugs. According to the literature, under normal conditions the cAMP:cGMP ratio in the rat gastric mucosa is approximately 8:10. Following prostacyclin administration, this ratio transiently decreases but later shows a strong elevation, indicating profound changes in the intracellular cyclic nucleotide balance. There is evidence that this elevation or 'shift' in the cAMP:cGMP ratio is linked, on a cellular or molecular level, to the anti-ulcerogenic, cyto-protective processes in the stomach.

The main therapeutic target is the control of gastric secretion using antacids, H_2 receptor blockers like ranitidine, famotidine, anticholinergics like pirenzepin, telezipine or proton pump blockers like omeprazole, lansoprazole, etc. (Bandyopadhyaya *et al.*, 2002a). Cimetidine and ranitidine (widely used H_2 receptor-blocking drugs) administered at doses that are too low to interfere with gastric acid secretion, cause an elevation in the cAMP:cGMP ratio, an effect that is also observed with other prostaglandin derivatives and anti-ulcerogenic drugs.

These drugs now used extensively to control gastric and duodenal ulcer, inflammation and pain have limitations and are not always affordable, the clinical evaluation showing intolerance, incidence of relapses and side-effects have made their efficacy questionable (Rao *et al.*, 2004). The development of novel nontoxic antiulcer drugs, including from medicinal plants, is therefore desired. The anti-ulcer potentials of most plants still remain largely unexplored, despite their prospects evidenced by their use as ethnomedicine (Maity *et al.*, 2009).

The foods that have been scientifically proved as anti-ulcerogenic either through animal or human trials have been discussed below.

Unripe Banana (*Musa sapientum*)

Green unripe *Musa sapientum* has been reported to have protective action against gastric mucosal injury in rats and assists in healing ulcer (Dunijic *et al.*, 1993). The medicinal properties of banana are part of the traditional folk medicine. There are a number of reports associating banana with anti-ulcerogenic properties (Elliot and Heward, 1976; Sanyal *et al.*, 1961; Hanszen, 1934) which appear to be due to its ability to stimulate the growth of gastric mucosa. The active factor(s) were water soluble and were concentrated by extraction to approximately three hundred times that in the dried banana powder. Interestingly, the ripe ones were inactive. (Best *et al.*, 1984). The active anti-ulcerogenic ingredient extracted from unripe plantain banana powder and identified as the flavonoid leucocyanidin and a purified synthetic leucocyanidin demonstrated a significant ($P < 0.05$) protective effect against aspirin-induced erosions (Lewis *et al.*, 1999; Lewis and Shaw, 2001; Prabha *et al.*, 2011). An indigenous drug like *M. sapientum* possessing fewer side-effects is the major thrust area of present day research, aiming at a better and safer approach for the management of peptic ulcer.

Goel *et al.* (1986) reported that banana powder treatment not only strengthened mucosal resistance against ulcerogens but also promoted healing by inducing cellular proliferation. The methanolic extract (50 mg/kg, twice daily for 5 days) showed significant anti-ulcer effect and anti-oxidant activity in gastric mucosal homogenates, by reversing the increase in ulcer index, lipid peroxidation and super oxide dismutase induced by stress. Banana pulp powder treated (0.5 g/kg orally, twice daily for 3 days) rats of either sex and showed, (i) a significant increase in the [3H] thymidine incorporation into mucosal cell DNA; (ii) a significant increase in the total carbohydrate (sum of total hexoses, hexosamine, fucose and sialic acid) content of gastric mucosa; (iii) a significant decrease in gastric juice DNA and protein; (iv) a significant increase in the total carbohydrates and carbohydrate/protein ratio of gastric juice confirming that banana powder strengthens mucosal resistance and promotes the healing of ulcers (Mukhopadhyaya *et al.*, 1987). The absence of anti-H pyloric activity of methanolic extract of banana *in vitro* and its anti-oxidant activity (Goel *et al.*, 2001) may be involved in its ulcer-protective activity. Mohan Kumar *et al.* (2006) also confirmed the ulcer protective effect of methanolic extract of unripe banana and this effect could be due to its predominant effect on mucosal glycoprotein, cell proliferation, free radicals and anti-oxidant systems.

Plantain banana thus, favoured wound healing thus ulcer healing activity probably due to its anti-oxidant effect and related wound healing biochemical parameters (Agarwal *et al.*,, 2009).

Whey Protein Concentrate

Among the major milk proteins, alpha-lactalbumin (alpha-LA) is demonstrated to have a marked protective effect against ethanol-induced gastric injury, with the same potency as that of the typical antiulcer agent, Selbex. Whey protein isolate (WPI), which contained 25 per cent alpha-LA, also protected against gastric injury, while casein showed no effect. Alpha-LA was about 4-fold more effective than WPI itself (Matsumoto *et al.*, 2001).

Whey protein concentrate (WPC) protected gastric mucosa from ethanol damage and that the protection depended on sulfhydryl compounds present in the WPC, including its capacity to stimulate glutathione synthesis (Rosaneli *et al.*, 2002). The authors reported that administration of a single dose of WPC resulted in 41 per cent inhibition of the ulcerative lesion index (ULI), and with repetitive doses 73 per cent inhibition was seen. Sub-chronic treatment for 10 days resulted in 64 per cent, inhibition. Further experiment by the same authors (Rosaneli *et al.*, 2004) showed that best inhibition of stomach ulcerative lesions was achieved in indomethacin model for repetitive or subchronic experiments by 50.1 per cent and 44 per cent, respectively. Castro *et al.* (2010) suggested from their experimental data, that gastrin, sulfhydryl compounds, and some mechanisms related to mucus production are all involved in gastric ulcer protection against ethanol. Bovine as well as porcine collagen hydrolysates presented a stronger effect on mucus production. And the effect of WPI was dependent on sulfhydryl compounds and when the two proteins were administered together the protective effect was much better.

Neem (*Azadirachta indica)*

Neem is known to have potent gastro-protective and anti-ulcer effects. Maity *et al.* (2009) on reviewing the studies available on the pharmacological and biochemical action of neem and their mechanism of action have concluded that neem bark extract has the potential for the development of novel medicines for the therapeutic control of gastric hyper-acidity and ulcer. Bandyopadhyay *et al.* (2002b) also reported that aqueous extract of neem bark has potent anti-secretory and anti-ulcer effects in animal models and has no significant adverse effect. They attributed the pharmacological effects to a phenolic glycoside. Bandyopadhyay *et al.* (2004) confirmed the anti-secretory and anti-ulcer effects of neem bark on human subjects. Raji *et al.* (2004) found the stem bark extract of neem probably acts via histamine H_2 receptor in inhibiting gastric secretion induced by histamine in rats.

The data obtained by Dorababu *et al.* (2006) suggested that the ulcer-protective effect of neem leaves may be due to its anti-secretary and proton pump inhibitory activity rather than on defensive mucin secretion. Further, with 2.5 g/kg dose of neem leaves have indicated no mortality in mice. Also when treated for 28 days with 1 g/kg dose of the extract, no significant alterations were seen in body or tissues weight, food and water intake, hematological profile and various liver and kidney function tests in rats.

Black Tea (*Camellia sinensis*)

While prior administration of tea extract for 7 days significantly reduced the incidence of ulcer, ulcer number and ulcer index produced by aspirin, indomethacin, ethanol, reserpine and cold restraint stress, it failed to inhibit the ulcers induced by serotonin and histamine. The hot water extract of black tea possesses anti-ulcer activity, probably mediated through prostaglandins (Maity *et al.*, 1995). Later, Maity *et al.* (1998) reported that glutathione plays a major role in cyto-protection against ulceration afforded by black tea extract. Still later in 2001, Maity's team provided evidence that nitric oxide plays a role in black tea extract mediated improvement in changes of intestinal motility and gastric emptying induced by diethyl maleate, diethyl maleate plus N-ethyl maleimide. Hamaishi *et al.* (2006) observed that tea catechin (50, 100 mg/kg twice orally, daily) markedly inhibited the increase in content of thiobarbituric acid-reactive substances in the ulcerated region of acetic acid-induced gastric ulcers and (100, 200 mg/kg orally) in the injured mucosa of rats treated with 50 per cent ethanol. It dose-dependently prevented the decrease in gastric mucosal hexosamine content induced by absolute ethanol too, but failed to inhibit the basal gastric acid secretion. Thus, tea catechin primarily protects gastric mucosa from acute gastric mucosal injury and promotes healing of chronic gastric ulcers by its anti-oxidant activity and gastric mucus-increasing actions.

Fish Oil

Pressure ulcers are an important source of morbidity and suffering for patients and a formidable burden on caregivers. While comparing fish oil and olive oil on indometacin-induced gastric lesions in rats, Guzel *et al.* (1995) found reduction in the ulcer index to 2.1 ±1.8 mm with fish oil, 13.7 ±1 5.4 mm with olive oil, and 14.6 ±2.4 mm with normal diet. Fish oil showed a potent healing effect on acute gastric erosions and ulcers induced by indomethacin and significantly enhanced the mucus content of the mucosa ($p < 0.05$). Al-Harbi *et al.* (1995) reported that fish oil, at a dose of 5 or 10 ml/kg body weight, provided significant protection in the various experimental models used. It produced a significant inhibition of gastric mucosal damage induced by pyloric ligation, NSAIDs, reserpine or hypothermic restraint ulcers. Fish oil also exerted a significant inhibitory action on gastric mucosal lesions produced by various necrotizing agents showing that eicosapentaenoic acid in fish oil possesses both anti-secretory and anti-ulcerogenic effects (Al-Harbi *et al.*, 1995). Manjari and Das (1998) also observed that polyunsaturated fatty acids (PUFAs) can inhibit the growth of *Helicobacter pylori* and heal the ulcer suggesting that free radicals, anti-oxidants, nitric oxide and PUFAs may play a significant role in the pathogenesis of duodenal ulcer. The same authors (2000) confirmed that PUFAs could prevent dexamethasone induced gastric ulceration.

Fish oil significantly reduced the severity of ulceration in gastric ulcers induced by aspirin, cold-restraint stress (CRS), alcohol, and pylorus ligation. Interestingly the results also indicated the potentiality of fish oil in maintaining the integrity of gastric mucosa by virtue of its effect on both offensive and defensive gastric mucosal factors. It decreased the offensive acid-pepsin secretion and augmented the defensive factors like mucin secretion, cellular mucus and life span of mucosal cells following pylorus ligation. There was a significant increase in the activity of anti-oxidant enzymes (catalase and glutathione peroxidase) and decrease in lipid peroxidation in gastric mucosa of CRS rats thus indicating the beneficial role of fish oil in gastric ulceration by inhibition of offensive mucosal factors and oxidative stress, and augmentation of defensive mucosal factors (Bhattacharya *et al.*, 2006).

According to Theilla *et al.* (2007) a diet enriched with eicosapentanoic acid and gamma-linolenic acid and vitamins A, C and E is associated with a significantly lower occurrence of new pressure ulcers in critically ill patients with acute lung injury. So, they (2012a) fed fish oil and micronutrient enriched formula to pressure ulcer patients and found the same to prevent worsening of pressure ulcers. They reported that this effect is mediated by an effect on adhesion molecule expression. Again Theilla *et al.* (2012b) observed that the mean levels of C-reactive protein and the mean score on the ulcer healing tool decreased significantly from day 0 to day 14 in the experimental group as compared to the control group in adult grade II patients. Thus, administration of a feeding formula enriched with fish oil was associated with decreased progression of pressure ulcers and a decrease in blood concentrations of C-reactive protein.

Manathakali (*Solanum nigrum*)

Solanum nigrum, a herbal plant is recommended in ayurveda for the management of gastric ulcers. Rajeswari and Subbulakshmi (2003) demonstrated that the leaves and fruits (aqueous extracts) of *Solanum nigrum* strongly inhibited ethanol induced gastritis, fruits being more potent than leaves. The hydroalcoholic extract of the fruits was also found to be effective in gastritis equivalent to fruit aqueous extract. The anti-ulcerogenic effect of this extract was not mediated through its antacid action. In this context, it is of considerable interest to note that certain prostaglandins are able to protect the gastric mucosal erosions induced by ethanol and strong acids, without affecting the gastric acid secretion (cytoprotection). Thus, the leaves and fruits failed to affect the volume of gastric juice, and offered significant protection in ethanol induced gastritis and aspirin induced pyloric ligated ulcers.

Tannins were acclaimed to be anti-ulcerogenic phytochemicals in recent times. Ezaki *et al.* (1985) demonstrated that the anti-ulcerogenic activity of *Linderae umbellatae* was due to the presence of condensed tannins. Tannins are local cicatrizant substances, not being absorbed by the gastro-intestinal tract and probably have anti-ulcer action in the plants in which they are present in high concentrations. According to de Jesus et al (2012) tannins react with the tissue proteins with which they come into contact. In gastric ulcers, this tannin-protein complex layer protects the stomach by promoting greater resistance to chemical and mechanical injury or irritation. This explains at least in part the anti-ulcer action of *Solanum nigrum* as the tannin content of leaves was 7.27 per cent (higher than that of fruits).

Jainu and Devi (2006) also confirmed these findings as the extract significantly inhibited H(+)K(+)ATPase activity and decreased the gastrin secretion in ethanol induced ulcer model. The histological studies showed the reduction of ulcer size by the *S. nigrum* extract. Toxicity studies also proved its safety.

Sundaikai (*Solanum torvum*)

Solanum torvum (Solanaceae) is a plant used in Indian as well as Cameroon ethno-medicine for the treatment of stomach ailments. Gastric ulcerations induced by HCl/ethanol, indomethacin, pylorus ligation and stress, were alleviated by about 96 - 98 per cent when treated with aqueous methanolic extract of *Solanum torvum* (750 mg/kg) thus supported the ethno-medical uses of the plant in the treatment of gastric ulcer (Nguelefack *et al.*, 2008).

Camel Milk

Camel milk fed to rats with ethanol–induced gastric ulcer, significantly ($P < 0.05$) reduced the number of long ulcers, average length of ulcers, ulcer index and the volume of gastric juice. The total protein was significantly ($P < 0.05$) increased and the pH of gastric juice was not significantly changed. The curative ratio was 70.70 per cent in camel milk treated group as compared to 45.12 per cent in ranitidine-treated rats.

Apart from the improved clinical course of the disease and the secretory and motor functions of the stomach in patients given mare, camel and cow's milk, there was a complete wound healing and remarkable decline of its size in 93, 90, and 70 per cent of patients respectively. The antacid properties as assessed by radiotelemetry were also more pronounced in mare and camel milk (Sharmanov *et al.*, 1981).

Ginger (*Zingiber officinale*)

Z. officinalis L. on gastric ulceration and secretion in rats indicated a significant protection against gastric ulcers induced by cold restraint stress, aspirin and pylorus ligation was studied by Agrawal *et al.* (2000). The proposed anti-ulcerogenic effects were augmentation of mucin secretion and decrease in cell shedding. Wu *et al.* (1990) reported that roasted ginger decoctions had an obvious inhibiting tendency on three gastric ulcer models except for the indomethacin induced model. On the other hand dry ginger showed no such effect.

While the exact mechanism of action is not clear, the plant contains active materials some of which have been identified to possess ulcer protective properties. 6-Gingersulfonic acid (Yoshikawa *et al.*, 1992) and three monoacyldigalactosyl glycerols including gingerglycolipids A, B, and C (Yoshikawa *et al.*, 1994) have been isolated from dried rhizomes of *Z. officinale* which are potent anti-ulcer constituents. 6-Gingerol and 6-shogaol are two other components mainly responsible for ginger pungency are less potent as ulcer-protective (Yamahara *et al.*, 1988; 1992). Minaiyan *et al.* (2006) concluded from their study that ginger hydroalcoholic extract was effective to protect against duodenal ulceration and for i.p. injection as well as chronic administration, the efficacy was comparable with ranitidine as reference drug. Anosike *et al.* (2009) found the ginger extract to show good protective effect against indomethacin-induced gastric ulcer in rats. Administration of the extract in doses of 100, 200 and 400 mg/kg evinced a significant ($p < 0.05$) reduction in the indomethacin-induced gastric erosion in all the experimental groups when compared to the control group. The per cent ulcer inhibition by the extract doses was comparable with that of ranitidine (100 mg/kg), the reference drug. These results confirm that ginger possess as good potential as an anti-ulcer agent.

Tulasi (*Ocimum sanctum/Ocimum suave*)

Ocimum sanctum (OS) is known to possess various therapeutic properties. OS was found to decrease the incidence and also enhance healing of ulcers (Dharmani *et al.*, 2004). The methanolic extract of leaves of *O. sanctum* with eugenol content of 5 per cent given in doses of 50-200 mg/kg, orally, twice daily for five days showed dose-dependent ulcer protective effect against cold restraint stress induced gastric ulcers. The extract also showed significant ulcer protection against ethanol and pyloric ligation-induced gastric ulcers, but was ineffective against aspirin-induced ulcers. Goel *et al.* (2005) found that the leaves inhibited the offensive acid-pepsin secretion and lipid peroxidation, and increased the gastric defensive factors like mucin secretion, cellular mucus, and life span of mucosal cells.

Kath and Gupta (2006) observed in ethanol treated rats, *Ocimum sanctum* leaf extract (100 mg/kg and 200 mg/kg) significantly decreased the levels of malondialdehyde to 2.45 ± 0.29 nmol/ml and 2.40 ± 0.14 nmol/ml respectively in comparison to 4.87 ± 0.06 in the diseased control. Similarly, in the histamine treated guinea pig group, the same doses of the extract significantly lowered the levels of malondialdehyde to 2.45 ± 0.12 nmol/ml and 2.37 ± 0.16 nmol/ml respectively when compared to 4.66 ± 0.11 in the diseased control. The extract (100 mg/kg and 200 mg/kg) also increased the levels of superoxide dismutase in pyloric ligated rats to 1.78 ± 0.12 U/ml and 1.89 ± 0.08 U/ml respectively when compared to 1.29 ± 0.06 U/ml in the diseased control. In the histamine treated guinea pig group also, the same doses of the extract produced a rise in the superoxide dismutase levels to 2.10 ± 0.11 U/ml and 2.20 ± 0.14 U/ml respectively when compared to 1.32 ± 0.07 in the diseased control. The lowered levels of malondialdehyde and increased levels of superoxide dismutase that signify anti-oxidant activity proved the beneficial effect of *Ocimum sanctum.*

At the dose of 250 mg/kg of the methanol extract of leaf of *Ocimum suave* there was complete inhibition of gastric lesions induced using the HCl/ethanol solution. In the pylorus ligated rats, the dose of 500 mg/kg completely inhibited lesion formation but with no effect on gastric acid secretion compared with the controls. But inhibition of HCl/ethanol-induced gastric lesions by the *Ocimum suave* extract was significantly reduced on pretreatment with indomethacin. The mucus secretion promoting effect of the extract was most significant when the gastric environment was highly acidic. This suggests this treatment with *Ocimum suave* does not require the use of antacids and anti-secretary agents (Tan *et al.*, 2002).

Cabbage (*Brassica oleracea* var. *capitata*)

Carvalho *et al.* (2011) validated the ethno-botanical claims regarding the use of cabbage in gastric disorders as evidenced by its significant inhibition in the formation of ulcers with a maximum of 99.44 per cent curation (250 mg/kg body weight) in acetylsalicylic acid-induced ulcers. According to Lemos *et al.* (2011) the anti-ulcer activity of *Brassica oleracea* extract is based on its ability to stimulate the synthesis of mucus, increased pH and decreased H^+ ions in the stomach.

Celery (*Apium graveolens*)

The phyto-chemical screening of celery showed the presence of flavonoids, tannins, volatile oils, alkaloids, sterols and/or tri-terpenes. Pre treatment with celery extract produced dose-dependent reduction in all experimentally induced gastric lesions. Al-Howiriny *et al.* (2010) observed that *Apium graveolens* extract significantly protected the gastric mucosa and suppressed the basal gastric secretion in rats, possibly through its anti-oxidant potential.

Parsley (*Petroselinum crispum*)

An ethanolic extract of parsley, (1 and 2 g/kg body weight) showed a significant anti-ulcerogenic activity in rats. Further, the depleted gastric wall mucus and non-protein sulfhydryl contents as a result of ethanol were replenished by pretreatment with Parsley extract. Acute toxicity tests showed a large margin of safety for the extract (Al-Howiriny *et al.*, 2003).

Spices

Diets containing black pepper (0.5 per cent), piperine (0.02 per cent), red pepper (3.0 per cent), capsaicin (0.01 per cent), and ginger (0.05 per cent) fed to groups of Wistar rats for 8 weeks significantly enhanced the activities of anti-oxidant enzymes–superoxide dismutase, catalase, glutathione reductase, and glutathione-S-transferase–in both gastric and intestinal mucosa, suggesting a gastro-intestinal protective role for these spices (Prakash and Srinivasan, 2010).

Cinnamon (*Cinnamomum tamala*)

Cinnamon is used traditionally in Indian System of Medicine as carminative, anthelmintic, diuretic, and used in colic, dyspepsia, and diarrhea. Eswaran *et al.* (2010) found a significant reduction in lesion index in ulcer-induced animals treated with cinnamon extract at different doses when compared with ulcerated rats in all models. In cinnamon fed rats, a significant decrease in the level of H(+)K(+)ATPase, volume of gastric juice, and acid output; and a significant increase in the gastric wall mucus level and pH could be seen probably due to its free radical scavenging activity. Tankam *et al.* (2013) reported that cinnamon powder significantly protected mice against ulceration by stress, ethanol, HCl and oral administration of aspirin but not against ulceration by subcutaneous administration of aspirin or indomethacin or oral administration of indomethacin.

Cumin/Black Cumin seeds (*Nigella sativa*)

Black seed or *Nigella sativa* (NS) has been reported to possess a large number of pharmacological activities including its anti-ulcer potential. In folkloric practices the seeds are taken as such, in the form of coarse dry powder or the powdered seeds are mixed with water. An aqueous suspension of black cumin seed significantly prevented gastric ulcer formation induced by necrotizing agents and significantly ameliorated the ulcer severity and basal gastric acid secretion in pylorus-ligated Shay rats. This anti-ulcer effect is either prostaglandin-mediated and/or through its anti-oxidant and anti-secretory activities (Al Mofleh *et al.*, 2008).

The black cumin seed oil and its constituent thymoquinone (TQ) were also found in an experimental model to protect gastric mucosa against the injurious effect of absolute alcohol and promote ulcer healing as evidenced from the ulcer index values and at least partly by their radical scavenging activity (Kanter *et al.*, 2005). This effect may also be related to the conservation of the gastric mucosal redox state (El Abhar *et al.*, 2003). Tayman *et al.* (2012) confirmed the significant reduction in the severity of intestinal damage in necrotizing enterocolitis by the seed oil.

According to Magdy *et al.* (2012) TQ has novel gastro-protective mechanisms via inhibiting proton pump, acid secretion and neutrophil infiltration, while enhancing mucin secretion, and nitric oxide production. Although TQ was found to protect gastric mucosa against the ulcerating effect of alcohol and mitigated most of the biochemical adverse effects induced by alcohol in gastric mucosa, the effect of TQ was found to be lesser than whole black cumin seed (Khaled, 2009).

Ramirez and Rao Jr. (2003) demonstrated that the tannins extracted from *S. cumini* have gastro-protective and anti-ulcerogenic effects. The healing effects on gastric ulcer was found to be 83 per cent for natural honey and 78 per cent for black cumin seeds as compared to 94 per cent for cimetidine a standard drug for ulcer treatment. In fact, 72 per cent, 78 per cent and 89 per cent of the animals showed recovery with honey, black cumin seeds and cimetidine respectively (Bukhari *et al.*, 2011).

Cloves (*Syzygium aromaticum*)

The hot aqueous extract of cloves was found to increase the gut muscle propulsion similar to the standard drugs carbachol and metoclopramide. Along with atropine, cloves produced a reduction in intestinal propulsion suggesting that cholinergic mechanism was involved in the action. The cloves extract significantly reduced the ulcer number and ulcer area in the ethanol and HCl-ethanol models ($p < 0.05$). In the indomethacin model, the extract, 700 mg kg(-1), compared favorably with misoprostol with an index of 0.20 ± 0.11 which was also found to be significant compared with the control (Agbaje, 2008).

Curry Leaves (*Murraya koenigii*)

Various doses of alkaloidal extract from *M. koenigii* leaves (10, 20 and 40 mg kg(-1), p.o) showed promising anti-ulcerogenic activity with protection against acute gastric ulcers induced by ethanol plus hydrochloric acid and aspirin models in a dose dependent manner (Mani *et al.*, 2013).

Anise/Fennel (*Pimpinella anisum*)

Anise significantly inhibited gastric mucosal damage induced by necrotizing agents and indomethacin. Al Mofleh *et al.* (2007) observed that the anti-ulcer/cyto-protective effect of aqueous suspension of anise is either prostaglandin-mediated and/or through its anti-secretory and anti-oxidative properties.

Jamun (*Eugenia jambolana*)

The gastro-protective properties of ethanolic extract of *E. jambolana* seed was reported to be mainly through promotion of mucosal defensive factors and anti-oxidant status and decreasing lipid peroxidation (Chaturvedi *et al.*, 2007). In diabetics its anti-hyperglycemic and mucosal defensive actions were found to be responsible for ameliorating gastric ulcers (Chaturvedi *et al.*, 2009 a). Jamun could also reverse the increased propensity to ulceration in diabetic rats. Surprisingly, the decrease in the acid-pepsin output was found to be even better than glibenclamide. This property of *Eugenia jambolana* seems to be due to its anti-diabetic and gastric anti-secretory effects (Chaturvedi *et al.*, 2009 b).

Bitter Gourd (*Momordica charantia*)

Momordica charantia (Cucurbitaceae) is a multipurpose herb cultivated in different parts of the world for its edible fruits. Fruits of *M. charantia* have been frequently used in folk medicine for rapid healing of cutaneous lesions and peptic ulcer, especially in Western Anatolia in Turkey. The olive oil extract as well as dried-powdered fruits of bitter gourd showed significant activity against HCl-EtOH induced ulcerogenesis in indomethacin-pretreated rats and diethyldithiocarbamate-induced ulcer models revealing its anti-ulcerogenic effect (Gürbüz *et al.*, 2000) with the effects of oily extract (10ml/kg) being similar to famotidine (Ozbaki° and Gürsan, 2005). Similarly, the healing of acetic acid induced gastric ulcer was increased by both doses 100 and 500 mg/kg of the extract. In pylorus-ligated rats, the extract showed significant decrease in ulcer index, total acidity, free acidity and pepsin content and an increase in gastric mucosal content. The extract also reduced the ulcer index in stress induced, ethanol induced and indomethacin induced gastric ulcers and cysteamine induced duodenal ulcer (Alam *et al.*, 2009).

Cluster Beans (*Cyamopsis tetragonoloba*)

Tender cluster beans (15 per cent freeze-dried powder fed to Wistar rats for 8 weeks) significantly enhanced the activities of anti-oxidant enzymes (superoxide dismutase, catalase, glutathione reductase, glutathione-S-transferase, and GPX) and the concentrations of anti-oxidant molecules in both gastric and intestinal mucosa indicating a significant gastro-protective effect. There was a much greater effect when combined with capsaicin (0.01 per cent) in terms of increased antioxidant status (Pande and Srinivasan, 2013).

Pumpkin (*Cucurbita pepo*)

The pretreatment of aspirin treated albino rats with *C. pepo* fruit pulp extract for 14 consecutive days resulted in an increase in alkaline phosphatase activity and mucosal thickness along with decrease in ulcer index. Thus, it is evident that pumpkin possesses gastro-duodenal protective and anti-ulcerogenic properties (Sarkar and Buha, 2008).

Amla (*Emblica officinalis/Phyllanthus emblica*)

Sairam *et al.* (2002) observed the ulcer protective potential of methanolic extract of *Emblica officinalis* in different acute gastric ulcer models induced by aspirin, ethanol, cold restraint stress and pyloric ligation. 10-50 mg/kg of the extract administered orally, twice daily for 5 days showed dose-dependent ulcer protective effects in all the above acute ulcer models. A dose of 20 mg/kg showed 59 per cent healing after 5 days and 65.5 per cent after 10 days of treatment with methanolic extract of amla in chronic gastric ulcers induced by acetic acid in rats. The authors observed that the same might be due to its effects both on offensive as well as defensive mucosal factors. Amla can be used as a gastro-protective agent in non steroidal anti-inflammatory drug (NSAID)-induced gastropathy as the healing effect was observed at 60mg/kg body weight (Chatterjee *et al.*, 2011). The effect was dose-dependent through the harmonization of the anti-oxidative property and modulation of anti-inflammatory cytokine level.

Papaya (*Carica Papaya/Carica candamarcensis*)

Latex from Caricaceae contains proteolytic enzymes localized in the fruit, which are used ethnopharmacologically to treat digestive disorders. Some of these proteins display proliferative properties when probed with mammalian cells, suggesting a role in the reconstruction of wounded tissue (Mello *et al.*, 2008). In experimental rodent models proteolytic fraction derived from *Carica candamarcensis* (P1G10) between 0.1 and 10 mg/kg protected indomethacin but not ethanol-induced gastric ulcers. The maximal protection attained was 67 per cent with 10 mg/kg of P1G10. The healing rate by 10 mg/kg of P1G10 using the acetic acid ulcerogenic model was similar to that of omeprazole (10 mg/kg) or ranitidine (100 mg/kg) probably mediated by an increase in the mucus content by 25 per cent and stimulation of angiogenesis by 64 per cent in a manner similar to growth factors.

Carica papaya extract significantly reduced the ulcer index, lipid peroxide levels and alkaline phosphatase activity in the rats. It also maintained the activity of the antioxidant enzyme, catalase in the gastric mucosa, to near normalcy when compared with water controls (Ologundudu *et al.*, 2008).

Mango (*Mangifera indica*)

Mangifera indica is a species of mango in the Anacardiaceae family. It is found in Indian forests and cultivated varieties have been introduced to other warm regions of the world. Mangiferin, a naturally occurring glucosylxanthone from *Mangifera indica*, (3, 10 and 30 mg/kg, P. O.) significantly attenuated the gastric damage induced by ethanol by 30, 35, and 63 per cent, and of indomethacin by 22, 23 and 57 per cent, respectively. When mangiferin (30 mg/kg) was applied intra-duodenally to 4-h pylorus-ligated rats, significant decrease in gastric secretary volume and total acidity was observed. In addition, mangiferin effectively prevented the ethanol-associated depletion of gastric mucosal non-protein sulfhydryl content in mice, suggesting an anti-oxidant action (Carvalho *et al.*, 2007).

Aloe vera

Tannins, one of the constituents of *Aloe vera* extract, form a pellicle over the lining of gastric mucosa to resist the attack of proteolytic enzymes (John and Onabanjo, 1990), and this might have helped in the restoration of glycoprotein moiety of gastric mucosa in *Aloe vera* treated ulcer rats. Flavonoids present in *Aloe vera* gel (Davis *et al.*, 1989) might play a role in stabilizing the antioxidant status of the gastric mucosa, which may have maintained its glycoprotein moiety. Thus, *Aloe vera* gel may have ameliorated glycoprotein abnormalities through its action on pepsin-mediated proteolysis.

Subramanian *et al.* (2007) observed that the treatment with *Aloe vera* gel extract antagonizes the aggressive factors, which play a crucial role in the pathogenesis of gastric lesions and augment defensive factors to protect the gastric mucosa from ulceration. The increase in the levels of glycoproteins, particularly sialic acid and hexosamine in the extract treated groups indicate the increase in the production of mucus, thereby possibly protecting the gastric mucosa in both ulcer models. The efficacy of the extract was more or less same in both the models and showed promising antiulcer activity more than that of ranitidine. Thus they established the gastro-protective nature of *Aloe vera* gel extract. The histological studies further established the ulcer curative properties of *Aloe vera* leaf gel extract.

Park *et al.* (2011) reported that mice treated with the polymer fraction of *Aloe vera* (150mg/Kg body weight) had significantly fewer gastric lesions than the controls as judged by matrix metalloproteinase (mRNA expression). They found the mRNA expressions of inducible nitric oxide synthase and neuronal nitric oxide synthase were each reduced by ~50 per cent in *Aloe vera* treated mice as against the controls thus protecting the gastric mucosa.

Russian Olive/Wild Olive (*Elaeagnus angustifolia* Fruits)

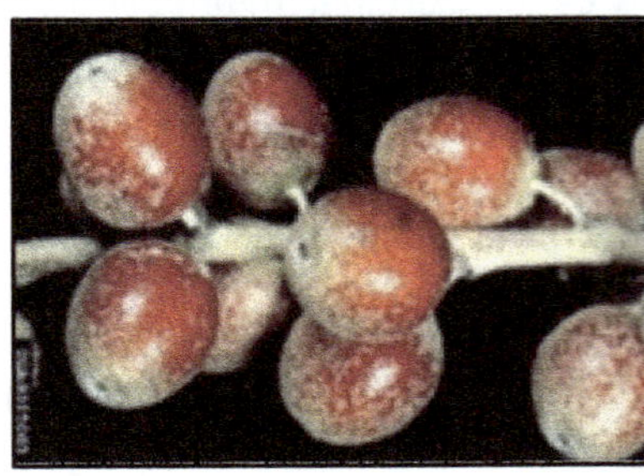

Extracts of the fruits of *Elaeagnus angustifolia* L. (Elaeagnaceae), fresh fruits of *Hibiscus esculentus* (Malvaceae), fresh roots of *Papaver rhoeas* L. (Papaveraceae), leaves of *Phlomis grandiflora* H.S. Thomson (Lamiaceae) and fresh fruits of *Rosa canina* L. (Rosaceae) exhibited statistically significant gastro-protective effect. Histopathological studies confirmed the results of the *in vivo* test (Gürbüz *et al.*, 2003).

Chicory (*Cichorium intybus*)

The decoction of chicory root showed significant protection against ulcerogenesis in the stomach of ethanol-induced gastric ulcer in rats. The anti- ulcerogencic protential was also confirmed using histo-pathological techniques (Gürbüz *et al.*, 2002).

Winter Melon/Ash Gourd (*Benincasa hispida*)

Benincasa hispida is recommended in Ayurveda for the management of peptic ulcers. Grover *et al.* (2001) reported that the oral feeding of different doses of the extract significantly reduced the ulcer index produced by various ulcerogens. The anti-ulcerogenic effect was dose-dependent in stress induced model of ulcer and not in other models. *B. hispida* probably has a CNS component in prevention of stress induced ulceration. However, antihistaminic, anti-cholinergic effects and prevention of disturbance in gastric micro-circulation as possible modes of action cannot be ruled out. Chronic toxicity studies carried out for 3 months revealed no deleterious effect of fresh juice of *B. hispida* on various hematological and biochemical parameters studied. Thus, extracts of *B. hispida* may be considered to be a drug of natural origin possessing anti-ulcer activity.

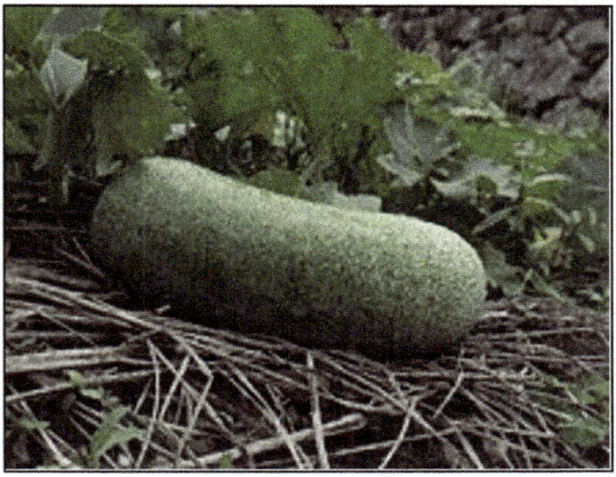

Winter Melon, also Called White Gourd, Winter Gourd, or Ash Gourd

Figs (*Ficus glomerata* Roxb)

Traditionally figs (*Ficus glomerata* Roxb, syn. *Ficus racemosa*) are used to treat anemia and gastro-intestinal disorders. Rao *et al.* (2008) reported that ethanolic extract of *F. glomerata* fruit (FGE) (50, 100 and 200 mg/kg body weight) twice daily for 5 days resulted in dose dependent inhibition of ulcer index in pylorus ligation, ethanol and cold restraint stress-induced ulcers in rats. FGE prevented the oxidative damage of gastric mucosa by blocking lipid peroxidation and by significant decrease in superoxide dismutase, H^+K^+ATPase and increase in catalase activity. Rao *et al.* (2008) opined that the gastro-protective activity might be due to gastric defence factors. The main constituents responsible for this activity might be phenolics. *Ficus asperifolia* extract also significantly increased gastric pH (Raji *et al.*, 2011).

Bael Fruit (*Aegle marmelos*)

Several anti-oxidant vitamins such as Vitamin A, Vitamin C, and Vitamin E have been isolated from Bael fruit (Ladaniya, 2008). In aspirin induced gastro-duodenal ulceration in albino rat, pretreatment with Bael fruit pulp extract for 14 consecutive days showed the reverse effects of aspirin suggesting its gastro-duodenal protective and anti- ulcerogenic properties through its anti-oxidant mechanism (Das and Roy, 2012).

Other Anti-Ulcerogenic Foods

Drumstick (*Moringa pterygosperma*)

Drumstick flower buds have shown some decrease in the ulcer index. (Akhtar and Ahmad, 1995).

Bay Laurel (*Laurus nobilis*)

The Methanol extract of the fruits of *Laurus nobilis* showed significant stomach protection against ulcerogenesis confirming the Turkish Folkloric Remedies accumulated in the Data Bank (Gürbüz *et al.*, 2002).

Guarana (*Paullinia cupana* Mart)

Guarana fruit is about the size of a coffee bean and due to the high caffeine concentration the seeds are used as a stimulant. Animals pretreated with Guarana (50 and 100 mg/kg p.o.) showed a significant reduction in the severity of gastric lesions induced by absolute ethanol the effect being similar to caffeine (20 and 30 mg/kg p.o.). While higher dose of guarana offered significant protection against gastric ulceration induced by indomethacin, caffeine was ineffective at the doses tested (Campos *et al.*, 2003).

Conclusions

It is encourageing to find that the Data Bank of Turkish Folk Remedies (TUHIB) has accumulated the data on herbal remedies. It is advisable to all the countries also to prepare a data bank of traditional remedies for various illnesses. Most of the research trials conducted so far have been on animal models and that too mostly on herbals from different countries. Hence there is a wide scope for future research on some of the foods *e.g.* drumstick leaves, cloves etc for their anti-ulcerogenic benefits. Moreover, there is also a simultaneous need for establishing clinical evidence in human patients and to suggest safe dosages.

References

Agbaje EO (2008). Gastrointestinal effects of *Syzigium aromaticum* (L.) Merr. and Perry (Myrtaceae) in animal models. Nig. Q. J. Hosp. Med. 18 (3): 137 - 41.

Agrawal AK, Rao CV, Sairam K, Joshi VK, Goel RK (2000). Effect of *Piper longum*, *Zingiber officianalis* and *Ferula* species on gastric ulceration and secretion in rats. Indian J. Exp. Biol. 38 (10): 994 - 98.

Agarwal PK, Singh A, Gaurav K, Goel S, Khanna HD, Goel RK (2009). Evaluation of wound healing activity of extracts of plantain banana (*Musa sapientum* var. *paradisiaca*) in rats. Indian J. Exp. Biol. 47 (1): 32 - 40.

Akhtar AH, Ahmad KU (1995). Anti-ulcerogenic evaluation of the methanolic extracts of some indigenous medicinal plants of Pakistan in aspirin-ulcerated rats. J. Ethnopharmacol. 46 (1): 1 - 6.

Alam S, Asad M, Asdaq SM, Prasad VS (2009). Anti-ulcer activity of methanolic extract of *Momordica charantia* in rats. J. Ethnopharmacol. 123 (3): 464 - 69.

Al-Harbi MM, Islam MW, al-Shabanah OA, al-Gharably NM (1995). Effect of acute administration of fish oil (omega-3 marine triglyceride) on gastric ulceration and secretion induced by various ulcerogenic and necrotizing agents in rats. Food Chem. Toxicol. 33 (7): 553 - 58.

Al-Howiriny T, Alsheikh A, Alqasoumi S, Al-Yahya M, ElTahir K, Rafatullah S (2010). Gastric anti-ulcer, anti-secretory and cyto-protective properties of celery (*Apium graveolens*) in rats. Pharm. Biol. 48 (7): 786 - 93.

Al-Howiriny T, Al-Sohaibani M, El-Tahir K, Rafatullah SAl-Howiriny T, Al-Sohaibani M, El-Tahir K, Rafatullah S (2003). Prevention of experimentally-induced gastric ulcers in rats by an ethanolic extract of Parsley *Petroselinum crispum*. Am. J. Chin. Med. 31 (5): 699 - 711.

Al Mofleh IA, Alhaider AA, Mossa JS, Al-Soohaibani MO, Rafatullah S (2007). Aqueous suspension of anise "*Pimpinella anisum*" protects rats against chemically induced gastric ulcers. World J. Gastroenterol. 13 (7): 1112 - 18.

Al Mofleh IA, Alhaider AA, Mossa JS, Al-Sohaibani MO, Al-Yahya MA, Rafatullah S, Shaik SA.(2008). Gastro-protective effect of an aqueous suspension of black cumin *Nigella sativa* on necrotizing agents-induced gastric injury in experimental animals. Saudi. J. Gastroenterol. 14 (3): 128 - 34.

Anosike CA, Obidoa O, Lawrence U, Ezeanyika S, Nwuba MM (2009). Anti-inflammatory and anti-ulcerogenic activity of the ethanol extract of ginger (*Zingiber officinale*). African Journal of Biochemistry Research. 3 (12): 379 - 84,

Balint GA (1998). A possible molecular basis for the effect of gastric anti-ulcerogenic drugs. Trends Pharmacol Sci. 19 (10): 401 - 403.

Bandyopadhyay D, Biswas K, Bhattacharyya M, Reiter RJ, Banerjee RK (2002a). Involvement of reactive oxygen species in gastric ulceration, protection by melatonin. Indian J. Exp. Biol. 40: 693 - 705.

Bandyopadhyay U, Biswas K, Chatterjee R, Bandyopadhyay D, Chattopadhyay I, Ganguly CK, Chakraborty T, Bhattacharya K, Banerjee RK (2002b). Gastro-protective effect of Neem (*Azadirachta indica*) bark extract: possible involvement of H(+)-K(+)-ATPase inhibition and scavenging of hydroxyl radical. Life Sci. 71 (24): 2845 - 65.

Bandyopadhyay U, Biswas K, Sengupta A, Moitra P, Dutta P, Sarkar D, Debnath P, Ganguly CK, Banerjee RK (2004). Clinical studies on the effect of Neem (*Azadirachta indica*) bark extract on gastric secretion and gastroduodenal ulcer. Life Sci. 75 (24): 2867 - 78.

Bhattacharjee M, Bhattacharjee S, Gupta A, Banerjee RK (2002). Critical role of an endogenous gastric peroxidase in controlling oxidative damage in *H. pylori*-mediated and non-mediated gastric ulcer. Free Radical Biol. Med. 3: 731 - 43.

Bhattacharya A, Ghosal S, Bhattacharya SK (2006). Effect of fish oil on offensive and defensive factors in gastric ulceration in rats. Prostaglandins Leukot. Essent. Fatty Acids. 74 (2): 109 - 116.

Best R, Lewis DA, Nasser N (1984). The anti-ulcerogenic activity of the unripe plantain banana (*Musa* species). Br. J. Pharmacol. 82 (1): 107 - 116.

Bukhari MH, Khalil J, Qamar S, Qamar Z, Zahid M, Ansari N, Bakhshi IM (2011). Comparative gastro-protective effects of natural honey, *Nigella sativa* and cimetidine against acetylsalicylic acid induced gastric ulcer in albino rats. J. Coll. Physicians Surg. Pak. 21 (3): 151 - 56.

Campos AR, Barros AI, Santos FA, Rao VS (2003). Guarana (*Paullinia cupana* Mart.) offers protection against gastric lesions induced by ethanol and indomethacin in rats. Phytother Res. 17 (10): 1199 - 202.

Carvalho AC, Guedes MM, de Souza AL, Trevisan MT, Lima AF, Santos FA, Rao VS (2007). Gastroprotective effect of mangiferin, a xanthonoid from *Mangifera indica*, against gastric injury induced by ethanol and indomethacin in rodents. Planta. Med. 73 (13): 1372 - 76.

Carvalho CA, Fernandes KM, Matta SL, Silva MB, Oliveira LL, Fonseca CC (2011). Evaluation of antiulcerogenic activity of aqueous extract of *Brassica oleracea* var. capitata (cabbage) on Wistar rat gastric ulceration. Arq. Gastroenterol. 48 (4): 276 - 82.

Castro GA, Carvalho JE, Tinti SV, Possenti A, Sgarbieri VC (2010). Anti-ulcerogenic effect of a whey protein isolate and collagen hydrolysates against ethanol ulcerative lesions on oral administration to rats. J. Med. Food. 13 (1): 83 - 90.

Chatterjee A, Chattopadhyay S, Bandyopadhyay SK (2011). Biphasic Effect of *Phyllanthus emblica* L. Extract on NSAID-Induced Ulcer: An Antioxidative Trail Weaved with Immuno-modulatory Effect. Evid. Based Complement. Alternat. Med. 2011: 146808.

Chaturvedi A, Bhawani G, Agarwal PK, Goel S, Singh A, Goel RK (2009 a). Ulcer healing properties of ethanolic extract of *Eugenia jambolana* seed in diabetic rats: study on gastric mucosal defensive factors. Indian J. Physiol. Pharmacol. 53 (1): 16 - 24.

Chaturvedi A, Bhawani G, Agarwal PK, Goel S, Singh A, Goel RK (2009 b). Antidiabetic and antiulcer effects of extract of *Eugenia jambolana* seed in mild diabetic rats: study on gastric mucosal offensive acid-pepsin secretion. Indian J. Physiol. Pharmacol. 53 (2): 137 - 46.

Chaturvedi A, Kumar MM, Bhawani G, Chaturvedi H, Kumar M, Goel RK (2007). Effect of ethanolic extract of *Eugenia jambolana* seeds on gastric ulceration and secretion in rats. Indian J. Physiol. Pharmacol. 51 (2): 131 -40.

Das SK, Roy C (2012). The protective role of *Aegle marmelos* on aspirin-induced gastro-duodenal ulceration in albino rat model: a possible involvement of antioxidants. Saudi. J. Gastroenterol. 18 (3): 188 - 94.

Davis, R.H., M.G. Leitner, J.M. Russo and M.E. Byrne, 1989. Anti-inflammatory activity of *Aloe vera* against a spectrum of irritants. J. Am. Ped. Med. Assoc. 79: 263 - 76.

de Jesus NZ, de Souza Falcao H, Gomes IF, de Almeida Leite TJ, de Morais Lima GR, Barbosa-Filho JM, Tavares JF, da Silva MS, de Athayde-Filho PF, Batista LM (2012). Tannins, peptic ulcers and related mechanisms. Int.J. Mol. Sci. 13 (3): 3203 - 28.

Dharmani P, Kuchibhotla VK, Maurya R, Srivastava S, Sharma S, Palit G (2004). Evaluation of anti-ulcerogenic and ulcer-healing properties of *Ocimum sanctum.* J. Ethnopharmacol. 93 (2-3): 197 - 206.

Dorababu M, Joshi MC, Bhawani G, Kumar MM, Chaturvedi A, Goel RK (2006). Effect of aqueous extract of neem (*Azadirachta indica)* leaves on offensive and diffensive gastric mucosal factors in rats. Indian J. Physiol. Pharmacol. 50 (3): 241 - 49.

Dunijic BS, Svensson J, Axelson J, Adler Creutz P, Bengmark S (1993). Green banana protection of gastric mucosa against experimentally induced injuries in rats a multi component mechanism. Scand. J. Gastroenterol. 28: 894 - 98.

El-Abhar HS, Abdallah DM, Saleh S (2003). Gastro-protective activity of *Nigella sativa* oil and its constituent, thymoquinone, against gastric mucosal injury induced by ischaemia/reperfusion in rats. J. Ethnopharmacol. 84 (2–3): 251 - 58.

Elliott RC, Heward GJ (1976). The influence of banana supplemented diet on gastric ulcers in mice. *Pharmacol. Res. Commun.* **8** (2): 167 - 71.

Eswaran MB, Surendran S, Vijayakumar M, Ojha SK, Rawat AK, Rao ChV (2010). Gastroprotective activity of *Cinnamomum tamala* leaves on experimental gastric ulcers in rats. J. Ethnopharmacol. 128 (2): 537 - 40.

Ezaki N, Kato M, Takizawa N, Morimoto S, Nonaka G, Nishioka I (1985). Pharmacological studies on *Linderae umbellatae* Ramus, IV. Effects of condensed tannin related compound on peptic activity and stress-induced gastric lesions in mice. Planta Med. 51 (1): 34 - 38.

Goel RK, Gupta S, Shankar R, Sanyal AKGoel RK, Gupta S, Shankar R, Sanyal AK (1986). Anti-ulcerogenic effect of banana powder (*Musa sapientum* var. paradisiaca) and its effect on mucosal resistance. J. Ethnopharmacol. 18 (1): 33 - 44.

Goel RK, Sairam K, Dorababu M, Prabha T, Rao ChV (2005). Effect of standardized extract of *Ocimum sanctum* Linn. on gastric mucosal offensive and defensive factors. Indian J. Exp. Biol. 43 (8): 715 - 21.

Goel RK, Sairam K, Rao CV (2001). Role of gastric antioxidant and anti-Helicobactor pylori activities in anti-ulcerogenic activity of plantain banana (*Musa sapientum* var. paradisiaca). Indian J. Exp. Biol. 39 (7): 719 - 22.

Grover JK, Adiga G, Vats V, Rathi SS (2001). Extracts of *Benincasa hispida* prevent development of experimental ulcers. J. Ethnopharmacol. 78 (2-3): 159 - 64.

Gürbüz I, Akyüz C, Ye°ilada E, Sener B (2000). Anti-ulcerogenic effect of *Momordica charantia* L. fruits on various ulcer models in rats. J. Ethnopharmacol. 71 (1-2): 77 - 82.

Gürbüz I, Ustün O, Yesilada E, Sezik E, Kutsal O (2003). Anti-ulcerogenic activity of some plants used as folk remedy in Turkey. J. Ethnopharmacol. 88 (1): 93 - 97.

Gürbüz I, Ustün O, Ye°ilada E, Sezik E, Akyürek N (2002). *In vivo* gastro-protective effects of five Turkish folk remedies against ethanol-induced lesions. J. Ethnopharmacol. 83 (3): 241 - 44.

Güzel C, Ulak G, Sermet A, Ciçek R, Ulak M (1995). Effect of fish oil on indometacin-induced gastric lesions in rats. Arzneimittelforschung. 45 (11): 1172 - 73.

Hamaishi K, Kojima R, Ito MHamaishi K, Kojima R, Ito M (2006). Anti-ulcer effect of tea catechin in rats. Biol. Pharm. Bull. 29 (11): 2206 - 213.

Hanszen A (1934). The bactericidal power of the stomach and some factors which influence it. Am. J. Dig. Dis. 1: 725 - 28.

Jainu M, Devi CS (2006). Antiulcerogenic and ulcer healing effects of *Solanum nigrum* (L.) on experimental ulcer models: possible mechanism for the inhibition of acid formation. J. Ethnopharmacol. 104 (1-2): 156 - 63.

John TA, Onabanjo AO (1990). Gastro-protective effects of an aqueous extract of *Entandrophragma utile* bark in experimental ethanol-induced peptic ulceration in mice and rats. J. Ethnopharmacol., 29: 87 - 93.

Khaled AAS (2009). Gastroprotective effects of *Nigella sativa* oil on the formation of stress gastritis in hypothyroidal rats. Int. J. Physiol. Pathophysiol. Pharmacol. 1: 143 - 49.

Kanter M, Demir H, Karakaya C, Ozbek H (2005). Gastroprotective activity of *Nigella sativa* L oil and its constituent, thymoquinone against acute alcohol-induced gastric mucosal injury in rats. World J. Gastroenterol. 11 (42): 6662 - 66.

Kath RK, Gupta RK (2006). Antioxidant activity of hydroalcoholic leaf extract of *Ocimum sanctum* in animal models of peptic ulcer. Indian J. Physiol. Pharmacol. 50 (4): 391 - 96.

Ladaniya MS (2008). Citrus fruit biology technology and - evaluation. Academic Press. Waltham, Massachusetts. pp. 1- 558.

Lemos M, Santin JR, Júnior LC, Niero R, Andrade SF (2011). Gastroprotective activity of hydroalcoholic extract obtained from the leaves of *Brassica oleracea* var. acephala DC in different animal models. J. Ethnopharmacol. 138 (2): 503 - 507.

Lewis DA, Fields WN, Shaw GP (1999). A natural flavonoid present in unripe plantain banana pulp (*Musa sapientum* L. var. paradisiaca) protects the gastric mucosa from aspirin-induced erosions. J Ethnopharmacol. 65 (3): 283 - 88.

Lewis DA, Shaw GP (2001). A natural flavonoid and synthetic analogues protect the gastric mucosa from aspirin-induced erosions. J. Nutr. Biochem. 12 (2): 95 - 100.

Magdy MA, Hanan el-A, Nabila el-M (2012). Thymoquinone: Novel gastro-protective mechanisms. Eur. J. Pharmacol. 697 (1–3): 126 - 31.

Maity P, Biswas K, Chattopadhyay I, Banerjee RK, Bandyopadhyay U (2009). The use of neem for controlling gastric hyperacidity and ulcer. Phytother. Res. 23 (6): 747 - 55.

Maity S, Vedasiromoni JR, Chaudhuri L, Ganguly DK (2001). Role of reduced glutathione and nitric oxide in the black tea extract-mediated protection against ulcerogen-induced changes in motility and gastric emptying in rats. Jpn. J. Pharmacol. 85 (4): 358 - 64.

Maity S, Vedasiromoni JR, Ganguly DK (1995). Anti-ulcer effect of the hot water extract of black tea (*Camellia sinensis*). J. Ethnopharmacol. 46 (3): 167 - 74.

Maity S, Vedasiromoni JR, Ganguly DK (1998). Role of glutathione in the antiulcer effect of hot water extract of black tea (*Camellia sinensis*). Jpn. J. Pharmacol. 78 (3): 285 - 92.

Mani V, Ramasamy K, Abdul Majeed AB (2013). Anti-inflammatory, analgesic and anti-ulcerogenic effect of total alkaloidal extract from *Murraya koenigii* leaves in animal models. Food Funct. 2013 Jan 29. [Epub ahead of print].

Manjari V, Das UN (1998). Oxidant stress, anti-oxidants, nitric oxide and essential fatty acids in peptic ulcer disease. Prostaglandins Leukot. Essent. Fatty Acids. 59 (6): 401 - 406.

Manjari V, Das UN (2000). Effect of polyunsaturated fatty acids on dexamethasone-induced gastric mucosal damage. Prostaglandins Leukot. Essent. Fatty Acids. 62 (2): 85 - 96.

Matsumoto H, Shimokawa Y, Ushida Y, Toida T, Hayasawa H (2001). New biological function of bovine alpha-lactalbumin: protective effect against ethanol- and stress-induced gastric mucosal injury in rats. Biosci. Biotechnol. Biochem. 65 (5): 1104 - 111.

Mello VJ, Gomes MT, Lemos FO, Delfino JL, Andrade SP, Lopes MT, Salas CE (2008). The gastric ulcer protective and healing role of cysteine proteinases from *Carica candamarcensis*. Phytomedicine. 15 (4): 237 - 44.

Minaiyan M, Ghannadi A, Karimzadeh A (2006). Anti-ulcerogeic effect of ginger (rhizome of *Zingiber officinale* Roscoe) on cystemine-induced duodenal ulcer in rats. DARU 14 (2): 97 – 101.

Mohan Kumar M, Joshi MC, Prabha T, Dorababu M, Goel RK (2006). Effect of plantain banana on gastric ulceration in NIDDM rats: role of gastric mucosal glycoproteins, cell proliferation, anti-oxidants and free radicals. Indian J. Exp. Biol. 44 (4): 292 - 99.

Mukhopadhyaya K, Bhattacharya D, Chakraborty A, Goel RK, Sanyal AK (1987). Effect of banana powder (*Musa sapientum* var. paradisiaca) on gastric mucosal shedding. J. Ethnopharmacol. 21 (1): 11 - 19.

Nguelefack TB, Feumebo CB, Ateufack G, Watcho P, Tatsimo S, Atsamo AD, Tane P, Kamanyi A (2008). Anti-ulcerogenic properties of the aqueous and methanol extracts from the leaves of *Solanum torvum* Swartz (Solanaceae) in rats. J. Ethnopharmacol. 119 (1): 135 - 40.

Ozbaki° Dengiz G, Gürsan N (2005). Effects of *Momordica charantia* L. (Cucurbitaceae) on indomethacin-induced ulcer model in rats. Turk. J. Gastroenterol. 16 (2): 85 - 88.

Ologundudu A,. Lawal AO, Ololade IA, Omonkhua AA, Obi FO (2008). The Anti-ulcerogenic Activity of Aqueous Extract of *Carica Papaya* Fruit on Aspirin – Induced Ulcer In Rats. The Internet Journal of Toxicology. 5 (2): DOI: 10.5580/481.

Pande S, Srinivasan K (2013). Protective effect of dietary tender cluster beans (*Cyamopsis tetragonoloba)* in the gastrointestinal tract of experimental rats. Appl. Physiol. Nutr. Metab. 38 (2): 169 - 76.

Park CH, Nam DY, Son HU, Lee SR, Lee HJ, Heo JC, Cha TY, Baek JH, Lee SH (2011). Polymer fraction of Aloe vera exhibits a protective activity on ethanol-induced gastric lesions. Int. J. Mol. Med. 27 (4): 511 - 18.

Prabha P, Karpagam TB, Varalakshmi A, Packiavathy SC (2011). Indigenous anti-ulcer activity of *Musa sapientum* on peptic ulcer. Pharmacognosy. Res. 3 (4): 232 - 38.

Prakash UN, Srinivasan K (2010). Gastrointestinal protective effect of dietary spices during ethanol-induced oxidant stress in experimental rats. Appl. Physiol. Nutr. Metab. 35 (2): 134 - 41.

Rajeswari M, Subbulakshmi G (2003). Effect of *Solanum nigrum* on gastritis and gastric ulcers. Proc. of the Nutrition Society of India. Hyderabad. India.

Raji Y, Ogunwande IA, Osadebe CA, John G (2004). Effects of *Azadirachta indica* extract on gastric ulceration and acid secretion in rats. J. Ethnopharmacol. 90 (1): 167 - 70.

Raji Y, Oyeyemi WA, Shittu ST, Bolarinwa AF (2011). Gastro-protective effect of methanol extract of *Ficus asperifolia* bark on indomethacin-induced gastric ulcer in rats. Niger. J. Physiol. Sci. 26 (1): 43 - 48.

Ramirez RO, Roa CC Jr (2003). The gastro-protective effect of tannins extracted from duhat (*Syzygium cumini* Skeels) bark on HCl/ethanol induced gastric mucosal injury in Sprague-Dawley rats. Clin. Hemorheol. Microcirc. 29 (3-4): 253 - 61.

Rao CH, Ojha SK, Radhakrishnan K, Govindarajan R, Rastogi S, Mehrotra S, *et al.* (2004). Antiulcer activity of *Utleria salicifolia* rhizome extract. J. Ethnopharmacol. 91: 243 - 49.

Rao CH, Verma AR, Vijayakumar M, Rastogi S (2008). Gastroprotective effect of standardized extract of *Ficus glomerata* fruit on experimental gastric ulcers in rats. J. Ethnopharmacol. 115 (2): 323 - 26.

Rosaneli CF, Bighetti AE, Antônio MA, Carvalho JE, Sgarbieri VC (2004). Protective effect of bovine milk whey protein concentrate on the ulcerative lesions caused by subcutaneous administration of indomethacin. J. Med. Food.7 (3): 309 - 314.

Rosaneli CF, Bighetti AE, Antônio MA, Carvalho JE, Sgarbieri VC (2002). Efficacy of a whey protein concentrate on the inhibition of stomach ulcerative lesions caused by ethanol ingestion. J. Med. Food. 5 (4): 221 - 28.

Sairam K, Rao ChV, Babu MD, Kumar KV, Agrawal VK, K Goel RK (2002). Anti-ulcerogenic effect of methanolic extract of *Emblica officinalis*: an experimental study. J. Ethnopharmacol. 82 (1): 1 - 9.

Sanyal RK, Das PK, Sinha S, Sinha YK (1961). Banana and gastric secretion. *J. Pharm. Pharmacol.* **13**: 318 - 19.

Sarkar S, Buha D (2008). Effect of ripe fruit pulp extract of *Cucurbita pepo* Linn. in aspirin induced gastric and duodenal ulcer in rats. Indian J. Exp. Biol. 46 (9): 639 - 45.

Sharmanov TSh, Kadyrova RKh, Salkhanov BA (1981). [Effectiveness of peptic ulcer diet therapy using rations containing whole mare's and camel's milk]. Vopr. Pitan. (3): 10 - 14. [Article in Russian].

Subramanian S, Sathish Kumar D, Arulselvan P, Senthilkumar GP, Mahadeva Rao US (2007). Evaluation of Anti-ulcerogenic Potential of *Aloe vera* Leaf Gel Extract Studied in Experimental Rats. Journal of Pharmacology and Toxicology, 2: 85 - 97.

Tan PV, Nyasse B, Dimo T, Mezui C (2002). Gastric cytoprotective anti-ulcer effects of the leaf methanol extract of *Ocimum suave* (Lamiaceae) in rats. J. Ethnopharmacol. 82 (2-3): 69 - 74.

Tankam JM, Sawada Y, Ito M (2013). Regular ingestion of *Cinnamomi cortex* pulveratus offers gastroprotectiveactivity in mice. J. Nat. Med. 67 (2): 289 - 95.

Tayman C, Cekmez F, Kafa IM, Canpolat FE, Cetinkaya M, Uysal S, Tunc T, Sarýcý SU (2012). Beneficial effects of *Nigella sativa* oil on intestinal damage in necrotizing enterocolitis. J. Invest. Surg. 25 (5): 286 - 94.

Theilla M, Schwartz B, Cohen J, Shapiro H, Anbar R, Singer P (2012a). Impact of a nutritional formula enriched in fish oil and micronutrients on pressure ulcers in critical care patients. Am. J. Crit. Care. 21 (4): e102 - 109.

Theilla M, Schwartz B, Zimra Y, Shapiro H, Anbar R, Rabizadeh E, Cohen J, Singer P (2012b). Enteral n-3 fatty acids and micronutrients enhance percentage of positive neutrophil and lymphocyte adhesion molecules: a potential mediator of pressure ulcer healing in critically ill patients. Br. J. Nutr. 107 (7): 1056 - 61.

Theilla M, Singer P, Cohen J, Dekeyser F (2007). A diet enriched in eicosapentanoic acid, gamma-linolenic acid and antioxidants in the prevention of new pressure ulcer formation in critically ill patients with acute lung injury: A randomized, prospective, controlled study. Clin. Nutr. 26 (6): 752 - 57.

Wu H, Ye D, Bai Y, Zhao Y (1990).Effect of dry ginger and roasted ginger on experimental gastric ulcers in rats]. Zhongguo. Zhong. Yao. Za. Zhi. 15 (5): 278 - 80, 317 - 18. [Article in Chinese].

Yamahara J, Hatayekama S, Taniguchi K, Kawamura M, Yoshikawa M (1992). Stomachic principles in ginger. II. Pungent and anti-ulcer effects of low polar constituents isolated from ginger, the dried rhizoma of *Zinger officinale* Roscoe cultivated in Taiwan. The absolute stereostructure of a new diaryheptanoid. Yakugaku. Zasshi. 112 (9): 645 - 55

Yamahara J, Mochizuki M, Rong HQ, Matsuda H, Fujimura H (1988). The anti-ulcer effect in rats of ginger constituents. J. Ethnopharmacol. 23 (2-3): 299 - 304.

Yoshikawa M, Hatakeyama S, Taniguchi K, Matuda H, Yamahara J (1992). 6-gingesulfonic acid, a new anti-ulcer principle, and ginger glycolipids A, B, and

C, three new monoacyldigalactosylglycerols, from *Zingiberis rhizome* originating in Taiwan. Chem. Pharm. Bull. (Tokyo). 40 (8): 2239 - 41.

Yoshikawa M, Yamaguchi S, Kunimi K, Matsuda H, Okuno Y, Yamahara J, Murakami N (1994). Stomachic principles in ginger. III. An anti-ulcer principle, 6-gingesulfonic acid, and three monoacyldigalactosylglycerols, gingerglycolipids A, B, and C, from *Zingiberis rhizome* originating in Taiwan. Chem. Pharm. Bull. (Tokyo). 42 (6): 1226 - 30.

Glossary

ADPRTL1 - ADP-Ribosyltransferase (NAD+; Poly (ADP-Ribose) Polymerase)-Like-1 - It is an enzyme that catalyzes the reversible addition of multiple branched chains of ADP-ribose to target proteins.

Aphrodisiacs - A substance that increases sexual desire.

Apoptosis - Programmed cancer cell death.

Azadirachtin - A chemical compound belonging to the limonoid group, is a secondary metabolitepresent in neem seeds.

Bax/Bcl-2 - Apoptosis regulator BAX also known as bcl-2-like protein 4 is a protein that in humans is encoded by the BAX gene.

CCD–18Co - human normal fibroblast colon cells.

CD31(+) - cluster of differentiation 31 (CD31) is a protein that in human is encoded by the *PECAM1* gene found on chromosome 17, plays a key role in removing aged neutrophils from the body.

Cip1/p21 - p21/WAF1 - also known as cyclin-dependent kinase inhibitor 1 or CDK-interacting protein 1 is a protein that in humans is encoded by the *CDKN1A* gene located on chromosome 6. functions as a regulator of cell cycle progression at G_1 andS phase.

cMyc - is a regulator gene that codes for a transcription factor.

COX-1, 2 and 3 - Cycloxygenage isozymes- prostaglandin-endoperoxide synthase (PTGS), are enzymes responsible for formation of important biological mediators called prostanoids, including prostaglandins, prostacyclin and thromboxane.

CTX - Carboxy-terminal collagen crosslinks, a marker of bone resorption.

CVD - Cardio Vascular Diseases.

DHPN - Di-hydroxypropyl)nitrosamine (DHPN), a potent carcinogen targeting the lung, liver, thyroid, and kidney.

DMBA - -Dimethylbenz(a)anthracene is an immunosuppressor and a powerful organ-specific laboratory carcinogen.

DNA methylation - A biochemical process involving the addition of a methyl group to the cytosine or adenine DNA nucleotides.

dUTP - is an enzyme belongs to the family of hydrolases.

EGCG - epigallocatechin-3-gallate, an antioxidant.

Emmenagogic activity - Promotion of menstruation.

Febrifuge - A medication that reduces fever; an antipyretic.

FITC - Fluorescein isothiocyanate (FITC) is a derivative of fluorescein used in wide-ranging applications including flow cytometry.

Gonadotrophic activity - Stimulation of the growth and activity of the gonads.

HCT-15 - Human colorectal carcinoma *HCT-15* cells.

HIV - Human Immunodeficiency Virus.

Hras - A transforming protein p21 is an enzyme that in humans is encoded by the *HRAS* geneGTPase HRas is involved in regulating cell division in response to growth factor stimulation.

IGFBP-3 - Insulin-like growth factor-binding protein 3, also known as IGFBP3, is a protein that, in humans, is encoded by the *IGFBP3* gene. It circulates in the plasma, prolonging the half-life of IGFs and altering their interaction with cell surface receptors.

IL-2: Inter Leukin-2 - A type of cytokine signaling molecule in the immune system.

IMR-90 - human normal lung cells.

Ki67-LI) - Antigen KI-67 is a nuclear protein that is associated with and may be necessary for cellular proliferation.

LNCaP - LNCaP cells are a cell line of human cells commonly used in the field of oncology.

Matrigel - is the trade name for a gelatinous protein mixture secreted by Engelbreth-Holm-Swarm (EHS) mouse sarcoma cell.

MCF-7 - Michigan Cancer Foundation-7, is a breast cancer cell line isolated in 1970 from a 69-year-old Caucasian woman.

MDA-MB-231 - Breast Cancer cell line.

NF-kappa B - is a protein complex that controls the transcription of DNA.

NF-κB - Transcription factor nuclear factor-κB (NF-κB).

NIK/IKK signaling - NF-kB-inducing kinase (NIK).

NNK - Nicotine-derived nitrosamine ketone (NNK), or 4-(methylnitrosamino)-1-(3-pyridyl)-1-butanone, is a nitrosamine present in tobacco that is a potent procarcinogen.

Nootropic agents - Memory/Neuro enhancers.

Nrf2 - Nuclear factor (erythroid-derived 2)-like 2, also known as NFE2L2 or Nrf2, is a transcription factor that in humans is encoded by the *NFE2L2* gene.

PAH - Polycyclic Aromatic Hydrocarbons - carcinogenic chemicals created by the burning of carbon based fuels including cigarette smoke.

PBMC - A peripheral blood mononuclear cell (PBMC) is any blood cell having a round nucleus. *e.g.*-Lymphocyte.

PC-3 - PC3 (PC-3) human prostate cancer cell lines.

PCA - Plate Count Agar.

Pro-Simbioflor - A preparation that contains the natural intestinal bacteria *Enterococcus faecalis* and *Escherichia coli*, in inactive form.

RhoA - Ras homolog gene family, member A (RhoA) is a small GTPase protein known to regulate the actin cytoskeleton in the formation of stress fibers. In humans, it is encoded by the gene *RHOA*.

RhoC - (Ras homolog gene family, member C) is a small (~21 kDa) signaling G protein (more specifically a GTPase), and is a member of the Rac subfamily of the family Rho family of GTPases.

RNA - Ribo Nucleic Acid.

ROS - Reactive Oxygen Species.

SKMEL-2 - Human Melanoma Cell Line.

SK-OV-3: ovarian carcinoma-derived cell-line SK-OV-3.

SOD - Antioxidant enzyme- Super Oxide Dismutase.

SREBP and PPARg - The transcription factors, peroxisome proliferator activated receptors (PPARalpha, PPARgamma1/PPARgamma2) and sterol regulatory element binding proteins (SREBP-1) regulate liver lipid metabolism.

STD - Sexually Transmitted Diseases.

Sudorific - An agent that causes or increases sweat.

Th1 - T helper cells (T_h cells) are a sub-group of lymphocytes, a type of white blood cell, that play an important role in the immune system, particularly in the adaptive immune system.

TPA - Tissue plasminogen activator (abbreviated tPA or PLAT) is a protein involved in the breakdown of blood clots.

Transforming growth factor beta (TGF-β) - is a protein that controls proliferation, cellular differentiation, and other functions in most cells. It is a type of cytokine which plays a role in immunity, cancer, bronchial asthma, heart disease, diabetes, Marfan syndrome, Parkinson's disease and AIDS.

TSNA - Tobacco-specific N-nitrosamines (TSNAs) are known to be some of the most potent carcinogens present in smokeless tobacco, snuff and tobacco smoke.

TUNEL - TUNEL is a common method for detecting DNA fragmentation that results from apoptotic signaling cascade.

VCAM-1 - vascular cell adhesion molecule 1 (VCAM-1) or cluster of differentiation 106 (CD106) is a protein that in humans is encoded by the *VCAM1* gene.

VEGFR2 - Receptor for **Vascular Endothelial Growth Factor-2.**

Wnt signaling - Wnt signaling pathway is a network of proteins that passes signals from receptors on the surface of the cell through the cytoplasm and ultimately to the cell's nucleus where the signaling cascade leads to the expression of target genes.

Wnt/beta-catenin - Wnt/β-catenin signaling is involved in a broad range of biological systems including stem cells, embryonic development and adult organs. Deregulation of components involved in Wnt/β-catenin signaling has been implicated in a wide spectrum of diseases including a number of cancers and degenerative diseases.

5-LOX -Arachidonate 5-lipoxygenase is a member of the lipoxygenase family of enzymes. It transforms EFAs into leukotrienes and is a current target for pharmaceutical intervention in a number of diseases.

Index

O

P

R

S

T

V

www.ingramcontent.com/pod-product-compliance
Lightning Source LLC
Chambersburg PA
CBHW071232230926
51849CB00001B/84
9789351301974